Fashions in Makeup

RICHARD CORSON

Fashions in Makeup

FROM ANCIENT TO MODERN TIMES

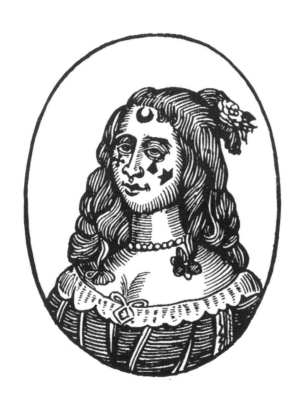

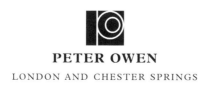

PETER OWEN

LONDON AND CHESTER SPRINGS

PETER OWEN PUBLISHERS
73 Kenway Road, London SW5 0RE

Peter Owen books are distributed in the USA by
Dufour Editions Inc., Chester Springs, PA 19425-0007

ISBN 0 7206 1195 4

A catalogue record for this book is available from
the British Library

Printed in Great Britain by
St Edmundsbury Press, Bury St Edmunds, Suffolk
Bound in Great Britain by
Woolnough Bookbinding, Irthlingborough, Northants

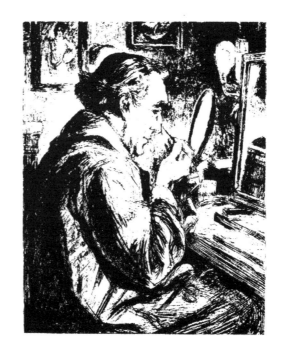

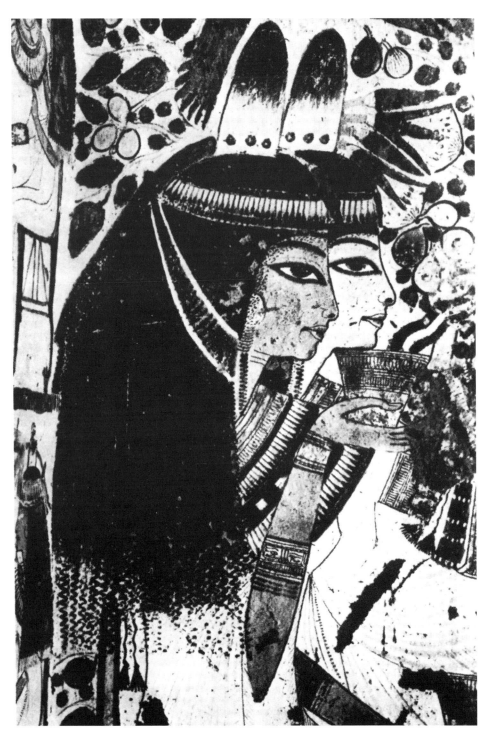

Egyptian women, their eyes painted with kohl.

Preface

There have been published, from time to time, books on the history of cosmetics — most of them limited in scope and sparsely illustrated. There is none, so far as I know, which treats the subject as fully as its historical importance would lead one to expect. Certainly there has never been gathered together in one volume a fraction of the illustrative material available.

The purpose of this book has been to determine as accurately as possible what men and women used on their faces, how they applied it, and what they looked like as a result. The available information — written descriptions, moral polemics, works of art, photographs, cosmetics containers, implements for applying makeup, and, occasionally, traces of the makeup itself, some of it thousands of years old — ranges from a mere smattering in the Dark Ages to an almost overwhelming abundance in the twentieth century. Although my intention has been to concentrate mainly on the Western world, I have occasionally included, for comparison, material from other countries. And though the book is primarily about makeup, it also touches upon such peripheral subjects as perfumes, bathing, hair styles, mirrors, and dressing-tables.

As with *Fashions in Hair* and *Fashions in Eyeglasses*, I have attempted to organize the material so as to provide a useful guide for actors, makeup artists, beauty consultants, illustrators, and writers whose work may at times require research in this relatively neglected field of study. I hope that the book may also prove enlightening – perhaps even entertaining – to others who may be merely curious about the fascinating and colourful history of makeup.

I am most grateful, once again, to Mr Mitchell Erickson for reading the manuscript and making many useful suggestions, to Miss Elizabeth Roth of the New York Public Library Prints Division for her invaluable assistance in finding illustrative material, and to the various museums which have given permission to reproduce works of art in their possession.

R.C., 1972

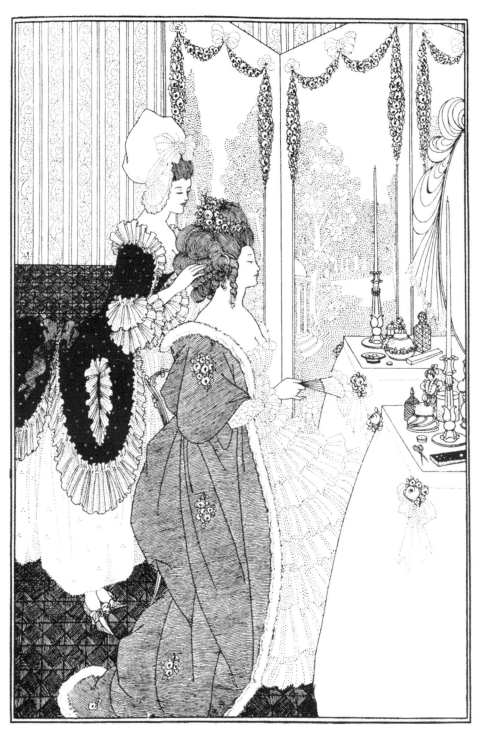

'The Toilet' by Aubrey Beardsley; illustration from *The Rape of the Lock*, 1896.

Contents

Contents

Illustrations

PLATES

FIGURES

The author wishes to thank the following for permission to reproduce the illustrations (figures) listed below:

Andrea Robb Corporation, New York, 244; the Earl of Bradford Collection, 82; the Trustees of the British Museum, London, 14, 24, 32, 38, 43, 52, 55, 94, 139, 153, 156; Government of India Tourist Office, 75; *Harpers and Queen,* 246; *Hygeia,* 229; the Metropolitan Museum of Art, New York — The Carnarvon Collection: Gift of Edward S. Harkness (1926), 16, Gift of H. Dunscombe Cott *(*1961), 47, Bequest of George Blumenthal (1941), 58, Fletcher Fund (1965), 70, Rogers Fund (1942), 132; the National Gallery of Scotland, Edinburgh, 126; the National Portrait Gallery, London, 80, 108; New York Public Library, Prints Division, 101, 105, 119, 123, 138, 140, 143, 144, 151, 154, 159, 160, 161, 166, 186, 197, 208; *New Yorker,* 225, 228; the Royal Scottish Museum, Edinburgh, 66; the Victoria and Albert Museum, London (Crown Copyright), 134, 157; *Vogue,* 214.

Fashions in Makeup

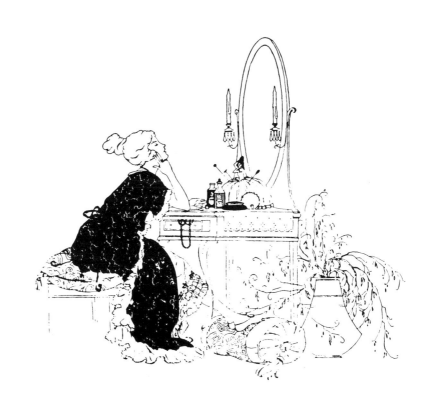

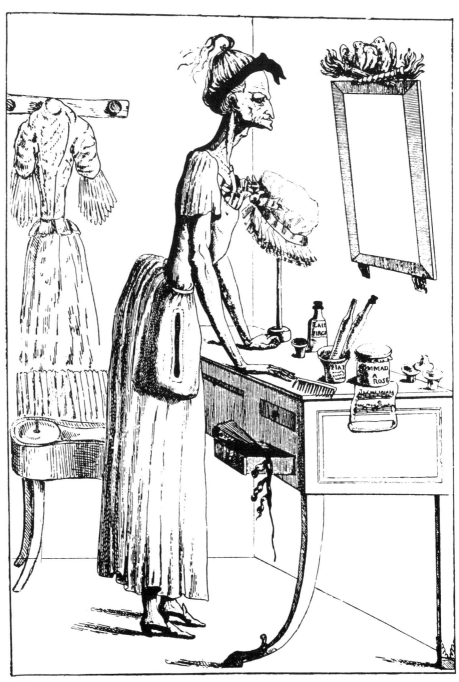

'J'aspire aussi moi'. Elderly coquette at her dressing table. French engraving, early nineteenth century.

BEAUTY AND FASHION

Says Beauty to Fashion, as they sat at the toilette,
'If I give a charm, you surely will spoil it;
When you take it in hand, there's such murth'ring and mangling,
'Tis so metamorphos'd by your fiddling and fangling,
That I scarce know my own, when I meet it again.
Such changelings you make, both of women and men.
To confirm what I say, look at Phryne, or Phillis,
I'm sure that I gave 'em good roses and lillies;
Now what have you done? — Let the world be the judge:
Why you daub 'em all over with cold-cream and rouge,
That, like Thisbe in Ovid, one cannot come at 'em,
Unless thro' a mud-wall of paint and pomatum.'

. . . .

    Thus Beauty begun, and Miss Fashion reply'd:
'Who does most for the sex? — Let it fairly be try'd,
And they that look round 'em will presently see,
They're much less beholden to you than to me;
I grant it, indeed, mighty favours you boast,
But how scanty your favours, how scarce is a toast?
A shape, a complexion, you confer now and then,
But to one that you give, you refuse it to ten;
In one you succeed, in another you fail,
Here your rose is too red, there your lilly's too pale;
Or some feature or other is always amiss:
And pray, let me know when you finish'd a piece
That I was not oblig'd to correct, or touch over.
Or you never would have either husband or lover?
For I hope, my fair lady, you do not forget,
Though you find the thread, that 'tis I make the net;
And say what you please, it must be allow'd,
That a woman is nothing unless à-la-mode;
Neglected she lives, and no beauty avails,
For what is a ship without rigging or sails;
Like the diamonds when rough, are the charms you bestow,
But mine is the setting and polishing too.
Your nymphs, with their shape, their complexions, and features,
What are they without me, but poor awkward creatures?

The rout, the assembly, the playhouse will tell,
'Tis I form the beau, and I finish the belle;
'Tis by me that their beauties must all be supply'd;
Which time has withdrawn, or which you have deny'd;
Impartial to all, did not I lend my air,
Both Venus and Cupid might throw up their trade,
And even your ladyship die an old maid.'

The London Magazine, 1762

1 · Fashions in Makeup

Loveliness shall sit at the toilet,
watching her oval face in the oval mirror.
Her smooth fingers shall flit among the paints and powder,
to tip and mingle them, catch up a pencil,
clasp a phial, and what not and what not,
until the mask of vermeil tinct has been laid aptly,
the enamel quite hardened. And, heavens,
how she will charm us and ensarcel our eyes!

MAX BEERBOHM

Throughout recorded history man has painted his face—at times decorating it boldly with elaborate coloured designs, again, touching it delicately with a little colour in the hope of regaining lost youth. A study of face painting among primitive tribes suggests that the first makeup may have been protective— possibly as a form of camouflage. Early tattooing appears to have been associated with puberty rites or to have had magical significance and dates back to ancient Egypt. It is also, among primitive tribes, a mark of status, as it has been from time to time among civilized peoples. Native chieftains sometimes have different facial markings from those used by other members of the tribe, or success in hunting may entitle one to use special markings. In the eighteenth century certain shades of rouge, being very expensive and difficult to obtain, might be considered status symbols.

Probably very early, face painting also came to be thought of as a method of beautification. Among civilized peoples makeup has always been looked upon as a beautifier of women and, from time to time, of men. Even the red-stained teeth of Hindu women and the black-stained teeth of the Japanese (Figure 1) have been considered to be a mark of beauty as were the high, shaved foreheads of the fifteenth century.

Among older women and some men, at least in the Western world, makeup has also been used in an attempt to recover the lost bloom of youth. Eighteenth-century dowagers caked their faces with thick white paint to conceal wrinkles and rubbed flaming scarlet rouge on to their sagging, whitened cheeks. And at least one Persian king always took his cosmetics case to the battlefield.

But the use of makeup has not always been so blatant. Sometimes, in fact, social pressures against it have been so great that it has had to be used with considerable skill and subtlety if it was to be used at all. Failure to do this could result in personal embarrassment, a tarnished reputation, or even, in the eighteenth century, as we shall see, nullification of one's marriage with full

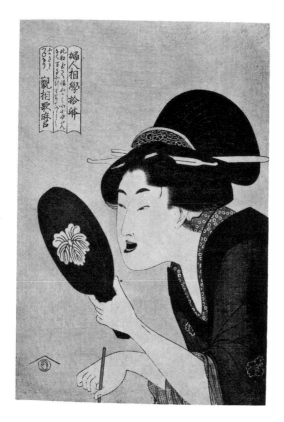

FIG. 1 : Blacking the teeth. Japanese
woodcut by Utamaro; *c.* 1796.

support of the law. The hypocrisy of what may best be called *restrictive* makeup
has never been more in evidence than in the nineteenth century when ladies
pinched their cheeks and bit their lips in order to provide the colour that the
restrictive moral climate would not permit them to achieve with paint.

Women, however, have seldom allowed themselves to be so stifled for very
long. The bolder ones, usually women of fashion, have always used makeup
surreptitiously with the intent of deceiving, gradually seducing their less
aggressive compatriots into following their lead until the deception becomes so
widespread and so much a matter of common knowledge that acceptance of the
artifice is forced upon a reluctant public, leading at first to tolerance, then to
permissiveness, and sometimes to wild abandon.

Such forthright use of makeup is indicative of a general permissiveness in
so-called moral behaviour and, in fact, may well be designated as *permissive*
makeup. During these periods of extremism, makeup gradually departs from
a representation of nature to ornamentation of the human face purely for
purposes of decoration. Curiously, highly decorative makeup tends to be used
only by primitive peoples and by civilized ones who have reached a certain

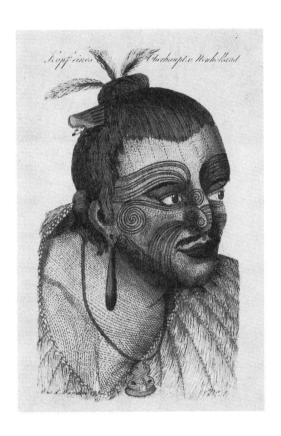

FIG. 2 : Tribal chieftain decorated
with tattooing.

level of sophistication. (See Figures 2 and 3.) In the Western world it has
flourished primarily among the ancient civilizations and among fashionable
women in the second half of the twentieth century. Orientals seem always to
have had a flair for it, actors use it as part of their art, and primitive tribesmen
seem drawn to it naturally.

But sociological changes are usually interlaced with economic, technological,
and psychological ones, as in the twentieth century, with supply following
increased demand brought about by a psychological need for youth and beauty.
We use makeup, and we have always used makeup, for what it can do for us
and to others. Although primitive man did at times use makeup to frighten
his enemies, it has usually been used to attract lovers and friends and to bolster
our own self-confidence. As our self-confidence increases, so does our willingness,
even eagerness, to use more makeup, resulting in an apparent reversal of the
natural law, with demand following supply as technology improves both the
quantity and quality of the product and the hucksters take over.

When the flamboyance has reached a peak beyond which it cannot reasonably
seem to go and beyond which no one really wants it to go, it subsides, at least

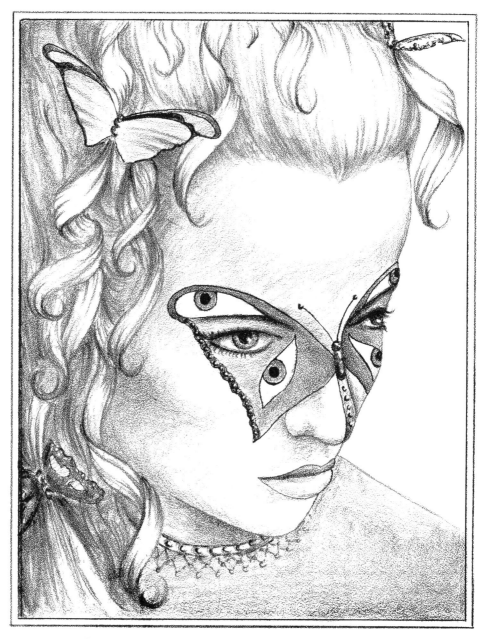

FIG. 3 : High-fashion party makeup, 1969. Such highly decorative makeup has been worn occasionally.

for a time, in favour of greater naturalness. This naturalness is always greeted with sighs of relief, which are then forgotten as a new peak of permissiveness eventually approaches. Anyone who tries to interfere with this natural rhythm of change, and many have, would do better by far to cultivate patience, secure in the knowledge that whatever women are doing to their faces today, tomorrow it will be something else.

Most notable among the interfering have been the moralists. Ensnared in their own theology and not always concerned with psychological needs or sociological changes, they have threatened hellfire and eternal damnation to those who dared defile God's handiwork with artificial colour. In 1583 Philip Stubbes, one of the most vehement of the breed, complained endlessly about Englishwoman who used 'certain oyles, liquors, unguents and waters' and flaunted God's will by colouring 'their faces with such sibbersauces' in a vain effort to improve their beauty. 'But who seethe not,' he warned, 'that their soules are thereby deformed, and they brought deeper into the displeasure and indignation of the Almighty, at whose voice the earth dooth tremble and at whose presence the heavens shall liquefie and melt away.'

Four centuries later American women were spending half a billion dollars a year on their sibbersauces.

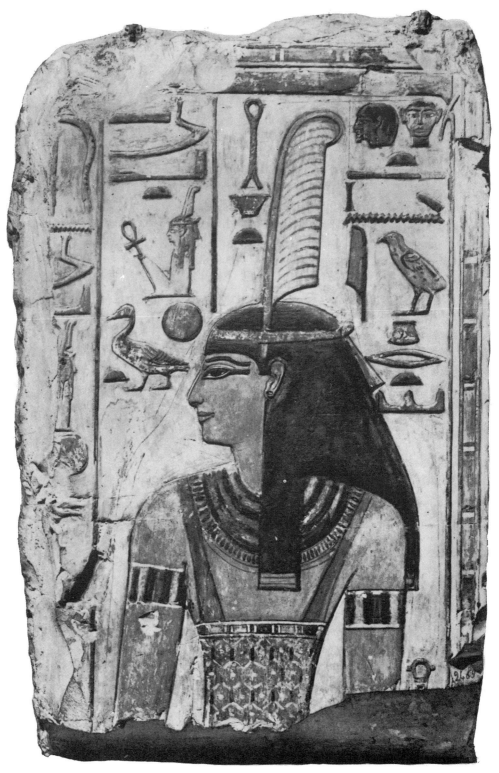

FIG. 4: Mayet, Egyptian goddess of Truth and Justice. The stylized eye makeup, common in Egyptian art, is probably an exaggeration of the makeup actually used. For more realistic representations, see Figs. 5 and 6.

2 · Ancient Civilizations

While you remain at home, Galla, your hair
is at the hairdresser's; you take out your teeth
at night and sleep tucked away in a hundred
cosmetics boxes — you have not even your own face
for a bedfellow. Then you wink at men
under an eyebrow you took out of a drawer
that same morning.

MARTIAL

A bald, bare-breasted woman, fresh from her bath, sits lazily holding a silver hand mirror, as her attendants remove from a wooden chest inlaid with mother-of-pearl, jars of skin cream, pots of rouge, and pottery tubes containing a variety of coloured pigments. As one of the attendants is pouring some ochre yellow powder out of one of the larger tubes into a shallow dish of water and blending the two into a thin yellowish liquid, the other is massaging the lady's face and neck with perfumed ointment from an alabaster jar.

After all of the excess face cream has been wiped away with a clean linen cloth, the first attendant dips another piece of linen into the yellow liquid and smooths it carefully over the lady's face, neck, and arms to lighten the skin and give it a fashionably yellow tint.

Meanwhile, the second attendant has spat into an ornate cosmetics spoon and mixed some green powder from a tiny black and gold pot with the saliva to form a thick liquid. While the yellow paint is still moist, she dips her finger into the green liquid and strokes it across the lady's eyelids, blending the edges of the green paint carefully into the yellow. When the green is dry, she wets a slender glass rod in her mouth and dips it into a blue pottery tube containing a black powder. With the blackened rod or stick, she then draws a heavy line across one of her mistress's eyelids, just above the lashes, extending it a bit beyond the outer corner of the eye. A similar line is drawn beneath the eye. She then paints on long and heavy eyebrows slightly above where the natural ones have been shaved off.

With her eyes completed, the lady is now ready to be rouged with a mixture of brownish red pigment and scented ointment, which the girl applies deftly with her finger tips to the cheekbones, blending it carefully into the yellow base. She then completes the makeup with the application of rouge to the lips.

Finally, when the attendants have helped their mistress into a diaphanous gown, tied a wide, ornately fashioned collar of semi-precious stones around her neck, and set a bulky black wig of oiled braids on her shaved head, our Egyptian lady is ready to greet her guests.

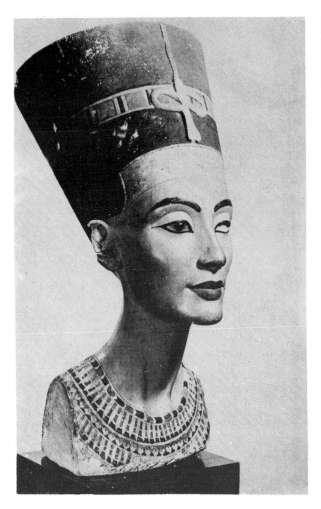

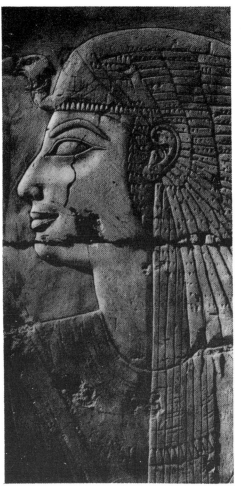

FIG. 5: Head of Nefertiti, Queen of Egypt. Painted lime-stone, first half of the fourteenth century B.C. Egyptians, both men and women, made up their eyes with kohl.

FIG. 6: The Egyptian Queen Akmet, mother of Hatshepsut. Stone relief, sixteenth century B.C. The painted brow and black eye lining are represented by high relief.

ANCIENT EGYPT

What man or woman first applied paint to the face or when it happened is lost in the mists of prehistoric times. Although archaeologists have unearthed Egyptian palettes for grinding eye paint, dating from about 10,000 B.C., most of the artifacts to be found in museums are less than half that old. All evidence indicates, however, that throughout their history, the Egyptians used obvious makeup, boldly applied, and had, in some form, most of the cosmetic aids which have ever been devised. They used perfumed oils and ointments to soften the skin and paints and dyes to colour it. Both men and women used makeup as part of their daily routine, and they went to their final resting place well supplied with cosmetics for the next world. Some of the cosmetics jars found in the tomb of Tutankhamun still contained a 3000-year-old skin cream composed of approximately nine parts of animal fat to one part of perfumed resin. (See Figure 7.)

In addition to rouging their cheeks and lips (5000-year-old samples of lip rouge have been found), they often stained their nails, the palms of their hands, and the soles of their feet a reddish orange with henna, accented veins on the breast and temples with blue, and sometimes even painted their nipples gold.

The skin might be lightened with a yellow ochre colour or darkened with an orange-tinted paint. The yellow was used by both sexes, the orange only by men. The pigment, mined in large chunks and ground by the cosmetics makers into a powder, was supplied in tubes, wooden boxes, and metal pots. Except for this yellow and orange base colour, the makeup of an Egyptian woman was not strikingly different from that of a fashionable woman of the 1960s, who usually placed exaggerated emphasis on the eyes, often to the point of complete stylization.

Whatever else the Egyptians did or did not do, they seldom failed to line their eyes heavily with kohl — a black, grey, or coloured powder made variously of powdered antimony (stibium), black manganese oxide, burnt almonds, lead,

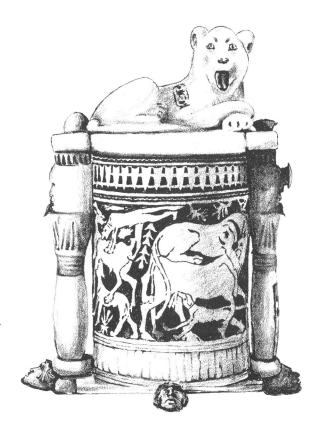

FIG. 7: Ancient Egyptian cosmetics jar. Made of calcite, hardstone, and ivory. Found in the tomb of Tutankhamun, it contained 3,000-year-old skin cream still in good condition.

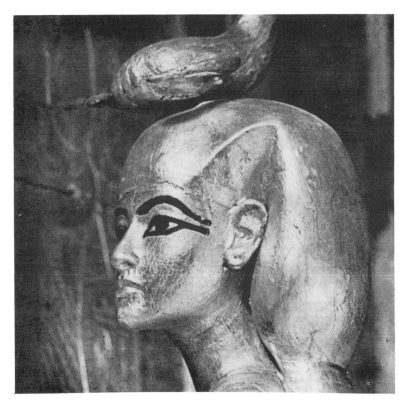

FIG. 8: The Egyptian goddess Selket. Made of yellow quartzite.
From the tomb of Tutankhamun, fourteenth century B.C.
Note the painted brows and black eye lining.

black oxide of copper, carbon, brown ochre, iron oxide, malachite, and chrysocolla, a green-blue copper ore. The powdered kohl was kept in pots and tubes (Plates 1–6 and Figure 11), moistened with saliva, and applied with a kohl stick of ivory, wood, silver, glass, or bronze (Plates 2 and 7). The kohl stick might be moistened and dipped into the tube or pot, or the powder might be poured into a cosmetics spoon or dish and moistened. (See Figures 9 and 10.) Small palettes were sometimes used for mixing the paint. Plate 1-A shows a very ancient one made of slate; Plate 1-C illustrates a small stone palette and pestle used for grinding the cosmetic powders. Kohl tubes or pots were made of faience, alabaster, wood, stone, glass, or metal; and the cosmetics boxes, dishes, and spoons, of ivory, faience, wood, alabaster, and bronze.

The kohl tubes were often double, triple, quadruple, or even quintuple. These multiple tubes (Figure 11 and Plates 2 and 6) were used for various colours of paint. Black, grey, and green were used for eye lining; and green, aqua, turquoise, terra cotta, black, and various shades of brown, for eyeshadow. Green malachite was one of the most popular pigments. When eyeshadow was used, it was always a different colour from that of the eye lining and was usually, though not always, applied to the lower lid as well as to the upper. When this was done, different colours were always used for the two lids. Cleopatra, it is said, used black on her brows and lashes, blue-black on her upper lids, and Nile green on her lower ones. The shadow above the eye was sometimes applied only to the lid itself, sometimes extended to the eyebrow. Colours used depended on personal preference and varied with the time of day.

Eyebrows were also darkened with kohl, though many women and some men shaved off their natural brows, usually replacing them with painted ones. It has been suggested that since containers for eye paint are inscribed with the dates between which their contents were to be used, the paint was intended to be to some extent medicinal as well as decorative, probably as protection against the glare of the sun and the dust and sand of the desert. This may have been so.

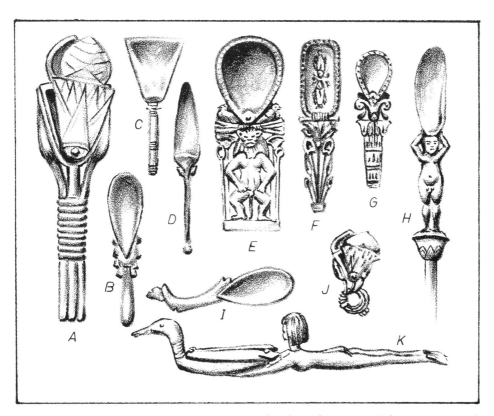

FIG. 9 : Ancient Egyptian cosmetics spoons. Made of wood, ivory, and faience. A, J, and K have swivel covers; the cover for K separates in the middle; the covers for E and G are missing. The date of the ivory spoon (H) is *c.* 1300 B.C.

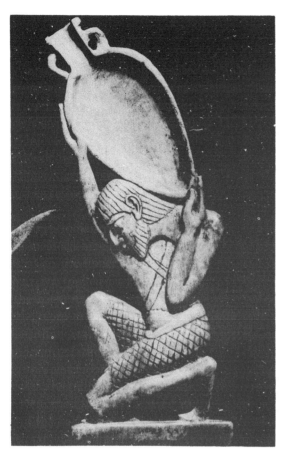

FIG. 10 : Egyptian toilet spoon of ivory.

There were, however, separate medicinal pastes used for such protection; and since they were sometimes kept in kohl tubes, it may be that the coloured paint protected the eye only against the sun, whereas the special paste provided the medicinal protection.

In addition to the various colours of powdered kohl and the cream rouges, the Egyptians sometimes made sticks of cosmetic paint by pouring a fatty mixture into the hollow stems of plants, which were then wrapped in leaves. Cosmetic pastes were also wrapped in leaves; and powders, pastes, and unguents were kept in jars and tubes. Black cosmetics from tombs at Achim have proved to be mixtures of lead sulphide and charcoal. A green eyeshadow in the British Museum contains verdigris and resin. Other green pastes have been found to be powdered silicates mixed with copper carbonate. Reddish brown paints were coloured with clays with a high iron content. All cosmetics were perfumed.

Both cosmetics and perfumes were compounded by professional cosmetics makers or, in earlier times, by the priests, who kept their formulas secret and sold their products to those who could afford them. One universally used cosmetic was perfumed oil or ointment, usually kept in bottles or jars of alabaster, glass, ivory, onyx, or bone. Nut oil and other vegetable (olive, palm, flax, almond, lettuce) and animal oils or fats were used and variously perfumed. The cheaper oil of castor-berry was also extensively used.

In the hot, dry, Egyptian climate, long before the invention of soap, these perfumed oils provided a means of cleansing the body and keeping the skin soft (Figure 13). Frequently, especially at dinners or parties, cone-shaped containers of a solid perfumed ointment (Figure 12) were placed on top of the wig. As the ointment melted and gradually trickled down, it cooled and perfumed the body. The perfumes and cosmetics contained such ingredients as frankincense, myrrh, spikenard, thyme, marjoram, origanum, balanos, and oils of almond, olive, and sesame.

A lady who was concerned about her complexion might be advised to wash her face with a concoction of bullock's bile, whipped ostrich eggs, oil, dough, refined natron, and hautet resin, combined with fresh milk. For wrinkles she might add to milk a mixture of incense, wax, fresh olive oil, and cyperus, crushed and ground, and apply it to her face for six days. One general beauty

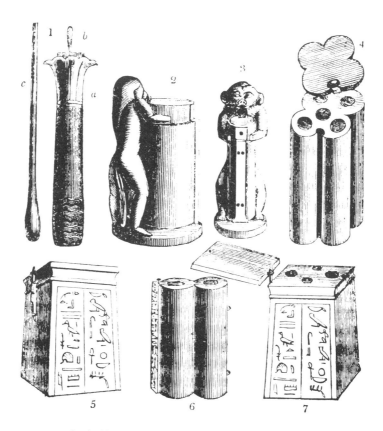

FIG. 11: Cosmetics containers for kohl. From Wilkinson's *The Ancient Egyptians*, 1854.

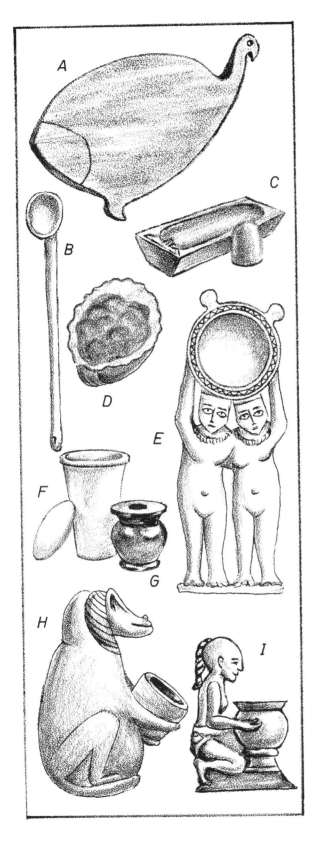

PLATE 1 : ANCIENT COSMETICS
IMPLEMENTS AND
CONTAINERS

A   Pre-Dynastic. Egyptian slate palette
used for mixing cosmetics. (*Metropolitan Museum of Art, New York*)

B   *c.* 3500 B.C., Egyptian. Small ivory
spoon, used for cosmetics. (*Metropolitan Museum of Art, New York*)

C   2000 – 1650 B.C., Egyptian. Small
stone palette and pestle for grinding
cosmetic paint. (*Dublin National
Museum*)

D   Sumerian shell containing cosmetic
paint. Those in the British Museum
contain terra cotta, apple green,
charcoal, and aqua.

E   Sumerian. Ivory cosmetics spoon.
(*British Museum*)

F   Egyptian, Middle Kingdom. Alabaster ointment jar and cover.
(*British Museum*)

G   Egyptian, Middle Kingdom. Hematite kohl-pot. (*British Museum*)

H   *c.* 1900 B.C., Egyptian. Ape holding
cosmetics jar. Burnished pottery.
(*British Museum*)

I   *c.* 1900 B.C., Egyptian. Cosmetics
pot held by kneeling girl. (*British
Museum*)

PLATE 2 : ANCIENT EGYPTIAN
COSMETICS CONTAINERS

A   c. 1900 B.C. Anhydrite kohl pot and lid with lugs in the form of cobra heads. About 1½ inches high. (*British Museum*)

B   Nineteenth century B.C. Rouge pot of obsidian and gold.

C   1800–1400 B.C. Cosmetics dish of blue-green faience. About 1½ inches in diameter. (*Royal Scottish Museum, Edinburgh*)

D   c. 1800 B.C. Covered jar of obsidian and gold, for oils and creams. Found in the tomb of Princess Sut-hathor-inunt. (*Metropolitan Museum of Art, New York*)

E   1580–1350 B.C. Ebony kohl tube and stick, from royal cosmetics set. (*Metropolitan Museum of Art, New York*)

F   c. 1250 B.C. Double kohl tube of acacia wood. The lid is kept in position by the kohl stick. (*British Museum*)

G   c. 1600 B.C. Quadruple kohl pot of glazed steatite, engraved with the name of the scribe l'Ahmase. (*British Museum*)

H   Fifteenth century B.C. Alabaster cosmetics dish. Fish and lotus blossom design. (*Metropolitan Museum of Art, New York*)

I   c. 1475 B.C. Multiple wooden kohl pot of the scribe Ahmose. It held 'good eye-paint for every day', and each tube contained a different colour for each season. The kohl stick can be seen protruding from the top. (*British Museum*)

J   c. 1360 B.C. Faience kohl tube, inscribed with the name of Tutankhamen and the Queen Anksenamun. (*British Museum*)

K   c. 1250 B.C. Glass kohl tube in the form of a palm column. Mustard and white stripes on black. (*British Museum*)

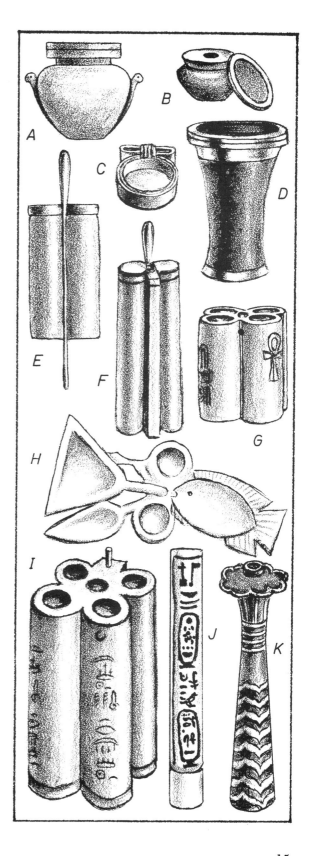

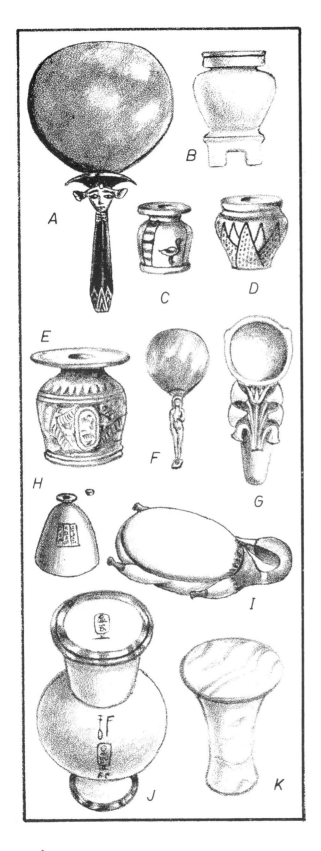

PLATE 3 : ANCIENT EGYPTIAN
COSMETICS POTS AND
IMPLEMENTS

A   1900–1840 B.C. Mirror of Sit-hat-hor-yūmet. Silver with handle of obsidian, inlaid with gold and precious stones. (*Cairo Museum*)

B   Cosmetics jar with cover. About 2½ inches high. (*Metropolitan Museum of Art, New York*)

C   Kohl pot.

D   Kohl pot.

E   Between the eighth and twenty-eighth Dynasty. Kohl pot.

F   Metal mirror.

G   Cosmetics spoon. Lotus design.

H   Alabaster vase for perfumed ointment. Stopper shown above. (*Alnwick Castle*)

I   1400–1350 B.C. Ivory cosmetics box in the form of a trussed duck. The duck's swivel back serves as a cover. About 3½ inches long. (*Metropolitan Museum of Art, New York*)

J   1490–1436 B.C. Steatite cosmetics jar belonging to a lady of the court of Thot-mosě III. About 3 inches high. (*Metropolitan Museum of Art, New York*)

K   1900–1840 B.C. Alabaster cosmetics jar, one of a set of eight found in a cosmetics chest belonging to Sit-hat-hor-yūmet. About 3½ inches high. (*Metropolitan Museum of Art, New York*)

PLATE 4 : ANCIENT EGYPTIAN
       COSMETICS CONTAINERS

A   *c.* 1900 B.C. Hematite kohl pot with band of gold foil. Shown without cover. (*British Museum*)

B   *c.* 1250 B.C. Diorite kohl pot with cover. Light grey-green with black markings. (*British Museum*)

C   *c.* 1250 B.C. Limestone hippopotamus with four kohl tubes drilled into its back. (*British Museum*)

D   *c.* 600 B.C. Glazed pottery ibex with cosmetics pot. (*British Museum*)

E   *c.* 300 B.C. Glazed toilet box and cover. Aqua designs painted in dark blue. (*British Museum*)

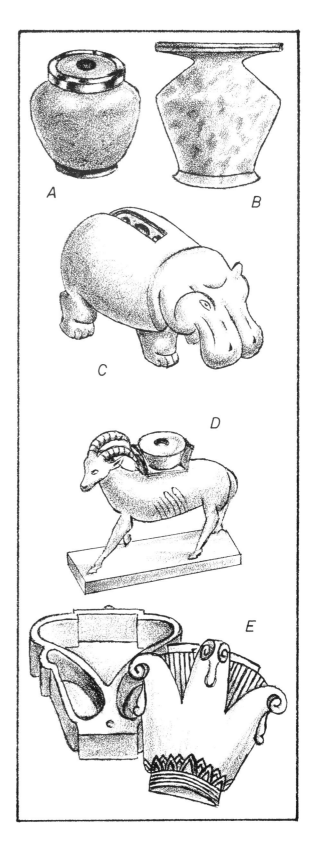

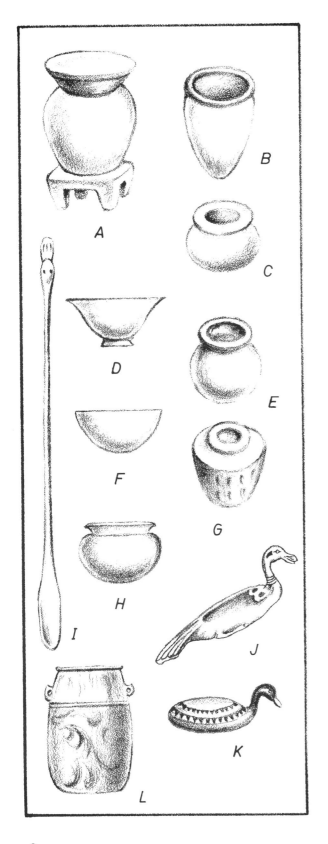

PLATE 5 : ANCIENT COSMETICS
CONTAINERS

A   *c.* 2000 B.C., Egyptian. Anhydrite cosmetics jar. About 4½ inches high. (*British Museum*)

B   *c.* 2000 B.C., Egyptian. Alabaster pot. About 4 inches high. (*British Museum*)

C   *c.* 2000 B.C., Egyptian. Small alabaster cosmetics pot. (*British Museum*)

D   *c.* 2000 B.C., Egyptian. Small anhydrite cosmetics container. (*British Museum*)

E   *c.* 2000 B.C., Egyptian. Alabaster cosmetics pot. (*British Museum*)

F   *c.* 2000 B.C., Egyptian. Rock crystal cosmetics container. About 2 inches in diameter. (*British Museum*)

G   Mesopotamian. Glazed cosmetics pot. About 2 inches in diameter. (*British Museum*)

H   *c.* 2000 B.C., Egyptian. Alabaster cosmetics container. About 2 inches in diameter. (*British Museum*)

I   *c.* 1250 B.C., Egyptian. Ivory toilet spoon. About 8 inches long. (*British Museum*)

J   Egyptian toilet box of wood in the form of a goose.

K   Egyptian toilet box of wood in the form of a goose.

L   Cosmetics container of bone. (*British Museum*)

PLATE 6 : ANCIENT EGYPTIAN TOILET
        BOXES

A   1370–1340 B.C. Ivory grasshopper
     painted in non-realistic style. The
     wings part to reveal a small cavity
     in the body for keeping eye paint.
     An item of great luxury. 2½ inches
     long. (*Brooklyn Museum*)

B   *c.* 1370–1340 B.C. Ivory ointment
     box representing a formal bouquet
     of pomegranate spray and lotus.
     8¼ inches long. (*Brooklyn Museum*)

C   *c.* 1225 B.C. Bag of green eye paint.
     Made of wood overlaid with plaster
     and gilded. Inscribed with the name
     of Ramses II. Probably used as a
     symbolic offering. (*British Museum*)

D   1570–1320 B.C. Multiple ivory con-
     tainer for eye paint. Design in
     brown. (*Brooklyn Museum*)

E   *c.* 300 B.C. One of a set of funerary
     ointment jars of sea green faience,
     each jar inscribed with the name of
     the chief ingredient. (*Brooklyn
     Museum*)

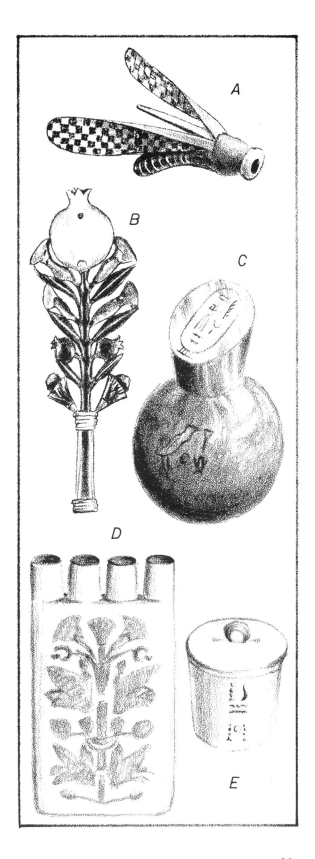

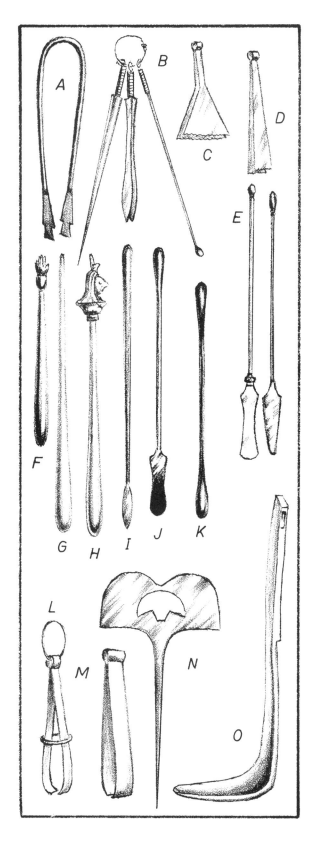

PLATE 7 : ANCIENT COSMETICS
IMPLEMENTS

A   *c.* 1300 B.C., Egyptian. Bronze tweezers. (*British Museum*)

B   Early Sumerian. Metal toothpick, tweezers, and ear scoop on wire ring. About 3 inches long. (*British Museum*)

C   Egyptian depilatory tweezers Similar ones used from the early Bronze age. (*British Museum*)

D   Egyptian depilatory tweezers. (*British Museum*)

E   Egyptian. Silver spatulas for applying cosmetics. About 6 inches long. (*British Museum*)

F   *c.* 1300 B.C., Egyptian. Black cosmetic stick. (*British Museum*)

G   *c.* 1300 B.C., Egyptian. Wooden kohl stick. About 5 inches long. (*British Museum*)

H   *c.* 1300 B.C., Egyptian. Metal kohl stick. (*British Museum*)

I   *c.* 1300 B.C., Egyptian. Black metal kohl stick. (*British Museum*)

J   Late Egyptian. Bronze kohl stick, blackened from kohl. (*Royal Scottish Museum, Edinburgh*)

K   Late Egyptian. Glass kohl stick. (*Royal Scottish Museum, Edinburgh*)

L   Roman period. Found in Scotland. Bronze tweezers. About 2½ inches long. (*Museum of Antiquities, Edinburgh*)

M   Roman period. Found in Scotland. Bronze tweezers. About 2½ inches long. (*Museum of Antiquities, Edinburgh*)

N   Late Bronze Age (after 1000 B.C.). Bronze razor, found in Ireland. About 4 inches long. (*Dublin National Museum*)

O   Roman period, found in Scotland. Bronze strigil, used for scraping the body after applying oil. (*Museum of Antiquities, Edinburgh*)

PLATE 8 : ANCIENT COSMETICS
CONTAINERS AND
IMPLEMENTS

A Seventh to sixth millennium B.C. Hoopoe-headed bone spatula from a Neolithic toilet set. (*Excavated in South Anatolia*)

B Seventh to sixth millennium B.C. Greenstone palette from a Neolithic toilet set.

C Seventh to sixth millennium B.C. Pronged bone fork from a Neolithic toilet set.

D Assyrian ointment box.

E Probably Babylonian. Cosmetics container. Ram in baked clay, with holes for cosmetics or ointments

F *c.* 3000 B.C. Bronze kohl stick from Mohenjo-Daro. 5 inches long.

G First century A.D., probably made in Yorkshire. Bronze mirror. Repoussé mounts at junction of handle and plate. About 8 inches in diameter. (*Royal Scottish Museum, Edinburgh*)

H *c.* 2500 B.C. Kohl pot from Mohenjo-Daro. Made of pink paste and ornamented with a petal design painted in polychrome. Neck and rim black. 5·2 inches high.

I *c.* 3000 B.C. Stone toilet jar from Mohenjo-Daro.

J *c.* 3000 B.C. Cosmetics jar from Mohenjo-Daro. 3 inches high.

K *c.* 2500 B.C. Cosmetics pot from Mohenjo-Daro. Cream and red. 1·72 inches high.

L *c.* 2500 B.C. Cosmetics pot from Mohenjo-Daro. 3·2 inches high.

M *c.* 2500 B.C. Bronze kohl pot from Mohenjo-Daro.

N Toilet jar from Mohenjo-Daro. Chocolate coloured with dark red bands. There are two holes in the neck for tying on the lid.

O *c.* 3000 B.C. Mohenjo-Daro. Back of cockle shell used to hold cosmetic paints.

P *c.* 2500 B.C. Toilet jar from Mohenjo-Daro.

Q *c.* 2500 B.C. Toilet jar from Mohenjo-Daro.

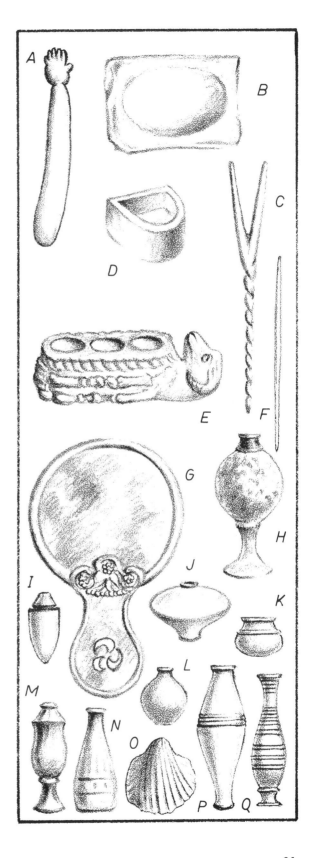

restorative required writing fluid, hippopotamus fat, and gazelle's dung; another contained, in part, phallus, vulva, and black lizard.

For greying hair, a very ancient recipe calls for the blood of a black cow, tortoise shell, and the neck of the gabgu-bird cooked in oil. Other hair-colouring preparations or treatments, according to Eifert, involved the horn of a fawn, warmed in oil; the bile of many crabs; dried tadpoles from the canal, crushed in oil; and the womb of a cat, warmed in oil with the egg of the gabgu-bird.

There was also a choice to be made in eyebrow dye -- 'crocodile earth with honey which has been dissolved in onion water' or, for variety, asses' liver warmed in oil with opium and made into little balls. In the third dynasty, a hair restorer prepared for Queen Schesch contained equal quantities of date blossoms, the heel of an Abyssinian greyhound, and asses' hooves, boiled in oil. Another early remedy for baldness required a mixture of fats taken from cats, snakes, horses, crocodiles, and ibexes.

Egyptian mirrors (Plates 3-A and Figures 14 and 15) were made of polished metal (usually bronze or silver, though gold and electrum may have been used as well), set into handles of wood, bronze, ivory, or faience. Sometimes gold or silver plating was used. Combs were of wood, alabaster, and ivory. These cosmetics and toilet articles were often kept in chests or boxes of wood, painted or inlaid (Figures 15 and 16), which were brought to the lady by her servants when she wished to do her makeup. There were no dressing tables as such, nor would there be until the Renaissance.

In a wooden toilet box belonging to Tutu, wife of the Scribe Ani, about 1400 B.C., there were found one terra-cotta and two alabaster vases containing unguents, pumice stone for smoothing the skin, an ivory comb with a carved back, a bronze shell for mixing unguents, a pair of gazelle-skin sandals, three red cushions for the elbows, a double stibium tube, bound with leather, and two stibium pencils, one of wood, the other of ivory. One of the tubes contained

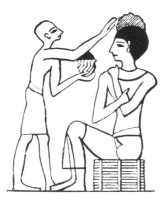

FIG. 12: Egyptian slave anointing a guest with perfume. From Rimmel's *Book of Perfumes*, 1865.

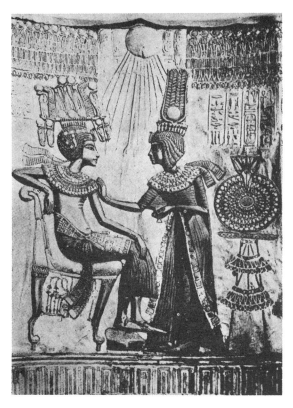

FIG. 13: Egyptian queen rubbing the body of the
Pharaoh with aromatic oils, fourteenth
century B.C.

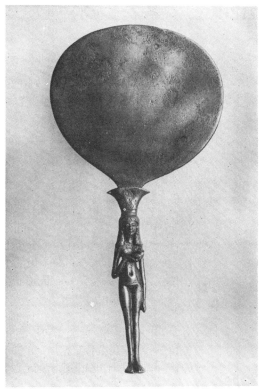

FIG. 14: Bronze mirror with handle in the shape of
a woman holding a duck. Egyptian, *c.* 1300
B.C.

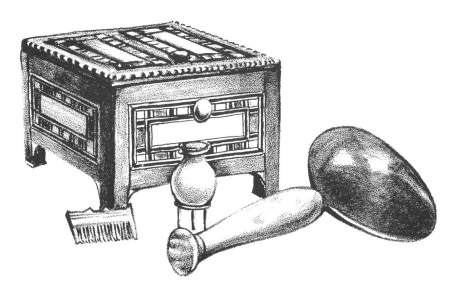

FIG. 15: Egyptian cosmetics box of painted wood, with mirror, comb, and covered cosmetics jar, *c.* 1250 B.C.

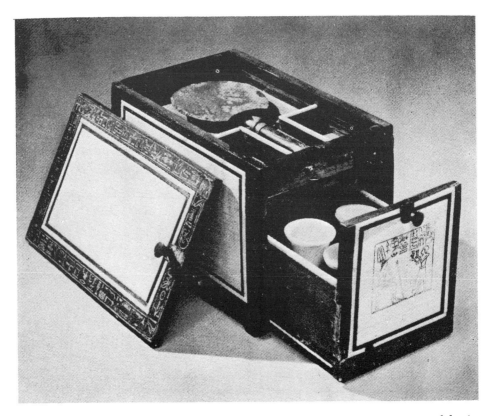

FIG. 16: Egyptian cosmetics chest of cedar, *c.* 1795 B.C. The drawer contains alabaster cosmetics jars similar to the one shown in Plate 3-K.

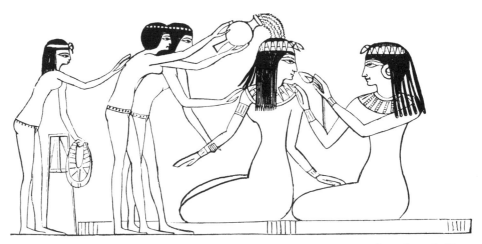

FIG. 17: Egyptian lady in the bath, with her attendants. The one on the right is holding a lotus bud and supporting the lady; those on the left are rubbing her arms, pouring water over her, and taking care of her ornaments. From Wilkinson's *The Ancient Egyptians*, 1854.

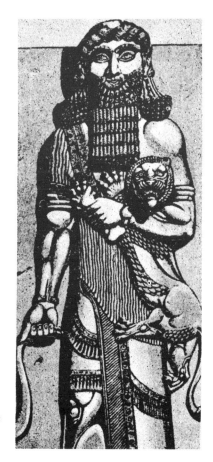

FIG. 18: Assyrian king. Eyes were lined, brows darkened, and false beards often worn by royalty.

stibium powder to be applied to the eyelids; the other, a medicinal paste to counteract the effects of dust and sand in hot weather.

THE MIDDLE EAST

The Assyrians equalled the Egyptians in their use of cosmetics, hair dyes, and curling tongs. Both men and women blackened their brows and lashes and lined their eyes with powdered antimony. Women, and sometimes men, often painted their faces with white lead, reddened their lips and cheeks and used henna on their nails and palms. King Assurbanipal, who lived in the seventh century B.C., was heavily rouged, painted, and perfumed. The perfumed bath was also an important part of the toilet.

In a 5000-year-old Sumerian tomb near Ur, archaeologists found a cosmetics pot of blue-green malachite and a tiny, shell-shaped gold cosmetics case with a

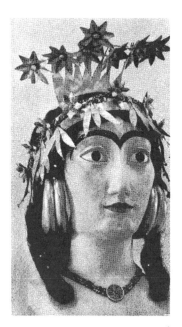
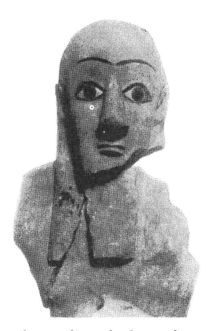

FIGS. 19 and 20: Sumerian portraits showing the prevailing style of eye makeup, *c.* 3200 B.C. The painted lady on the left is Queen Schub-ad of Ur.

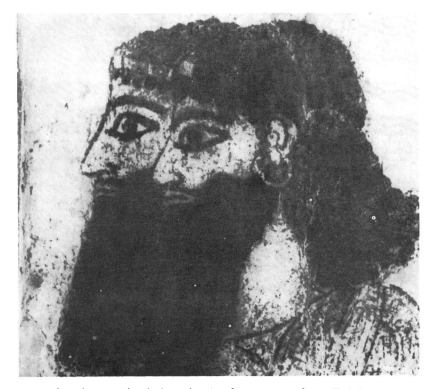

FIG. 21: Assyrian mural painting, showing heavy eye makeup. Eighth century B.C.

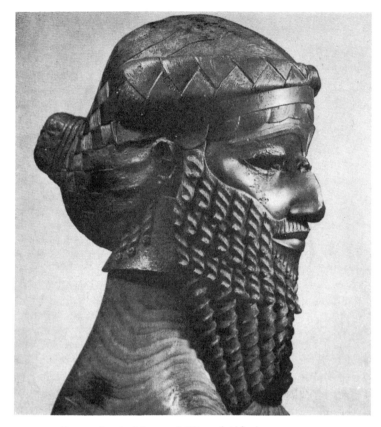

FIG. 22 : Bronze head of Sargon I, King of Akkad, *c.* 2200 B.C.

miniature cosmetics spoon, tweezers for removing superfluous hair from the eyebrows, and a metal rod for pushing down cuticle. In the British Museum there are small Sumerian shells still filled with cakes of coloured paint (apple green, aqua, terra-cotta, charcoal) used for making up the eyes (Plate 1-D). There is also a set of metal cosmetics instruments (toothpick, ear scoop, tweezers) hanging from a circle of wire (Plate 7-B) and a cosmetics spoon carved out of ivory (Plate 1-E). Lip rouges, believed to have been used by Queen Schub-ad more than four thousand years ago, have also been found at Ur.

Babylonians — young men, as well as women — painted their faces with white lead and vermilion and lined their eyes with stibium. They curled and perfumed their hair, kept their skin smooth with pumice stone, and scented their bodies with precious perfumes. Both hair and body were annointed with oil, which softened the skin and destroyed the vermin.

Cosmetics and rich perfumes were also used by the Medes. According to Xenophon, Astyages, King of the Medes, made up heavily with coloured paint, lined his eyes with black, and wore a magnificent wig of flowing ringlets. There

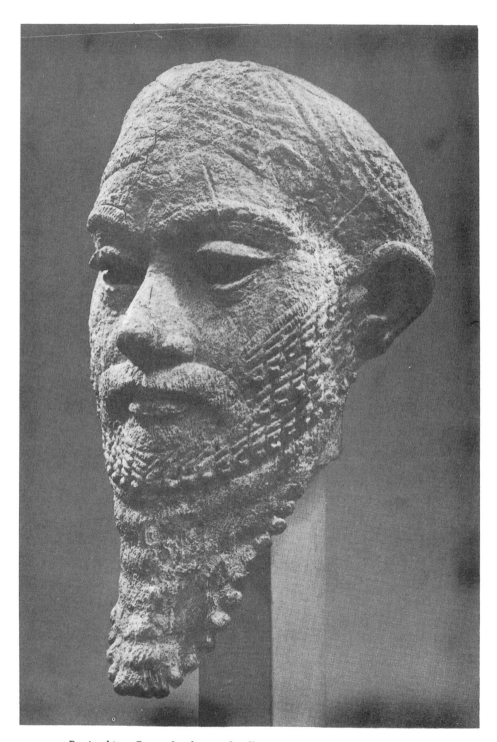

FIG. 23 : Persian king. Copper head, second millennium B.C.

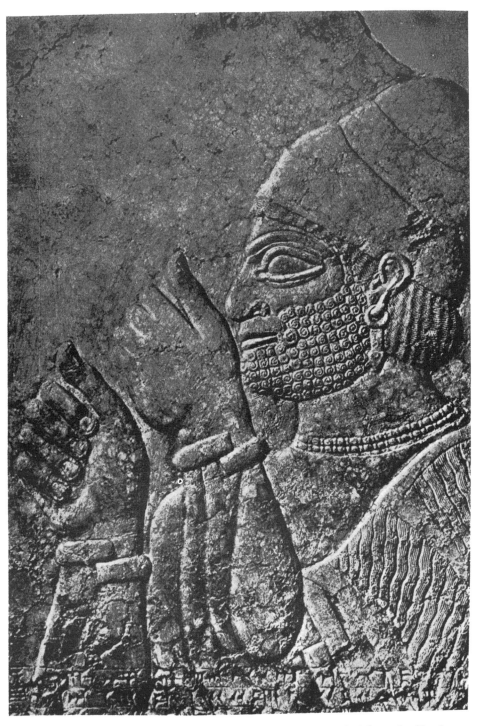

FIG. 24: Noble Phoenician with curled beard and lined eyes. Relief from the Northwest Palace at Nimrud, ninth century B.C.

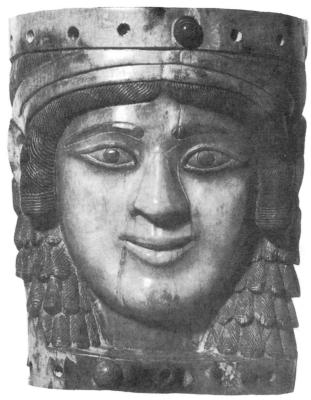

FIG. 25: Phoenician head, possibly of the goddess Astarte. Ivory sculpture, showing fully lined eyes, heavy brows, and elaborately curled wig.

is a frequently repeated story about a courageous warrior named Parsondes, who, having observed that Nanarus, governor of Babylon, shaved himself, lined his eyes with stibium, and painted his face with white lead, tried to persuade the king to install him as governor in place of Nanarus, whom he considered to be less manly than himself and therefore less worthy of the position. This the king refused to do. Nanarus, having heard of Parsondes's attempt to replace him, had the manly warrior brought before him, swearing he would completely feminize him. He had him shaved, bathed twice a day, his skin rubbed with pumice stone, and his eyes lined with stibium. His hair was plaited in the female style, and he was taught to sing and play the harp.

The final test of the success of the experiment came when an emissary from the King, on an official visit, was allowed to choose the most beautiful and accomplished among the governer's harem. After carefully observing the more than a hundred women, the emissary finally made his choice—the exquisitely groomed and painted Parsondes, who was then set free and allowed to return home with the emissary.

In Persia, after the fall of the Medes, both men and women used perfumes and cosmetics lavishly, particularly face creams and eye makeup, though little rouge. The King always took his cosmetics case to war. Excavations of graves at Susa and El-'Ubeid have brought forth small conical vases containing remnants of a green eye paint. It is believed that in addition to the protection this afforded the eyes, certain colours were thought to have magical powers. Men stained their beards, hair, and eyebrows with henna. Beards were curled and oiled and sometimes extended with fake hair.

The Syrians were also exceedingly fond of perfumes, and it is reported that at games held at Daphne by the King, there were two hundred women sprinkling perfume from golden watering-pots, processions of boys bearing golden dishes of frankincense, myrrh, and saffron, enormous incense burners covered with gold, and fifteen golden dishes of different perfumes with which the guests were anointed as they arrived. They departed with crowns of myrrh and frankincense. The Syrian men wore a moderate amount of makeup, including eye paint and some rouge.

Upper-class Scythian women painted their faces, and both men and women used perfumes which, Pliny tells us, were made from cinnamon, saffron, spikenard, crocus, lotus, thyme, marjoram, and other herbs and spices.

Even though the Hebrews were forbidden to make graven images, they did sometimes paint their faces. (See marble cosmetics palettes in Figure 26.) Jezebel, according to the Old Testament (2 Kings IX 30), 'painted her face, and tired her head, and looked out at a window'. It is possible that she painted only her eyes, which was certainly not unusual, but in any event, she did use cosmetics.

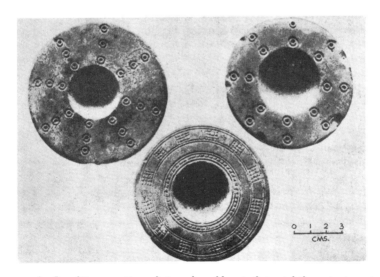

FIG. 26: Israelite cosmetics palettes of marble, ninth to eighth centuries B.C.

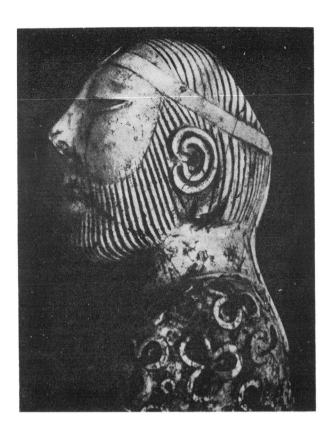

FIG. 27: Limestone head of a man from Mohenjo-Daro. Indo-Sumerian, 3000–2000 B.C.

THE INDUS VALLEY

Excavations in the Indus Valley, particularly at Mohenjo-Daro, have turned up numerous 4500–5000-year-old cosmetics pots of clay, stone, ivory, faience and alabaster, in a variety of shapes, most of them only two or three inches high with very small openings. Many of these are believed to have been kohl pots, though some may have been for precious oils or unguents. Galena and probably lamp black mixed with fat was used for eye makeup. It appears that *terre verte* was used instead of malachite for green eye paint.

Other kohl pots and jars, most of them with spouts, some blackened on the inside, have been found. Presumably the black makeup was poured on to a palette to be moistened for use. The kohl sticks, averaging about five inches in length, were sometimes made of copper or bronze but probably more frequently of wood. Both ends were rounded and were similar to the Egyptian kohl sticks shown in Plate 7-K. The cosmetics are believed to have been placed on small four-legged pottery tables when in use. Polished bronze mirrors were used in applying makeup.

Lumps of red ochre, presumably used for rouge, have been found in small shells very much like the Sumerian shells containing eye paints, illustrated in

Plate 1-D. Sticks of rouge have also been discovered, as well as a green makeup used as eyeshadow. Carbonate of lead may have been used to whiten the face. Probably both men and women used cosmetics, and certainly both used small razors as well as bronze mirrors with wooden handles.

In ancient India there were elaborate public baths. Rasps and scrapers of various types were used for cleansing and stimulating the body. Most of them were evidently made of clay mixed with sand, though at least one of sandstone has been found. Some were barrel-shaped and hollow, some flat, some pointed, some triangular.

Much later, around the fourth and fifth centuries B.C., during a period of opulence and luxury, the king's toilet was taken care of by his barber, who bathed and perfumed him and dressed his hair with tweezers and curling tongs of gold. The less exalted bathed in rivers, wells, or tanks. They scraped their bodies, often using perfumed powder, with a wooden hand-shaped instrument, crocodile teeth, the jawbone of an ox, a twisted cloth, or by other means. Often they rubbed themselves against trees or columns to stimulate the circulation. Both hot and cold baths were available.

Upon entering a steam bath, one had to smear the face with wet clay and wet the rest of the body or cover it as a protection against the intense heat of the open fire. The first user of the bath was required to sweep out the ashes, clean the bathroom, pound the scented powders, fill the water jar, and moisten the clay with water. The last person out was expected to clean the floor, put out the fire, arrange the bath chairs properly, and close the door. Women of the world used scented bath powder instead of unscented clay and the red powder from rice husks.

Among the cosmetics employed in this period were collyrium and antimony (for the eyes), vermilion, realgar, yellow orpiment, and lamp soot. These cosmetics were perfumed with sandalwood, black zedoary, tagara, and an essence made from bhaddamuttaka, a kind of grass. The cosmetics were kept in special boxes and applied with cosmetics sticks, which, in the case of the wealthy, were often made of gold and silver. Nuns, along with laymen, were permitted to have cosmetics boxes of ivory, horn, bamboo, reed, wood, and shells.

Women used perfumed powders and ointments and painted their bodies. Heavy, exotic perfumes were used lavishly, sandalwood being one of the most popular. The eyes were enlarged and accented with paint applied with cosmetics sticks. Designs were often painted on the cheeks, and the skin of the face was creamed and powdered. The most curious practice was the staining of the tips of the fingers and soles of the feet with the coppery red lac-dye. This is referred to in the fourth act of *Śakoontalá* by a hermit arriving with bridal gifts after passing through a mysterious forest:

> Straightway depending from a neighbouring tree
> Appeared a robe of linen tissue, pure

> And spotless as a moonbeam — mystic pledge
> Of bridal happiness; another tree
> Distilled a roseate dye wherewith to stain
> The lady's feet.

Another reference is to be found in an Indian ode entitled *Megha-dúta*:

> The rose hath humbly bowed to meet
> With glowing lips her hallowed feet,
> And lent them all its bloom.

Beards were trimmed with razors and scissors, and chest and pubic hair was shaved. Hair on the belly was sometimes cut in patterns. Women wore their hair long. The hair was dressed with the aid of combs, fingers, beeswax, and ointments.

During this period highly polished mirrors of gold with ivory handles were used by royalty and others who could afford them. The less affluent used more ordinary mirrors or even bowls of water.

The fingernails were worn long and often polished, though polishing, like many other things, was forbidden to nuns. The nails were trimmed with special nail-cutters or sometimes torn or chewed off or rubbed against rough walls.

During the first, second, and third centuries B.C., life in the palace became even more luxurious, and large sums were spent on perfumes and cosmetics. Sandalwood was still the source of much of the perfume, and it was available in a great variety of scents and colours. Various kinds of perfumes were described

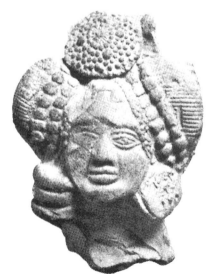

FIG. 28: Terracotta head of a woman. India, third century B.C. or earlier.

PLATE 9 : ANCIENT HAIR STYLES OF
INDIA

A Very ancient men's style with chignon supported by a fillet.
B Dancing girl, very ancient style.
C Pre-Christian period. Topknot worn with turban.
D Women's plaited style.
E Pre-Christian. Men's topknot style worn with turban.
F Early Christian era. Men's topknot style.
G Early Christian era. Men's style.
H Early Christian era. An unpāsaka hairdo with a separate bow of hair at the crown.
I Women's spiral hairdo, Gandhāra.
J Women's topknot hairdo, Gandhāra.
K Women's topknot hairdo, Gandhāra.
L Women's spiral hairdo, Gandhāra.
M Early Christian era. Women's pigtail hairdo, decorated with net and rosettes, Gandhāra.
N Early Christian era. Women's hairdo with chaplet, tied at back. Ghandāra.
O Early Christian era. Women's pigtail hairdo. Ghandāra.

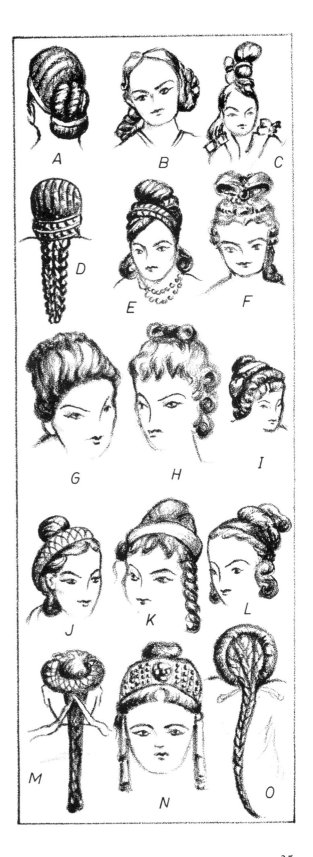

as smelling like damp earth, fish, lotus flowers, or goat's urine, and they were coloured dark red, greenish yellow, black, or brown. Aloes-wood was also extensively used for perfumes and incense and was to be found in various colours and scents, one of which is described as reminiscent of jasmine. The penetrating and long-lasting odour was particularly suitable for incense but was also used for body oils. Powders and pastes were made by pounding leaves and flowers.

Women painted their faces with suns, moons, flowers, stars, and birds, as well as geometric designs; and eye paint, along with other cosmetics, continued to be used.

The long hair was arranged in various ways. Since Indian coiffures are not covered in *Fashions in Hair*, a page of sketches is included here (see Plate 9). In the ancient Indus Valley men wore short beards, with the upper lip sometimes shaved, as in Sumer, and sometimes not. The hair was pulled back and either cut short or gathered in a knot or chignon at the back, with a fillet of beaten gold or, more commonly, of cotton or other fabric, worn around the head.

Luxurious living continued into the early Christian era, the most notable change being that now the use of cosmetics and care of the body in general was considered important for preservation of health and vigour. It was thought proper for a man, upon rising, to brush his teeth with the split ends of a twig and a paste made from honey, fruit, leaves, or spices. He then washed his eyes and his mouth with a solution often made by soaking the bark of the ksira tree in milk. After this he would make up his eyes with collyrium and antimony and chew a few betel leaves to sweeten the breath. The collyrium, in addition to beautifying the eyes, was supposed to stop burning and itching, clean the eyes, and improve the vision. It was probably applied with the fingers. Antimony, when used, was applied with special rods.

Before bathing, the man rubbed oil into his hair, massaged his body with oil, then exercised. The most common oil was derived from scented sesame seeds; richer oils were obtained from saffron, cinnamon, and myrrh. The bath might be taken in one's home or at wells, rivers, or open tanks. Those who could afford it often bathed in scented water, perfumed with saffron, oleander, camphor, or aromatic herbs and spices, often with musk added. Body scrapers, usually of terra-cotta, were still in use.

After the bath, the man used a scented paste on his body and put on gems and flowers along with his clean clothes. The perfumed powders and pastes which were applied to the body served as deodorants and were usually obtained from flowers, resins, and aromatic woods. Sandalwood was frequently used. The scented pastes were also believed to counteract fatigue and perspiration, improve the complexion, increase the strength, and give one a general feeling of well-being. Applied to the face, the pastes were supposed to steady the eyes, beautify the cheeks and the mouth, improve the contours, ward off skin eruptions, and produce a glow 'like that of a lotus flower'.

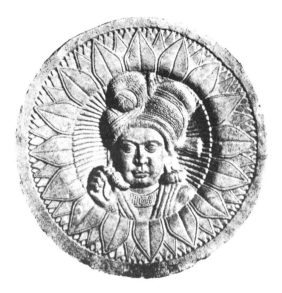

FIG. 29: Royal head on medallion. Northern India, second century B.C.

Lastly, the man perfumed his face and sometimes stained his lips with a lac-dye or a red mineral paint. The chin and the upper lip were shaved every fourth day.

Women in this early Christian period equalled and even surpassed the men in their use of perfumes, cosmetics, and ornamentation. It was considered a moral obligation, in fact, for a wife who wished for a long life for her husband, to make regular use of saffron, turmeric, red lead, and collyrium in her toilet, as well as to decorate herself with ornaments and arrange her hair attractively. She either kept her teeth very white or stained them a lotus red. She might still, as in former days, paint designs on her face and shoulders. Lac-dye was often used for the painting. Sometimes designs were cut from papyrus or betel leaves. Part of the design might be cut out and stuck on and the rest of it drawn on with a red paint stick. Rouge was also used for the lips and cheeks, and a tiny slate container of rouge has been found in Mohenjo-Daro. Lac-dye was still applied to the hands and feet, and in some areas in the south the breasts were painted with a vermilion paste.

The toilet depended to some extent on the season -- oil, saffron, musk, and aloes-wood smoke being considered suitable in the winter, and a body-paste of camphor, sandalwood, aloes-wood, and saffron in the spring. In the hot summer a man of the upper classes might remain inside, shower frequently, wear camphor garlands and necklaces scented with sandalwood, fan himself with a moistened palm-leaf fan, and sleep on a bed decorated with plantain leaves and flowers.

Street vendors, especially in the seaports, sold all sorts of perfumes and cosmetics — red, yellow, and black paints, bath powders, cooling pastes, flowers, incense. Many exotic scents and costly ointments were imported from Arabia and Somaliland. Perfumes were dispensed from small bottles or from sprinklers. These had tiny holes in the bottom of the flask, and the flow could be regulated by placing a finger over the opening at the top.

ANCIENT GREECE

Homerian Greeks are believed to have used little makeup, but later Greek women used paints and washes for colouring the skin. We know that by the fourth century B.C. the use of makeup was well established. Barthélémy describes 'one of the prettiest women of Athens' as being painted rose colour and white. The white, unfortunately, was sometimes white lead, which for more than two thousand years would whiten women's faces, destroy their complexions, and even result in premature death. The rouge was sometimes of vermilion, more often of vegetable substances, such as mulberry, seaweed, and *paederos*, a root similar to alkanet. Later, cinnabar (red sulphide of mercury) was used as well as white lead. Orpiment, a compound of arsenic, was used as a depilatory.

In Xenophon's *Good Husbandry*, Ischomacus, referring to his fifteen-year-old wife, says:

'When I found her one day painted with rouge . . . I pointed out to her that she was being as dishonest in attempting to deceive me about her looks as I should be were I to deceive her about my property. I told her that although her artifice might deceive others, it could not mislead one who saw her regularly. I was sure to catch her in the morning before her cosmetics had been applied, or tears would betray her, or perspiration, or the bath.'

The cream rouge, sometimes a more earthy red than the rose colour described by Barthélémy, seems to have been applied to the cheekbone area in a more-or-less round pattern, though there were undoubtedly personal variations. Rouged cheeks were normally accompanied by rouged lips, though sometimes the lips alone were coloured. Fragrant oils were used in the hair, and grey hair was sometimes darkened by both men and women.

A painted marble head dating from about 530 B.C. (see Figure 32) shows clear traces of the paint which represented the woman's makeup, presumably the fashionable makeup of the day. The eyebrows are painted black and are fairly close together. The eye makeup is astonishingly like that of the late 1960s. The upper lid is shadowed with a reddish brown and the lower edge of the bone above with a sort of jade green. The upper lid only is lined with the same green, which extends beyond the eye at both corners. The lips are painted with a brownish red, and the whole cheek is rouged with the same shade of red.

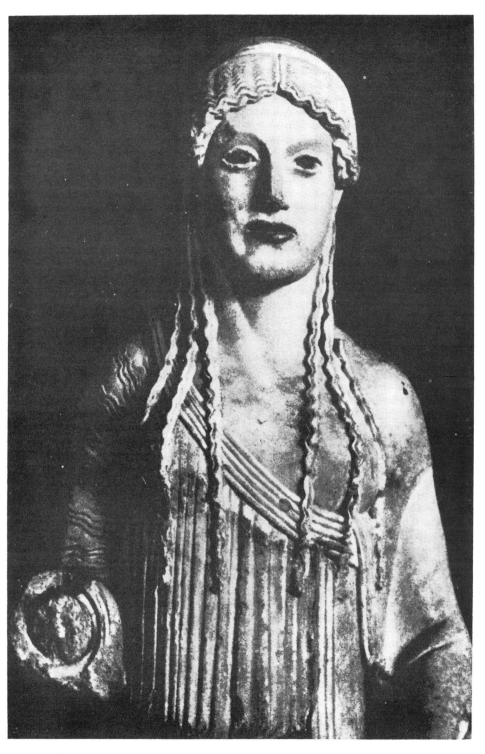

FIG. 30: *Kore* of Euthydicos. Marble sculpture from the Acropolis, Athens, *c.* 480 B.C.
Note the heavily painted lips.

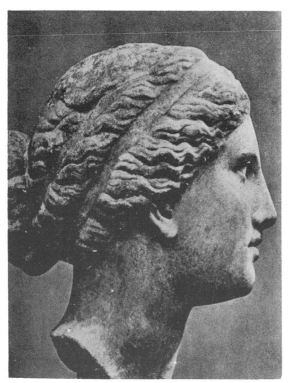 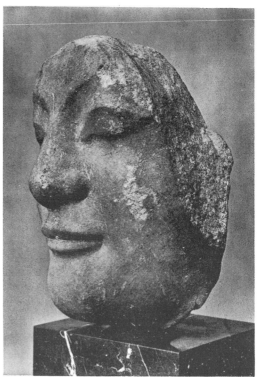

FIG. 31: Marble head of Aphrodite by Praxiteles, using Phryne as his model, fourth century B.C.

FIG. 32: Marble head of a Greek woman, *c.* 530 B.C. From the Temple of Artemis at Ephesus. The painted eye and cheek makeup still remain.

Lower class working women did not, so far as is known, wear makeup. But a travelling entertainer is described as having a brownish red cream rouge spread generously over her cheeks and lips. The rouge, kept in a box with a tight-fitting lid, was somewhat thicker than the usual consistency of cold cream. The black paint which she applied thickly with a kohl stick to her brows and lashes, was melted over a flame.

Egyptian kohl and sometimes ordinary soot or lampblack was used in eye makeup. Some women wore false eyebrows. Petronius mentions a lady taking her eyebrows out of a little box. But real or false, the Greeks favoured eyebrows which met above the nose. Anacrion's mistress had just such brows:

> Taking care her eyebrows be
> Not apart, not mingled neither,
> But as hers are, stol'n together,
> Met by stealth, yet leaning too
> O'er the eyes their darkest hue.

Nearly three hundred years later Theocritus wrote of a young cowherd who relates that:

> Passing a bower last evening with my cows,
> A girl look'd out — a girl with meeting brows.
> 'Beautiful! Beautiful!' cried she. I heard,
> But went on, looking down, and gave her not a word.

Plutarch tells us that Lycurgus banished cosmetics from Sparta as a flatterer of the senses and 'forbade the city to all who used the art of painting the body, for evil arts corrupted men's manners'. Probably Lycurgus objected only to what was clearly visible and not to the face-packs of meal which were applied at night and removed with milk in the morning.

Both men and women liked blond hair and often took considerable pains to get it. 'The sun's rays,' wrote Menander, 'are the best means for lightening the hair, as our men well know. After washing their hair with a special ointment made here in Athens, they sit bareheaded in the sun by the hour, waiting for their hair to turn a beautiful golden blond. And it does.'

The Greeks usually cleaned their teeth carefully and scraped their bodies with curved strigils (Figure 35) after the bath to remove the cleansing powders and oils and to stimulate the circulation. They used perfumes lavishly, sometimes even using different scents for different parts of the body, as described by Antiphanes, writing of a typical Athenian dandy, who bathes

> In gilded tub, and steeps his feet
> And legs in rich Egyptian unguents;
> His neck and chest he rubs with oil of palm
> And both his arms with sweet extract of mint,
> His eyebrows and his hair with marjoram,
> His knees and face with essence of wild thyme.

The scent of violets was also popular. Fashionable young men carried the use of scents to such an extreme that Solon went so far as to promulgate a law prohibiting the sale of fragrant oils to Athenian men. According to Pliny, Lucius Plotius, in hiding in Salerno, was flushed out by the authorities, who found him by following their noses to his strong and distinctive perfume.

Oils for cosmetics, massage, and medicinal purposes were obtained from various sources. For a good quality of olive oil, the unripe fruit was used; and when the olives could not conveniently be picked from the tree, they were beaten down with canes. They were then crushed in stone mills and the pulp placed in a wicker basket and weighted with stones. The oil thus forced out of the olives ran out through the wicker of the basket and was caught in another vessel. Later, a wooden-frame press was used instead of the wicker baskets. Similar methods were used for extracting oil from sesame, almonds, palm, and

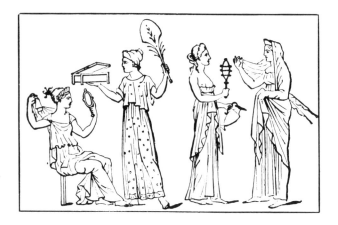

FIG. 33: **Greek** ladies at their toilet. From Rimmel's *Book of Perfumes*, 1865.

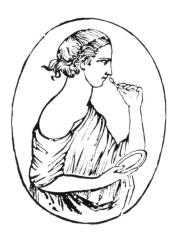

FIG. 34: Greek woman painting her lips. From Rimmel's *Book of Perfumes*.

other sources. Salt, gum, resin, and sometimes honey, vinegar, and fennel were added to preserve the oils.

According to Pliny, oil was obtained from wool (the modern-day lanolin) by heating the newly shorn wool in a bronze container of water. When it had cooled, the oil or fat which had risen to the top was removed, washed, strained through a cloth, and left in the sun until it was transparent. Unfortunately, it

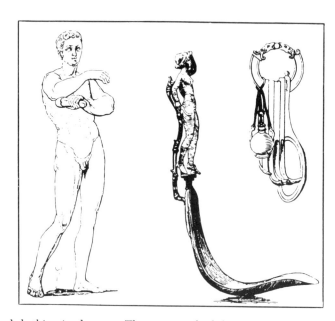

FIG. 35: Greek bathing implements. The man on the left is scraping himself with a strigil. In the centre is an unusually decorative strigil; on the right, a ring containing an ampulla of scented oil, strigils, and a spoon. From Rimmel's *Book of Perfumes*.

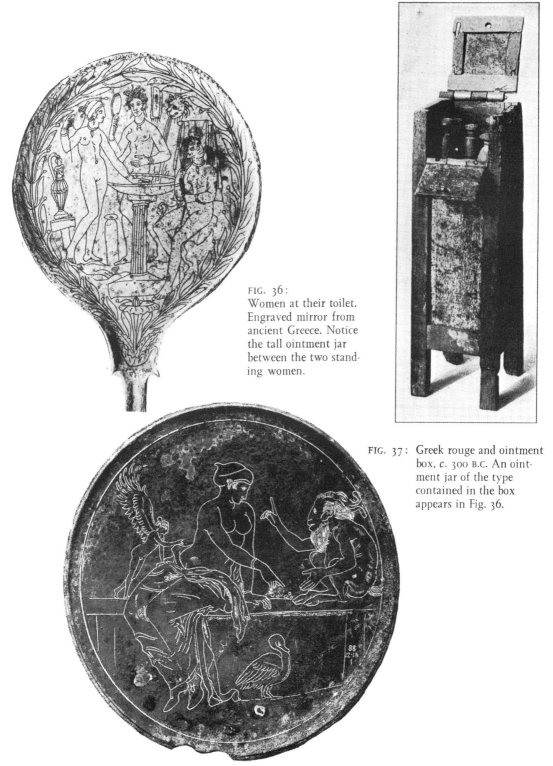

FIG. 36:
Women at their toilet.
Engraved mirror from
ancient Greece. Notice
the tall ointment jar
between the two stand-
ing women.

FIG. 37: Greek rouge and ointment
box, *c.* 300 B.C. An ointment jar of the type
contained in the box
appears in Fig. 36.

FIG. 38: Aphrodite and Pan playing dice. Engraved mirror cover, allegedly from Corinth,
fourth century B.C.

43

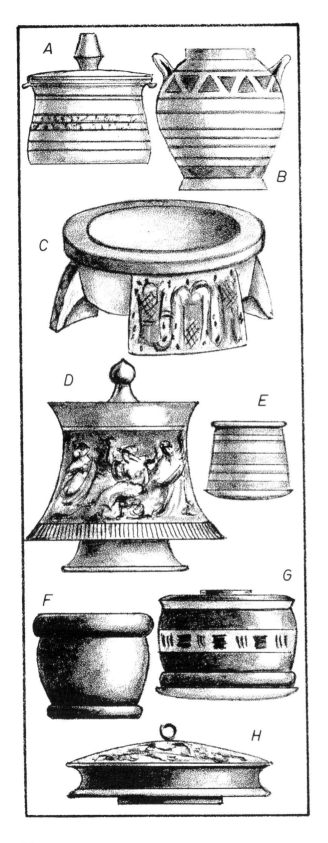

PLATE 10 : ANCIENT GREEK COSMETICS
CONTAINERS

A 675–640 B.C., Proto-Corinthian.
Made of clay. (*Metropolitan
Museum of Art, New York*)

B 575–550 B.C., Corinthian. (*Metropolitan Museum of Art, New York*)

C 575–550 B.C., Corinthian. Made of
clay. (*Metropolitan Museum of Art,
New York*)

D *c.* 460 B.C., Attic. Black and tan.
About 5 inches high. (*Metropolitan
Museum of Art, New York*)

E Late sixth century B.C., Corinthian.
Clay. About 1½ inches high.
(*Metropolitan Museum of Art,
New York*)

F *c.* 510 B.C., Attic. Black with decoration in top of lid. Inscribed, 'Ly-
sikles is fair'. About 3 inches in
diameter. (*Metropolitan Museum of
Art, New York*)

G Fifth century B.C., Attic. Black and
tan. About 4 inches in diameter.
(*Metropolitan Museum of Art, New
York*)

H *c.* 400 B.C., Attic. Bronze ring in lid.
About 7 inches in diameter. (*Metropolitan Museum of Art, New York*)

PLATE 11 : ANCIENT GREEK
COSMETICS CONTAINERS

A   *c.* 700 B.C. Perfume jar from Camae. About 2 inches high. Inscription reads, 'I am Tataie's scent bottle. Whoever steals me shall go blind.' (*British Museum*)

B   Sixth century B.C., Corinthian. Cosmetics jar — tripod style, with lid. About 3½ inches in diameter. (*Metropolitan Museum of Art, New York*)

C   Mid-sixth century B.C., Attic. Cosmetics pot with swans. About 2 inches in diameter. (*British Museum*)

D   Fifth century B.C., Attic. Black cosmetics jar. About 2 inches in diameter. (*Metropolitan Museum of Art, New York*)

E   Fourth century B.C. Bronze cosmetics pot, said to be from Tarentum. About 3 inches in diameter. (*British Museum*)

F   About fourth century B.C. Black and tan clay cosmetics pot, containing traces of rouge. About 2½ inches in diameter. (*British Museum*)

G   *c.* 465–450 B.C. Cosmetics pot of painted clay. 'Judgment of Paris.' (*Metropolitan Museum of Art, New York*)

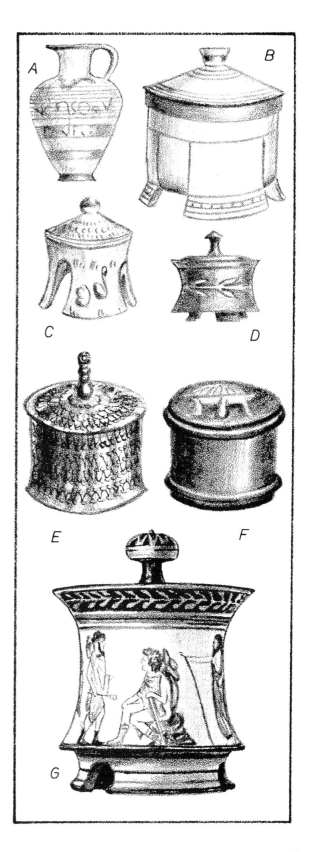

tended to decompose and to develop an evil smell. Other animal fats, goose fat, and butter were also used, especially in cosmetics.

William Alexander reported that the Scythians 'never washed themselves, lest it should spoil the beauty of their skin, but they used a *succedaneum*: they pounded Cypress and Cedar with incense, infused the powder in water, made it into a paste, and spread it over their faces; when it came off, it is said not only to have smoothed and beautified, but even to have perfumed the part upon which it was laid.'

In this seventeenth-century translation, the Greek physician Galen, the inventor of cold cream, warns about the dangers of poisonous cosmetics:

'The excellencie of this Mercurie sublimate is such that the women who often paint themselves with it, though they be very young, they presently turne old with withered and wrinkeled faces like an Ape, and before age come upon them, they tremble (poor wretches) as if they were sicke of the staggers, reeling and full of quick-silver, for so are they: for the Soliman and quick-silver differ only in this, that the Soliman is the more corosive and byting; insomuch that being applied to the face, it is true, that it eateth out the spots and staines of the face, but so, that with all, it drieth up, and consumeth the flesh that is underneath, so that of force the poore skin shrinketh.'

Physicians and writers were to continue the warnings, largely unheeded, for the next fifteen hundred years.

THE ETRUSCANS

The highly civilized Etruscans lined their eyes and probably painted their eyebrows, bringing them fairly close together at the nose (Figures 39 and 41). There is no evidence that the men used colour on their faces, though some of them may well have done so. But the women presumably did. Elaborate toilet boxes (Figure 42) and ornate mirrors (Figure 43) still exist. Rouge and lip rouge were commonly used during this period, and using a wash of colour over the entire face was not unknown. Men wore curled beards, with or without moustaches. The women's hair was waved or curled and allowed to hang in long curls or braids (Figure 40) over the shoulders. The men's hair was sometimes curled in ringlets over the forehead and hung over the shoulders in long curls like the women's. Sometimes, as in Figure 41, it was worn short.

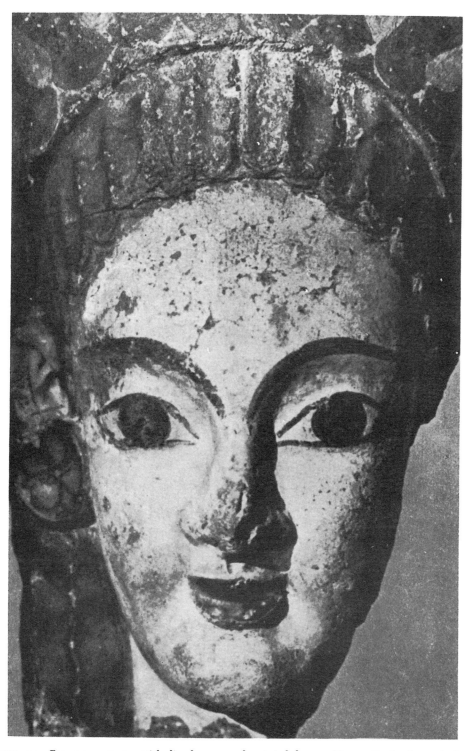

FIG. 39: Etruscan woman with lined eyes and painted brows. Terracotta head, *c*. sixth century B.C.

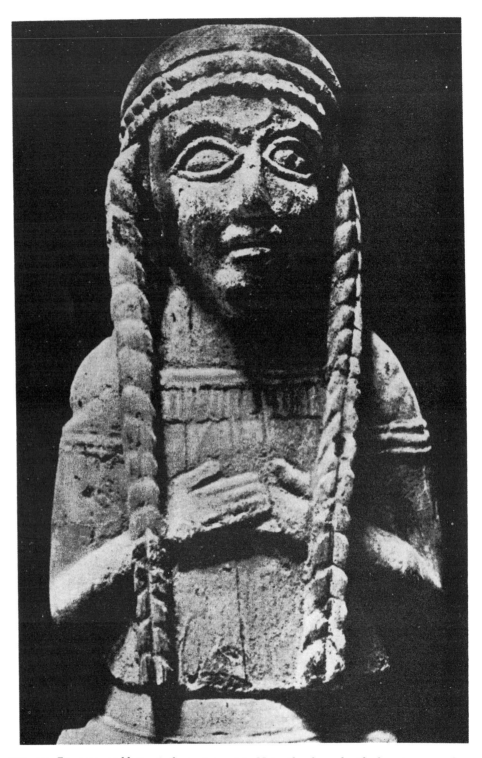

FIG. 40: Etruscan goddess, sixth century B.C. Note the long braids hanging over her shoulders.

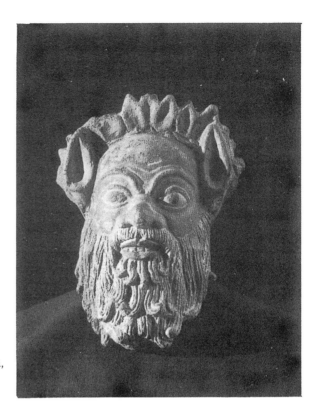

FIG. 41 : Etruscan head of Silenus, in terracotta, early fifth century B.C. Brows are painted and eyes are lined.

ANCIENT ROME

'Paint,' wrote Plautus, 'is not for the young, nor white lead, quince ointment, or any other cosmetic.' But elsewhere he has two girls from Carthage arguing for and against the need for makeup, one insisting it was necessary for beauty, the other declaring that good food needs no seasoning. This was answered, in turn, by a remark that a woman without makeup is like food without salt. Cornelius Gallus was in favour of makeup for women and encouraged his mistress to use more of it.

Ovid recommended light vermilion to supply the colour denied by nature, and Horace reported that women used three kinds of paint — red lead, carmine, and an extract of crocodile dung. But Tibullius asked, 'What's the use of lighting up your cheeks with a sparkling paint?' And Propertius insisted that the best face was still the natural face. Clement I lashed out at painted women 'who use crocodiles' excrement . . . blacken their eyebrows with soot, and paint their faces with white lead.' The crocodile excrement was used as a mud-pack.

Light complexions were considered essential for fashionable women, and the more sympathy the woman wanted, the whiter the makeup. White lead and chalk were both used to whiten the skin. Martial points out that Fabula feared the rain because of the chalk on her face, and Sabella took pains to avoid the

49

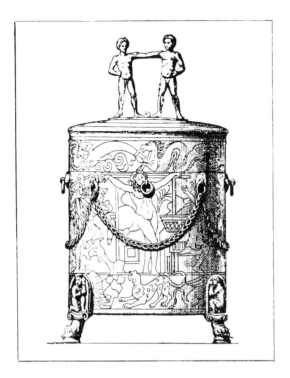

FIG. 42: Etruscan toilet box. From
Ménard's *La Vie Privée
des Anciens*, 1880.

sun because of the ceruse on hers. Augustus restricted the use of ceruse (white paint) to patrician ladies, but the restrictions did not hold for long.

In *The Art of Love* Ovid addresses himself to women on the subject of their makeup:

'You know how to whiten your skin with wax and to supply with carmine the rosy blush of Nature. You have the art to fill the space between your eyebrows, if that be necessary, and with makeup to conceal the telltale marks of the advancing years. You do not hesitate to increase the brightness of your eyes with powdered ash or with saffron gathered on the banks of the Cydnus. . . . But on no account let your lover come upon you surrounded by the accoutrements of your cosmetic art. Your artifice should go unsuspected. Who could help but feel disgust at the thick paint on your face melting and running down onto your breasts? How can one describe the obnoxious smell of the oesypum, even though it comes from Athens, of that oil extracted from the fleece of sheep. . . . Do not use the marrow taken from deer or clean your teeth in front of others. I realize that all of this can heighten your charms, but it is nonetheless unpleasant to watch. . . . If we arrive before you've finished your toilet, have the servants tell us you are still asleep. You will seem all the lovelier when you do appear. Why do I need to know what gives your skin its whiteness? Shut

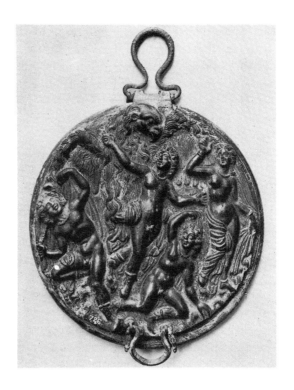

FIG. 43 : Ganymede and the Eagle.
Etruscan folding mirror
of bronze, *c.* 200 B.C.

your door, and let me not see the work till it's complete. There are many things we men had best know nothing of. Most of these artificial aids we'd find distressing if you let us see them. . . . Rare, however, is the face without a fault. Hide these blemishes with care. . . . If you are sallow, put on a little rouge; if you are swarthy, see what the fish of Pharos will do for you.'

In *The Art of Beauty* Ovid is more specific :

'When you are well rested from a night of sleep and your body is refreshed, let me teach you how to make your skin a dazzling white. Take the barley which our ships bring back from Libyan fields and strip it of its straw and husks. Take of this two pound and of vetches an equal quantity and with ten eggs mix them well. Dry this mixture in the open air, then let it be ground by a mill-stone worked by the patient ass.' He then instructs the reader to pulverize one sixth of a pound of hartshorn into a fine powder and pass it through a sieve, after which one is to add a dozen skinned narcissus bulbs, pounding the mixture in a marble mortar. The recipe is completed by the addition of 'two ounces of gum and Tuscan wheat and nine times as much of honey. Any woman who uses this cosmetic paste,' Ovid assures his readers, 'will have a face more shining than her mirror.'

Another recipe requires baking some lupins and beans: 'Take six pounds each and grind it all in the mill. Add to that white lead and the scum of red nitre and Illyrian iris. All this must then be kneaded by strong, young arms. When all are duly mashed, an ounce should be the proper weight. If you add to this the mud with which the Halcyon cements its nest, you will have a certain cure for spots and pimples. An ounce applied in equal parts is the dose I recommend. To make the mixture more adhesive and easier to apply, add honey from the honeycombs of Attica. . . .

'A mixture of incense and nitre will help get rid of blackheads. Take of each four ounces, adding an ounce of gum from bark and a small cube of oily myrrh. Crush all together and force through a sieve. Mix the resulting powder with honey to bind it. Some recommend that fennel be added to the myrrh — nine scruples of myrrh and five of fennel. Add to this a handful of dried rose-leaves, sal-ammoniac, and frankincense. Pour barley water over it, and let the weight of the incense and the sal-ammoniac equal the weight of the roses. A few applications of the mixture will give you a beautiful complexion.'

Ovid said that he had seen used, as a substitute for rouge, poppies soaked in cold water and rubbed on the cheeks.

Whenever makeup has become excessive according to conservative standards, there have been critics to point out to women, and occasionally to men, the folly of their painted ways. The Roman satirists usually criticized with greater wit and a finer cutting edge than most of those who followed, but still without any notable success.

'Galla,' wrote Martial, 'you are but a composition of lies. Whilst you were in Rome, your hair was growing on the banks of the Rhine; at night, when you lay aside your silken robes, you lay aside your teeth as well; and two thirds of your person are locked up in boxes for the night; the eyebrows with which you make such insinuating motions are the work of your slaves. Thus no man can say, I love you, for you are not what he loves, and no one loves what you are.'

Polla, a Roman matron, who, according to Pliny, spent her sixtieth birthday in a 'poultice of honey and wine lees with finely ground narcissus bulbs', was the object of one of Martial's many plaints:

> Leave off thy paint, perfume, and childish dress,
> And Nature's aging honestly confess;
> Twofold we see those faults which art would mend;
> Plain, downright ugliness would less offend.

Lycornis's cosmetic habits warranted only a passing mention:

'Lycornis, who is blacker than the colour of the ripe mulberry, considers herself beautiful when she paints her face with white lead.'

Although Ovid approved of cosmetics for women when they were skillfully applied, he did not consider them appropriate for men:

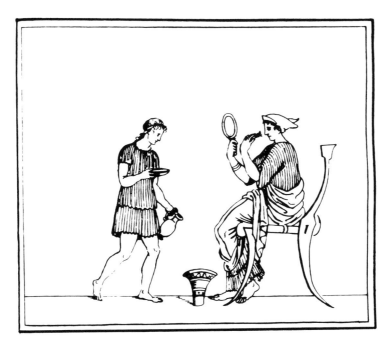

FIG. 44: Roman lady applying makeup. From Ménard's *La Vie Privée des Anciens*, 1880.

'And don't, I beg of you, let your hair be curled or use powder on your face. Leave all such foppery to the effeminate priests. . . . Theseus won Ariadne without concerning himself unduly about his hair. Phaedra fell in love with Hippolytus, who most assuredly was not a dandy. . . . Don't let your hair stick out in tufts; be sure that both hair and beard are neatly trimmed. See also that your nails are neat and clean; don't let hair grow out of your nostrils; be sure that your breath is pleasant, and don't go about smelling like a goat. All other refinements of the toilet leave to women and effeminate dandies.'

Juvenal also objected to the beautification of men, as in this vivid portrait of a contemporary flirt:

> But tell me yet — this thing, thus daubed and oiled,
> Poulticed, plastered, baked by turns and boiled,
> Thus with pomatums, ointments, laquered o'er,
> Is it a face, Usidius, or a sore?

In his second satire Juvenal lashed out at the priests and generals for their vanity and use of cosmetics:

> With jet-black pencils one his eyebrows dyes,
> And adds new fire to his lascivious eyes. . . .
> Another thinks a general must kill,

But as a courtier, uses all his skill
To keep his skin from tan; before the fight
He paints and sets his soiled complexion right.

Martial was equally unsympathetic and directed his venom at several men who painted:

TO PANNICUS

I would not have you curl your hair, nor yet would I have
you throw it into disorder. Your skin I would have neither
over-sleek nor neglected. Your beard should be neither that
of an effeminate Asiatic nor that of an accused person. I
alike detest, Pannicus, one who is more and one who is less
than a man. Your legs and breasts bristle with shaggy hair;
but your mind, Pannicus, shows no sign of manliness.

TO OLUS

Thy beard is hoary; but thy locks are black;
To tinge the beard thou hast not yet the knack.

TO PHOEBUS

You manufacture, with the aid of unguents, a false head of
hair, and your bald and dirty skull is covered with dyed
locks. There is no need to have a hairdresser for your head —
a sponge, Phoebus, would do it better.

Both Nero and Poppaea used cosmetics. Her routine of beautification was so elaborate that she required, or thought she did, a hundred slaves to help her. Her nightly face-mask, made of moistened and perfumed meal, which dried into a hard mask, was washed off in the morning with asses' milk. She also bathed in asses' milk to preserve the beauty of her skin, which she then covered with chalk and poisonous white lead. She used fucus, a red or purplish paint, to rouge her cheeks and lips, antimony to darken her lids, lashes, and brows, and blue paint for her veins. 'Dragon's blood' mixed with sheep fat served to colour her nails. In addition, she had depilatories for stray hairs, meal paste and lemon juice to bleach her freckles, pumice stone to whiten her teeth, barley flour and butter for pimples, and Hessian soap, as it was later called, to bleach her hair. The effect of the makeup was hardly subtle, and keeping it intact required considerable care, but nonetheless it became extremely popular with women of Rome. Curiously, this painted or plastered face, popularly known as the 'domestic face' since it was worn at home, seemed to be intended for the husband and was frequently, according to Juvenal, the only one he ever saw:

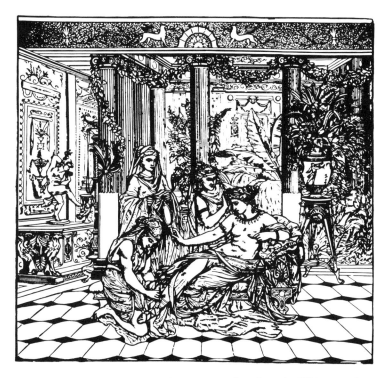

FIG. 45 : Roman lady at her toilet. Drawing based on the Elkington plaque.

She duly, once a month, renews her face;
Meantime, it lies in dawb, and hid in grease;
Those are the husband's nights; she craves her due,
He takes fat kisses, and is stuck in glue.
But to the loved adult'rer when she steers,
Fresh from the bath, in brightness she appears;
For him the rich Arabia sweets her gum;
And precious oils from distant Indies come.
How haggardly soe'er she looks at home,
Th'eclipse then vanishes; and all her face
Is opened, and restored to ev'ry grace,
The crust removed; her cheeks as smooth as silk,
Are polished with a wash of asses' milk;
And should she to the farthest north be sent,
A train of these attend her banishment.
But hadst thou seen her plaistered up before,
'Twas so unlike a face, it seemed a sore.

There is ample evidence of the use of rouge in the rock crystal pots of it uncovered at Herculaneium. The Greek and Roman rouge was usually rose-coloured, made of white chalk dissolved in a purple dye and precipitated twice. The second precipitate was the rouge.

Like the Greeks, the Romans considered eyebrows which met over the nose a mark of beauty (see Figure 46). For blackening the eyebrows, the Romans used preparations made from antimony, lead, or soot. Pliny recommends certain hair pomades and warns against the harmfulness of others. He also gives a recipe for a popular hair dye:

'Take a pint of leeches and two quarts of pure vinegar; pound them into a pot and ferment for sixty days. At the end of this time rub into the scalp in the sunlight and the hair will become beautifully black. Do not forget during the operation to hold oil in the mouth, without which your teeth will take the same tint.'

Martial, on the other hand, warns Galla to stop dyeing her hair before she has none left to dye. Superfluous hair was removed with depilatory plasters. Cleaners and whiteners for the teeth and even false teeth were available. The skin, when it wasn't covered with paint, was carefully washed and perfumed.

Small, round beauty marks, called *splenia*, were used by Roman women, evidently in some profusion since Martial says of one woman, 'A number of beauty spots covered her superb forehead'; and Ovid, of another, 'Few spaces are without spots'. It is said that Regulus, a Roman lawyer, used to wear a patch on the right or left side of his forehead, depending on whether he was pleading for the defendant or the plaintiff.

The Romans had as much trouble with wrinkles as anyone else and used an astringent called *tentipellium* to try to prevent them. Constantin James mentions, among the Roman lady's cosmetic aids, 'the cataplasma made from large beans cooked in butter; and', he adds, 'as these treatments invariably left a rancid odour, she tried to remove it with a pure water followed by the use of alenium, the base of which was the milk of the she-ass, or by lomentum made of wheat and perfumed with the Myrrh of Judea.' As a remedy for blackheads and pimples, the Roman lady often used a sort of gum gathered from certain birds' nests. Ladies who could afford to, used cosmetics prepared from ashes of date pits, spikenard, or rose leaves.

The luxury-loving Romans tended to use perfumes excessively. Patricians anointed themselves three times a day with perfumed oils which they carried to the baths in exquisitely decorated gold vessels. Nero is said to have used more than a year's supply of Arabian perfumes at Poppaea's funeral, and entire open amphitheatres were sometimes perfumed by censers. In order to conserve the supply of perfumes, all of which were imported from Arabia, Licinius Crassus restricted the use of perfumes for non-religious purposes.

Along with his many satiric verses, Martial presented a long list of 'Presents

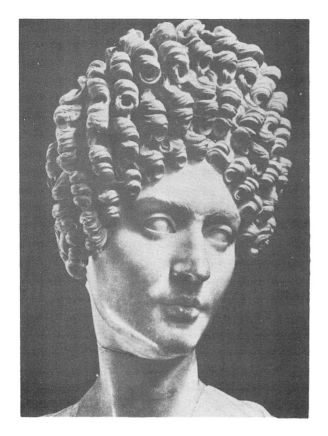

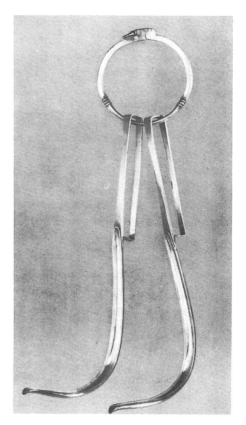

FIG. 46: Roman beauty with meeting eyebrows and *orbis* headdress. Late first century A.D.

FIG. 47: Roman strigils of silver, first century B.C. Used for scraping the body.

Made to Guests at Feasts'. Although paints were not mentioned specifically (perhaps they were not considered suitable gifts), other cosmetics and cosmetic implements were:

A GOLDEN HAIRPIN. That your oiled tresses may not injure your splendid silk dress. Let this pin fix your twisted hair and keep it up.

COMBS. Of what use will be this piece of boxwood, cut into so many teeth, and now presented to you, seeing that you have no hair?

POMATUM. My caustic influence reddens the hair of the Germans; by my aid you may surpass your slaves' tresses.

MATTIAC BALLS. If you desire, Octogenarian, to change the colour of your venerable hair, accept these Mattiac balls. But to what purpose, for you are bald?

BARBERS' INSTRUMENTS. Some of these instruments are adapted for cutting the hair; one is useful for long nails, another for rough chins.

STRIGILS, FOR SCRAPING THE SKIN IN THE BATH. Pergamus sent these; scrape yourself with the curved iron, and the scourer will not so often have to cleanse your linen. [See Figure 47.]

TOOTH POWDER. What have I to do with you? Let the fair and young use me. I am not accustomed to polish false teeth.

BALMS. Balm delights me; it is the perfume for men. Ye matrons, scent yourselves with the essences of Cosmos.

A PILLOW. Rub your hair with the nard of Cosmos, and your pillow will smell of it. When your hair has lost the perfume, the pillow retains it.

The Baths. The bath was an important part of the Roman toilet and eventually of the social life as well. During the early years of the Republic, labourers washed the arms and legs daily, usually in the Tiber or one of its tributaries, and bathed the entire body only once every ninth day. But after water was brought into the city by means of the aqueducts, public baths began to be built. They rapidly increased in size, number, beauty, and complexity until, by some estimates, there were nearly eight hundred of them in Rome. The baths of Caracalla contained 1600 marble seats and could accommodate 2300 bathers at one time.

In using the public baths, the bather, after undressing, went first into the *unctuarium*, where his body was anointed with oil from large jars, then into another room, when he was covered with sand or powder before engaging in wrestling or other physical exercise. Following this he would sit on a marble bench in the hot baths and scrape his body or have it scraped by a slave, using a strigil of silver, bronze or ivory (Figures 47 and 48). He might also swim in the pool if he wished. After having vases of clean water poured over him, he proceeded to the tepid baths and then to the cold. Before leaving the baths, he had his body lightly oiled and might, if he wished, have superfluous hairs removed. Those who wanted the body to be perfumed went again to the *unctuarium*.

Originally the baths were open only from two to five during the afternoon. Then Nero had them opened at noon, and eventually they remained open from dawn to dusk. Bathing twice a day became the usual thing, and some men remained at the baths all day, meeting their friends and discussing news, politics, philosophy, or merely gossiping. At times there were regulations about who might not bathe with whom; at other times everyone, both men and women, bathed together.

Even with the extensive and elaborate public baths, elegant and often very large private baths, richly decorated, became commonplace. According to Seneca, those of the upper classes had 'a procession of statues, a number of columns supporting nothing, placed as ornaments merely because of the expense, the water murmuring down steps, and the doors of rare and costly stones.'

In spite of the baths, deodorants seem to have been a problem with the Romans, and Thais evidently had not solved her problem successfully:

'Cunningly wishing to exchange her disagreeable odour for some other, she,

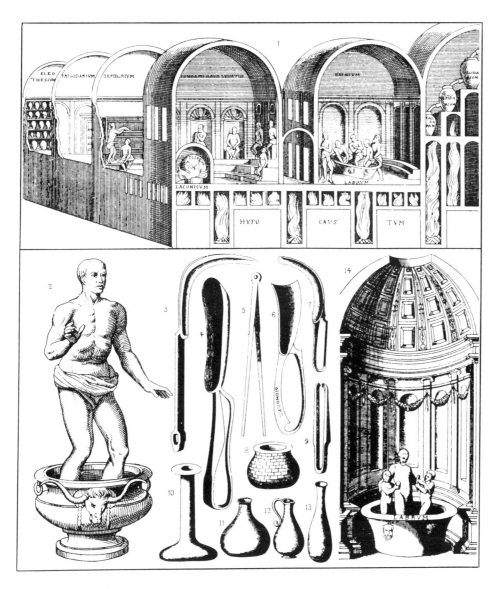

FIG. 48: Roman bath. At the top is a cross-section of a public bath, showing the various rooms; below, in the centre, are oil bottles, tweezers, and strigils for scraping the skin. From Racinet's *Le Costume Historique*, 1888.

on laying aside her garments to enter the bath, makes herself green with a depilatory or conceals herself beneath a daubing of chalk dissolved in acid or covers herself with three or four layers of rich bean-unguent. When by a thousand artifices, she thinks she has succeeded in making herself safe, Thais still smells of Thais.'

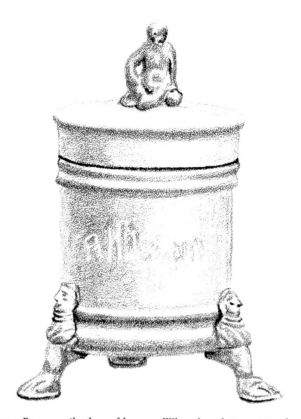

FIG. 49: Roman toilet box of bronze. When found, it contained mirror, rouge pot, hairpins, combs, strigils, and other cosmetics implements.

The Lady's Toilet. Lucian describes in some detail the scene of a Roman lady's toilet:

'She must, these days, use powders, pomades, paints . . . each chambermaid, each slave carries one of the essential objects for the toilet. One holds a silver basin, another a chamber pot, a third a water pot; still others the mirror and as many boxes as one could find in a pharmacy: and all these boxes contain only things she would not want anyone to see. In one are teeth and drugs for the gums; in other, eyelashes and eyebrows and the means of restoring faded beauty. But it is especially on the coiffure that they use the most art and spend the most time. Several women who fancy changing their black hair to blonde or even golden, rub the hair with a pommade which they then dry in strong sunlight. Others, whose black hair still pleases them, spend their family fortune on ointments scented with all the perfumes of Arabia. They heat irons to make curls which nature has denied them. The hair must fall over the forehead nearly to the eyebrows. . . . The curls behind hang very low on the shoulders.'

In more recent times, Carl Boettiger, in his *Sabina*, gives his version of the Roman lady's toilet:

'In the evening, before going to bed, she had spread on her face, following the fashion of her time, a paste made of bread softened in asses' milk, an invention of the notorious Poppaea, wife of Nero. . . . This coating dried during the night, and Sabina, at the moment of rising, seemed to have a plaster head covered with creases and fissures. . . . Let us add that Sabina, in going to bed, had left with her other clothes certain essential parts of the human face, such as eyebrows, teeth, hair, and so on. . . .'

In the morning, 'Sabina, upon entering the chamber, where she finds a crowd of slaves who have been waiting for her for several hours, makes a sign to the one who has been in charge of guarding the entrance to her antechamber and tells him which of the merchants, soothsayers, purveyors of toilet articles, letter carriers, she wishes to let in. Sabina is sick or still abed for all other visitors; and what woman, during all these preparations, would allow herself to be seen by profane eyes until she is once again adorned with all her charms!'

Each slave has been assigned a specific task, is responsible for a single jewel, a certain garment, or a particular part of the body. And each is expected to carry out her task to perfection. A mischance with a single curl can result in a severe beating. For greater efficiency, the slaves are organized into troops which arrive and leave instantly on command:

'First come those who carry the makeup, who apply the rouge and the white paint, those who comb the eyebrows, those who clean and polish the teeth. . . . Scaphion, holding a basin full of warm asses' milk, with a sponge carefully removes the crust which covers the face of her mistress. Phiole is the name of the second slave, who, when her mistress's face is clean, applies the rouge and the white paint. But before beginning this cosmetic operation, she breathes on a metal mirror which she presents to Sabina. This scents it, indicating by the odour if the saliva of the slave is healthy and perfumed and if she has chewed during the morning the pastilles which were prescribed for her, because it is with the saliva that Phiole must grind the paint before applying it to the cheeks of her mistress.

'The little boxes, the shells, and all the implements with which, as Hamlet says, women spoil the most beautiful work of the creator, were closed up again in two little containers of ivory and crystal which were one of the most precious furnishings of the lady's toilet. . . . Except for the white lead, which is a caustic that was extensively used in those times, all of the other paints were derived from the animal or the vegetable kingdoms.

'While Phiole is busy with the painting, the third slave, Stimmi, is waiting, holding in her left hand a shell full of powdered lead diluted in water, which resembles soot . . . and in the right hand a sort of quill or hair pencil. Black eyelashes and well-arched eyebrows which terminate at the root of the nose and nearly come together, are considered necessary to the beauty of a woman. The slave was called Stimmi, a word which in Greek meant black for the eyes and

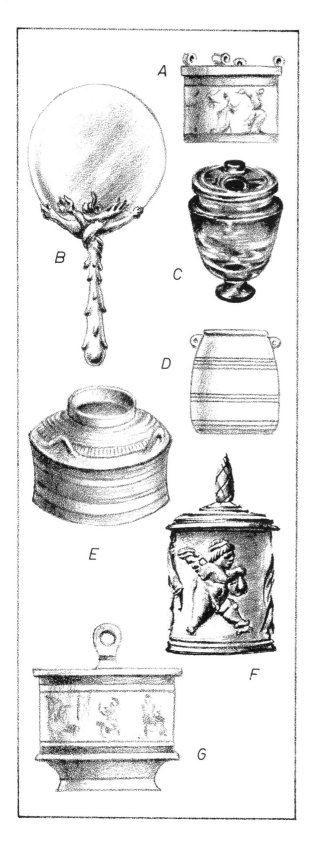

PLATE 12 : ANCIENT GREEK AND ROMAN
COSMETICS CONTAINERS
AND MIRRORS

A   460–450 B.C., Greek. Clay toilet box.
About 5 inches in diameter. (*British Museum*)

B   First century A.D., Roman. Silver
mirror with handle in the form of
the club of Hercules, decorated
with his lion skin. (*Royal Scottish Museum, Edinburgh*)

C   Roman cosmetics pot of rock crystal.
About 2 inches high. (*British Museum*)

D   *c*. 600 B.C., Greek. Bone cosmetics
pot with holes for cord. (*British Museum*)

E   Thirteenth century B.C., Greek.
Clay ointment jar. About 6 inches
high. (*British Museum*)

F   Third century, Roman. Cosmetics
pot of ivory. 2 inches high. (*British Museum*)

G   460–50 B.C., Greek. Clay toilet box.
About 6 inches in diameter. (*British Museum*)

which the Romans, with a slight alteration, had made *stibium*. It was a powder made of lead, antimony, or bismuth.' As a matter of fact, the word was used to refer to any makeup, even rouge.

'Already the facile hand of Stimmi . . . has transformed her mistress into a Juno with cow-eyes, and she is replaced by Mastiche, another slave who takes care of the teeth. This one first gave Sabina the gum which women chew each morning. In addition to the transparent, yellowish drops of this gum, Mastiche carries on a golden tray a small onyx phial filled with the urine of a young boy, with which to dilute the crushed pumice stone, giving to this mixture all sorts of colours by adding to it some marble dust; but all that is only sham; the teeth which the slave carried in a beautiful little box have been placed by her in the gums, and those certainly had no need of being cleaned; as for the two or three large teeth which still remained in Sabina's mouth, nothing in the world could have polished or whitened them. The false teeth of ivory, set into the gums with gold, are an invention so old that the first laws of Rome, those of the Twelve Tables, expressly refer to it, and we conclude, based on an epigram of Martial, that the use of false teeth was general in his time.'

After Sabina has been made up and her teeth put in, she is ready for the unveiling of her head. Having had no success with various pomades and corrosive soaps intended to bleach her black hair to a fashionable reddish blonde, she had decided to cut her hair and have a wig made by a merchant who had recently received some hair from the banks of the Rhine. But most women did not ordinarily resort to wigs except as a disguise or in cases of absolute necessity since they were easily dislodged or disarrayed when attending the baths. Fortunately, one of her hairdressers had discovered, a few days earlier, at a Gallic perfumer's near the Circus Maximus, a new pomade, which was to be rubbed into the hair after it had been washed with lye-water. The hair was then allowed to dry in the sun. After this had been done, Sabina's hair was curled, powdered, and confined in a sort of caul. Now, at last, the results of the experiment are unveiled:

' "Ah, the beautiful red! The hair of Aurora is not of such a brilliant blonde!" cry all the slaves at once, as if someone has given them the signal; and Sabina, enchanted by their approval, expects to see in her mirror the confirmation of their longed-for astonishment. She smiles with pleasure and seats herself with a triumphant air in her chair in order that her four women may complete the edifice of her coiffure. While Calmis, with a curling iron she has heated in a silver heater, arranges the hair at the temples and on the forehead . . . Psecas, with a dexterity which one acquires only by long experience, perfumes with spikenard and precious scents from the Orient, which she has put in her mouth, her mistress's hair, which retains throughout the day a sweet smell of ambrosia. . . . The Greeks tell that a king of Persia often gave to his wives the entire revenue from a wealthy village for the purchase

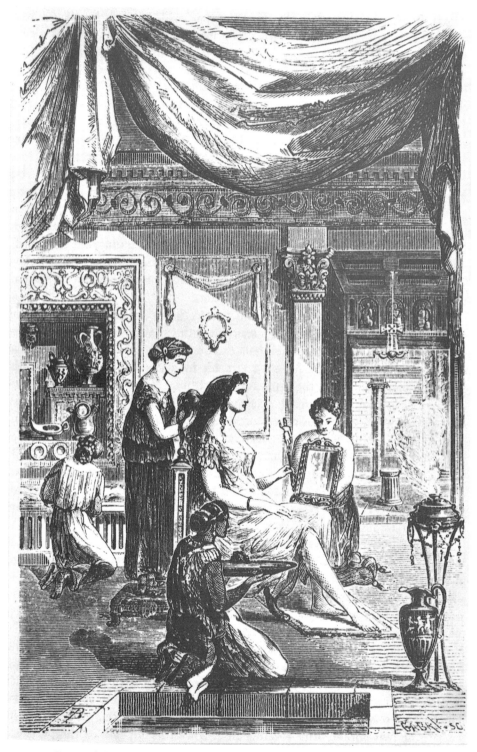

FIG. 50: Roman lady's dressing-room. Nineteenth-century engraving. From Rimmel's *Book of Perfumes*.

of their perfumes, and Sabina certainly needs a similar sum for this single article of her toilet. . . .

'As soon as Psecas has finished her service, Cypassis presents herself. She is a pretty and skillful negress who shows great intelligence and finesse in secret commissions for her mistress, who, on her side, has a special affection for her and knows how to appreciate and reward the services which she renders. Cypassis is charged with the most important matter of this part of the toilet. When the hair has been well combed and perfumed, she dresses the hair at the back of the head and collects all of it on the forehead in a sort of cushion, forming a coiffure to which has been given the generic name of *nodus*, but which can be varied in a hundred different ways. . . .

'The first and most facile of Sabina's hairdressers puts the final touch on the work of her companions. Her mistress had instructed her in all the theory of the coiffure, how it must be in harmony with the face, with the shape of the head, even with the rest of the appearance. It is now necessary to decide if today Sabina will encircle her head with a diadem, letting a few curls of hair float down on both sides, or if she will have on her forehead the great knotted foretop. . . . It was a question of having a great golden metal plate or a ribbon decorated with pearls and gold which would allow only a few curls on the forehead. Sabina today wishes less to inspire respect than to please and make conquests, so she decides on the knot. Made with the hair itself, this formed a sort of foretop which ordinarily was accompanied by curls falling on both sides.'

To the slave Latris falls the unenviable task of presenting Sabina with the mirror — in this case, one of silver and gold surrounded by precious stones and attached to an elegant ivory handle. There are sponges for polishing and cleaning the metal reflecting surface. If Sabina is pleased with her reflection, all will be well; if not, someone will be punished. And if, the Gods forbid, Latris should drop and break the mirror, which cost more than she herself did, Sabina's cruel temper would know no bounds. But the reflection pleases, and if the rest of the toilet goes well, the slaves are safe for another day.

EARLY CHRISTIAN PERIOD

Most of our information about makeup in this period comes from the writings of churchmen who objected to it. There was a great procession of men of the church who preached and wrote against artificial aids to beauty, both hair and paint. None of this had any noticeable effect. Tertullian said that 'they sinne against the Lord, which bespot their cheekes with red colours, and dye their eyes'. Clement of Alexandria, who declared that when wig-wearers were blessed,

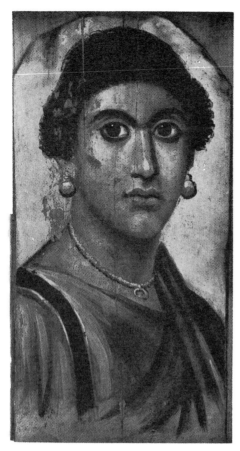

FIG. 51:
Portrait of an Egyptian woman painted
in encaustic, from Hawara, early second
century A.D. The front hair is arranged
in curls around the forehead; the back
hair is swept up in a coil.

the blessing remained on the wig and did not penetrate to the wearer beneath,
found, in this seventeenth-century translation, the use of cosmetics no less
immoral:

'The women which are exercised in frizling their haire, in anointing their
cheekes, in painting their eyes, and dying their haire, and following other
wantonnesse with unlawfull artes, doe seeme to me to draw on unhappy lovers:
but if any man shall open the vaile of the Temple, I meane their dressing,
colouring, dying, and those things, that are plaistered on them, thinking to find
true beautie, I wot well he will grow into a lothing and detestation. . . . They
are not once, but thrice worthy to perish, which dawbe their browes, and weare
their cheekes with their painted stuffe.'

St Cyprian followed the same pattern:

'The very Devils first taught the use of colouring the Eye-brows, and clapping
on a false and lying Blush on the Cheeks, so also to change the very natural
Colour of the Hair and to adulterate the true and Naked Complexion of the
whole Head and Face with those cursed Impostures. . . . God hath said, come
let us make men after our own Image. And does any one dare to alter or correct

66

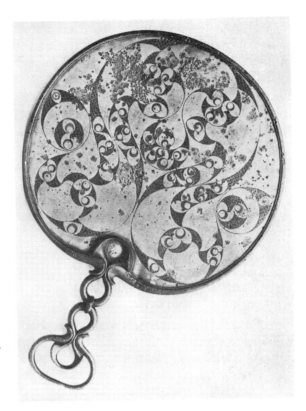

FIG. 52 : The Desborough Mirror. Decorated back of a bronze mirror of the British Iron Age, early first century A.D.

what he hath made? They do but lay violent hands upon God while they strive to mend or reform what he hath so well finished already. Do they not know that the Natural is God's, but the Artificial is the Devil's? . . . Dost not thou tremble to consider that at the Resurrection thy Maker will not acknowledge thee as his own Creature? Canst thou be so Impudent to look on God with those Eyes which are so different from those Himself made?'

In the latter part of the fourth century, St Ambrose is quoted (again in a seventeenth-century translation) as speaking out against the immorality of cosmetics:

'Painting is deceitful . . . lasts but awhile, and is wiped off with either rain or sweat. It deceives and beguiles, can not please him whom thou desirest to please, who perceiveth this pleasing beauty to be none of thine, but borrowed. And thou also displeaseth thy maker, who seeth his work to be defaced. . . . O woman, thou defacest the picture if thou daubest thy countenance with materiall whitenesse or a borrowed red. . . . Do not take away God's picturing and assume the picture of a harlot.'

At about this same time St Jerome wrote in a similar vein :

'Shee paints her selfe by a glasse, and to the contumely of her Creator laboureth to be fayrer then shee was borne . . . what makes this purple and white stuffe in the face of a Christian woman, the inflamers of youth, the nourishers of lust, and tokens of an unchast soule? . . . Those women are matter of scandall to Christian eies, which doe paint their faces and eyes with certaine artificiall colours, whose faces being plaistered and deformed with too much brightnesse, are counterfeits of Idols. . . . How can shee weep for her sinnes when her teares will make furrowes in her face.'

In his treatise on the education of young women, he instructed:

'Accustom her not to wear Pendants in her Ears, nor to Paint, nor to load her Neck and Head with Pearles; neither let her change the Colour of her Hair nor Curle or Crisp it up with bows, least it prove a prediction of infernal Flames.'

Thus, thanks to the Christian Fathers, we know that for three or four centuries after the birth of Christ, some women whitened their faces, necks, and breasts with a thick, water-soluble paint, reddened their cheeks and lips with a purplish rouge, coloured their eyelids, blackened their eyebrows, and dyed their hair. The purplish rouge was probably magenta — a colour which can often be seen in flakes of paint still clinging to ancient Greek sculpture.

But the Jews were painting as much as the Christians. Suppose, for example, we are in the second century A.D., watching a Palestinian woman at her morning toilet. After the serving girl has cleansed her mistress's face with an abrasive powder rubbed on the skin with a damp linen cloth, she empties a small container of starch, powdered white lead, and crimson pigment into a basin of warm water. After stirring this until it is smooth and fairly thick, she takes up some of the resulting pale pink liquid on a linen cloth and smooths it over the lady's face and neck. While the paint is still wet, she uses her forefinger, which she has dipped into a thick, blue-green liquid, to shadow the lady's eyelids. On other days the shadow may be green, brown, or grey. For evening wear it may even be black, just as the base colour may be slightly more salmon in colour than a true pink.

When the unblended shadow is dry, the girl dips a slender wooden kohl stick into a pottery tube of liquid black eye paint and lines the lady's upper lid, extending the line slightly beyond the outer corner of the eye. The same black paint is applied with the kohl stick to the eyebrow, following the natural line.

From a tiny bronze pot the girl then pours out a bit of bright red pigment into a small, shallow dish of water, stirring it in with a kohl stick to make a thin, red liquid. Dipping a linen cloth into the liquid rouge, she smooths the colour carefully on to the lady's cheekbones and blends the edges as best she can into the pink foundation. The lips are reddened with moist rouge from a small grey pot. Today she may choose a bright red-orange lip rouge and tomorrow a deep raspberry, almost purple, shade. The makeup completed, she

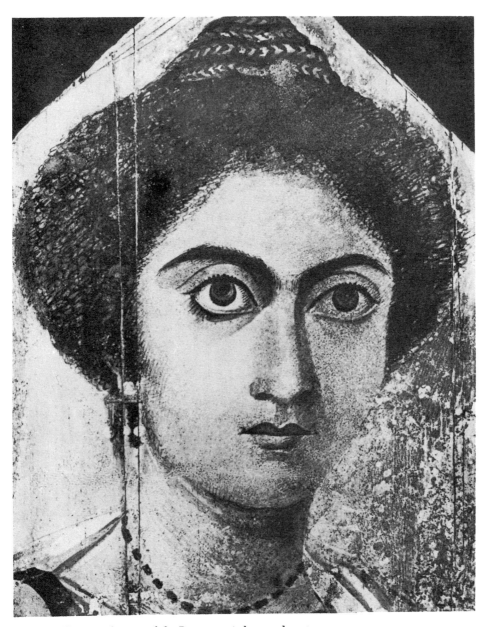

FIG. 53 : Egyptian beauty of the Roman period, second century A.D.

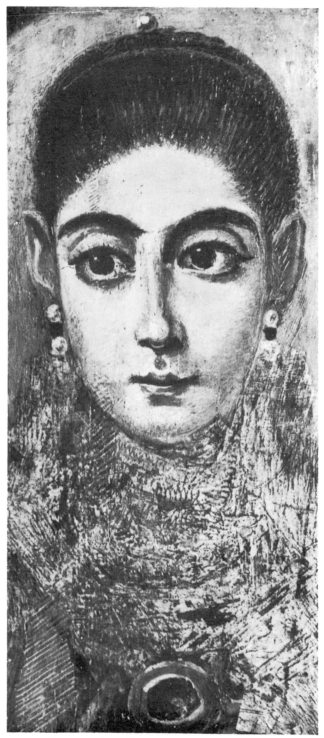

FIG. 54: Portrait of an Egyptian woman from a mummy case, encaustic on wood, third century A.D.

studies her blatantly painted face in a bronze hand mirror and smiles with pleasure at the result. Her maid, like other young girls of the lower class, lines her own eyes with black paint but uses no other makeup. The girl's mother also wears eye lining but adds a bit of rouge.

The thick, opaque face paint was sometimes white rather than pink; and when the shoulders and the bosom were exposed, they were painted along with the face and neck. Sometimes both eyelids were lined, sometimes only the upper one, and the black powder used for the lining was probably much like the Egyptian kohl. The placement of the shadow seems to have depended on personal preference. Eyebrows were sometimes plucked and toenails stained the colour of henna.

Since all of this painting was presumably not done with any great subtlety, perhaps there really was something for the Church fathers to complain about after all.

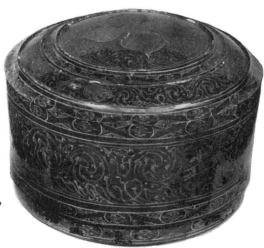

FIG. 55 : Chinese toilet box of painted lacquer, with silver inlaid animals, third century A.D.

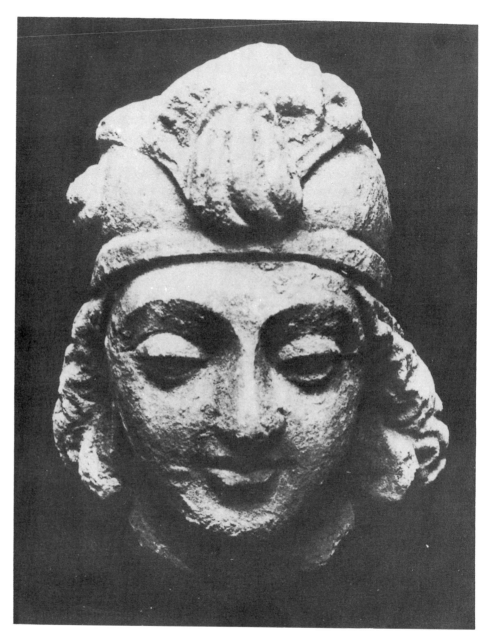

FIG. 56: Gothic-Buddhist head, *c*. fourth century A.D.

3 · The Middle Ages

Full small y-pulled were here browes two,
And they were bent, and blake as any sloo.
                                    GEOFFREY CHAUCER

Information on the use of cosmetics in the Middle Ages is sketchy at best, consisting mostly of illuminated manuscripts, art objects, occasional archaeological finds, and remarks, casual or outraged, about women who painted. We know that women and often men throughout the world did paint their faces and even their bodies, though in Britain body painting and tattooing seem to have disappeared after the Norman Conquest. We also know, in some cases, what they kept their paint in and the implements used to apply it. And we know, in general, what they wanted to look like and sometimes what they actually did look like.

PAINTS AND WASHES

Almost without exception, so far as we know, upper-class European women in the Middle Ages wanted to be pale, and frequently they achieved this by being either bled or painted. Those who lived in the towns and villages obtained their makeup at the workshops of the cosmetics makers; others had to rely on itinerant merchants, probably not unlike the sixteenth-century one shown in Figure 81 (see p. 104).

A thirteenth-century French verse lists some of the requirements of a lady's toilet supplied by such a travelling merchant:

> I have all the various things
> A woman needs who would be fair:
> Razors, forceps, mirrors too,
> Combs and irons for her hair,
> Picks and brushes for her teeth,
> Bandeaux or a fancy pin,
> Cotton to apply her rouge,
> White enamel for her skin.

Water-soluble paints were used for lightening and smoothing the skin. In sixth-century Spain they were pink in colour and were used almost exclusively by prostitutes. Upper-class women used a white powder. Three centuries later, in Germany, the paints were still pink but were used, though

73

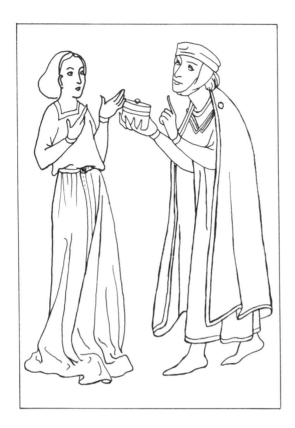

FIG. 57: Lady visiting a makeup specialist, who is trying to sell her a box of cosmetic paint. After a late thirteenth-century miniature.

probably not widely, by lower class women who were not necessarily prostitutes. In eleventh-century Britain paint was still used by prostitutes but appears to have been white rather than pink, perhaps because the women were already pink and wanted to be something else.

Although many women throughout the Middle Ages did paint their faces and dye their hair, it was, as usual, natural beauty which was admired by most men and certainly by the poets. 'Nor was she painted or disguised,' says one of them, 'for she had no need.' Gautier de Coinsi, a religious poet of the early thirteenth century, describes a modest and prudent maiden who does not:

> ... associate with those
> Who go together pair by pair,
> Who paint themselves to counterfeit youth
> And incessantly comb their hair.

As usual, neither poets nor prelates had much effect on women's painting. In Italy at this time makeup was worn extensively by all classes but with an attempt, not usually successful, to make it look natural. The face paint was

PLATE 13 : MEDIEVAL COSMETICS
DISHES AND ACCESSORIES

A   Thirteenth-fourteenth century, Chinese. Cosmetics box and cover. Lung-Ch'üan ware. Porcelain with carved decoration under a celadon glaze. Grey-green. About 4 inches in diameter. (*Victoria and Albert Museum*)

B   Twelfth-thirteenth century, Korean. Toilet box and cover with inlaid decoration. Light grey-blue-green celadon glaze. About 2½ inches in diameter. (*Victoria and Albert Museum*)

C   Twelfth-thirteenth century, Korean. Toilet box and cover with inlaid decoration. Grey-blue-green celadon glaze. (*Victoria and Albert Museum*)

D   Fifth to eighth century, Frankish. Bronze tweezers. (*Metropolitan Museum of Art, New York*)

E   Thirteenth century, Korean. Oil bottle. Grey-green celadon glaze. (*Victoria and Albert Museum*)

F   Late fifteenth century. Ivory mirror, back and front. Hung from girdle or carried in pocket. Used by both men and women. (*Louvre*)

G   Eighth to Tenth century, Viking. Double bone comb. About 4 inches long. (*Edinburgh Museum of Art*)

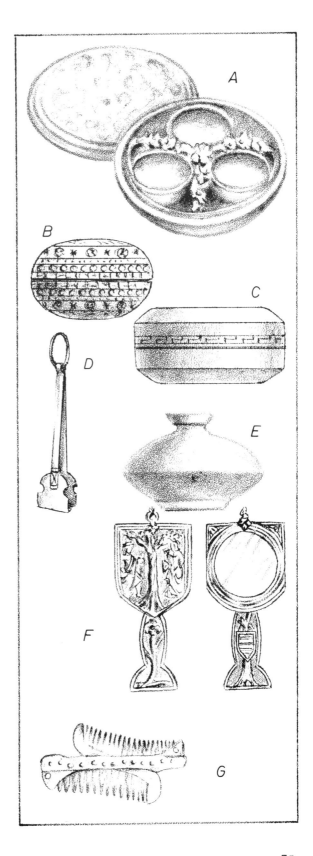

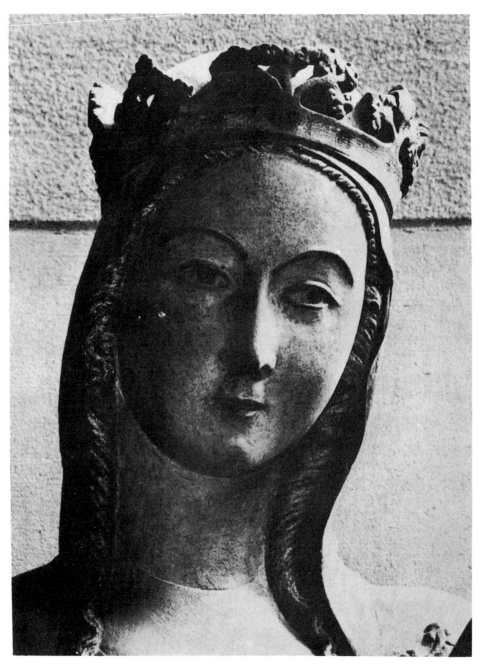

FIG. 58: Gothic sculptured madonna from Spain, fourteenth century. The eyes are lined, the eyebrows plucked and painted, and the lips and cheeks rouged.

pink or flesh in colour and often darker than the natural skin. It was supplied in powder form, made into a paste with water, and applied with the fingers.

Although a fourteenth-century manuscript gives directions for making the face white and red, an early satirist of the same period speaks deprecatingly of a woman:

> Who puts false hair upon her head and paints herself
> To please the world.

In France in the fifteenth century a water-soluble paste, usually white, sometimes flesh-coloured, was commonly used to colour the face by upper-class women. In preparing the paste, the lady would spoon some dry pigment into a flat dish, mix it with water, then apply it to her face with the fingers.

For alleviating skin problems, a good many of which undoubtedly arose as a result of the paint used, there was a special medication available — asparagus roots, wild anise, and the bulbs of white lillies in the milk of asses and red goats. This was aged in warm horse manure before being filtered through felt. The lady rubbed her face with pieces of soft bread dipped into the filtered liquid, and she did this 'for as long as it takes to say the credo thrice'.

An intriguing formula for a cosmetic water in an ancient French perfumery book entitled *Les Secrets de Maîstre Alexys de Piedontois* instructs one to 'take a young raven from the nest, feed it on hard eggs for forty days, kill it, and distill it with myrtle-leaves, talc, and almond oil'.

Under Charles VIII, who was crowned King of France in 1483, dress became more extravagant and the use of paint even more widespread. Claudius Marius, a clergyman, violently attacked the women of Marseille for painting their faces; and Oliver Maillard also preached against what he considered women's excesses: 'And you, my ladies, who are painted, who carry your tail lifted up, and you, gentlemen, who suffer your daughters to wear tails, do you believe then that people go into paradise with such dresses!'

In deciding whether or not he wished to pursue the possibility of marriage to the Queen of Naples, Henry VII of England instructed his ambassadors to note, among other things, 'whether she be painted or not' and 'the clearness of her skin'. She did not appear to be painted, reported the ambassadors, and her skin, what they could see of it, was clear.

ROUGE

In general, during the Middle Ages, rouge seems to have been used less frequently by upper class women than by prostitutes. Customs varied, however, from country to country, and from century to century. Aldhelm describes Anglo-Saxon women as having 'their cheeks dyed red with *stibium*' (a general term

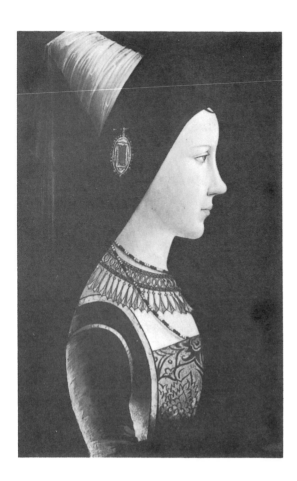

FIG. 59 : Mary of Burgundy, Dutch or French painting, *c.* 1470–75. The eyebrows are plucked and side hair has been shaved.

often used for any coloured face paint other than the white or pink foundation). In Spain in the sixth century a moist rouge for cheeks and lips was used by the lower classes, sometimes with the makeup base, sometimes without. This early Spanish rouge was rose-coloured. A few centuries later, in Germany and Britain, it was more orange in hue, evidently made from earth colours, and was applied in a more-or-less round pattern. In the thirteenth century rouge was used by all classes but less frequently than the makeup base. In Tuscany upper class women wore a fairly bright pink colour, whereas the lower classes used a less expensive earthy red. A French poet of the time admired lips which were plump and 'redder than cochineal'.

Full lips were also preferred in the fourteenth century. Chaucer described such lips in *The Court of Love*:

> With pregnant lippès thin, not fat, but ever lean,
> They serve of naught; they be not worth a bean;
> For if the base be full, there is delight.

But Chaucer's women whitened their cheeks whereas some of their continental contemporaries reddened theirs. A young man begged Lydia :

> Bare, oh, bare, thy cheeks of rose,
> Dyed with Tyrian red that glows.

Fifteenth-century French women (prostitutes more often than the upper classes) painted their lips and their cheeks with a crimson rouge, usually applied in a round spot, reasonably well blended.

EYE MAKEUP

Eyeshadow in various colours — green, blue, grey, brown — was used to some extent throughout the Middle Ages, from sixth-century Spain to fifteenth-century France. In Tuscany in the thirteenth century eye makeup was common among upper-class women. The upper lids were sometimes lined with a black liquid, applied with a stick, and shadowed with brown, grey, blue-green, or violet. At this time azure eyes were preferred by the French and grey by the English. A century later Roman women were lining their eyes with black, usually only on the upper lid, and sometimes shadowing them with green, blue-green, brown, or grey. In fifteenth-century France only prostitutes, it appears, used eye makeup — green, blue-green, brown, or grey shadow and black liner on the upper lid. The liner, like the Egyptian kohl, was made by mixing black pigment with saliva and applying it with a small stick.

But the greatest change occurred with the eyebrows, which were usually natural until the fourteenth century. A thirteenth-century English poet describes a lady's brows as 'white between and not too near', and a French one admires brows which are 'brownish, narrow, and delicate'.

The admiration for narrow brows evidently increased, for in the fourteenth and fifteenth centuries fashionable women plucked their eyebrows into a thin line (see Figures 59 and 63). In England, it appears, even lower-class women plucked their brows — like the carpenter's wife in Chaucer's *Canterbury Tales*:

> Full small y-pulled were here browes two,
> And they were bent, and blake as any sloo.

But the fact that women's brows were plucked did not necessarily make the practice acceptable to men. The Knight of La Tour Landy, who abhorred all things unnatural, including plucking and painting, advised his daughters to 'takithe ensaumple, and holde it in your herte that ye put no thinge to poppe, painte, and fayre youre visages, the which is made after Goddes ymage, otherwise thanne your Creatour and nature hath ordeined; and that ye plucke no browes, nothing temples, nor forhed; and also that ye wasshe not the here of youre hede in none other thing but in lye and water.' The Knight also asked the rhetorical question, 'whi take women none hede of the gret love that God hathe yeve hem

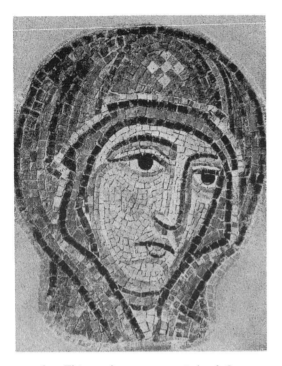

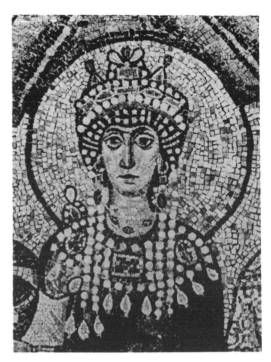

FIG. 60: Thirteenth-century mosaic head, San Marco, Venice. The heavy eye-lining is typical of the period.

FIG. 61: Empress Theodora. Sixth-century Byzantine mosaic from San Vitale, Ravenna. The eyes are heavily lined.

to make hem after hys figure? and whi popithe they, and paintithe, and pluckithe her visage otherwise than God hath ordeined him?' And he told of a sinful woman who had done these things and as a result was tortured in hell, where the devil held her 'bi the tresses of the here of her hede, like as a lyon holdithe his praie . . . and thruste in her browes, temples, and forehede hote brenninge alles and nedeles.' And all of this came as a result of her having 'plucked her browes, front and forehead, to have awey the here, to make her selff the fayrer to the plesinge of the worlde.'

HAIR

Hair styles have usually changed more rapidly than styles in makeup, and the changes have been easier to delineate. They have also more frequently been subject to legal restrictions. According to Thomas Wright, early Frankish laws specified that 'if a free man squeezed a free woman's arm below the elbow, he was liable to a penalty of twelve hundred denarii; if it was above the elbow, the fine was raised to fourteen hundred denarii.' But if he were to disarrange a woman's hair to such an extent that her obbo (a sort of cap) fell to the ground, the fine was fifteen solidi. Free men and women both wore the hair long, and cutting off a woman's hair was a very serious matter. According to the Burgundian law, a free man cutting off the hair of a female slave was subject to a penalty. A slave cutting off the hair of a free woman was put to death. Unmarried girls wore their hair loose, and of unmarried ladies it was said that they 'remained in their hair'. Married women did up their hair in braids or fillets and sometimes curled it with irons and painted their faces.

The Anglo-Saxons, for some reason, had an affinity for blue hair. Since the hair of both men and women is consistently painted blue in illuminations of the period, we assume that in life it was coloured with dye or powder. According to Caesar, the early Britons coloured their faces blue with woad, evidently as a sort of war paint. As with the Franks, the hair of the Anglo-Saxons hung loose before marriage and was bound up afterwards. In early times the married woman's hair was cut short to symbolize her servitude, but this practice was later abandoned. In the late seventh century, Aldhelm described Anglo-Saxon women of the world as arranging 'delicately their waving locks, curled artificially by the curling-iron'. Tweezers, frequently found in the graves of Anglo-Saxon women, were probably used for plucking their eyebrows and superfluous hairs. A pair of Frankish tweezers is shown in Plate 13-D.

Women of the Middle Ages, it is reported, decorated their hair with a mixture of swallow droppings, grey succinum, burnt bear claws, and lizard tallow. Ivor Griffith quotes an ancient Celtic recipe for restoring hair:

'With mice fill an earthen pipkin, close the mouth with clay and let it be buried beneath the hearth-stone, but so as the fire's too great heat reach it not. So be it for one year, at the end of which take out whatever may be there. For baldness it is great. But it is urgent that whoever shall handle it have a glove on his hand, lest at his fingers ends the hair come sprouting forth.'

In the latter part of the eleventh century, contemporary historian Ordericus Vitalis denounced the young Normans for their effeminacy. 'They parted their hair,' he wrote, 'from the crown of the head on each side of the forehead and let their locks grow long like women. . . . The forepart of their heads is bare, after the manner of thieves, while behind they nourish long hair, like harlots. . . . Their locks are curled with hot irons, and instead of wearing caps, they bind their heads with fillets.' He objected to their modes of dress as well, especially to their shoes with turned-up points.

At the end of the thirteenth century false hair was often used by women to provide the projecting rolls of braids over the ears. These false pieces, called *atours*, early in the fourteenth century were shaped like horns (Figure 63), which upset the clergy even more than the use of paint. The horns, filled out with flax or hemp, are mentioned in *Le Roman de la Rose*:

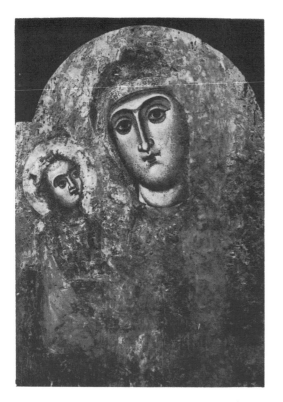

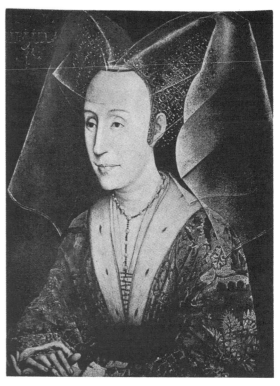

FIG. 62: Thirteenth-century icon, Dubrovnik, Yugoslavia.

FIG. 63: Portrait of a lady, by Rogier van der Weyden. This mid-fifteenth-century portrait, with the fashionable plucked eyebrows and the very high shaved forehead, is thought to be of Isabella of Portugal.

> Over her ears she wears such horns
> That stag or ox or unicorns,
> If they came face to face with her,
> Could not o'ercome her horns.

Another satirist says:

> They have horns with which to kill the men;
> They pile up other people's hair upon their heads.

> . . . .

> The bishop is aware
> Of all the horns and hair,
>   And in his sermon duly notes
> That he will give his solemn blessing
> To those who'll mock this sort of dressing
>   By shouting loudly, 'Push, you goats!'

In 1417, despite threats and warnings from the clergy of cataclysmic disasters, the horns were bigger than ever. According to Juvenal des Ursins, 'the ladies and demoiselles of the queen's household displayed great and excessive pride, and wore horns wonderfully high and broad, and had on each side, instead of pads, two great ears, so large that when they had to pass through the door of the chamber, they were obliged to turn sideways and stoop, or they could not pass'. But simpler head-dresses were also worn, and the horns soon gave way to the hennin.

Bathing

Cleanliness was relative in the Middle Ages, and bathing facilities varied considerably. The Anglo-Saxons had hot baths, but in the reign of King Edgar both warm baths and soft beds were forbidden as encouraging effeminacy. Presumably cold baths were acceptably masculine. Young men at the time tended to be meticulous in their grooming — often, according to Thomas Wright, even more so than the ladies. This seems also to have been true of the Danish invaders, who, 'following the custom of their country, used to comb their hair every day, bathed every Saturday, often changed their clothes, and used many other such frivolous means of setting off the beauty of their persons.'

Perfumes were little used in the Dark Ages; but by the fourteenth century saffron had become one of the favourite scents, though there were very few to choose from, none of them particularly subtle or exotic, at least by modern standards.

Bathing was evidently becoming more popular. An inventory taken after the death of Charles V in 1380 listed twenty-four gold wash basins, a number of similar ones of silver, and one foot basin which weighed forty-seven silver marcs. In Paris, however, as in ancient Rome, bathing was usually done in the public baths, which were open twenty-four hours a day, making it possible for one to spend the night. They were closed on Sundays and holidays. In homes which had bathing facilities it was customary to bathe before meals, even if one were a guest, and to go directly from the bathroom to the dining room.

The public baths were scattered about Paris. There was one in a passage off what is now the rue de l'École-de-Médecine, another in the famous rue du Chat-qui-pêche (which now seems no more than a dark alley), and one for women only, called The Silver Lion, in a house in the rue Beaubourg.

But it would seem, judging from a list of precepts for the behaviour and appearance of women, published in 1483 by Jean Sulpice, that in spite of baths and paints, the basic principles of cleanliness had not quite been grasped by the populace:

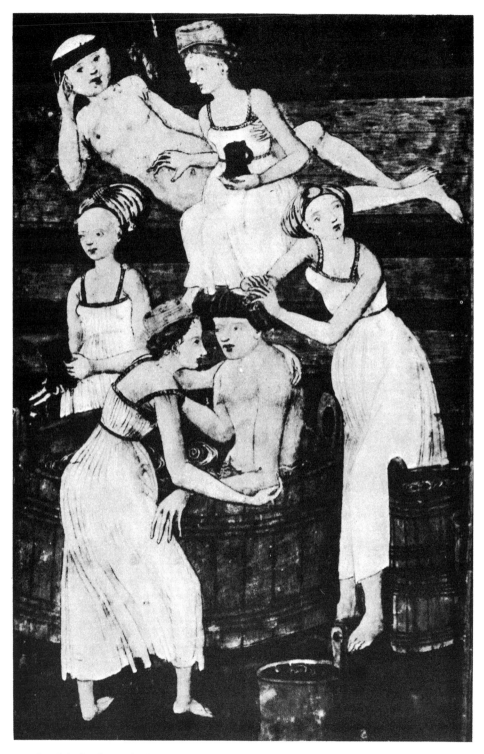

FIG. 64: Monks being bathed in a public bath house. From the Jena Codex, early sixteenth century.

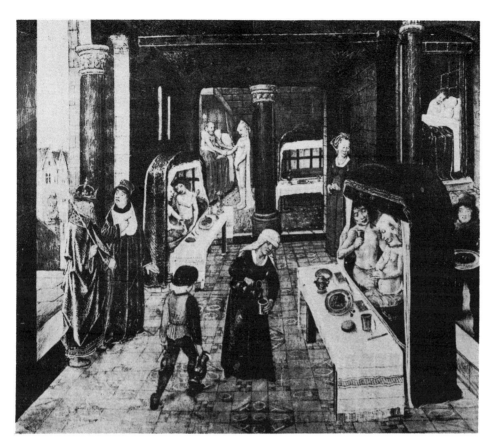

FIG. 65: French bath house, fifteenth century. Ladies are available in and out of the bath. Miniature from the *Memorable Deeds and Sayings* of Valerius Maximus.

'Your dress should be clean and without filth.

'Do not let your face or your hands be dirty.

'Take care that no drippings from the nose hang there like icicles that one sees hanging from the rafters and eaves of houses in winter.

'Your fingernails should not be too long or full of filth.

'Make sure that your hair is well combed and that your headdress is not full of feathers or other trash.

'Your shoes should be clean and not dirty or muddy.

'Your tongue should not be covered with filth.

'Have your teeth clean and without rust — that is to say, without the yellow matter attached to them as a result of insufficient cleansing.

'Understand that it is improper and discourteous to scratch your head at the

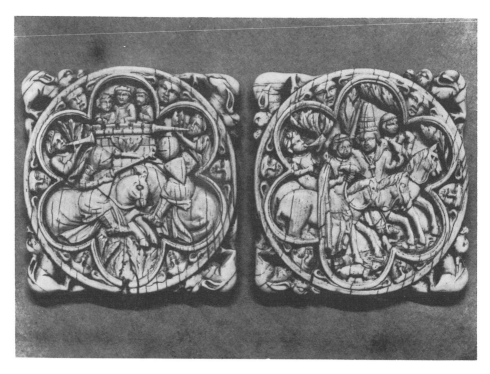

FIG. 66: Ivory mirror case, front and back. French, fourteenth century.

table; to remove from your neck fleas or other vermin and kill them in front of others; to scratch or pull at scabs in whatever part of the body they may be.

'If you have to blow your nose, you should not remove the excrement with the fingers, but in a handkerchief. And if you spit or cough, you need not swallow what you have already drawn into the throat, but spit on the ground or into a handkerchief or napkin.

'If you are forced to belch, do so as quietly as possible, always averting the face.'

MIRRORS

At the beginning of the Dark Ages women were seeing their makeup reflected, perhaps not too clearly, in mirrors of silver. Glass mirrors, backed with silver or tin, were first mentioned by Isidore, who died in 636. Both men and women often wore mirrors suspended from the girdle, and men sometimes wore them

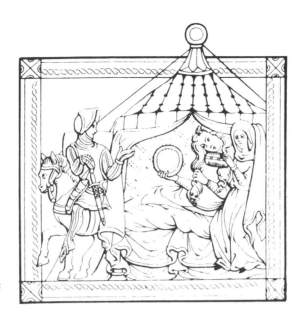

FIG. 67 : Lady at her toilet, early
fourteenth century.
Engraving from Rimmel's
Book of Perfumes, 1865.

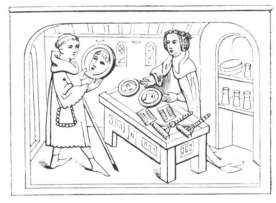

FIG. 68 : Perfumer's shop, late
fourteenth century.
Engraving from Rimmel's
Book of Perfumes, 1865.

Von eyner edlen frowen wie
die vor eym spiegel stund/sich mutzend/vnnd sy in den spiegel
den tüfel sach jr den hyndern zeigend/

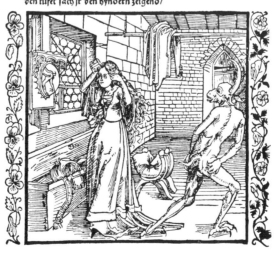

FIG. 69 : Swiss noblewoman at her
toilet, 1493. She sees more
than she bargained for.

in their hats. Mirror cases were often elaborately carved, like the ivory one in Figure 66.

Figure 67, which shows a metal hand mirror in use, is engraved from an illustration in a manuscript of French prose romances. Sir Gawain 'comes to a pleasant prairie, in the midst of which he discovers a rich pavilion. Under the pavilion was a couch, on which reposed a beautiful damsel, her hair spread over her shoulders and a maid standing by, combing it with a comb of ivory set in gold.'

In Figure 68, engraved from a fourteenth-century manuscript illustration, we see a perfumer's shop, in which Agyographe, an allegorical lady, is showing the pilgrim a mirror which flatters the person using it, making him appear more handsome than he really is. But he chooses one which does just the reverse. Glass mirrors were in general use at the time. The lady shown in Figure 69 is using a wall mirror of glass and evidently seeing more than she bargained for.

ASIA AND AFRICA

European makeup fashions showed a degree of consistency, even during the Middle Ages, but elsewhere makeup practices were often traditional and unchanging, showing little similarity to the makeup of other countries. Fashionable Japanese ladies, like the Chinese, used white face paint, rouge, and nail colouring. Sometimes they also gilded the lower lip. They blackened their teeth, shaved their eyebrows, and designed new ones with paint. They had, it is reported, fifteen choices for the style of the hair in front and twelve for the back. Men of fashion also used rouge and carried mirrors about with them. Said Lady Sei Shonagun in A.D. 991, 'I lowered my head and hid my face with my sleeve lest I brush away my powder and appear with a spotted face.'

In Africa cosmetics have been used for centuries by both men and women. The men probably did it first in order to frighten their enemies and possibly to attract the women. Fellatah women stained their fingers and toes by wrapping them with henna leaves, shadowed their eyelids with sulphide of antimony, dyed their hair with indigo, and stained their teeth yellow, purple, and blue.

Although the use of perfumes died out in Europe during the Dark Ages, the art was kept alive elsewhere. In the tenth century Avicenna, an Arabian physician, was teaching others the art of preparing fragrances from leaves, and in the twelfth century Saladin had the walls of the mosque of Omar washed with rose water to celebrate his triumphal entry. The Arabs introduced additional cosmetics and perfumes into Spain in A.D. 711.

But it was primarily the Crusaders who once again brought Oriental perfumes

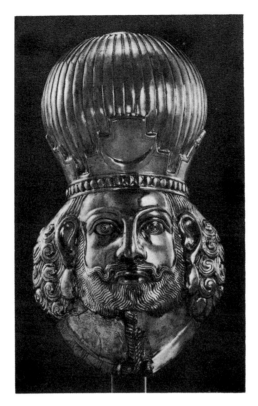 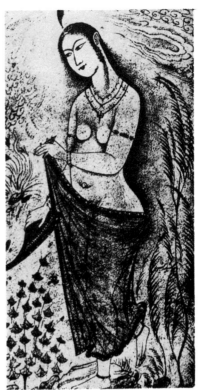

FIG. 70: Persian king of the Sassanian Dynasty, A.D. 224–642. The upper part of the crown represents a pleated silk covering for the king's sacred topknot.

FIG. 71: Persian lady with meeting brows.

into Europe, especially Italy and France, where new scents began to be developed. Catherine de' Medici, it is said, liked to combine her perfumes with poisons.

During the Dark Ages in Europe, the civilization in the Indus Valley, led by the Gupta emperors, was passing through a golden age in its culture, accompanied by great prosperity and a flourishing of art and literature. Both men and women continued to use cosmetics, fragrant oils, and perfumes.

Bathing was still a ritual of great importance. King Śūdraka had in his bathroom a golden basin filled with perfumed water. As the King sat on a crystal stool in the middle of the basin, female attendants rubbed a special paste into his hair and emptied vessels of water perfumed with saffron and sandalwood over his head. There were usually several attendants, both male and female, including water-carriers and unguent bearers.

In the toilet room, after the bath, the King's body would be smeared with a paste of sandalwood, musk, camphor, and saffron. After the morning meal he would chew betel leaf. Even when going into battle he did not neglect the morning toilet.

A fashionable young man of the period is described as having his hair coiffed with clusters of curls and a cornet of white flowers, his forehead smeared

89

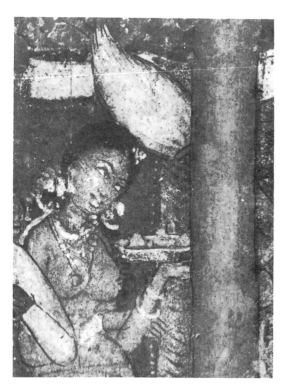

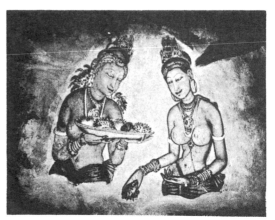

FIG. 73 : Asparsas and attendant. Ceylon, late
fifth century. Frescoes on rock above
palace at Sigiriya.

FIG. 72 : Lady with toilet tray. India, sixth or
seventh century. Ajanta cave
painting.

with red arsenic, his breath perfumed with mango, kakkola fruit, cloves,
camphor, and coral trees, his arms decorated with painted designs, and his chest
powdered with camphor dust. Men also lined their eyes with a collyrium stick,
and heightened their lip colouring with betel. Sometimes they painted designs
on the face, chest, and arms.

Women coloured their lips with lac-dye, lined their eyes with a collyrium
stick (Figure 75) and also painted designs on the face, usually with sandalwood
paste and musk, in red, white, and black. They smeared their bodies with
sandalwood paste and painted their arms and breasts with designs in black,
white, yellow, or red, the designs being made with the fingers, with stick paint,
or with a brush. Sometimes they were cut from leaves and pasted on. Women
also stained the bottoms of their feet with lac and the tops with saffron, and
painted their loins with sandal. Even the lowest classes painted and perfumed
themselves and wore flowers.

A special ritual was followed by a woman on her wedding day. After her
bath, a lady of high position would have various pastes and unguents applied
to her body, and her hair perfumed by the smoke from the fire which dried it.
Her eyes were lined with collyrium, and ornamental designs were painted on
her face. The bride's mother, using a yellow unguent of orpiment and realgar,
made a special mark on the girl's forehead. All festive occasions were

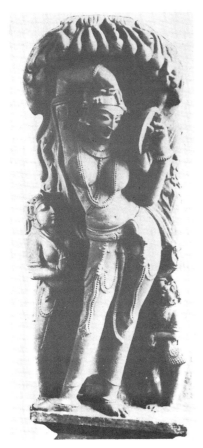 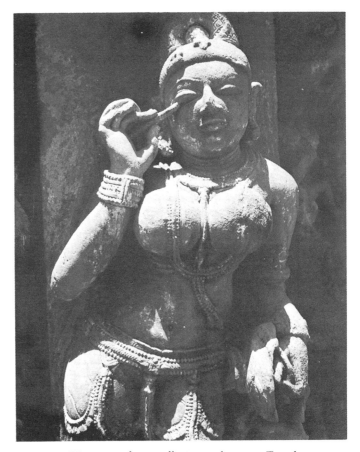

FIG. 74: Woman at her toilet, India, eleventh century. Standing under a tree, she is placing vermilion at the parting of her hair. Sandstone sculpture.

FIG. 75: Woman applying collyrium to her eyes. Temple sculpture from Khajuraho, India, *c*. eleventh century.

accompanied by an increased use of perfumes and cosmetics. Sometimes women would squirt diluted coloured dyes on each other with golden syringes.

But in general there were no rigidly set patterns followed in the use of cosmetics. Women liked variety and changed their perfumes and toiletries with the seasons. And in different parts of the country different customs were observed.

PRIMITIVE TRIBES

Makeup among the aborigines is often applied to the body as well as the face and includes both painting and tattooing. Columbus reported, with some surprise, that native men in the New World used cosmetics, painting themselves 'white and red or other colours, sometimes the whole body or only the face, the eyes, or the nose'. The skin was lubricated with deer's or bear's fat before the vegetable and mineral colours were applied. Columbus seemed to think that the paints might be protective rather than decorative.

Virginia Eifert reports that Australian men carried boxes of red, yellow, and white paint to retouch their makeup, which was simple on ordinary days, elaborate on special occasions. Women were permitted to paint their faces but not their bodies. Men of the New Hebrides also carried makeup boxes with yellow ochre, coral, lime, and purple ashes. For head-hunting ceremonies they painted themselves all over with yellow ochre, leaving circles of dark skin around the eyes, nose, and mouth. When the white traders came, the natives were able to obtain more sophisticated ingredients for their paints.

In areas where red clay is plentiful, as it is among the Bantus, it is still used as a cosmetic. Mixed with oil, it is rubbed on both skin and hair, primarily as a protection from the elements. Other tribes, in making their cosmetics, use such ingredients as soot, leaves, dung, butter, antelope blood, and blue mica-schist. Tattooing and deliberate scarring of the skin in patterns were and still are commonplace.

Darwin points out that 'not one great country can be named . . . in which the aborigenes do not tattoo themselves'. Although the tattooing may have social and religious significance, beautification seems always to be the predominant purpose. And the natives undergo considerable physical pain in the process, which involves repeated puncturing of the skin and introducing of blue paint into the wounds. In the Mayan civilization the art of tattooing was developed to a high degree, with very elaborate patterns, even animals and mythical figures. The front teeth were sometimes filed to points, holes drilled in them, and precious stones inserted.

4 · *The Italian Renaissance*

It is not to be believed, that any simple women
without a great inducement and instigation of the divel,
would ever leave their natural and gracefull countenances
to seeke others that are suppositions and counterfeits,
and should goe up and downe whited and sised over
with paintings laied one upon another, in such sort
that a man might easily cut off a curd or cheese-cake
from either of their cheekes.

ANDREAS DE LAGUNA

In 1548 Firenzuola, an Italian monk and man of letters, published a volume entitled *Dialogo delle Bellezze delle Donne* (Dialogue on the Beauty of Women) from which one can form a fairly accurate picture of the ideal Renaissance beauty. 'It is fitting,' wrote Firenzuola, 'that the cheeks should be fair; and such fairness is in things which, beside whiteness, have a certain glow, like ivory; but whiteness, is that which hath no such glow, as snow. And whereas the cheeks to be beautiful must be of this fairness, the bosom must be white.... The hair ... should be fine and fair, in the similitude now of gold, now of honey, and now of the bright and shining rays of the sun; waving, thick, abundant....

'The forehead must be spacious [Figure 85], that is, wide and high, fair and serene.... The height ... must be equal to half the width.... And we have said it must be fair, since it must not be of an over dull whiteness, without any lustre, but should shine after the manner of a mirror, not by wetness or by painting, or by foul washes, like that of Bovinetta, which an it were fish to fry, might be worth a farthing a pound more as not needing to be floured; howbeit it is not to be sold or fried.

'The line of the brow should not be all flat, but curved like an arch toward the crown of the head, so gently that it is scarce to be perceived; but from the boss of the temples it should descend more straightly.' The monk favoured ebony eyebrows of 'soft, short hairs' and dark tan or nut-brown eyes. 'Deep black is not much to be commended, since it tends to a somewhat gloomy and cruel gaze; and nut brown, if dark, gives a soft, bright, clear, and kindly gaze.' He liked the eyes to be large and full to give an impression of sweetness and modesty. The lashes should be 'thin and not over long and not white ... nor would I have them very black, which makes the gaze fierce.

'The socket which surrounds the eye is not to be very deep, nor too large, nor different in colour from the cheek; and let ladies who paint be on their guard — those, I would say, who are known, since this part is very often not apt to take the paint or the plastering by reason of its hollow shape, or to retain it

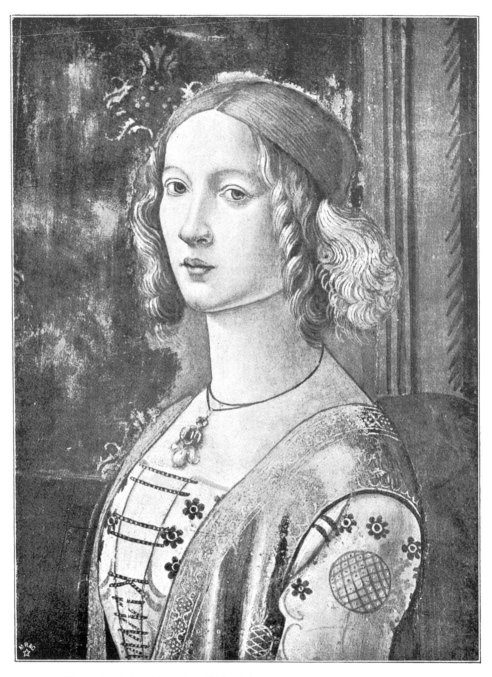

FIG. 76: Florentine lady. Fresco by Ghirlandaio, 1490. The eyebrows are still plucked, but the forehead appears to be unshaved.

by reason of the motion of the eyelashes, and thus makes a division which looks very ill.'

For the ears he suggested the colour of pale rubies bordered with a transparent roll the colour of pomegranate seeds. The temples were to be white and flat, not hollow, and neither too full nor too narrow.

He preferred cheeks to be not so white as the forehead, with a patch of sunset vermilion. The nose should be of proper size, more narrow than wide, slightly turned up at the tip, and coloured but not red. The mouth was to be small with medium lips, vermilion in colour and not to show more than five or six teeth — uppers only — when parted. He liked the tip of the tongue — 'neither pointed nor square'—to be scarlet. Although he favoured a long, slender neck, he considered a slight double chin a mark of beauty.

Firenzuola evidently relied on God to provide his ideal beauty, for like other men of the Church, he considered artificial aids an abomination not to be tolerated.

PAINTS AND WASHES

But in spite of the Church, the Renaissance brought with it a revival in personal decoration. A variety of paints and washes was available and widely used. Burkardt suggests that the extensive use of cosmetics may have been due partly to the custom of masking and painting at the Mysteries. In any case, women in both city and country used cosmetics freely, unaffected by satires and sermons and the unfortunate effects of poisonous ingredients. Venetian ladies even formed a society (and elected officers) for learning and testing new discoveries in the cosmetic arts. Isabella Cortese was president at one time, and Catherine de' Medici was an honorary member.

Whatever new discoveries may have been made by the society, the ladies continued to whiten their faces with poisonous white lead, often applying one coat over another, either to avoid the trouble of removing the paint each day or in order to fill in wrinkles. Usually the paint was applied to the neck and the bosom as well as the face. In any case, whether thickly applied or not, it was obviously unnatural. And though it evidently must have given the women some satisfaction, it clearly did not enhance their beauty in the eyes of men — at least the men who took the trouble to write about it. Andreas de Laguna, Spanish physician to Pope Julius III, insisted that the white face paint had been invented by the devil in order to make women 'ugly, enormous, and abominable'. (See Figure 106.) And Firenzuola, the monk who dreamed of the ideal natural beauty, complained of the cosmetics which were 'used to paint and whiten the whole face, just as lime and plaster cover the face of a wall; and peradventure

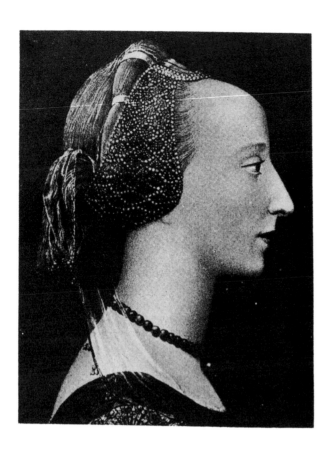

FIG. 77: Portrait of a lady. Painting by Pollaiuolo, showing the plucked eyebrows and high shaved forehead fashionable in the mid-fifteenth century.

those foolish maids believe that men, whom they seek to please, do not discern this foulness, which I would have them to know wears them out and makes them grow old before their time, and destroys their teeth, while they seem to be wearing a mask all the year through. Look now at Mona Bettola Gagliana — what do you think of her? The more she paints and the more she dresses up the older she seems; nay, she is like a gold ducat that hath lain in aqua-fortis. And it would not be thus if she had not used washes so much when she was young.'

Physicians in general, it appears, warned women against using poisons on their skin — not only white lead, but mercury sublimate, which was frequently used to remove imperfections in the skin and make it smooth. De Laguna referred to the dangers of the mercury as 'infamous inconveniences which . . . might be somewhat more tollerable if they did sticke and stay onely in them who use it, and did not descend to their offspring. For this infamy' he warned, 'is like to original sinne and goes from generation to generation, when as the child borne of them, before it be able to goe, doth shed his teeth one after another, as being corrupted and rotten, not through his fault, but by reason of the vitiousnesse and taint of the mother that painted her selfe, who, if she loath and abhorre to heare this, let her forbeare to do the other.'

To avoid the horrors of lead or mercury poisoning and the wrath of God at the same time, Firenzuola suggested that it was permissible to make their faces smoother by using 'barley water or the water of Lupines, or the juyce of Lymons, and infinite other things, which Dioscorides prescribes as cleanly and delicate to cleare the face, and not goe continually with rank smelles of ointments and plaisters about them.'

Rouge, when it was used by upper class women, was applied more subtly than was the white and is infrequently mentioned, though de Laguna refers to colourful complexions which are clearly not natural and perhaps not intentional. 'There are many,' he fumed, 'who have so betard their faces with these mixtures and slubber-sauces, that they have made their faces of a thousand colours: that is to say: some as yellow as the marigold, others a darke greene, others blunket colour, others as of a deepe red died in the wooll. . . . Thus the use of this ceruse, besides the rotting of the teeth and the unsavourie breath which it causeth, being ministred in paintings, doth turne faire creatures into infernall Furies. Wherefore let all gentlewomen & honorable matrons, that make price of their honesty and beauty, leave these base arts to the common strumpets, of whom they are fittest to be used, that by the filthiness they may be known and noted.'

In the fifteenth century the eyebrows of fashionable women were still being plucked into a thin line (Figures 76 and 77), but eye makeup was not commonly used. By the end of the sixteenth century the brows had returned to their natural fullness. Beauty spots were occasionally worn.

TEETH AND HAIR

Teeth were not well cared for, and the use of poisonous paints on the face evidently speeded their decay. But though there was no toothpaste, there were recipes for tooth care for any who might be interested. Giambattista della Porta, an Italian philosopher and scientist, supplied one 'for white and pearly teeth'. The reader was instructed to take 'three handfuls each of flowers and leaves of sage, nettle, rosemary, mallow, olive, plantain, and rind of walnut roots; two handfuls each of rock rose, horehound, bramble-tops; a pound of flower and a half a pound of seed of myrtle; two handfuls of rosebuds; two drachms each of sandalwood, coriander, and citron pips; three drachms of cinnamon; ten drachms of cypress nuts; five green pine cones; two drachms each of mastic and Armenian clay', reduce all of them to a powder, infuse them in 'sharp black wine', and macerate them for three days, during which time she might presumably take a well deserved rest. After pressing out the wine, she was then supposed to distill the residue 'on a gentle fire' with two ounces of alum. In using the concoction, she was to fill the mouth with it and rub the teeth with

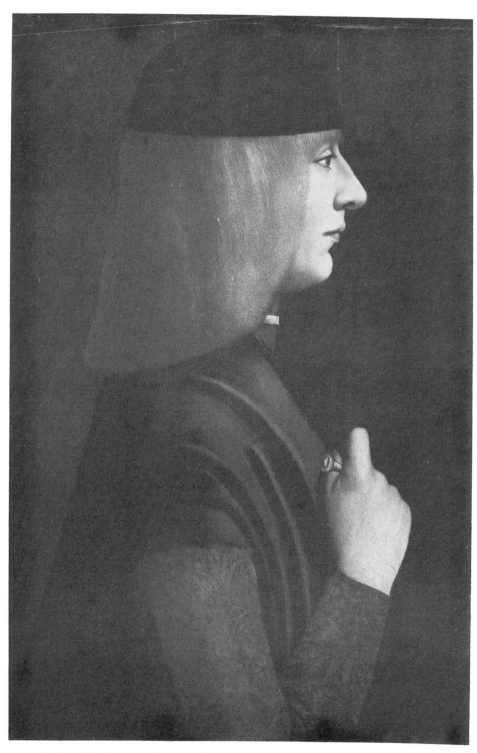

FIG. 78: Portrait of a man. Painting by Ambrogio da Predis, late fifteenth century. Hair is probably either bleached or false.

a finger wrapped in fine linen. False hair — some of it real, some made of white or yellow silk — was worn, though not universally, by both men and women. Blonde hair was in fashion, and women spent hours in the sun bleaching their own (see *Fashions in Hair*, pp. 172–4). Laws were passed; preachers ranted; false hair, along with other trinkets bespeaking personal vanity, was burned in the public squares. But fashionable men and women continued wearing false hair and bleaching and dyeing their own until the fashion died a natural death. Women also continued to shave the front hair (Figure 77) as they had done in the fourteenth century. By the end of the fifteenth century, however, the custom had virtually disappeared (Figure 76).

Della Porta included two recipes for the hair :

'*To dye the hair yellow*. Add enough of honey to soften the lees of white wine and keep the hair wet with this all night. Then bruise the roots of celandine and greater olivers-madder, mix them with oil of cummin seed, box shavings, and saffron; and keep this on the head for four and twenty hours, when it should be washed off with a lye of cabbage-stalks and ashes of rye-straw.

'*To make the hair thick and curly*. Boil maiden hair with smallage seed — in wine and oil; or roots of daffydillies, or dwarf-elders, boiled in wine and oil.'

BATHING AND PERFUMES

Bathing at this period in history had become infrequent and was considered of little importance. But since the results could hardly have gone unnoticed, perfume became increasingly necessary. In 1508 the monks of the Dominican Brotherhood in the Convent of Santa Maria Novella in Florence established what was to become one of the most celebrated perfumeries in Europe. It was patronized by the Medicis and the popes, who gave generous donations to the convent. Throughout the centuries each new director of the perfumery would add his own favourite recipes to the original ones. Pope Innocent XI contributed a recipe to cure burns, thereafter called Balsam Innocenziano. In their catalogue one can find listed such specialities as quina elixer, long life elixer, rhubarb elixer, melissa water, and Regina water (the invention of a Medici queen). Their orris powder was used to perfume linen, brush the teeth, and dust on to the skin after bathing.

Perfumes were, in fact, as lavishly used as they had been in ancient Rome, often being liberally applied to animals and inanimate objects as well as to people. Pietro Aretino, in a letter to Cosimo I, thanked him for a perfumed roll of money. It is said that some of these objects which have come down to us still bear traces of their original scent.

The moralists complained about the use of perfumes but not about the filth.

And the Church itself seemed more concerned with paint than with the dirt that it covered. Usually the complaints had little or no effect, but so great was the influence of Savonarola in the late fifteenth century that he actually persuaded the women of Florence to give up the use of cosmetics and publicly to pitch their paints into the fire. But then Savonarola made the crucial mistake of arranging to have his successful exhortations backed up with a direct prohibition by the Medici. The women rebelled, as could surely have been predicted, and the cosmeticians were back in business.

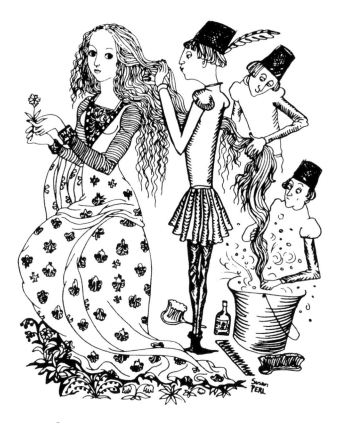

FIG. 79: Lucrezia Borgia having her hair touched up on the way to her wedding, *c.* 1493. *New York Times Magazine* illustration by Susan Perl, 1955.

5 · Elizabethan Days

It must needs be graunted, that the dying and colouring
of faces with artificiall colours and unnatural
Oyntments is most offensive to God, and derogatorie
to his Majestie: for do they think that the
God of all glorie, and who only decketh and adorneth
the Sun, the Moon, the Starres and all the hoast of
heaven with unspeakable glorie and incomparable
beautie, canot make thee beautiful and faire enough
(if it please him) without their sibbersauces?

PHILIP STUBBES, 1583

Makeup became more permissive under Elizabeth I, who introduced 'sweet coffers' containing paint, powder, and patches. Richard Puttenham, in drawing a verse portrait of Queen Elizabeth, published in 1589, carefully refrained from making it clear that her colouring was not entirely natural:

Two lips wrought out of *rubie* rocke,
Like leaves to shut and to unlock.
As portall door in prince's chamber,
A golden tongue in mouth of amber.
Her bosom sleek as *Paris plaster*
Held up two balls of *alabaster*.

But Puttenham was less tactful about Her Majesty's female subjects in a chapter entitled 'Of Ornaments Poeticall', in which he suggested that 'if our colours in Our Art of Poesie (as well as in other mechanicall artes) be not well tempered, or not well layd, or be used in excesse, or never so little disordered, or misplaced, they not only give it no manner of grace at all, but rather to disfigure the stuffe, and spill the whole workmanship, taking away all bewtie and good liking from it, no less than if the crimson tainte which should be laid upon a ladies lips, or right in the center of her cheekes, should by some oversight or mishap be applied to her forhead or chinne, it would make (ye would say) but a very ridiculous bewty.'

PAINTS AND WASHES

Along with her red wigs, Elizabeth wore the fashionable red and white paint on her exposed skin, and the older she got, the more she painted. According to Ben Jonson, she 'never saw herself after she became old in a true glass; they

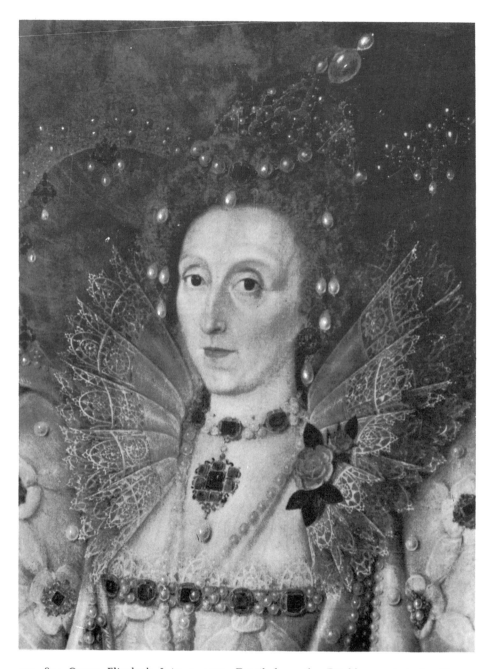

FIG. 80: Queen Elizabeth I in *c.* 1592. Detail from the Ditchley portrait by Marens Gheeraerts the Younger.

painted her, and sometymes would vermilion her nose.' The French ambassador
noted that her face appeared 'to be very aged, and her teeth are very yellow
and unequal compared with what they were formerly, and on the left side less
than the right.'

White lead was used for the paint, though powdered borax was preferred by
some women. Ochre and mercuric sulphide were both used for cheek rouge of
various shades; cochineal, blended with gum arabic, egg white, and fig milk
provided rouge for the lips. Cosmetics were also manufactured from pigeon's
wings and claws, Venetian turpentine, eggs, honey, lillies, shells, camphor,
ground mother-of-pearl, musk, and ambergris.

Edward de Vere, Earl of Oxford, introduced a number of foreign cosmetics
and perfumes into the court of Elizabeth. In Guiana Sir Walter Raleigh observed
'divers berries, that die a most perfect crimson and Carnation; and for painting,
all France, Italy, or the east Indies, yeild none such: For the more the skyn
is washed, the fayrer the cullour appeareth.' Michel de Montaigne reported
seeing some women 'swallow gravel, ashes, coals, dust, tallow candles, and for
the nonce, labour and toil themselves to spoil their stomach, only to get a pale-
bleak colour.'

Women who preferred not to use paint to whiten their skin and conceal
roughness were advised to 'wash in your own Urine, or with Rose-water mix'd
with Wine, or else make a Decoction of the Rinds of Lemon.' Some women
merely washed their faces in water in which beans had been boiled. Diane de
Poitier, noted for her beautiful complexion, is said to have used no cosmetic other
than rain water. And Catherine de' Medicis' physician instructed her, if she
would have a fair complexion, 'to go into the royal gardens at dawn and gather
dew-drenched peach blossoms, which should then be crushed with oil of almonds
by the light of the moon.' Catherine is credited with having spread the art of
face painting from Italy into France, where she insisted on its use at court. The
clergy threatened, but the ladies preferred to listen to Catherine. In 1582 Jean
Liébaut, a medical doctor in Paris, published a 463-page book entitled
L'Embellissement et Ornement du Corps Humain, which included instructions
and recipes for making various forms of cosmetics and lotions, bleaching and
dyeing hair, and caring for the skin and hair. Many of his recipes were copied
in books published during the next century or so.

Since the use of cosmetics had become general, especially among the upper
classes, somebody had to manufacture them. In *The Country Ferme*, published
in 1600, Richard Surflet advised the country wife to achieve some skill in making
'fukes & such things as are apt for the decking and painting of the body . . . not
that she should make use of them herself, but that she may make some profit &
benefit by the sale thereof, unto great Lords and Ladies & other persons that may
attend to be curious and paint up themselves.' It should be noted that lords were
included as well as ladies. For the country wife who wished to try out her own

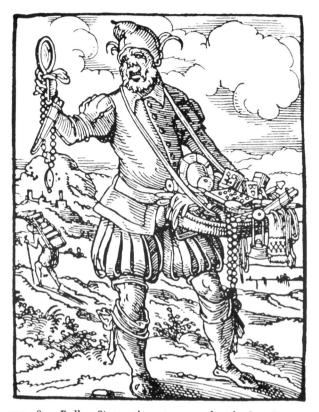

FIG. 81: Pedlar. Sixteenth-century woodcut by Jost Amman.

cosmetics and needed a mirror, there were itinerant pedlars (Figure 81) who could supply them.

In 1602 Hugh Plat, who invented, among other things, children's alphabet blocks, secret inks, a gamblers' finger ring with a reflecting sphere, and revolving spits for roasting meat, wrote a small book called *Delightes for Ladies, to advance their Persons, Tables, Closets, and Distillatories: with Beauties, Banquets, Perfumes & Waters*. He included a few recipes aimed toward beautification of his readers. The following are taken from the edition of 1627:

'*A white fucus or beauty for the face.* The jaw bones of a Hog or Sow well burnt, beaten, and searced thorow a fine Searce, and after, ground upon a porphyrie or serpentine stone, is an excellent fucus, being laid on with the oyle of white poppy.

'*To take away spots and freckles from the face or hands.* The sappe that issueth out of a Birch tree in great abundance, being opened, in March or Aprill, with a receiver of glasse set under the boring thereof to receive the same, doth perform the same most excellently & maketh the skin very cleer. This sap will dissolve pearle; a secret not known unto many.

'*An excellent Pomatum to cleer the skinne*. Wash Barrows grease ofte times in Maydeaw, that hath beene clarified in the Sunne, till it bee exceeding white: then take Marshmallow rootes, scraping off the outsides: then make thin slices of them, and mix them: set them to macerate in a seething Balneo, and scumme it well till it bee thorowly clarified, and will come to rope: then strain it and put now and then a spooneful of May-dew therein, beating it till it bee thorow cold in often change of May-dew: then throw away that dew and put it in a glasse, covering it with May-dew: and so reserve it to your use. Let the mallow roots be two or three daies dried in the shade before you use them. This I had of a great Professor of Art, and for a rare and dainty Secret, as the best fucus this day in use.'

Hartman, in *The True Preserver*, gives the recipe for 'A Cosmetick Water used by Queen Elizabeth:

'Take the whites of two new layd eggs, beat the shells of them to powder & put them in a quart bottle with the whites & let them be beaten together for three hours; then put into it four ounces of burnt Allum in fine powder, beat it two hours longer; then put into it three ounces of white Sugar candy in powder, beat it also for two hours, then put in it four ounces of Borax also in powder, & beat it also; then take a pynte of water that runs from under the wheel of a mill, & put into it four ounces of white Poppy seeds well beaten, mix them well together, so that it be like milk, then pour that into the quart bottle with the other things . . . beating it every time the space of two hours; then strain it through a fine white linnen cloath; & having put it into the bottle again let it be beaten for two or three hours longer. And to know when it is well made & well beaten is when it froths the breadth of three fingers above it. It will keep a twelve month, it is a very good cosmetick, it whitens, smooths, & softens the skin, use it only three times a week.'

Egg whites were used to give a fashionable glaze to the skin.

Artificial aids to beauty are mentioned from time to time in Shakespeare's plays. Hermia calls Helena a painted maypole, and Hamlet accuses Ophelia of painting her face: 'God hath given you one face and you make yourself another.'

In *The Silent Woman*, first performed in 1601, Ben Jonson had Clerimont complain of being kept waiting till a woman had 'painted and perfum'd and washt and scour'd'. True-wit defended the making up, insisting only that it be done in private, but that having been done, it should be freely acknowledged. 'Is it for us,' he asked, 'to see their perukes put on, their false teeth, their complexion, their eyebrows, their nails?' He had, in fact, he said, 'once followed a rude fellow into a chamber, where the poor madam, for haste, and troubled, snatch'd at her peruke to cover her baldness; and put it on the wrong way. . . .

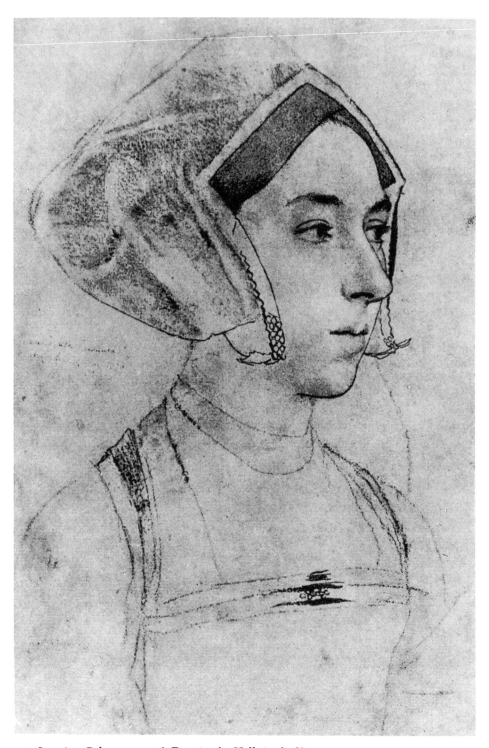

FIG. 82: Ann Boleyn, 1505–36. Drawing by Holbein the Younger.

And the unconscionable knave held her in compliment an hour with that reverst face, when I still look'd when she should talk from the t'other side.'

But women did not always do their own makeup unaided. In *The Malcontent* Dr Plasterface is described as 'the most exquisite in forging of veines, sprightning of eyes, dying of haire, sleeking of skinnes, blushing of cheekes, surphleing of breastes, blanching and bleaching of teeth, that ever made an old lady gracious by torchlight.' Another of Marston's characters complains of a lady friend 'so steept in lemons juyce, so surphuled, I cannot see her face'.

The moralists, even more than the poets, were outraged by the spreading popularity of painting. One of the most famous polemics against everything new, pleasurable, or man-made, was written in 1583 by Philip Stubbes and entitled *The Anatomie of Abuses*. It contained, according to the title page, *a Discoverie, or Briefe Summarie of Such Notable Vice and Imperfections, as now raigne in many Christian Countreyes of the Worlde: but (especiallie) in a verie famous lande called Anglia: Together, with most fearfull examples of Gods Judgments, executed upon the wicked for the same, as well in Anglia of late, as in other place, elsewhere. Verie Godley, to be read of all true Christians, everie where: but most needefull, to be regarded in Englande.*

According to Stubbes, 'The greatest abuse, which offendeth God moste . . . is the execrable sinne of Pride'. Stubbes goes into exhaustive detail about what the various kinds of pride involve, but we are concerned here with only one small element, which upset him to about the same degree that everything else worldly upset him. 'The Women of Anglia,' he tells us, 'use to colour their faces with certain oyles, liquors, unguents and waters made to that end, whereby they think their beautie is greatly decored; but who seethe not that their soules are thereby deformed, and they brought deeper into the displeasure and indignation of the Almighty, at whose voice the earth dooth tremble and at whose presence the heavens shall liquifie and melt away. . . . Thinkest thou that thou canst make thy self fairer then God who made us all? These must needes be their inventions, or else they would never go about to colour their faces with such sibbersauces.'

All of the moralists had much the same approach; but despite the similarity of their arguments, they seemed never to lack a publisher and, presumably, a reading public. At mid-century there was published in London *The Booke in Meeter of Robin Conscience: against his Father Covetousnesse, his Mother Newgise, and his Sister Proud Beautye* — a book which was, so the author would have us believe, 'very necessary to be read and marked of all Maydens that seeke the vaine glory of this world, and the uncomly tricked therein, that they may avoide the dangers thereof: for feare of condemnation.' In this case the girls' own brother (Robin Conscience) is condemning her. Having noticed that sometimes her colour fades, he asks if she thinks she can be fairer than God has made her. Being a woman of the world, Proud Beautye answers:

If God make my face as browne as a berry,
I can painte it white and ruddish withall;
And if God make me looke as red as a Cherry,
I can drie up my blood with Chalke in a wall;
If God make me grosse, I can pent my selfe small.
To be faire and feate, nice and neate, is a gay thing:
To colly and kisse, my pleasure it is, for all your new learning.

The author, lest the reader somehow miss the point, has added a marginal comment: 'The prattises and motions of Sathan and are used of those that be his fathers darlings now a dayes.' He repeats the sentiment marginally from time to time throughout the dialogue.

Later in the century the French poet Guillaume Du Bartas composed a cynical picture of painting women which should have given any woman pause had she believed him:

But besides all her sumptuous equipage,
Much fitter for her state, then for her age,
Close in her closet with her best complexions,
Shee mends her faces wrinkle-full defections.
Her cheeke she cherries, and her eye she cheeres,
And faines her fond as wench of fifteene yeeres.

. . . .

Chaste Lady maides here must I speake to you,
That with vile painting spoile your native hue.
Not to inflame younglings with wanton thirst,
But to keepe fashion with these times accurst.

. . . .

Shall I take her, that will spend all I have,
And all her time in pranking proudly brave?
How did I dote? The golde upon her head,
The lillies of her breast, the Rosie red
In either cheeke, and all her other riches,
Wherewith she bleareth sight, and sense bewitches,
Is none of hers: it is but borrowed stuffe,
Or stolne, or bought, plaine counterfeite in proofe.
My glorious idoll, I did so adore,
Is but a vizard newly varnished ore

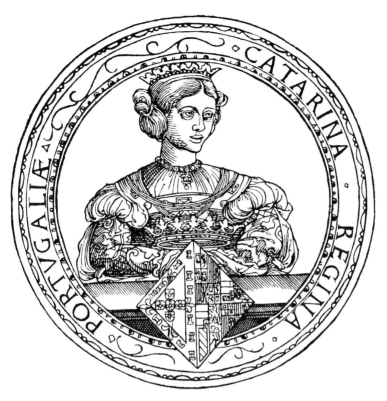

FIG. 83 : Catherine of Portugal, 1540. Woodcut by an unknown artist.

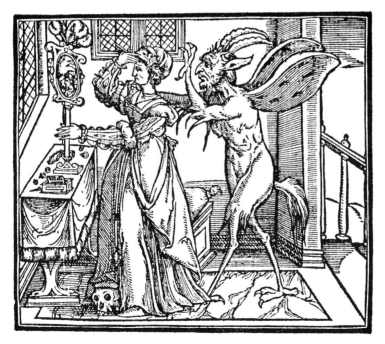

FIG. 84 : The Sin of Pride, 1570.

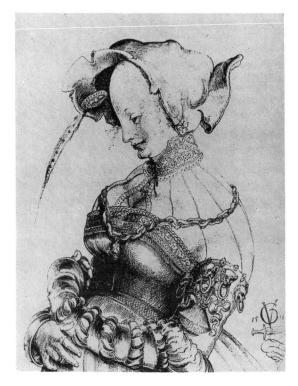

FIG. 85: Young woman with plucked eyebrows and shaved hairline. Drawing by Urs Graf, 1518.

With spauling rheumes, hot fumes, and ceruses.
Fo, fy, such poisons one would lothe to kisse,
I wed, at least I ween, I wed a lasse,
Young, fresh, and faire; but in a yeare and lesse,
Or at most, my lovely, lively bride,
Is turn'd a hagge, a fury by my side.
With hollow yellow teeth, or none perhaps,
With stinking breath, swart cheeks, & hanging chaps,
With wrinkled neck, and stooping, as she goes,
With driveling mouth, and with a sniveling nose.

Despite all of the criticism from men, be they moralists, poets, or husbands, more and more women painted, and their painting was at least tolerated by the public. In Marston's *Dutch Courtesan*, first performed about 1603, Mistress Mulligrub, speaking of Master Burnish, says that his wife 'has been as proper a woman as any in Cheap; she paints now, and yet she keeps her husband's old customers to him still'. In Paris even the nuns were to be seen in the streets painted, rouged, and powdered.

PATCHES

The end of the sixteenth century saw the beginning of a new era in patching, thus providing the clergy with one more sin to preach against. The custom of wearing little black beauty spots to set off the whiteness of the skin is believed to have begun with use of black velvet or taffeta court plasters on the temples for relief of the toothache, a practice touched upon by Joseph Hall in writing of Gallia, who:

> ... wore a velvet mastic-patch
> Upon her temples when no tooth did ach;
> When beauty was her rheum I soon espied,
> Nor could her plaster cure her of her pride.

Thus, women began using the patches to improve their beauty instead of their teeth, and the fashion was launched. Since customs may be accidentally revived from time to time and seem quite original, this may very well have happened. But the fact remains that the ancient Romans had used patches, with or without the excuse of a toothache, many centuries earlier.

HAIR

Women's hair styles came in for as much criticism as their painting, both of which, the moralists assumed, could have only one purpose — to tempt men into immoral behaviour. 'For what meaneth else,' asked William Averell in 1588, 'the daintie trimming of their heads, the laying out of their hayres, the painting and washing of their faces, the opening of their breasts, and discovering them to their wastes, their bents of Whale bone to beare out their bummes, their great sleeves and bumbasted shoulders, squared in breadth to make their wastes small, their culloured hose, their variable shooes?'

Alberti was another complainer who was incensed by women's 'gadding abroad with frizled lockes, embroidered garments, & other open marks of their lightnesse, onely but to procure their owne scorne and derision,' and he warned his readers (whom he addressed as 'deare Sisters') that neither 'golde, pearles, periwigs, nor painting' would win the love that could better be achieved through a 'faire & comely demeanour, humanities, gentlenesse, and modestie'.

Stephen Gosson, rector of St Botolph, Bishopgate, from 1600 until his death in 1623, seems to have prepared for the job at the rectory by writing poetry in complaint of women's vanity. His *Pleasant Quippes for Upstart Newfangled Gentlewomen*, published in 1595, was aptly subtitled, *A Glasse to view the Pride of vain-glorious Woman; containing a pleasant invective against the*

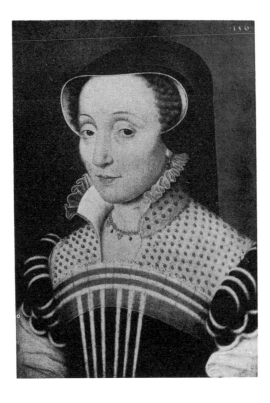

FIG. 86: Claudia of Beaune. School of Clouet, 1568. The eyebrows are plucked and the hairline is shaved.

fantastical forreigne Toyes daylie used in Women's Apparell. Only one verse of the nine-page poem refers specifically to hair styles and cosmetics:

These flaming heads with staring haire,
 these wyers turnde like hornes of ram:
These painted faces which they weare,
 can any tell from whence they cam?
 Dan Sathan, Lord of fayned lyes,
 All these new fangeles did devise.

The 'flaming heads' were presumably dyed to match Elizabeth's red wigs. Hair dyes were in use at the time, and in 1602 Hugh Plat instructed his readers 'How to colour the head or beard into a chestnut colour in halfe an houre:

'Take one part of lead calcined with Sulphur, and one part of quicklime: temper them somewhat thin with water: lay it upon the hair, chafing it well in, and let it dry one quarter of an hour or thereabouts; then wash the same off with fair water divers times: and lastly with sope and water, and it will be a very natural hair-colour. The longer it lyeth upon the haire, the browner it groweth. This coloureth not the flesh at all, and yet it lasteth very long in the hair.'

In *The Booke of Robin Conscience* Robin's sister flippantly defies her brother's moral chiding:

> Tush, I can dye my haire; be it never so black,
> I can make it shine like golde in a little space:
> Also to tire up my head I have such a knack,
> That some maides will delight to follow my trace.
> I can lay out my haire to set out my face:
> Oh, to be faire and feate, nice and neate, is a gay thing:
> To colly and kisse, my pleasure it is, for all your new learning.

These words, the author warns us, lest we inadvertently be taken in, are the 'workes of the devill'. Robin, evidently speaking for the author, gives the expected response:

> To dye and to fleare your haire so abroad,
> Surely, sister, you doo it shamefully use:
> For with the Scriptures it dooth not accord,
> That maides nor wives their haire should so abuse;
> Cover it for shame: it is the use of the studues.
> Therefore measure your pleasure by God's woord and will,
> And you shall finde that your minde is whorish and ill.

And the dialogue goes on about sweet-smelling pomanders, golden chains, and stomachers; and at the end the author regretfully comes to a conclusion which, had it been reached earlier, might have saved him a great deal of trouble:

> To talke well with some women dooth as much good,
> As a sicke man to eate up a loade of greene wood.

Teeth

It appears that Elizabethan teeth were seldom the rows of shining pearls the poets used to write about. They were usually neither very healthy nor very clean, and frequently they were missing. Joseph Hall, later Bishop of Norwich, closes his sixth book of *Satires*, published in 1598, when he was twenty-four, with a jaundiced look at women:

> As witty Pontan in great earnest said,
> His mistress' breasts were like two weights of lead.
> Another thinks her teeth might liken'd be
> To two fair ranks of poles of ivory,

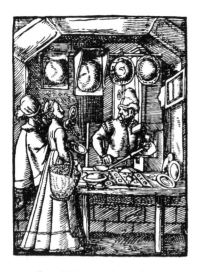

FIG. 87: Mirror-maker's shop, late
sixteenth century.
Woodcut by Jost Amman.

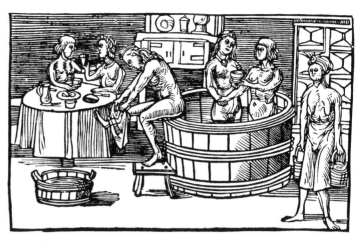

FIG. 88: Bathing in Antwerp, 1514. Woodcut from the popular
medical treatise, *Regimen Sanitatis*. It was customary
to go directly from the bath to the table.

> To fence in sure the wild beast of her tongue,
> From either going far, or going wrong;
> Her grinders like two chalk-stones in a mill,
> Which shall with time and wearing wax as ill
> As old Catilla's, which wont every night
> Lay up her holy pegs till next daylight,
> And with them grind soft-simpering all the day,
> When lest her laughter should her gums betray
> Her hands must hide her mouth if she but smile;
> Gain would she seem all frixe and frolic still.
> Her forehead fair is like a brazen hill
> Whose wrinkles furrows which her age doth breed,
> Are daubed full of Venice chalk for need.

But dental disasters did not result entirely from ignorance. There were instructions available for what may seem to us rather casual dental care. Hugh Plat, in his *Delightes for Ladies*, gives a recipe 'To keep the teeth both white and sound.

'Of hony take a quart, as much vinegar, & half so much white wine; boyl them together, and wash your teeth therewith now and then.' At the end of another recipe for cleaning the teeth, Plat adds that, 'if your teeth bee very scaly, let some expert Barber first take off the Scales with his instrument, and then you may keep them cleane by rubbing them with the aforementioned roules.'

BATHS AND PERFUMES

In England there were no bathrooms as such in private dwellings. Baths were taken in a portable wooden tub placed near the bedroom fire. The water was scented with herbs, and perfumed soap was often used. In France and Belgium men and women bathed together before meals in a large wooden tub, then immediately sat down to dinner, still in the nude (see Figure 88). An engraving after Jost Amman shows a Dutch family bathing together in small wooden tubs (Figure 89).

As in other countries (see Figure 90), there were also public baths. Steam baths, known as *hothouses* or *hummums*, their Persian name, were especially popular with women, who liked to assemble there for food and gossip. Ben Jonson mentions sweating in hothouses, and a character in *The Puritan*, referring to some particularly exhausting work, says, 'Marry, it will take me much sweat; I were better go to sixteen hothouses'. Eventually the baths became so notorious for illicit intrigues that they fell into disuse.

In France the public baths (see Figure 65), which had suffered from a bad reputation since the fourteenth century, came more and more under criticism by the clergy and suffered the same fate as the English hothouses. Then, having lost the habit of frequenting the public baths, people also lost the habit of washing at all. Even Marguerite of Navarre saw nothing out of the way in noting casually that she had not washed her hands for a week—and this at a time when one ate with the fingers and blew one's nose in one's hand (though it was not considered proper to do it in the same hand one used for holding meat). Erasmus, in 1530, suggested the use of the handkerchief but added that it was not forbidden to use the fingers provided one put one's foot upon what fell to the ground.

Soap was in use at the time, and in *The Good Huswifes Jewell*, a book of recipes 'imprinted at London by John Wolfe for Edward White, dwelling at the little North doore of Paules at the signe of the Gunne, 1587', the author Thomas Dawson includes a recipe for making it:

'First you must take halfe a strike of Asshen Asshes, and a quarte of Lime, then you must mingle both these together, and then you must fil a panne full of water and seeth them well, so done, you must take fower pounde of Beastes tallowe, and put it into the Lye, and seeth them together untill it be hard.'

The book also contains, among its scores of recipes for foods and medicines, one intriguingly headed 'To make a strong broth for fickle men'.

But since soap was infrequently used and sanitation was poor, perfumes helped to make life bearable. A recipe for Queen Elizabeth's Perfume was used for several centuries:

'Take eight spoonfuls of compound water, the weight of twopence in fine

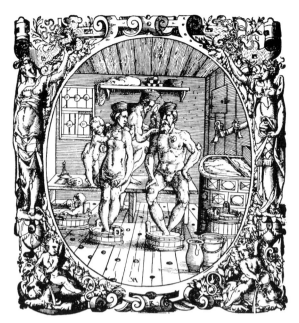

FIG. 89: Dutch bathroom, late sixteenth century. Cupping-glasses are being applied to the man. Woodcut by Jost Amman.

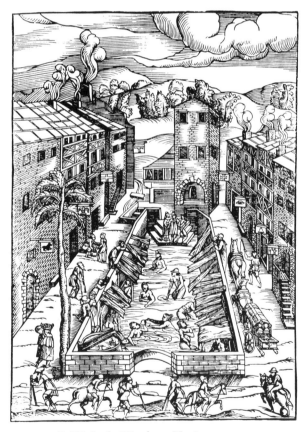

FIG. 90: Public bath. Woodcut, Venice, 1553.

powder of sugar, and boil it on hot embers & coals softly & half an ounce of sweet marjoram dried in the sun, the weight of two pence of the powder of Benjamin, this perfume is very sweet & good for the time.'

Men matched the women in their use of perfumes. Nicolas de Montau objected to the Ladies 'making use of every perfume—cordial, civet, musk, ambergris, and other precious aromatic substances—for perfuming their dresses and linen, nay, their whole bodies.' Fans, used by both men and women, were scented, and jewelery was designed with cavities for holding scent. Jeanne d'Albret, mother of Henri IV, is said to have been poisoned by perfumed gloves from Italy.

But the moralists objected to perfumes, poisoned or not, and seemed to feel that the less bearable life was, the greater would be the rewards thereafter. Philip Stubbes, whose *Anatomie of Abuses* has already been mentioned, was still harping on 'the sinne of Pride' when he wrote:

'Is this not a certen sweete Pride, to have cyvet, muske, sweete powders, fragrant Pomanders, odorous perfumes & such like, whereof the smel may be felt and perceived not only all over the house or place where they be present, but also a stones cast of, almost, yea the bed wherein they have layed their delicate bodies, the places where they have sate, the clothes and thinges which they have touched shall smell a weeke, a moneth, and more after they be gon. But the Prophet Elaias telleth them, instead of their pomaunders, musks, civets, balmes, sweet odours and perfumes, they shall have stench and horrour in the nethermost hel. Let them take heed to it and amend their wicked lives.'

Presumably they at least took heed, for the book was a sixteenth-century best seller, and two years later the third edition, revised and expanded, was published. But the book, in any of its editions, had no appreciable effect on the use of perfumes or, probably, on the Sinne of Pride.

MEN

Men occasionally used makeup, and those who did came in for their share of criticism. The moralists also complained about their hair styles, as they have from time to time for the past two thousand years, and the poets wrote satiric verses about them. One of these, by Joseph Hall, was directed at the problems of a fashionable gentleman of the period on venturing out in a high wind:

> Fie on all court'sy and unruly winds,
> Two only foes that fair disguisement finds.
> Strange curse! but fit for such a fickle age,
> When scalps are subject to such vassalage.

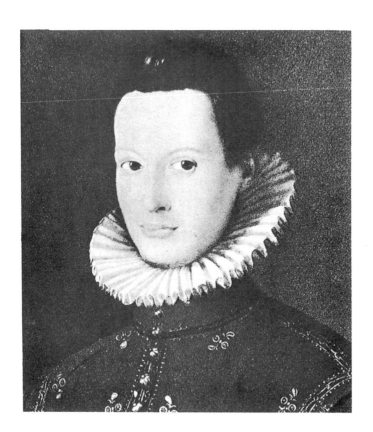

FIG. 91 : Giovanni de' Medici.
Painting from the work-
shop of Bronzino, late
sixteenth century. The
eyebrows have evidently
been plucked in the
feminine style.

Late travelling along in London way,
Me met, as seem'd by his disguis'd array,
A lusty courtier, whose curled head
With abron locks was fairly furnished.
I him saluted in our lavish wise :
He answers my untimely courtesies.
His bonnet vail'd, ere ever he could think,
The unruly wind blows off his periwinke.
He lights and runs, and quickly hath him sped,
To overtake his overrunning head.
The sportful wind, to mock the headless man,
Tosses apace his pitch'd Rogerian :
And straight it to a deeper ditch hath blown;
There must my yonker fetch his waxen crown.
I look'd and laugh'd, whiles in his raging mind,
He curs'd all court'sy and unruly wind.
I look'd and laugh'd, and much I marvelled,
To see so large a causeway in his head,
And me bethought, that when it first begon,
'Twas some shrewd autumn that so bar'd the bone.

Is't not sweet pride, when men their crowns must shade,
With that which herks the hams of every jade,
Or floor-strew'd locks from off the barber's shears?
But waxen crowns well 'gree with borrow'd hairs.

In a later satire Hall wrote again about fashions and affectations of men:

I wot not how the world's degenerate,
That men or know, or like not their estate;
Out from the Gades up to th' Eastern morn,
Not one but holds his native state forlorn.
When comely striplings wish it were their chance
For Caenis' distaff to exchange their lance,
And wear curl'd periwigs, and chalk their face,
And still are poring on their pocket-glass.

Frenchmen who chose to paint their faces at least had a royal example for a time. Henri III went about the streets of Paris 'made up like an old coquette', as Franklin puts it, his face plastered with white and red, his hair covered with perfumed violet powder. But even so, the use of cosmetics by men was not generally looked upon with favour by either sex.

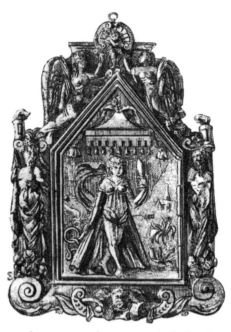

FIG. 92a : Sixteenth-century pocket mirror of gilted and enamelled silver.

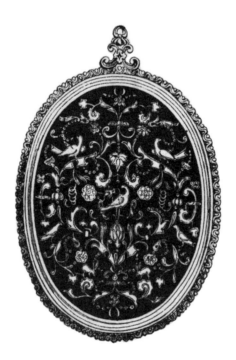

FIG. 92b : Back of small steel mirror, sixteenth century.

6 · The Early Seventeenth Century
1603-1625

She hath a fair hair, if it be her own,
a rare face, if it be not painted,
a white skin, if it be not plastered,
a full breast, if it be not bolstered.

A STRAUNGE FOOT POST, 1613

The use of paint became more discreet during the reign of James I but was still sufficiently evident, among the lower classes as well as the aristocracy, to be written about and openly discussed. The moralists and the clerics continued to use the humourless, heavy-handed, sledge-hammer approach to criticism. In their monumental outrage they usually managed to invoke the name of the devil, as in *Quips Upon Questions*:

Where's the Devill?
He's got a boxe of women's paint —
Where pride is, thers the Divell too.

But the playwrights and the poets, well aware that more could be accomplished through laughter than invective, took a slyer approach.

In *Lingua: or, the Combat of the Tongue and the Five Senses for Superiority*, an early seventeenth-century play, Phantastes says, 'If her face be naught, in my opinion, the more view it the worse. Bid her wear the multitude of her deformities under a mask, till my leisure will serve to devise some durable and unstained black of painting.'

But few writers were so open-minded about painting. In *Wit Restored* Sir John Mennis wrote of 'a Painted Madam':

Men say y'are fair; and fair ye are, 'tis true,
But (hark!) we praise the painter now, not you.

He felt equally strongly about 'a Painted Curtezan':

Whosoever saith thou sellest all, doth jest,
Thou buy'st thy beauty, that sels all the rest.

Also in *Wit Restored* Sir John Mennis and Dr James Smith took another jibe at painted women in 'Will Bagnalls Ballet', believed to have been written during the reign of James I:

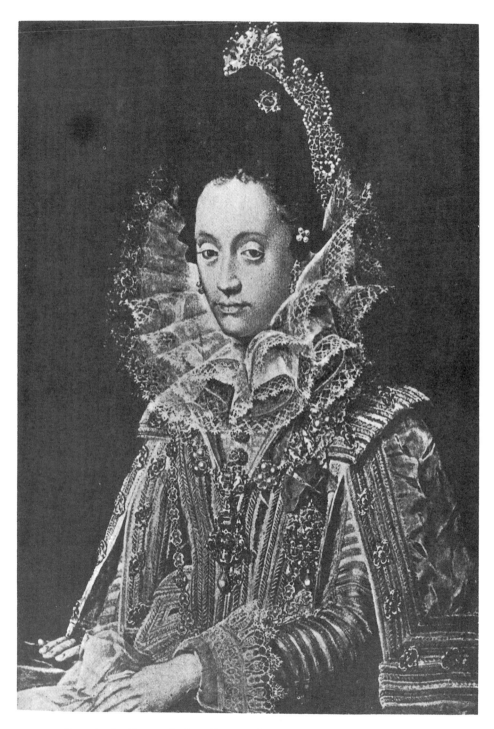

FIG. 93 : Portrait of a German duchess. Painting by Peter Candido, 1613.

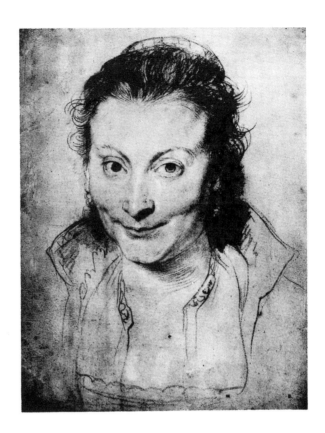

FIG. 94: Elizabeth Brand. Drawing by Peter Paul Rubens, early seventeenth century.

> Your faces trict and painted be,
>   Your breasts all open bare,
> So farre, that a man may almost see
>   Unto your lady-ware.
> And in the church to tell you true,
> Men cannot serve God for looking on you.
>   *O Women, monstrous women,*
>   *What do you meane to do?*

What some men thought they meant to do is suggested in two lines by Edward Tylman:

> *Fucus* is paint, and *fucus* is deceit,
> And *fucus* they use, that doe mean to cheat.

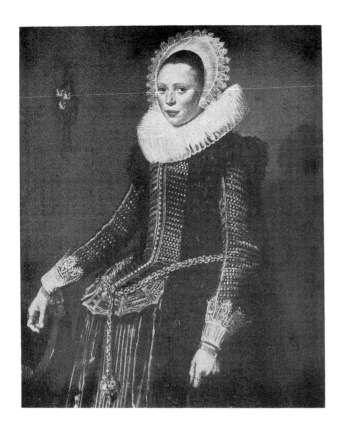

FIG. 95 : Portrait of a woman. Painting by Frans Hals, early seventeenth century.

THE IDEAL BEAUTY

What the women actually meant to do was presumably to achieve the ideal beauty described by Robert Herrick:

> Black and rowling is her eye,
> Double chinn'd, and forehead high:
> Lips she has, all Rubie red
> Cheeks like Creame Enclaritèd:
> And a nose that is the grace
> And Proscenium of her face.

But judging from the barbs that various writers directed at the painted ladies, they succeeded only fitfully.

George Chapman, who died in 1634, compares women to the temples of Egypt:

> With alabaster pillars were those temples
> Upheld and beautified, and so are women;
> Most curiously glazed — and so are women;
> Cunningly painted too — and so are women.

Elsewhere a character of Chapman's describes a lady as being 'very faire, I think that she bee painted'.

In John Suckling's 'Ballad Upon a Wedding' it's not quite clear whether or not the bride is painted:

> Her cheeks so rare a white was on,
> No daisy makes comparison;
> Who sees them is undone;
> For streaks of red were mingled there,
> Such as are on a Cath'rine pear,
> The side that's next the sun.

The author of 'How to Choose a Wife' clearly expected her endowments to be completely natural:

> Good sir, if you will shew the best of your skill
> To picke a vertuous creature,
> Then picke such a wife, as you love a life,
> Of a comely grace and feature;
> The noblest part, let it be her heart,
> Without deceit or cunning,
> With a nimble wit, and all things fit,
> With a tongue that's never running,
> The haire of her head, it must not be red,
> But faire and brown as a berry;
> Her fore-head high, with a christall eye,
> Her lips as red as a cherry.

PAINTS AND POWDERS

Despite the voluble complaints of clergymen and writers, men in general accepted the painted faces with resignation — as a foolish conceit, perhaps, but hardly a mortal sin.

Ceruse, as the pale makeup base was called, was a white, flesh, or pink paint worn exclusively by upper-class women, though many women preferred to use a white powder instead. The paint was sometimes applied quite thickly to help conceal wrinkles. Since it was usually used only on the face and neck and sometimes only the face, the line of demarcation was often fairly obvious. The slight sheen of the enamel was in marked contrast to the matte finish of the powdered faces.

In Ben Jonson's *The Devil is an Ass*, first performed in 1616, Wittipol, a young gallant, expounds to Lady Taile-Bush on some of the disadvantages of painting:

> They say that painting quite destroys the face. . . .
> Corrupts the breath; hath left so little sweetness

> In kissing, as 'tis now us'd but for fashion;
> And shortly will be taken for a punishment.
> Decays the fore-teeth that should guard the tongue;
> And suffers that run riot everlasting!
> And (which is worse) some ladies when they meet,
> Cannot be merry and laugh, but they do spit
> In one another's faces! . . .
> Then, they say, 'tis dangerous
> To all the fal'n, yet well dispos'd mad-dams,
> That are industrious, and desire to earn
> Their living with their sweat! for any distemper
> Of heat and motion may displace the colours;
> And if the paint once run about their faces,
> Twenty to one they will appear so ill-favour'd,
> Their servants run away too, and leave the pleasure
> Imperfect, and the reckoning als' unpaid.

But women painted anyway, and since they frequently made their own paints, they were avid collectors of new recipes. Lady Taile-Bush says she understands that the Spanish fucuses or paints contain:

> Water of gourds, of radish, the white beans,
> Flowers of glass, of thistles, rose-marine,
> Raw honey, mustard-seed, and bread dough-bak'd,
> The crums o' bread, goats-milk, and white of eggs,
> Camphire, and lily-roots, the fat of swans,
> Marrow of veal, white pigeons, and pine-kernels,
> The seeds of nettles, purseline, and hares-gall;
> Limons, thin-skin'd. . . .

But Wittipol assures her that those are the *ordinary* Spanish fucuses. There are much rarer ones containing:

> Your allum scagliola, or pol-dipedra;
> And zuccarino; turpentine of Abezzo,
> Wash'd in nine waters; soda di levante,
> Or your fern ashes; benjamin di gotta:
> Grasso di serpe; porceletto marino;
> Oils of lentisco; ducche mugia; make
> The admirable vernish for the face,
> Gives the right lustre; but two drops rubb'd on
> With a piece of scarlet, makes a lady of sixty
> Look as sixteen. But above all, the water
> Of the white hen, of the lady Estifania's.

He then describes how to make the water of the white hen, which, to judge from the tiny amount prescribed, must have been an extraordinarily powerful cosmetic:

> Madam, you take your hen,
> Plume it, and skin it, cleanse it o' the inwards;
> Then chop it, bones an all; add to four ounces
> Of carravicins, pipitas, sope of Cyprus,
> Make the decoction, strain it. Then distil it,
> And keep it in your gally-pot well glidder'd:
> Three drops preserves from wrinkles, warts, spots, moles,
> Blemish, or sun-burnings, and keeps the skin
> *In decimo sexto*, ever bright and smooth,
> As any looking-glass; and indeed is call'd
> The virgins milk for the face. . . .

The enamelled ladies used a moist rouge, presumably applied directly with the fingertips, whereas the powdered ladies, when they coloured their cheeks at all, used a dry rouge applied and blended with a cloth. The dry rouge, in various shades of rose, was purchased as a powder, then mixed with water and allowed to harden into a cake. The moist rouge, sometimes used on the lips as well, was a brighter cherry red. Both were usually applied generously over a large area of the cheek. Lower class women used a cheaper ochre red and tended to apply it excessively.

Rosy cheeks and lips were considered desirable, and the lower lip was supposed to be fuller than the upper. Sir John Suckling wrote of a lovely lady he admired, that:

> Her lips were red, and one was thin
> Compared with that was next her chin,
>   Some bee had stung it newly.

Sir John did not seem to be particularly concerned as to whether or not the colour was natural.

Eyebrows were occasionally darkened, and a cream eyeshadow in blue, brown, or grey was sometimes worn by upper-class women. It was usually concentrated on the upper lid near the eye but might occasionally, in a burst of enthusiasm, be allowed to creep up toward the eyebrow.

At the beginning of the century Marston had pointed out in his play *Antonio and Mellida* that male courtiers sometimes used makeup — 'The fifth paints and has always a good colour for what he speaks'. Fitzgeffrey was also distressed about the vanity of men, especially when flaunted in public:

> W'ant it for Women we shu'd all be men.
> I cannot present better instance, then
> In you Spruse *Coxcombe*, you Affecting *Asse*,
> That never walkes without his Looking-glasse,
> In a Tobacco box, or Diall set,
> That he may privately conferre with it.

Men's makeup, which was considered effeminate, was almost always deceptive, whereas women's had been growing increasingly less so. Makeup for men consisted of cheek rouge, pink or flesh powder, and sometimes a touch of lip rouge.

A TREATISE AGAINST PAINTING

To Thomas Tuke ('Minister of God's Word at Saint Giles in the Fields'), paint was unacceptable on either sex. In 1616 he wrote *A Treatise Against Painting and Tincturing of Men and Women: Against Murther and Poysoning: Pride and Ambition: Adulterie and Witchcraft. And the Roote of all these, Disobedience to the Ministery of the Word. Whereunto is Added the picture of a picture, or, the Character of a Painted Woman.* The tract was printed in London 'for Edward Merchant, dwelling in St. Pauls Church-yard, neere the Crosse'.

Tuke begins his book in a flurry of verse. A poem by Arthur Dowton goes directly to the point with commendable brevity:

> TO WOMEN THAT PAINT THEMSELVES
> A Lome wall and painted face are one;
> For th' beauty of them both is quickly gone.
> When the lome is fallen off, then lathes appeare,
> So wrinkles in that face fro th' eye to th' eare.
> The chastest of your sex contemme these arts,
> And many that use them have rid in carts.

Thomas Draiton, equally surly, requires two poems to say the same thing:

> OF THE ORIGINALL OF PAINTING THE FACE
> Describe what is faire painting of the face,
> It is a thing proceedes from want of grace:
> Which thing deformitie did just beget,
> And is on earth the greatest counterfet.

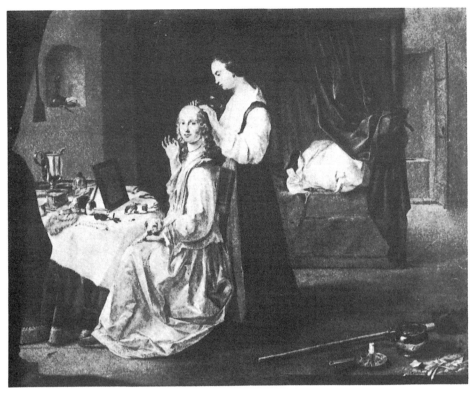

FIG. 96: A Dutch lady at her toilet. Painting by Ochtervelt, late seventeenth century.

OF TINCTURING THE FACE

To what may I a painted wench compare?
Shee's one disguized, when her face is bare.
She is a sickly woman alwaies lying.
Her colour's gone, but more she is buying.
She is a raine bow, colours altogether,
She makes faire shew, and beares us all faire weather:
And like a bow: shee's flexible to bend,
And is led in a string by any friend.
She is Medea, who by likelihood
Can change old Aeson into younger blood,
Which can old age in youthfull colours bury,
And make Prosperpine of an hagge, or furie,
Shee's a Physitian well skild in complexions,
The sickle will soone looke well by her confections. . . .
And to conclude, sheele please men in all places:
For shee's a Mimique, and can make good faces.

129

Tuke then quotes endlessly from the early Christians and anyone else who agrees with him and adds a little invective of his own:

'What a pride it is that thou canst not bee content to appear in thine owne likenesse and to seeme that to others which thou art in thy selfe? The bird appears in her owne feathers, the Peacocke shewes himselfe in his owne colours, the sheepe is seene in her own fleece and likenesse, white or black; the tree hath her own rinde, appears in her owne blossomes and fruits; and shall it be horrible to a woman to seeme to be, as she is indeed, displeasing to her to appeare in her owne likenesse, her owne haire, her owne complexion? She was borne in her owne, nature would shew itself in her proper colours; she was not borne painted in this world . . . neither shall she ride painted in the next world, and I thinke she would be loth die painted, why then should she live painted, why should she love it? . . . A painted face is a *superfluous* face. It were well if the world were well rid of all such superfluous creatures.'

PATCHES AND PATCHING

Although the fashion of patching was beginning to take hold in the late sixteenth century, it did not really blossom until the seventeenth—*par excellence*, the century of patches. (See Figures 103, 107, 111, 113, 115.) The clergy predictably continued its outcry against them. Colbert, Archbishop of Montpellier, aware, as were other clergymen, that their preaching was having no effect, announced to his parishoners that in the future he would tolerate patches out of sympathy for the poor unfortunates who were obliged to wear them to hide blemishes. This was immediately followed by a marked reduction in patching in Colbert's diocese, though not in others.

Patches provided a never-ending source of material for satires, which evidently accomplished nothing at the time but add considerably to our knowledge of what the ladies did and what the men thought about it. In 'Dr Smith's Ballet', a sequel to 'Will Bagnall's Ballet' from *Wit Restored*, we find four frequently quoted lines describing ladies' excessive patching and the shapes of their patches:

> Their faces are besmear'd and pierc'd,
> With severall sorts of patches,
> As if some cats their skins had flead
> With scarres, half-moons, and notches.

This was followed by still another poetic jibe at patched and enamelled women, reflecting *Upon the Naked Bedlams, and Spotted Beasts, we see in Covent Garden*:

When *Besse*! she ne're was halfe so vainly clad,
Besse ne're was halfe so naked, halfe so mad.
Again, this raves with lust, for love *Besse* ranted,
Then *Besses* skin was tan'd, but this is painted:
No, this is Madam Spots, 'tis she, I know her;
Her face is powdred *Ermin*, I'le speak to her;
How does your most enammel'd ladyship?
Nay, pardon me, I dare not touch your lip.
What kisse a leopard! he that lips will close,
With such a beast as you, may lose his nose.

．．．．．．．．．．．．．．．．．．．．

But dapl'd ladies, if you needs must show
Your nakednesse, yet pray why spotted so?
Has beauty, think you, lustre from these spots?
Is paper fairer when 'tis stain'd with blots?
What, have you cut your mask out into sippets,
Like wanton girles, to make you spots and tippets;
As I have seen a cook, that ever-neat,
To garnish out a dish, hath spoil'd good meat?
Pride is a plague, why sure these are the sores,
I will write (*Lord have mercy*) on your doors.

．．．．．．．．．．．．．．．．．．．

Come, tell me true, for what these spots are set,
Are they decoyes to draw fools to your net?
Are they like ribbons in the mane and taile,
Of an old wincing mare that's set to sale?

．．．．．．．．．．．．．．．．．．

Take my advice to be secure from jeers,
Wash off your stinking spots with bitter teares,
  O you sweet rurall beauties who were never
Infected with this ugly spotted feaver,
Whose face is smoother then the wory plaine,
Need neither spots from France, nor paint from Spaine.

．．．．．．．．．．．．．．．．．．．

In 1616 court ladies in Berlin were observed to be heavily patched. And somewhat later Johann Moscherosch reported seeing 'a group of women looking as if their faces had been scratched, pecked, and cut, for on those parts to which they wished to attract special attention, they had stuck small black plasters which looked like gnats and fleas of every imaginable shape and size, as well as other singular lures to finger and eye.' Although patching was an upper-class affectation, women of the lower classes sometimes wore patches but in less profusion.

The wearing of patches by men, though apparently unusual at this time, is mentioned by Angelina in *The Elder Brother*:

> 'Tis not a face I only am in love with;
> Nor will I say your face is excellent,
> A reasonable hunting-face to court the wind with!
> No, nor your visits each day in new suits,
> Nor your black patches you wear variously,
> Some cut like stars, some in half moons, some lozenges,
> All which best show you still a younger brother.

But this was only the beginning. Patching continued to increase in popularity throughout the century.

PERFUMES

Perfumed gloves were greatly esteemed in Elizabethan days. The following recipe (clearly intended for ladies with time on their hands) appears in Gervase Markham's *Countrey Contentments*, published in 1623:

'Take Angelica-water and Rose-water, and put into them the powder of Cloves, Amber-greece, Muske and Lignum Aloes, Benjamine and Callamus Aramattecus; boyle these till halfe bee consumed; then straine it, and put your Cloves therein; then hang them in the Sunne to drie, and turne them often; and thus three times wet them, and drie them againe: or otherwise, take Rosewater and wet your gloves therein, then hang them up till they be almost drie; then take halfe an ounce of Benjamine, and grind it with Oyle of Almons, and rub it on the Gloves therein, then hang them up till it be almost dried in: then take twentie graines of Amber-greece, and twentie graines of Muske, and grind them together with Oyle of Almons, and so rub it on the Gloves, and then hang them up to drie, or else let them drie in your bosome, and so after use them at your pleasure.'

Markham also included instructions for making wash-balls:

'To make very good washing balls take Storax of both kindes, Benjamine,

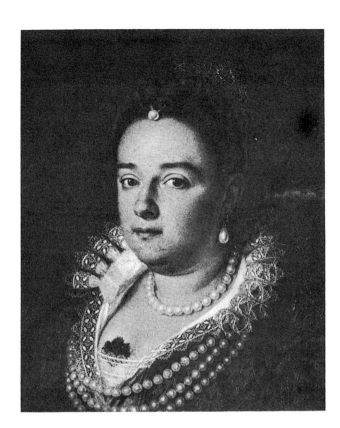

Calamus Aromaticus, Labdanum of each alike; and bray them two powder with Cloves and Arras; then beate them all with a sufficient quantity of Sope till it be stiffe, then with your hand you shall worke it like paste, and make round balls thereof.'

A good perfume was a little more complicated:

'To make an excellent sweet water for perfume, you shall take of Basill, mints, Marjorum, Corn-flagge roots, Isop, Savory, Sage, Balme, Lavender, and Rosemary, of each one a handfull, of Cloves Cinamon and Nutmegges of each halfe an ounce, then three or foure Pome-citrons cut into slices, infuse all these into Damaske-rose water the space of three daies, & then distill it with a gentle fire of Charcole, then when you have put it into a very clean glasse, take of fat Muske, Civet, and Amber greece of each the quantity of a scruple, and put into a ragge of fine Lawne, and then hang it within the water: this being either burnt upon a hot pan, or else boiled in perfuming pannes with Cloves, Bay-leaves and Lemmon-pils, will make the most delicatest perfume that may be without any offence, and will last the longest of all other sweet perfumes, as hath been found by experience.'

For a combination herbal and milk bath one was advised to 'Take Rosemary, Featherfew, Orgaine, Pellitory of the wall, Fennell, Mallowes, Violet leaves and Nettles, boil all these together, and when it is well sodden, put to it two or three gallons of milk, then let the party stand or sit in it an hour or two, the bath reaching up to the stomach, and when they come out, they must go to bed and sweat, and beware taking of cold.'

Asia and Africa

Styles of makeup were very different from the European in other parts of the world. In *Purchas his Pilgrimes* we are told that in 1610 Moorish women were observed 'with their chinnes distayned into knots and flowres of blue, made by pricking of the skinne with Needles, and rubbing it over with Inke and the Juyce of an herbe, which will never weare out againe.' In 1613 the voyagers found Japanese women 'attired in gownes of silke, clapt the one skirt over the other, and so girt to them, bare-legged, only a paire of halfe buskins bound with silke riband about their instep: their haire very blacke and very longe, tyed up in a knot upon the crowne in a comely manner: their heads no where shaven as the mens were. They were well-faced, handed, and footed; cleare skind and white, but wanting colour, which they amend by arte.' And we further learn that in 1620 in the Turkish seraglio the virgin chosen by the sultan 'hath all the art that possible may be shewen upon her by the Cadun, in attiring, painting, and perfuming her.'

7 · The Mid-Seventeenth Century
1625-1659

I say (and not without reason)
that a woman the more curious she is about her face,
the more carelesse about her house,
the repairing of the one being the ruining of the other.

ANTHROPOMETAMORPHOSIS, 1650

In seventeenth-century Italy it was possible to find, among ladies' cosmetics, a colourless preparation of liquid arsenic called Aqua Toffana (after Signora Toffana, who concocted it) or sometimes Aquetta di Napoli or Manna of St Nicholas di Bari. In lieu of printed information about its use, private instructions were given to the lady at the time of purchase. It was not until more than six hundred husbands had died of arsenic poisoning that Signora Toffana was arrested and executed as the most prolific poisoner of the century.

Life for husbands was less perilous in England — they had only to live with the knowledge that their wives' complexions were not their own or that any day they might impetuously decide to follow the advice of the Duchess of Newcastle and, like snakes in moulting season, remove their old skin (with oil of vitriol) so that it might be replaced by a new one.

But there were others whose advice was less drastic and usually highly moralistic in tone. John Bulwer, who objected to anything unnatural, wrote that 'our English ladies, who seeme to have borrowed some of their Cosmeticall conceits from Barbarous Nations, are seldome known to be contented with a Face of Gods making, for they are either adding, detracting, or altering continually, having many Fucusses in readinesse for the same purpose. Sometimes they think they have too much colour, then they have to make them look pale and faire. Now they have too little colour, then Spanish paper, Red Leather, or other Cosmeticall Rubriques must be had. Yet for all of this, it may be, the skins of their Faces do not please them: off they go with Mercury water, and so they remaine like peeld Ewes untill their Faces have recovered a new Epidermis.'

Bulwer also expresses his disapproval of Spanish women: 'When they are married, they have a priviledge to weare high shoes and to paint, which is generally practised there; and the Queen useth it her selfe; which brings on a great decay in the Naturall Face: For it is observed that women in England look as youthfull at fifty as some there at twenty five. This, saith Muster, is to be reproved in your Spanish women, that they now and then deforme their face with washes of Vermilion & Ceruse, because they have lesse native colour

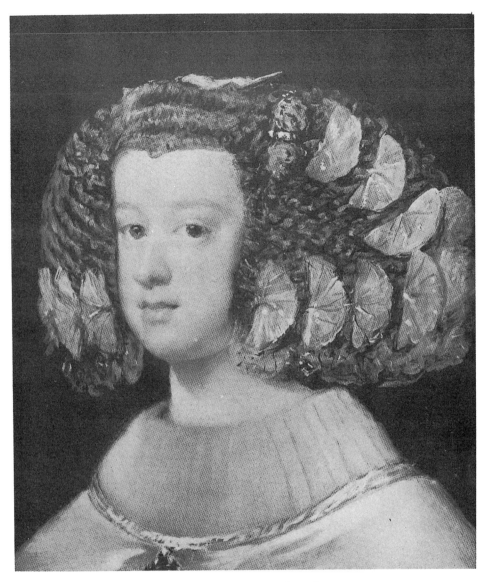

FIG. 98 : The Infanta Maria Theresa, *c.* 1653. Painting by Velasquez.

than your French women; and indeed other nations learnt from them the use of Spanish paper.' He had heard that Venetian women were very fair but that, alas, all of them, young and old, were painted.

Bulwer warned women of all nations that in the end their colours would moulder and their old 'mapel' faces would appear *au naturel*, and they would be 'sufficiently laught at by all, besides the harme that paint hath done; for, that Face which was bad enough is hereby made worse, there being a venomous quality in the paint which wrinkleth the Face before its time, it dims the Eyes, and blacks the Teeth; with false colours they spoile their Face, and gaine nought but contempt and hatred of their Husbands. . . . This adulterate decoration by Painting and Ceruse is well worthy the imperfections which attend it, being neither fine enough to deceive, nor handsome enough to please, nor safe and wholesome to use. And this attempt is not only inconvenient, but very vaine and ridiculous; for, while by washes, paintings, and such slibber-slabbers, they presume by the Ministry of Art to overcome Nature, they faile in their Designe; for Art, as experience teacheth us, cannot surmount Nature. . . . I say (and not without reason) that a woman the more curious she is about her face, the more carelesse about her house, the repairing of the one being the ruining of the other.'

THE ENGLISH GENTLEWOMAN

In 1631 Richard Brathwait published a detailed treatise for the guidance of women, setting forth precise specifications as to what they should and should not wear, do, and be. It was called *The English Gentlewoman drawne out to the full Body: Expressing what Habilliments doe best attire her, what Ornaments doe best adorne her, what Complements doe best accomplish her.*

We are told at the outset that the English gentlewoman 'hath learned better things than to foole her selfe in a painted disguise'. As with most writers of tracts setting forth rules for proper behaviour of other people, Brathwait then sighs for the past. 'Time was,' he says, when 'the face knew not . . . what painting was, whose adulterate *shape* takes now acquaintance from the *shop.* Then were such women matter of scandall to Christian eyes, which used painting their skinne, powdring their hayre, darting their eye. . . . Fashion is now ever under saile: the Invention ever Teeming; Phantasticke wits ever breeding. More time spent how to *abuse* time and corrupt licentious youth than how to addresse employment for the one or to rectifie the distempers of the other. . . . Sacrificing more houres to their Looking glasse, than they reserve minutes to lament their defects. . . . Miserable is the condition of that creature who, so her skin be sleake, cares not if her soule be rough. So her outward habit be pure and without blemish, values little her inward garnish. Such an one hath made a firm Contract with vanity, clozing her contemptuous age with a fearfull Catastrophe.'

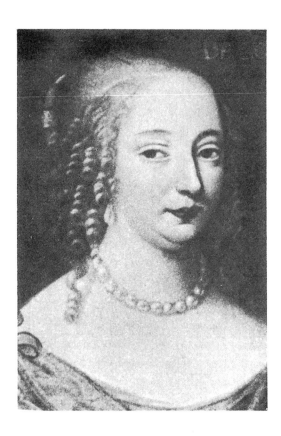

FIG. 99: Seventeenth-century portrait, possibly
Marie d'Orléans, Demoiselle de Longue-
ville. Except for her light hair, she
exhibits most of the attributes of the
ideal beauty of the period.

PARADOXES AND PROBLEMES

Then, almost as an antidote to Brathwait, came John Donne's scandalous
Paradoxes and Problemes, probably written before 1600 but first published in
1632. Donne proposed in his *Paradoxes* 'That it is possible to find some vertue
in Some Women. . . . That Nature is our worst Guide', and 'That Old men are
more fantastike than Young', and 'That Women ought to Paint':

'Foulnesse is Lothsome: can that be so which helpes it? . . . What thou lovest
in her *face* is *colour*, and *painting* gives that, but thou hatest it, not because it
is, but because thou knowest it. Foole, whom ignorance makes happy; the
Starres, the Sonne, the Skye whom thou admirest, also have no *colour*, but are
faire, because they seeme to bee coloured: If this seeming will not satisfy thee in
her, thou hast good assurance of her *colour*, when thou seest her *lay* it on. If her
face bee *painted* on a Boord or Wall, thou wilt love it, and the Boord, and the
Wall: Canst thou loath it then when it speakes, smiles, and kisses, because it
is *painted*? Are wee not more delighted with seeing Birds, Fruites, and Beasts
painted then wee are with Naturalls? And doe wee not with pleasure behold the
painted shape of Monsters and Divels, whom true, wee durst not regard? Wee
repair the ruines of our houses, but first cold tempests warnes us of it, and bytes
us through it; wee mend the wracke and staines of our Apparell, but first our
eyes, and other bodies are offended; but by this providence of women, this is

138

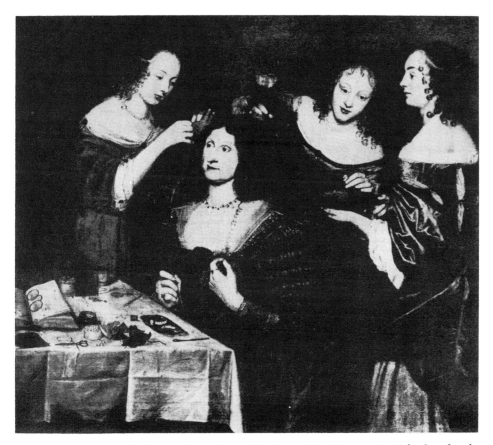

FIG. 100: Elizabeth of Bohemia being dressed by her maids. Group portrait by her daughter, Princess Louisa Hollandina, mid-seventeenth century. There are false teeth
and cosmetics containers on the dressing-table.

prevented. If in *kissing* or *breathing* upon her, the *painting* fall off, thou art
angry; wilt thou be so, if it sticke on? Thou didst love her; if thou beginnest to
hate her, then 'tis because she is not *painted*. If thou wilt say now, thou didst
hate her before, thou didst hate her and love her together, bee constant in
something, and love her who shewes her great *love* to thee, in taking this paines
to seeme *lovely* to thee.'

Donne's treatise, it is said, sold extremely well.

THE COMPLEAT WOMAN

In *The Compleat Woman*, published in 1639, Jacques DuBoscq seems at first to
be treading a sensible and tolerant middle road:

'It is certain that in what fashion soever we be apparelled, we hardly please all sorts of persons. Either the yong or olc' will finde somewhat to carp at, and it is almost impossible to avoid either the laughter of the one or the censure of the others. There are such sowre spirits that will not let men follow the fashion, holding it intolerable, if they prove it not to be invented a thousand yeares agoe. . . . It is a lesse vanity to follow the fashions received then to keep ones selfe unto the old. Verily fooles invent them, but the wise accomodate themselves unto them instead of inveighing against them. Habit as well as words should be conformable to the times.'

But Monsieur DuBoscq's open-mindedness has its limits, especially where painted women are concerned:

'Let them not think that I here go about to excuse these paintings. . . . These dishonest attires adde nothing to beauty, and nothing diminish foulenesse and deformity, since by the opinion of Pythagoras, a foule woman painted makes the heavens laugh and the earth to weep. When all is done, they have nothing that you find not in shops, they glory in a thing that is none of theirs, he that should marke them well, should perceive it to be nothing but a Picture, and they that deceive the eyes, as those old guilded Images which are eaten with wormes, and nothing but rottennesse within.'

QUEEN OF HUNGARY WATER

But there were those whose aim was to help the ladies achieve the beauty they so much desired. For more than two centuries nearly every book on cosmetics, cooking, or home remedies contained a recipe for Queen of Hungary Water, which, judging from the Queen's Book of Hours (dated 12 October 1652), must have been remarkably potent, though it sounds deceptively simple:

'Take what Quantity you please of the Flowers of Rosemary, put them into a Glass Retort, and pour in as much Spirit of Wine as the Flowers can imbibe. Close the Retort well, and let the Flowers macerate for six Days; then distil in a Sand-Heat.'

The Queen added her own enthusiastic endorsement of the recipe:

'I, Isabella, Queen of Hungary, when seventy-two years old, gouty and infirm, used a flask of this water, and it had such wondrous effect that I seemed to grow young and beautiful. So the king of Poland wished to marry me, and I did not refuse him, out of love to our Lord, who I doubt not sent me this flask by the hands of an angel in the garb of the old hermit from whom I had it.'

A century later LeCamus wrote that he could 'give good Proofs that the Queen of Hungary had this Receipt from a Faquir that serv'd in the Seraglio and had read the manuscript which he (LeCamus) was now translating.

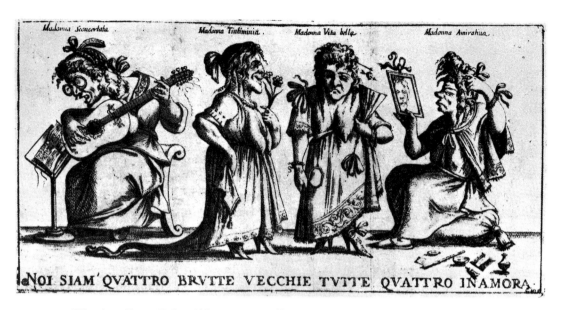

FIG. 101: 'We Are Four Ugly Old Women, All Four in Love.' Seventeenth-century engraved caricature by Mitelli. The fourth lady's cosmetics are on the floor beside her.

THE PAINTED FACE

In a bitter satire on women, entitled *A Woman's Birth*, based on the proposition that Hymen in a drunken fit begat the first human female, the unknown author could not resist a jab at the widespread use of the inconstant white lead paints, which often turned an embarrassing grey or black:

> Flora bestow'd upon her cheeke a hue
>> Of red and white, to make her feature pleasant,
> That she the easier might the heart subdue
>> Of king, prince, courtier, cittizen, or peasant;
> But he that trusts her faith, it is so slacke,
> Her red and white to willow turnes, and blacke.

Even the God of Love was enamoured of the female child and made his contribution:

> He prank't it up in fardingals and muffs,
> In masks, rebatos, shapperowns, and wyers,
> In paintings, powd'rings, perriwigs, and cuffes,
>> In Dutch, Italian, Spanish, French attires:
> Thus was it born, brought forth, and made Love's baby,
> And this is that which now we call a lady.

141

In *Wishes to His Supposed Mistress*, Richard Crashaw also makes it quite clear that his ideal woman is allowed no hint of artifice:

> A Face that's best
> By its own beauty dressed,
> And can alone commend the rest.
>
> A Face, made up
> Out of no other shop
> Than what Nature's white hand sets ope.
>
> . . . .
>
> A Cheek, where grows
> More than a morning rose,
> Which to no box its being owes.
>
> Lips, where all day
> A lover's kiss may play,
> Yet carry nothing thence away.

In 1641 Henry Peacham pointed out that 'For a Penny, a chambermaid may buy as much red ochre as will serve seven years for the painting of her cheeks' and in the early 1650s Izaak Walton wrote of 'Artificial Paint or Patches' in which women prided themselves. In fact, paint was never very far from the minds of men satirizing women in the seventeenth century.

In the American colonies cosmetics and perfumes were not widely used and then only by the upper classes, who imported them, mostly from England. But rouge, powder, creams, lotions, pomatum, patches, and various forms of scent were not unknown. As was customary in Europe at the time, women often used home-made lotions, creams, powders, and even rouges. One of the least attractive of these do-it-yourself cosmetic practices, surely to the lady's husband anyway, was the application of strips of bacon to the face before retiring in order to keep the skin soft and smooth.

SPOTS AND PATCHES

The painting went on, and so did the patching. Patches, essential to the fashionable, were to be had in a variety of shapes and sizes (Figures 103, 107), worn by both men and women. In Glapthorne's *Lady's Privilege*, a play of 1640, we find the line, 'Look you, signor, if't be a lover's part you are to act, take a

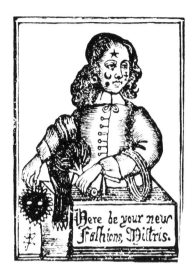

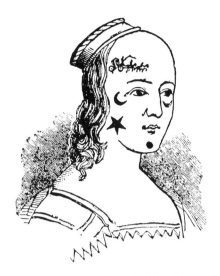

FIG. 102: Woodcut showing an English pedlar displaying his wares, which include a variety of black patches. From *The Boursse of Reformation*, 1640.

FIG. 103: A well-patched English lady of about 1650. After a woodcut from Bulwer's *Anthropometamorphosis*.

black spot or two. I can furnish you; 'twill make your face more amorous and appear more gracious in your mistress' eyes.' A broadside printed six years later, and entitled 'The Picture of an English Anticke', portrays an exquisite, or fop, his face spotted with patches.

By 1649 the custom of patching had evidently infiltrated the ranks of the clergy, for an edict of that year threatened with God's anger those abbots who were 'frizzed and powdered, their faces covered with patches'. Madame de Mazarin, even in her retirement in a convent, continued to wear her patches and refused to take them off despite the firm insistence of her husband—not that she wished to be stubborn about it, but so as to make it perfectly clear that in wearing them she meant no offence to God.

Patches, along with other cosmetics, were often sold by itinerant salesmen, as illustrated in Figure 102 and described in 'The Boursse of Reformation', part of which follows:

> Heer patches are of every cut,
>   For pimples and for scarrs,
> Here's all the wandring planett signes,
>   And some oth' fixed starrs,

> Already gum'd to make them stick,
>   They need no other sky,
> Nor starrs for *Lilly* for to vew
>   To tell your fortunes by,
>   Come lads and lasses, what do you lack
>   Here is weare of all prices
>   Heres long & short; heres wide & straight;
>   Here are things of all sizes.

In 1650, at the Black-Spread-Eagle in London's Duck Lane, John Bulwer's *Anthropometamorphosis: Man Transform'd; or, the Artificial Changeling* was published. It was evidently successful, for in 1653 an enlarged edition with drawings was brought out by another publisher. The purpose of the book seemed to be to glorify the human body (especially the Caucasian one and more especially the English) in its natural form and to describe and deprecate both natural and unnatural variations from Bulwer's ideal. The descriptive subtitle sets the tone:

> *Historically Presented*. In the mad and cruel Gallantry, Foolish Bravery, ridiculous Beauty, Filthy Finenesse, and loathsome Lovelinesse of Most Nations, Fashioning & altering their Bodies from the Mould intended by Nature. With a Vindication of the Regular Beauty and Honesty of Nature and An Appendix of the Pedigree of the English Gallant.

In due time Bulwer got around to patching:

'Our Ladies here have lately entertained a vaine Custome of spotting their Faces, out of an affectation of a Mole to set off their beauty, such as Venus had, and it is well if one black patch will serve to make their Faces remarkable; for some fill their Visages full of them, varied into all manner of shapes and figures. This is as odious and senselesse an affectation as ever was used by any barbarous Nation in the World. . . .'

What Bulwer and others could not do by invoking the wrath of God, Cromwell did, briefly and only in England, by invoking the power of the government. He disapproved of patching and forbade its practice. But following the Restoration, patches flourished in greater profusion than ever before, and both men and women painted.

MAKEUP FOR MEN

If Bulwer was censorious of women who patched and painted, he was outraged by 'the like prodigious affectation in the Faces of effeminate Gallants, a bare-headed sect of amorous Idolaters, who of late have begun to wear eye patches and beauty-spots, nay, painting, with the most tender and phantasticall Ladies. . . .

Painting,' he raged, 'is bad both in a foule and faire woman, but worst of all in a man; for if it be the received opinion of some Physicians, that the using of Complexion, and such like slibber-slabbers, is a weaknesse and infirmity in itselfe, who can say whether such men as use them be sound or not? it being a great dishonesty, and an unseemly sight to see a man painted, who perchance had a reasonable good naturall complexion of his own, that when he hath by nature those colours proper to him, he should besoot his Face with the same paintings, or make such slight reckoning of those faire pledges of Natures goodnesse, and embrace such counterfeit stuffe, to the ill example of others; so that his face, which he thinks doth so much commend him, should be made of ointments, greasie ingredients, and slabber-sawces, or done by certaine powders, Oxe-galls, Lees, Latherings, and other such sluttish and beastly confections. . . .'

Jacques DuBoscq took much the same approach, finding it 'a shamefull thing to see that men are more addicted to these superfluities then women', and adding that, 'Hortensius the Roman Oratour spent halfe the day in beholding and dressing himselfe instead of studying his Orations: And without looking back so far, we live in an Age where men make profession of this vicious curiosity more than ever; and I assure my selfe that if they well examined this intolerable vanity and sprucenesse of many men, they would give the stile of Aristagoras, who took such pains to play the spruce Gallant till at last they cald him Madame at every word.'

AROUND THE WORLD

Bulwer's moral concern was not only for his own English flock, but for men and women all over the world. 'The People of Candou Island,' he notes, 'put a certaine blackness upon their Eye-lids.' He is more specific about the Turks, who, he says, 'have a black powder made of Mineral called Alchole, which with a fine pencill they lay under their Eye-lids, which doth colour them black, whereby the white of the Eye is set off more white: with the same powder also they colour the haires of their Eye-lids, which is practised also by the women. And you shall finde in Xenephon that the Medes used to paint their Eyes.'

Going further afield, he notes that 'In the 49 degree of the South Pole, there are Gyants, who have red circles painted about their Eies, among other notes of their fearfull bravery. They of Cape Lopos Gonsalves, both Men and Women, use sometimes to make one of their Eyes white, the other red or yellow. The Guineans use to paint one Eye red many times, the other white or yellow. The women in the Northern Islands, about Greenland, have blew stroaks about their Eyes.'

Bulwer concludes that 'All endeavour of Art pretending to advance the Eye above its naturall Beauty is vaine and impious, as much derogating from the

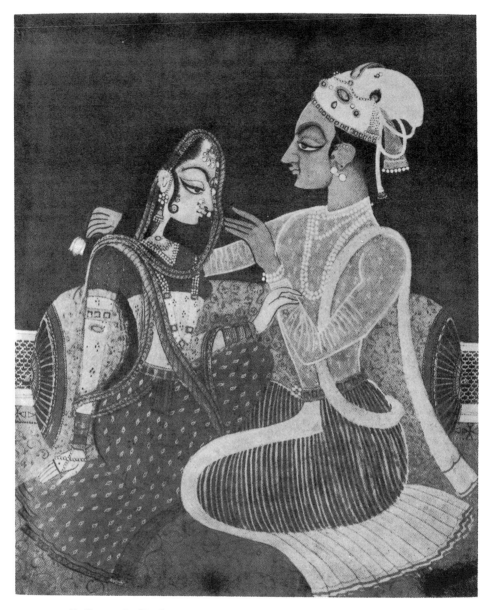

FIG. 104: **Radha** with Krishna. Painting showing the heavy eye-lining and blackened brows typical of Indian makeup.

wisdome of Nature. Art indeed, where Nature sometimes failes and prove defective, may helpe to further her perfection; but where shee appeares absolute, there to add or detract is instead of mending to marr all. Yet perchance the Turks in painting the haire of their Eye-lids, might be excused if they did it to a Naturall end (which I doubt they doe not, but in a Phantasticall bravery), for some think that the haire of the Eye-lids doe cast a shadow upon the Eye, helping thereby the blacknesse of the thin membrane Charion, the first that covereth the Optique Sinew, and prohibits the diffusion of the splendour of the Christal-line: which as Montalto saies, is better done when they are black, which he sheweth by the example of one, who having gray Eyes and somewhat white Haires on his Eye-lids, as often as he blackt them with Ink, he saw better.'

Tattooing, though it was not called that, received its share of Bulwer's disapproval: 'The Virginian women pounce and rase their Faces and whole Bodies with a sharp iron, which makes a stampe in curious knots and drawes the proportions of Fowles, Fishes, or Beasts; then with painting of sundry lively colours they rub it into the stamp, which will never be taken away, because it is dried into the flesh.'

Bulwer then proceeded to painting in general, pointing out that the 'Arabian women, before they go unto their husbands, either on the marriage day or any other time, to lye with them, paint their Faces, Breasts, Armes, and Hands, with a certaine azured colour, thinking that they are very handsome after this manner, and they hold this custome from the Arabians which first entred into Africk, and these learned it from the Africans; yet at this day the town of Barbery, inhabited by them of the country, do not imitate this custome, but their wives love to maintaine their naturall complexion. It is true that they have sometimes a certaine black painting, made of the smoake of Galls and Saffron, with the which they make little spots upon their cheekes, and they paint their Eyebrows of a Triangular forme, and they lay some upon their chin, which resembles an Olive leaf. . . . But you must understand that these women dare not weare this painting above two or three daies, nor shew themselves before their Kinsmen in this equipage, for that it favours something of a whore; they only give the sight and content thereof unto their husbands to incite them to love, for that these women desire the sport much, and they think that their beauty receives a great grace by this painting.'

Bulwer mentions, without explanation, that the 'Native Socotorans paint their Faces with Yellow and black spots, loathsome to behold'. A West Indian custom is even more intriguing: 'If any of them maketh love, he shall be painted with red or blue colour, and his Mistris also. . . . But when they are sad or plot some Treason, then they overcast all their Face with black, and are hideously deformed.' Persian women's pale complexions were reddened and their cheeks were 'fat and painted'. And as a moral lesson to all of them Bulwer noted that 'they offer violence to God when they strive to deforme and transfigure that which he hath formed, not knowing that everything that is borne is the worke of God, and what ever is changed is the worke of the Devill.'

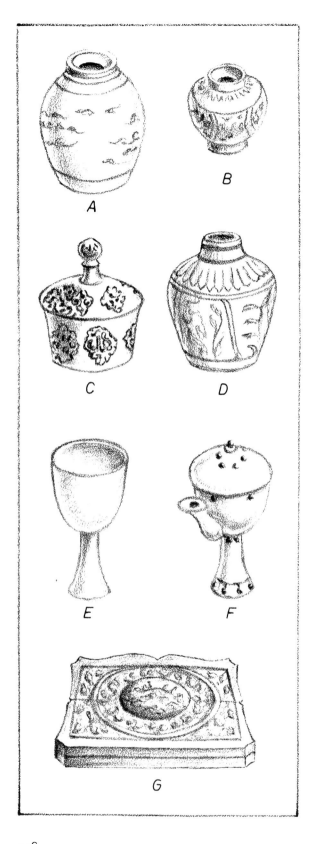

PLATE 14 : SIXTEENTH- AND
SEVENTEENTH-CENTURY
COSMETICS CONTAINERS

A   Probably sixteenth century Chinese cosmetics jar. Blue on off-white. About 2½ inches high. (*Victoria and Albert Museum*)

B   Seventeenth century. Chinese cosmetics jar. (*Victoria and Albert Museum*)

C   Probably sixteenth century, Turkish. Ivory kohl pot and cover, with black mastic fillings. Inscribed, 'He who insists succeeds'. About 2 inches high. (*Victoria and Albert Museum*)

D   Sixteenth or seventeenth century. Chinese cosmetics jar. Blue on glazed yellowish white pottery. About 2½ inches high. (*Victoria and Albert Museum*)

E   Seventeenth century, Mughal. Jade cup for cosmetics. About 2½ inches high. (*Victoria and Albert Museum*)

F   Seventeenth century, Mughal. Jade cup for cosmetics with rubies in gold setting. About 2½ inches high. (*Victoria and Albert Museum*)

G   Seventeenth century, French. Patchbox of carved wood. (*Victoria and Albert Museum*)

THEATRICAL MAKEUP

In the seventeenth century makeup for the theatre was strong and obvious. Even in small, travelling theatres with the audience crowded around the stage, the makeup was applied with a heavy hand. The skin was darkened with a thick paste, and a bright red dry rouge was applied to the cheeks and lips with a cloth and blended into the still damp base colour. The eyes were lined with black, probably applied with a stick; the eyebrows were blackened and, for female characters, the eyelashes as well; and the eyes were shadowed with coloured paint and highlighted with white. Blue was a popular colour for the eyeshadow. Aging was done by drawing on lines of water paint with a stick.

HAIR AND TEETH

Throughout history the length of men's hair has been a bone of contention, but never more so than in the seventeenth century, when the short-haired Puritans or Roundheads pointed self-righteous fingers of shame at the Cavaliers with their flowing locks. The Puritans on arriving in America, published a manifesto attempting to impose their views on the entire male population, proclaiming it 'an impious custom and a shameful practice, for any man who has the least care for his soul to wear long haire'. They prohibited the wearing of long hair in churches and declared that those persons who persisted in spite of the prohibitions would 'have both God and man at the same time against them'.

A parody entitled *Dialogue Between Captaine Long-Haire and Alderman Short-Haire* refers to the Cavaliers and the Roundheads:

C.L.   Ask me no more why I do waire
       My haire so far below mine eare;
       For the first man that e'er was made
       Did never know the barber trade.

A.S.   Aske me no more where all the day,
       The foolish owle doth make her stay;
       'Tis in your locks, for tak't frome me,
       She thinks your haire an ivy-tree.

C.L.   Tell me no more that length of haire,
       Can make the visage seem less fair;
       For know, howe'er my hair doth sit,
       I'm sure that yours comes *short* of it.

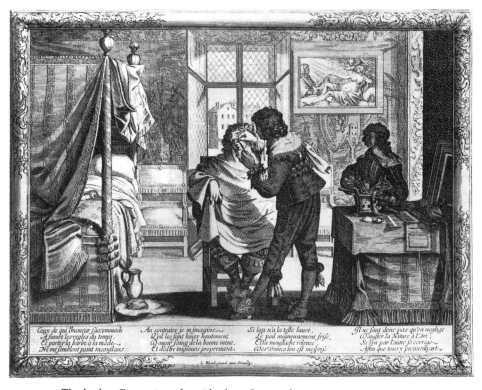

Ceux qui l'humeur s'accommode / A suivre les regles du temps, / Et porter la barbe à la mode, / Ne me semblent point inconstans. · Au contraire je m'imagine / Qu'il les faut louer hautement, / Qu'avoir soing de la bonne mine, / Et d'estre tousiours proprement. · Si l'on n'a la teste lauee, / Le poil mignonnement frisé, / Et la moustache relevee, / Des Dames l'on est mesprisé. · Il ne faut donc pas qu'on neglige / D'aiuster la Nature à l'Art : / Si l'eu par l'autre se corrige, / Afin que tous y prennent part.

le Blond excud. aux Princlys

FIG. 105 : The barber. Engraving after Abraham Bosse, 1635.

A.S. Tell me no more men wear long haire
To chase away the coldest ayre;
For by experience we may see,
Long hair will but a backwind be.

C.L. Tell me no more that long hair can
Argue deboystness in a man;
For 'tis religious, being inclined,
To keep the temples from the wind.

A.S. Tell me no more that roarers waire
Their hair extent below their ear;
For having morgaged theyr land,
They'd faine obscure th'appearing band.

C.L. Ask me no more why hair may be
Th'expression of gentility;
'Tis that which, being largely grown,
Derives its pedigree from the crown.

In the *Verney Memoirs* we are told of the inconveniences Sir Ralph had to endure in France, during his stay at Blois, with wearing a periwig, a fashion not yet widespread in England. There were endless bills for the wigs themselves, for the ribbons, the pomade, and the powder. Ralph sent detailed instructions about length, style, and thickness and enclosed a sample lock of hair with a note of instruction: 'Let it be well curled in great rings and not frizzled, and see that he makes it handsomely and fashionably, and with two locks and let them be tyed with black ribbon . . . let not the wig part behind, charge him to curl it on both sides towards the face.' The wig cost twelve livres. Good hair powder being hard to obtain, Sir John Cooke sent along with the instructions 'a small phiole of white Cyprus powder, which I beseech you to present to my Lady as an example of the best Monpelier affords, for I saw it made myself. It must be mixed with other powder, else it will bring the headache. There is a powder cheaper, but not so proper for the hair.'

In 1649 an English friend asked Sir Ralph to obtain for him some 'little brushes for making cleane of the teeth, most covered with sylver and some few with gold and sylver Twiste, together with some Petit Bouettes.' These were evidently difficult to obtain in England.

BATHS AND PERFUMES

Despite the urging of Sir John Harington in *The Englishman's Doctor* 'to be cleane and well apparelled', the inconvenience of bathing proved a discouragement for many people, who preferred to substitute perfumes for cleanliness. A ballad of the period entitled 'The Worst is Past' lists a variety of situations or conditions, which, when corrected, indicate hope for the future. Each verse ends with essentially the same line. It is interesting to note that personal cleanliness rates inclusion in the list:

> When as Joan Slattern cleanly growes,
> Doth cut her nails, and pare her toes,
> And will turn cleanly at the last,
> *Why then, I think, the worst is past.*

Although 'batheing rooms' were rare, there was one at Chatsworth, according to Celia Fiennes, of blue and white marble and a bath with 'two locks to let in one hott, ye other Cold water to attemper it as persons please'.

In view of the wide use of perfumes by both men and women, it is not surprising that a number of recipes have come down to us. One is entitled 'King Philip his Perfume', with no very clear indication of which Philip it was. In any case, the recipe called for 'six spoonfuls of Rosewater, of Ambergreece & Civet two

Barley Corns weight of either, a little Musk & two penny weight of sugar beaten fine; beat these together & mould them up with a little Gum Dragon steeped in Rose-water, & so dry them & keep them to burn in a Perfumery Pan.'

About 1640, in the Laws of Gallantry, it was recommended that the entire body be bathed occasionally, that the hands be washed every day, the face almost as often, and the head from time to time. Gallants were permitted to wear round and long patches and even large black plasters, 'the sign of the toothache', on the temples.

THE SIN OF PAINTING

Thomas Hall, an English pastor, was one of many clerics who looked upon paint and patches as the work of the devil and who tried, with little success, to save women from their own folly. Since Hall's book, first published in 1653, was entitled *The Loathsomnesse of Long Haire*, presumably he was distressed primarily about men's hair. He states confidently that 'where one wicked man weare short haire, there is a thousand weare long', and he discusses the matter at exhausting length. But beards are quite another thing and receive his unqualified support. Having at last finished with the men, he appears to realize that he has chastised only half the sinners and adds an appendix directed to the women, which begins, '*Gentlewomen*, Lest you should think yourselves wholly forgotten, having done with the long Locks of Men, I shall now adde a word, and but a word, concerning the Vanities and Exorbitancies of many Women, in painting, patching, spotting, and blotting themselves. I shall do nothing out of any soure or discontented humour, but soley and singly out of love to your soules, wishing you eternall welfare &c.' Having wished them well, Hall then blasts them with five pages of invective designed to terrify them into abject conformity with his interpretation of God's wishes.

He begins by pointing out that some women paint their 'faces, breasts, *et cetera*' (the *et cetera* is never explained) in order to 'ensnare others, and to kindle a fire and flame of lust in the hearts of those who cast their eyes upon them', thus destroying both themselves and their neighbours. 'This practice of artificial painting and colouring the body,' Hall warns, 'is sinfull and abominable.' Why? Because 'it was the Devil (say the ancient Fathers) who did at first teach lewd women this art of painting and colouring their haire and faces' and '*Jerom* says, that the painted face is not a member of Gods *making*, but of the Devils *marring*.'

The root of the problem seemed, as always, to lie with excessive vanity, which resulted in an affront to God's workmanship and therefore displeasing to Him. 'It is the badge of an harlot,' Hall fumes. 'Rotten posts are painted, and gilded Nutmegs are usually the worst. . . . It's contrary to the simplicity of the Gospell,

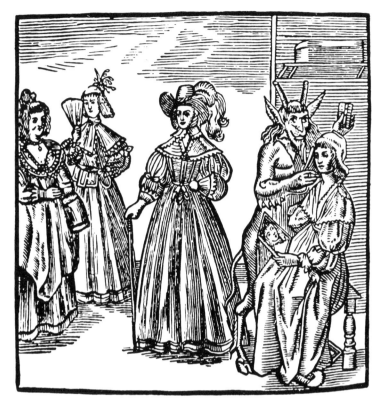

FIG. 106: The Devil mending God's work. English woodcut, early
seventeenth century.

which forbids all gayish attire and sinfull guises. . . . Lying is unlawfull; but this
painting and disguising of faces is no better than dissimulation and lying; they
teach their faces to lye, and to shew what it is not; and so by deceiving others,
at last they deceive themselves, getting deformity instead of beauty, losing that
true beauty which they have by Nature, by their Medicines and Mineralls, oft
making their faces to wrinkle, their colour pale, ofte poyson their skin, and
dimme their ey-sight.'

In addition to all this, it is 'scandalous, and of evill report amongst Gods
people' because nowhere 'in all the book of God' can one read 'of any saint that
did ever thus paint and spot themselves' and people had therefore better be content with what God has given them, accepting their natural complexion, whatever it may be, for better or for worse. And Hall's clinching argument is that
such painting 'will not be able to endure the fire of Gods wrath . . . especially
it will off at the fire of the great day'.

Playing the Devil's advocate for a moment, Hall then points out that defend-
ers of painting and patching claim that they do it to make themselves more

alluring—either to get husbands or to please the ones they already have. In answering this argument, of which he is clearly contemptuous, he insists that 'They are but sorrily adorned who adorne themselves with sinne, as if one should go tumble in some filthy kennell, thinking thereby to make himselfe more comely: now sinne is called mire, filth, a blot, pollution, dung, death, &c.'

It is all right with Hall for women to please their husbands so long as it is done lawfully, honestly, and modestly, but painting is none of these. Women who paint to get husbands are mere cheaters and deceivers, and only foolish men would judge the fitness of wines by their outward appearance. In fact, Hall goes on, 'Painting is so farre from making honest Husbands love their Wives, that it makes them loath them: and if men cannot love their Wives because God commands them so to do, much lesse will they love them for their painting and patching.'

This word to the women is followed by eleven pages of *Arguments against naked Backs and Breasts, &c.* and, more to the point in our present discussion, *Seven Arguments against Spots and Black-patches (worn for pride) on the Face, &c.*:

'As for Spots and Black-patches on the Face, Back, Breast, &c., which some call Beauty-spots (the Devil loves to put fine names on foule things) we may call them base and Beastly-spots, the spots of the proud, wanton, idle Droans of the world. Let such consider, That those spots are not the spots of Gods children. . . . These are not spots of Infirmity, but spots of Malignity and Rebellion; they are proud, and they will be so; they are spotted, and spotted they will be, in despight of all the Ministers in the world. These are Leprosie-spots not Beauty-spots, spots that defile and debase, but no whit adorne the wearers of them. Such spots, many times, are the husbands blots.' Women would do better, Hall advises, to follow the example of Mary, who was unspotted, rather than 'the fashion of every vaine fantastick person.

'Consider, if the Plague-spots appear on a person, or a garment be infected with it, we will not come nigh them; but these spots are worse, for those are but spots of Punishment, by which God is glorified; but these are spots of Pride and Vanity, by which God is dishonoured, his Name blasphemed, and Religion scandalized.'

The next four paragraphs warn against fashion, evil, vanity, pride, and the possible loss of one's chastity. Then, lest his readers have not taken his warnings seriously, Hall adopts an even more threatening tone:

'This monstrous pride is ever a forerunner of destruction, as we see in the woman of *Judah* a little before the Captivity. . . . God is the same still and hates pride as much in *England* as ever he did in *Israel*. He that punished painted *Jesabel*, who was cast out at a window in the midst of her pride and eaten up with doggs, will not suffer the proud Dames of our time to go unpunished, unlesse by speedie humiliation and amendment they prevent it.'

Gathering his forces for a rousing climax, Hall then describes what will happen to the painted and patched who fail to repent and mend their wicked ways:

'Instead of their costly perfumes and sweet smells, they should have stinke; to wit, most noysome and loathsome favours in their siege, and in the cabins and holes, whither they that escaped should be thrust in their Captivity, or where they should be glad to hide themselves. Instead of their brave and costly girdles, they should have rends; that is, they should go in tatters and raggs, as poore beggars having never a whole coat to their backs. Instead of dressing of haire, to wit, all of their frizling, crisping, curling, laying out their haire, their perukes, the hanging downe of their locks, or tufts, or whatsoever they had, they should have baldnesse, when they had torne off their haire through the extremity of misery. . . . That beauty of theirs, which they had so abused, it should now be painted with another die; it should be tanned and burnt with the sun, like the hue of the Black-moores.'

According to biographical notes, Hall lived 'a retired and obscure life and never looked farther than his beloved Kings Norton'. He was said to be 'of a free and liberal heart, just, and one that lived much by faith, of humble deportment and carriage'.

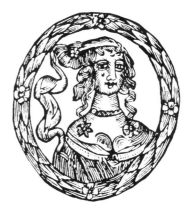

FIG. 107: Patched lady, *c.* 1640. English woodcut.

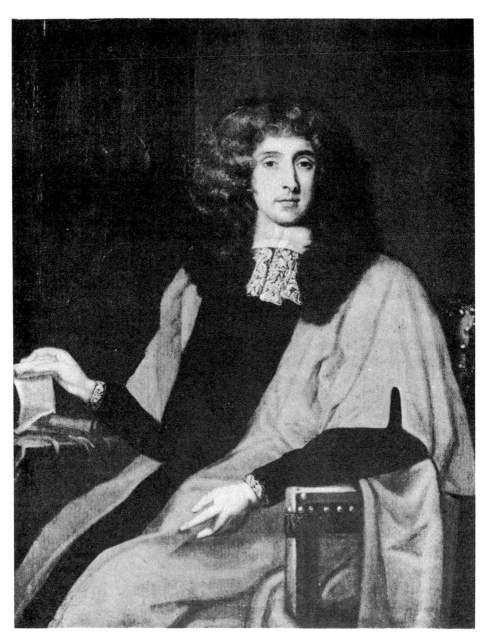

FIG. 108: Judge Jeffreys, *c.* 1678–80. Painting attributed to William Claret. Jeffreys, Lord Chancellor of England and notorious for his conduct of the 'bloody assizes', is said to have been flagrant in his use of makeup.

8 · *The Restoration 1660-1685*

Not ten among a thousand weare
Their own Complections nor their haire.

SAMUEL BUTLER

During the first half of the seventeenth century, the change from deceptive to permissive face painting had taken place; and by the Restoration, obvious make-up was firmly established among women, particularly at court. By the end of the reign of Charles II, men were using makeup openly.

DECENCY IN CONVERSATION AMONGST WOMEN

Just as there were, in the seventeenth century, some clergymen who set themselves up as moral arbiters of men's fashions, there were others who appeared to derive equal satisfaction from doing the same thing for women. One of these was Robert Codrington, who wrote what was surely intended to be the definitive work on the subject. The title is both explicit and comprehensive: *The Second Part of Youths Behaviour, or Decency in Conversation Amongst Women; Containing Excellent Directions for the Education of Young Ladies, Gentlewomen, and other Persons, and Rules of Advice how at the first to deport themselves, and afterwards govern the Affairs of a Family.* It was published in London in 1664, just ten years after Thomas Hall's diatribe against long hair for men.

The work was written in the form of a letter, entitled *The Letter of one Lady to another, condemning in her own Judgment the common practice of embelling the Complexion of the Face with the helps of Art, and giving many Reasons for it.* The reasons, primarily, are that it is un-Christian (being condemned in the Scriptures) and that it betokens pride. The first lady writes:

> But grant it were not scandalous nor sinfull nay grant it were not absolutely unlawfull, yet the offence it giveth to pious Men is a sufficient Argument that it ought not to be practised. Is it not much safer to want a little Complexion in the Cheek than to grieve the Heart of any tender Christian. Although many things may be permitted in themselves, yet they become evil and are to be forborn when others are offended at them. And this (as I am often told) should be Argument enough to deter all modest and good Women from laying any new Complexion on their Faces.

157

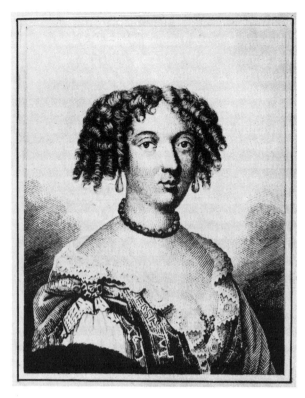

FIG. 109: Madame de Monte-
span (1640–1707),
mistress of Louis XIV.
Engraved portrait.

Neither is this All, for the very name of a painted Face doth destroy the
Reputation of her that useth it, and doth expose Her to all manner of
Reproaches. It ought therefore altogether to be eschewed. . . . There is no
Person but may conclude that if God threatens to punish strange Apparrel,
he will not spare to punish strange Faces.

The answer must surely have delighted Codrington's readers:

I shall not deny but that sundry Reverend and Learned Persons are of a
Judgement opposite to my own, which have prevailed much on the easie
Credulity of many young Ladies, and did at first upon my own, untill I
began to examine the grounds of their opinions. . . . And indeed it seems
very strange to me that if this Artificiall Beauty to enliven a pale Complexion . . . be so great a Sin, that these Divines cannot produce any Reasons
of force out of the Scripture expressly to forbid it. . . .
   Now where it is objected that Jezabel was devoured by Dogs because she
painted her Eyes, if your Ladiship be pleased to look again upon the His-

tory, you shall find that the painting of her Face, or Eyes, was thirteen or fourteen years after that the Prophet Elisha did presage it, and it was no more the cause of her dreadfull Death than was the dressing of her Head or her looking out the Window, which was at one and the same time, and one of them as innocent as the other. If all that Jezabel did is to be avoided as a Sin, we may not call a solemn Assembly, nor keep a Fast, because that Jezabel did so, as appeareth by the same History, we may not embrace or kiss a Friend, because Joab did so when he killed Abner, and Judas when he betrayed his Master. And as for Herodias dancing . . . which was the Cause of John Baptists Death, we may find in the Gospel that she danced alone, which is allowed by the austerest Divines, and by the precisest Matrons in the education of their Children; she danced not with Herod, but before Herod; it was not the decent motion of her feet, but the disorderly affections of her heart, and the perverseness of her Spirit to the Baptists Doctrine that was the occasion of his murther. . . . Believe me Madam, there is not in the whole Scripture any morall Command to be found that expressly doth forbid it as a Sin. We may observe that Queen Esther made use of sweet perfumes, of gorgeous habiliments and beautiful colours, and whatsoever was then in fashion the more to attract the Eyes and affections of the King until her, and this was in her so far from a Sin, that it were almost a Sin in her not to have done it. . . . Neither is it any new invention for Ladies to use artificiall Helps for the advancement of their Beauties, it is as generall as ancient, and there is no Nation but doth practise it without any Reproach or Pride or Vanity. . . . And although in this Nation a commendable Discretion is used in powdering, curling, and gumming the Hair, and in quickening the Complexion, yet beyond the Seas, it is everywhere frequently done, and as freely owned. It is strange methinks that Supplies should be allowed of for bodily defects and deformities; the Shoomaker is imployed and commanded for making the Body higher, and the Tailor for making of it straiter, and must we account it a sin or scandall to advance the Beauty of the Face? The Face is the Seat of Beauty, and every part of the Body is to contribute to the Honour and the comeliness of it.

Madam,

Your most humble and most devoted Servant

Codrington warns his readers of the danger of seeing too many plays and tells of a young woman who went to the theatre every night and as a result (he implies) fell ill, had fits of madness, and died. Young ladies are also warned to be wary of strangers, servants, privacy, vanity, idleness, licentious pamphlets, idle songs and ballads, and being seen too often in public.

THE FASHIONABLE LOOK

Between 1670 and 1685 wide, fleshy faces were in fashion—faces with full, red lips, prominent eyes, dark eyebrows, dark hair, and double chins.

The seventeenth-century gentleman did not prefer blondes—or redheads either. Only black or brown hair with a suitable complexion was in real demand. A ballad entitled 'The Young Man's Counsellour; or, The Most deserved praise of those sweet Complexioned Damosels of the Black and the Brown' sets forth reasons for the preference. The published version is prefaced by a four-line verse:

> The pleasant Blacks and modest Browns,
>   their loving Husbands please;
> Now if I had ten thousand pounds,
>   I'd marry one of these.

The ballad itself enlarges upon the premise:

> Beware of a Lass that's too kind,
>   whose Visage is Swarthy and Pale;
> For most of that sort you will find
>   are subject to play with their Tale
> And count it a very small Crime
>   to dally with every Mate:
> Then Young-men take warning in time,
>   for fear you repent it too late.
> *But as for the Black and the Brown,*
>   *they are the cream of the Town;*
> *For loe, here behold, they never can scold,*
>   *nor give you so much as a Frown.*
>
> Now she that is freckl'd and fair,
>   she'll baffle thy money in pride;
> Black patches and powdered Hair,
>   nay, wanton and lazy beside;
> She'll plunder and pillage thy Purse;
>   all this by experience I know.
> Whoever is plagu'd with this Curse,
>   he needs no more sorrow I trow.
> *But as for the Black, &c.*
>
> Beware of thin Lips, and sharp Nose,
>   whose Hair is the colour of Gold;

If ever you marry with those,
    you're fitted, I' faith, with a Scold.
Whenever she wants of her will,
    then down flows her Crockadile's Tears;
But when her Top Tippit is up,
    she'll Ring you a Peal in your Ears.
But as for the Black, &c.

Now as for the Locks which are Gray,
    such Women are both old and tuff;
They'll hold a brisk youngster in play,
    and think they have never enough;
For if with a Damosel you jest,
    and tho' but in innocent mirth,
Streight jealousie Reigns in her Breast:
    now this is a Hell upon Earth.
But as for the Black, &c.

The Flaxen hath no good Report,
    tho' many may fancy the same;
I know that most of that sort
    are notable Girls of the Game:
They'll Gossip and Junket about;
    nay, tipple Wine, Brandy, and Beer,
Spend more in a day, without doubt,
    then ever they earn in a year.
But as for the Black, &c.

The Sandy and Swarthy I'll sware,
    she has the good name of a Slut;
And you must take very good Care,
    or else she will poyson your Gut:
Her Beauty will never forsake you;
    you may have it always in sight;
There's no man a Cuckold will make you,
    except he does it for spight.
But as for the Black, &c.

The Yellow is none of the best,
    they are for Contention and Strife;
That poor man is happily blest,
    that hath such a one to his Wife.
At night when he comes to his home,
    she'll call him both Cuckold and Fool,
And proffer his Noddle to comb
    sometimes with a three-legged Stool.
But as for the Black, &c.

. . . .

The Carrots I'd like to've forgot,
    which is the worst colour of all;
If such a one fall to thy Lot,
    thy Blessing and comfort is small.
All Blessings will bid thee farewell,
    the very first night you are Wed,
Her Carrots will cast such a smell,
    you'll never endure her in Bed.
But as for the Black, &c.

You Young-men that hear me this day,
    and would with a loving Wife speed,
Remember this Counsel I pray,
    and then you're happy indeed :
If you mean to marry with any,
    pray buy this New Song, without doubt,
You'll find it to be the best Penny
    that e'er you was known to lay out.
As for the Black and the Brown,
    they are the cream of the Town;
For loe, here behold, they never can scold,
    nor give you so much as a frown.

PAINTS AND WASHES

Ladies of the court of Charles II painted freely. According to Lola Montez, they used a face wash prepared by boiling gum benzoin in spirits of wine, then adding fifteen drops of the tincture to a glass of water. This was supposed to draw

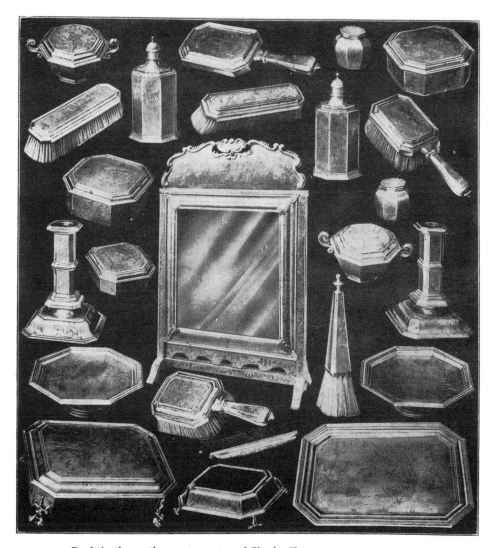

FIG. 110: English silver toilet service, reign of Charles II.

the blood to the surface and give the skin a rosy glow. Lola Montez recommended it nearly two hundred years later. Herbalist George Wilson is reported to have provided James II with a skin lotion made of coriander, vanilla pods, nutmeg, cloves, storax, benzoin-gum, lemon rind, and honey.

For whitening the skin some women dusted the pulverized ash of the jawbone of a pig over a light coating of poppy seed oil. Margaret Cunliffe-Owen, writing in 1897, highly recommended a flesh-coloured powder called *Poudre d'Amour*, the recipe for which had been handed down in her family from an ancestress at the court of Louis XIV:

'Scrape six juicy raw carrots and half a pink beet-root, squeeze the juice out through a muslin bag and put it aside. Take 3 ounces finely powdered corn-starch, mix it with the carrot and beet juice, expose it to the sun and stir occasionally until the fluid evaporates, leaving the tinted starch dry. Sift through a piece of silk gauze and add:

Powdered Venetian talc, 300 grains
Powdered lycopodium, 300 grains
Powdered bergamot, 45 grains
Powdered bismuth, 7 grains

Sift again and keep in a sandalwood box.'

In his *Love in a Wood* Wycherly refers to a girl who 'betwixt pomatum and Spanish red, has a complexion like a Holland cheese'. And Samuel Butler wrote in *Hudibras* that

'Tis in vain to think to guess
At Women by Appearances;
That paint and patch their Imperfections
Of intellectual Complections,
And dawb their Tempers o'er with Washes
As artificial as their Faces.

Later Butler referred to women

That, like their watches, weare their faces
In delicate Inammeld cases,

and insisted that

Not ten among a thousand weare
Their own Complections nor their haire.

Nonetheless, Mary Beatrice of Modena, wife of James II, detested rouge and wore it only because the king insisted. When Father Seraphine, her confessor, noticed it for the first time, he told Her Majesty bluntly that he would rather see her yellow or green than *rouged*.

Men were also using cosmetics. From about 1680 to 1710, according to Carrington, men of fashion used makeup openly. In the National Portrait Gallery in London there is a portrait (see Figure 108), painted about 1680, of the elegant, painted Judge Jeffreys, Chief Justice of the King's Bench and Lord Chancellor, notorious for his brutality, especially during the Bloody Assizes.

SPOTS AND PATCHES

On the thirtieth of August, 1660, Samuel Pepys's wife wore patches for the first time—and at breakfast at that. Pepys does not record having expressed his dismay to Mrs Pepys, but he does record his surprise at hearing Lord Sandwich mention that he would like his wife and his daughter to wear black patches. This was in October. By November Pepys had so completely accustomed himself to the idea that he decided to give his wife permission to do what she had been doing since August, whereupon he confided to his diary, 'My wife seemed very pretty to-day, it being the first time I had ever given her leave to wear a black patch'.

His admiration for the patch grew; and after seeing his wife standing near Henrietta, Duchess of Orleans, who was visiting her brother, Charles II, Pepys wrote, 'The Princess Henrietta is very pretty . . . but my wife . . . with two or three black patches on, and well dressed, did seem to me much handsomer than she'. But patches worn by women of a lower class were quite another matter. In October, two years later, while strolling about the Exchange, Pepys observed 'one very pretty Exchange lass, with her face full of black patches, which was a strange sight'. He also said that the Duchess of Newcastle wore many patches 'because of pimples around her mouth'. Lady Castlemaine, whom Pepys mentioned from time to time, decreed that when in mourning all the ladies should dress in black 'with their hair plain and without spots'.

The French called patches *mouches* or flies. In La Fontaine's fable *The Fly and the Ant*, the fly boasts:

> I increase by a tint the natural white,
> And you'll find that the very last thing to rise
> To the face of a lady pursuing a man
> Is her hand in adjusting her borrowed flies.

In Racine's *Athalie*, the Queen, referring to her mother, says:

> Even she had need of paint to the ears
> In order to repair the damage of the years.

And Molière's *Précieuses*,

> To assure their beauty'd be unmatched,
> Appeared with faces thoroughly patched.

A French poet provided in 1661 his version of the origin of patches. We find, in the beginning, Cupid lolling about on a beautiful afternoon with his mother. Cupid is chasing flies, which seems to annoy Venus. But he only laughs:

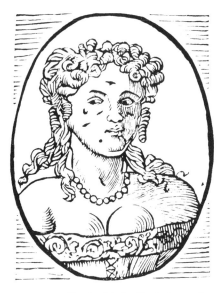

FIG. 111 : Patched lady. English woodcut,
late seventeenth century.

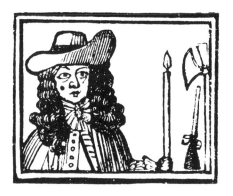

FIG. 112 : Patched presbyter. English
woodcut, *c.* 1680.

> And to avoid his mother's wrath
> Cupid traps a fly which hath
> Alighted on her breast, and he
> Doth hold it there so all can see
> How suddenly the breast seems quite
> A dazzling, bright, effulgent white,
> As 'round a cloud of blackish hue
> The sky becomes a brighter blue.

The goddess is delighted with the effect and promises her son two turtle-doves as a reward.

> Industrious Cupid then cuts out
> From black material, about
> A thousand flies, and just one fly
> He places near his mother's eye,
> (It's not entirely clear which might
> Have here been meant — the left or right),
> And then another on her breast
> (Perhaps, who knows, at her behest)
> And on her cheek another goes
> And on her forehead, chin, and nose.

And thus, implies the poet, began the custom of patching—a more gallant explanation, certainly, than the one about its being invented to hide pimples.

In the days of Louis XIV patches served a purpose beyond pure decoration. A patch near the lip, called a *coquette*, was considered tantalizing and flirtatious, whereas a round (*assassin*) or heart-shaped patch on the temple was considerably more dignified and serious. On the left cheek a heart-shaped patch served as a warning that the wearer was already engaged and therefore not available; after she was safely married, she transferred the patch to the right. A patch at the corner of the eye was known as *la passionnée*, in the middle of the forehead as *la majestueuse*, in the middle of the cheek as *la galante*, on the nose (never the tip, however), as *l'impudent* or *l'effrontée*, on the nasolabial fold as *l'enjouée*, on the lower lip as *la discrète*, beside the mouth as *la baiseuse*, between the mouth and the chin as *la silencieuse*, and covering a mole or a pimple as *la voleuse* or *la receleuse*. Great ladies, according to Lacroix, usually wore seven or eight of them and always carried their patch boxes with them to replace any which might fall off or to satisfy any sudden urge for an additional one. A seventeenth-century patch box is shown in Plate 14-G.

Tucked into Robert Codrington's pages of advice on rules of conduct for young women, there is a firm condemnation of patching:

'But whiles . . . I have given some allowance of liberty to young Gentlewomen in their Habits, for it is impossible there should be Youth without some vanity, yet I know not how to excuse the vain Custom now so much in Fashion, to deform the Face with black Spots, under a pretence to make it appear more beautifull: It is a Riddle as well in Nature as in Reason, that a Blemish should appear a Grace, and that a Deformity should adde unto a Beauty; I have seen a Face so spotted with half Moons and Stars, that my young Lady might not only seem a stranger to others, but to her self also. There is a native modesty in the gallantry of Attire, as there is in Gesture, and which doth more fully become, and would more absolutely accomplish a young Lady, than to cover the face with Love-spots, as if she would keep her self from the sight of her own Vanity.'

Codrington continues the subject of patching by quoting a supposed letter from *A Lady to Her Daughter, desiring her to wear no more Spots or black Patches in her Face*:

DAUGHTER,

The indulgence which I bear unto you, and the wellcome intelligence which every day I do receive how carefull you are to deserve it, doth invite me to be the more tender over you. . . . Nevertheless . . . I am to my great grief enformed that although you seem an Enemy to the Vices of this Age, you are addicted too much to the Fashions of it, and that lately you have been seen abroad with those Deformities on your Face which give them

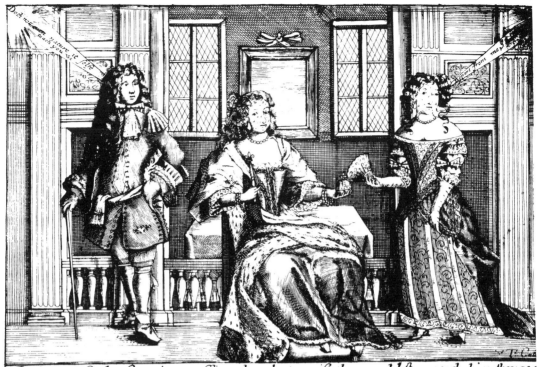

Doth not Gods Creation suffice thee but as if thou woldest exceed him thougoe about to mend it Chrisost: Hom: 4.in.1.ad Tim:

At yᶜ Resurrection thy maker will not acknowledge thee August: Tom 10. ser: 24

London Printed for I: Dunton at the black Rauen in the Poultery. 1683

FIG. 113: Patched ladies, 1683. Illustration from *England's Vanity.*

their proper Name are called *Black Patches.* A Fashion till of late never practised either in Rome or Venice or the Seraglio of the Turk, nor ever read of in all the Histories of the Vanities of Women. It appeareth strange to me that young Gentlewomen should lose their Reason with their Modesty and think that they do add until their Beauty by Subtracting from it. I must deal plainly with you, I am afraid that the Black Oath of *God damn me* in the Mouth of a Ranter, and the Black Patch in the Face of a Gentlewoman are near of kin to one another. I shall therefore assume that freedom of power which is due until me as to command you to wear them no more till I am better satisfied in their decency or their lawfullness. . . .

Your loving and care ful Mother,
M.C.

The daughter dutifully answers:

MADAM,

It is as well Religion as Duty in me to render you all observances, and I do make it as much my Delight as my Imployment. . . . I perceive some idle tongue hath been so busie with my Face, as to enform you that there hath lately been seen some Black Spots upon it. And I must confess, it leaveth some Impression upon my Spirit that I should be so unhappy to incurre your displeasure for following a Fashion that hath so much Innocence to plead for its Excuse, and so much Custom for its Authority. You may see every day some little Clouds in the Face of the Sun, yet the Sun is not ashamed that it hath attracted them; you may behold the Moon, in the fullness of all her Beauty to have some remarkable Spots in the Face thereof, and by these Spots it is that she gaineth her greatest Reputation, for she is inconstant in all things else, but in this only. . . . When I do put on my Mask (which is no more nor better than one great Black Patch) you do commend me for it And, will you be displeased at me for the wearing of a few black Spots in my face, which, if they are cut into Stars do represent unto me whither I would go, or if into little worms, whether I must go, the one of them testifying in me the sense of my unworthiness, to increase my humility, and the other the height of my Meditations, to advance my Affections. It is the unhappinesse of the most harmless things to be subject to the greatest misconstruction. . . . Nevertheless, according to the obligation of my Duty . . . I am determined to wear them no more . . . that by the fruits of my obedience you may perceive what an absolute power your Commands have over her who is,

 Madam,
  Your most humble and obedient Daughter
          A.C.

ENGLAND'S VANITY

In 1683 John Dunton of London published an anonymously written volume called *Englands Vanity: or the Voice of God Against the Monstrous Sin of Pride, in Dress and Apparel: Wherein Naked Breasts and Shoulders, Antick and Fantastick Garbs, Patches, and Painting, long Perriwigs, Towers, Shades, Curlings, and Crispings, with an Hundred more Fooleries of both Sexes, are condemned as Notoriously Unlawful*. The title page is reproduced in Figure 114.

The author uses some of the popular representational patches as symbols of the fate of those who wear them:

'And methinks the Mourning Coach and Horses (all in black) and plying in their Foreheads, stands ready harness'd to whirl them to Acheron, though I pity poor Charon for the darkness of the Night, since the Moon on the Cheek is all in Eclipse, and the poor Stars on the Temples are clouded in Sables. And no Comfort left him but the Lozenges on the Chin, which if he please he may

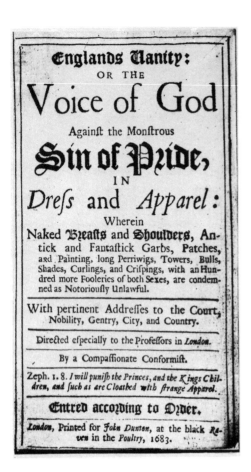

FIG. 114: *England's Vanity*. Title-page of the book published 1683.

pick off for his Cold; But will find as little comfort in them as they that wore them, and lesser in the whole voyage, when opening their mouths, he shall find no silver there for his Fare, and will discover them (as we) but Patches still.'

The coach and horses, stars, moons, and lozenges can all be seen in Figures 102 and 103.

The anonymous author is equally unrelenting about painting. 'The French,' he reminds us, 'have a good Lituny. . . . From Beef without Mustard, a Servant which overvalues himself, and from a woman which Painteth, Good Lord deliver us. . . .

'Lewis the Eleventh, King of France in his Melancholy Humour, strongly fancied that every thing stunk about him, all the odoriferous Perfumes, or fragrant Savours his officers could get for him, did by no means drive away the conceit, but still he smelt a filthy stink. And surely all the Perfumes of Arabia, Reader, were they gathered into Bags and Hung under their Armholes, will never take away the rankness and fulsomness of those unsavoury Creatures, who stink alive, as they move about, infecting the very Air, and bringing the Plagues upon us, Nauseous Fumes into the very Nostrils of God and his Holy Angels. I could collect an University of Writers that have all damn'd this impudent and graceless practice to the Pit of Hell, but I hasten from the scent of them. For I begin already to feel the power of Lewis his Imagination arising from my very Pen, and am affraid I have mistaken the Complexion-pot for my Standish.

'Behold! to what purpose is all this daubing and smearing the Face that is so pretty already? What do the ladies mean by it? What is their end? Why, to appear desirable and to win the repute of a Celebrated Beauty. A glorious Conquest! . . . But is this all the Plot? Can those Ruby Cheeks be satisfied with the Aeiry Bloomes of Report and Reputation? Wind is but a poor report for an hungry Stomack, sure there is something more at the bottom. Yes, to win a Gallant; very well, and what then? Will one content her? Will she leave daubing then? No, then she daubs to keep him. But this is uncharitable, cannot an honest Lady Paint? Ask God himself, *Ezech.* 29. 40. . . . And there is the depth of the Plot. . . . These painted Jezebels enter into the very Houses of the (Married) Gallants, Where their poor Wives are forced to lock themselves up and cry to God against them with bitter tears.'

Painting, then, according to our author, leads inexorably to prostitution, which in turn he blames for most of England's ills, including the Plague. He rants against 'these Moabitish Wenches sent in on very purpose to ruine us with their bewitching eyes and Painted Cheeks, and Gallavanting it so shamelessly in our streets; this I confess, England, looks like the kindly effects of the Execrable Councel of the Sorcerer, who knows no other way to confound us, but by whores.'

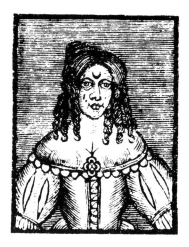

FIG. 115: Lady with topknot and patches. English woodcut, *c.* 1680.

9 · The Late Seventeenth Century
1685-1700

I have a Wife, the more's my care,
  Who like a gaudy peacock goes,
In top-knots, patches, powder'd hair;
  Besides she is the worst of shrows;
This fills my heart with grief and care
To think I must this burden bear.

THE INVINCIBLE PRIDE OF WOMEN

'To make a perfect Beauty is required a Smooth Complexion, white and red, and each colour to be truly placed, and lose themselves imperceptibly the one in the other; which some Ladies would express by the new French Phrase, *demeslee*. Full Eyes, well made of a dark or black colour, graceful and casting a lustre. A Nose well made, neither too big nor too small — A little Mouth, the upper-Lip resembling a Heart in shape, and the under some what larger, but both of a vermilion colour, as well in Winter as Summer; and on each side two small dimples easily to be discern'd in their moving upwards, which look like a kind of constant smile. — White Teeth, very clean, well ranged in order, of an equal bigness, neither short nor long, but very close. — A forked Chin, not too long, and hanging double. A full, round, or oval Visage. The Temples high rais'd. — As for the colour of the Hair, opinions are various.

One the fair hair, another brown admires,
A third a colour between both desires.
But herein all concentre and do rest,
The colour o' th' lov'd object is the best.

'Therefore 'tis indifferent to me which of the three they be, provided the Hair be very long, and thick, loose, cleanly kept, and a very little frizz'd or curl'd in rings; but above all that it be not red, nor come near that tincture. For it were disadvantageous to them to have all the other species of Beauty if they are of that colour. I have a natural antipathy against it, insomuch that I oftentimes betake myself to my heels when I spy it; not but they are usually accompanied with a pure skin, for which I have a great inclination; but the aversion I have for the one makes me abandon the other.'

THE LADIES DICTIONARY

The Ladies Dictionary, from which the paragraphs above were taken, was published in London in 1694 and described as 'A General Entertainment for the Fair-Sex' and 'A Work Never Before Attempted in English'. It provides an extraordinary view of customs and attitudes of the day. The anonymous authors, who are in frequent disagreement, have scattered references to cosmetics throughout the large volume under various headings. The first comes under *Beautifying, Reasons and Arguments for its Lawfulness, and that it is not discommendable in itself*, &c. The section begins with the usual argument that one cannot serve the Lord and please Men at the same time and that therefore women must not paint.

'This,' counters the first author, 'seems to us a little odd, and quite beside the true meaning of the Text, for if it be granted that by being the Lord's Servants, we cannot please Men: Then Wives consequently may not please their Husbands, Children their Parents, Subjects their Prince, Servants their Masters, nor Trades-men their Customers.' He feels, on the other hand, that there 'is a comely Decency in adorning and attiring the body'. And as for the objection that 'beautifying is in use with Harlots and therefore ought to be avoided by modest and virtuous ladies', he replies that there can be no objection in virtuous Women using those things which dishonest women use since the one wears apparel, and so does the other, the one eats & drinks, and so does the other'. It is their intentions which really make the difference. 'Women,' he insists, 'were never design'd for Deformity; and where any such thing happens by defect, it is but reasonable Art should repair it.'

This refreshing attitude, curiously enough, appears to be lost in conventional doctrine by the time we reach the letter P. Under *Painting the Face*, the author (evidently not the same one who wrote about *Beautifying*) states forthrightly:

'I think those that paint their Faces ought to be severely reproved. This wicked trade and practice of painting has been much censured by the Fathers.' He follows this with quotations from St Cyprian and others who the author of the Bs suggested ought to meddle more with ladies' hearts and less with their faces. Then he goes on:

'Imagine one of our forefathers were alive again and should see one of those his Gay Daughters walk in Cheap-side before him, what do you think he would think it were? . . . Sure he could not but stand amazed to think what new Creatures the times had yielded since he lived; and then if he should run before her, to see if by the foresight he might guess what it were, when his eyes should meet with a powdred Frizzle, a painted Hide shadowed with a Fan not more painted, Breasts displayed, and a Loose Lock over her shoulders betwixt a painted Cloth and Skin, how would he more bless himself to think what mixture in Nature could be guilty of such a Monster.'

The author, outraged by the moons, stars, crosses, lozenges, and coach and horses women wore on their cheeks, remarked that if they had been born with them, they would have been registered among 'the prodigious and Monstrous births. Fashion brought in Painting and Antick dress. . . . When God shall come to Judge the quick and the dead, he will not know those who have so defaced that Fashion which he hath Erected. . . . And it should be considered that as some . . . are always carining the vessel of the body with physick, washing and following with external applications till they sink it; so are many tampering continually to mend the feature and complexion, which God made very well, because it pleased him to make them no other, till they utterly spoil them.'

Becoming increasingly incensed with each paragraph, the author expresses 'a kind of itching desire to go and rub their cheeks . . . to give them to understand the artifices wherewith they endeavour to abuse them. For I phancy,' he adds primly, 'no beauty but what is natural . . . and am an enemy to those kind of disguises that in vain strive to imitate the naturals.'

For the lover who suspects his lady of using paints, the author suggests that he take a good look at her when she gets up in the morning. If this is impractical or if, by chance, she has had the foresight to paint before going to bed, the only alternative is to slip the lady's maid a few guineas, which he guarantees will unlock any secrets the lady may have.

PAINT, POWDER, AND PATCHES

In the 1690s the fashionable face became longer and more oval, with the hair moving upwards. The nose also grew longer, but the full red lips remained much as they had been. And fashionable women of all ages painted and patched. Misson reported, based on his travels, that 'In England the young, old, handsome, ugly, are all bepatch'd till they are bed-rid. I have often counted fifteen Patches, or more, upon the Swarthy wrinkled phiz of an old Hag three-score and ten and upwards.'

Schopenhauer's mother, Johanna, would have found the very idea of patching incredible had she not seen with her own eyes the gummed patches of black silk, cut into 'tiny full and half moons, little stars and hearts, which were intended, when attached to the face with taste and discernment, to increase its charms and enliven the facial expression. A series of moons increasing in size from the tiniest to the largest, affixed at the outer corner of the eye, served to make the eyes appear larger and to heighten their lustre; a few stars at the corner of the mouth were supposed to give the smile a roguish charm; a *mouche* in the right place on the check suggested a dimple. There were also patches of a larger size — suns, doves, cupids even. These were called *assassins*, presumably because of their devastating effect on the hearts.'

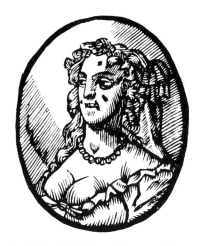

FIG. 116: Patched lady. English woodcut, *c.* 1680.

Nevertheless, the painted lady was still suspect among the unsophisticated or even among sophisticated men who preferred women with simple, natural charms. A ballad called 'The Country Miss new come in Fashion' begins:

> Give me the Lass that's true Country bred,
> With paragon gown, straw Hat on her head;
> Feeding upon good Bacon and Beans,
> But who never knew what jilting means.
>
> What though her skin be tawny and coarse,
> Flocks she lyes on, she'l kiss ne'r the worse;
> Shame she ne'r had, like Miss of the Town,
> That's painted and patcht, and lyes up and down.

In *The London Lasse's Lamentation*, published the same year, we hear from one of the painted and patched:

> As fine as the Queen of May, I flourish with gallantry,
> I wear my Top-knot, e'ery day, *yet cannot be married, not I.*
>
> I paint and I powder still, to tempt all that I come nigh,
> But Fortune she has sent a frown, *I cannot be married, not I.*

In still another ballad on the same theme, entitled 'The Innocent Country-Maid's Delight', a milkmaid compares country girls with city girls:

> Each Lass she will paint her face,
> To seem with a comely grace,

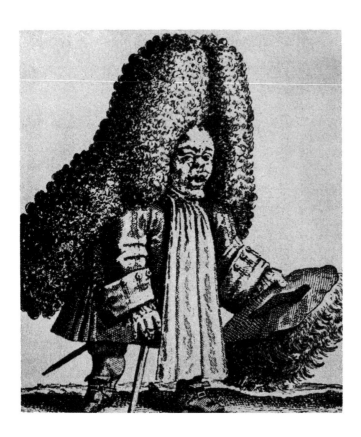

And powder their hair,
To make them look fair,
That Gallants may them embrace:
But every morning,
Before their adorning,
They're far unfit for sale;
But 'tis not so, with we that go,
Through frost and snow, when winds do blow,
To carry the milking-payl.

Even many Frenchmen felt the same way. Jean de La Bruyère, in his
Caractères, wrote:

'If it is the men whom the women wish to please, if it is for them that they
make themselves up or colour themselves . . . I say to them, on behalf of all
men or of most of them, that white paint and rouge makes them frightful and
disgusting, that rouge alone ages them and disguises them; that men hate as
much to see women with paint on their faces as with false teeth in their mouths
and balls of wax in their jaws; that they seriously object to all of the artifice
which women use to make themselves ugly.'

But men themselves were still using cosmetics. In 1689 the Earl of Bedford paid
out two pounds and fourpence for orange flower water, Queen of Hungary's

water, essences, washballs, and powder for hair, hands, and linen. Tooth powder was an additional ten shillings. The Earl's dressing table, according to Gladys Scott Thompson, was covered with pale blue silk with a pincushion and comb-bags to match. Scented powder was sprinkled on the dressing table and among the linen or used in little bags for the same purpose. The scented waters were used primarily as after-shave lotions.

Poisonous paints were evidently not the only dangers women encountered in their pursuit of beauty. In October 1689 Madame de Sévigné wrote to her daughter:

'It had never entered my brain to accuse certain iron wires of the head-dress of being the cause of long faces. . . . I had heard they were very friendly; but no, quite the contrary. These two little wires press against the temples, prevent the circulation of blood, and cause abscesses. Some die in consequence. They may consider themselves fortunate whose faces are only lengthened an ell, and who become pale as death; but young people, who are more hardy, may recover in time. I am very much inclined to place this story in the class with some others, formerly related to me by the good Princesse de Tarente; however, it is not amiss to know everything.'

Mundus Muliebris

But after 1690 the man who did wish to know could always consult John Evelyn's *Mundus Muliebris: or, The Ladies Dressing Room Unlock'd and Her Toilette Spread*, a satiric piece in rhymed couplets, actually written by his daughter Mary, a brilliant and learned young lady, who died when she was nineteen. It is subtitled *A Voyage to Marryland* and lists, for the benefit of a man about to marry, those things he will have to provide for his wife. The list, needless to say, is very long. The items pertaining to hair can be found in *Fashions in Hair*; those having to do with cosmetics include:

> Some of chicken skin for night,
> To keep her hands plump, soft, and white;
> *Mouches* for pushes, to be sure,
> From Paris the *très-fine* procure,
> And Spanish paper, lip and cheek,
> With spittle sweetly to belick:
> Nor therefore space in the next place,
> The pocket sprunking looking-glass;
> *Calembuc* comb in *pulvil* case
> To set and trim the hair and face:

> And that the cheeks may both agree,
> *Plumpers* to fill the cavity;
> Washes, unguents, and cosmeticks;
> A pair of silver candlesticks;
> Snuffers and snuff-dish; boxes more,
> For powders, patches, waters store,
> In silver flasks, or bottles, cups
> Cover'd, or open, to wash chaps;
> Nor may Hungarian queen's be wanting,
> Nor store of spirits against fainting :
> Of other waters, rich and sweet,
> To sprinkle handkerchief is meet;
> *D'ange*, orange, *mill-fleur*, myrtle,
> Whole quarts the chamber to bequirtle.

To this was appended the *Fop-Dictionary, or, An Alphabetical Catalogue of the Hard and Foreign Names and Terms of the Art Cosmetick, &c., together with their Interpretations, for Instruction of the Unlearned.* Again, only the cosmetic items are listed below :

COSMETICS. Here used for any effeminate ornament; also, artificial complections and perfumes.

MOUCHES. Flies, or black patches, by the vulgar.

PLUMPERS. Certain very thin, round, and light balls, to plump out and fill up the cavities of the cheeks, much us'd by old Court-Countesses.

POLVIL. The Portugal term for the most exquisite powders and perfumes.

SPANISH PAPER. A beautiful red colouring which the ladies, &c. in Spain paint their faces withal.

RECIPES FOR BEAUTY

For those willing to make their own cosmetics, there was published in 1685, in an English translation, a volume of miscellaneous recipes entitled *Curiosities of Art and Nature*, written by Nicolas Lémery, apothecary to Louis XIV. These recipes, according to the title page, were 'Extracted out of the Cabinets of the most Eminent Personages of the French Court'. Although there were no recipes for rouge, there were several for various lotions and pomatums. One of Lémery's more dramatic recipes was designed *To Take away wrinkles from the Face:*

'Take a Fire-shovel and heat it; and cast thereon the Powder of Myrrh; putting the Face over it, to receive the Fume, having a course Cloth about the Head, the better to receive the Fume; do this thrice; then heating the Fire-shovel again, take some White-wine in your mouth and besprinkle the Shovel therewith, receiving the Fume that rises, doing this like wise thrice, continuing it morning and evening, as long as you will, and you will see wonders.' Unfortunately, we have no record of what wonders the ladies saw. The same recipe appeared in another collection nearly a century later.

For the Redness in the Face Lémery suggested:

'Upon a pound of Veal put six new laid Eggs; heat them together, and add half a pint of White-wine-Vinegar, and an handful of wild Tansy, distill them in *Balneo Marioe*, and wash the Face therewith.' There was also a recipe for *A Water to whiten the Face* and one for ox-gall mixed with alum, 'Salt of Glass', sugar candy, and borax, then stirred for a fortnight and filtered. ' 'Tis us'd,' said Lémery, 'to preserve Persons from being Sun-burnt, in putting it upon the Face, when you would go in the Country, washing them at night with common Water, and this will take off all the gross Tan.'

One of his more exhaustive recipes was for *A Water to Beautifie the Face and to take away the Wrinkles:*

'Take River Water, and strain it through a white Linnen Cloth; put it into a new glaz'd earthen Pot, with an handful of Barley well wash'd and cleans'd from dust, and boyl it over a Charcoal fire till the Barley be broken; then take it from the fire and let it stand, and then strain it through a Linnen Cloth, into a glass Bottle, that it be a quarter empty, to which add three drops of white Balsam, or Balsam of Peru, the first is the best, to a quart of water; and then shake the Bottle for ten or twelve hours without intermission till the Balsam be intirely incorporated into the said Water, and the Water remain a little troubled, and a little whitish, and then it hath arriv'd to its perfection; It wonderfully embellishes the Face, and preserves it young and fresh: it takes away wrinkles also in Time, in using it once a day. Note, you must wash your Face with River, Rain, or Fountain-water, before you use this water.'

For whitening the face the book contained a recipe for *A most excellent Spanish White:*

'Take the Seeds of Oriental Pearl, white or pale Coral, of each two ounces, beat them apart, then put them into a Matras, and add as much Aq. fort. as you shall think fit, Juice of Citron is better: then you must have another Matras, wherein you must put Tin-Ice 8 ounces; having first beaten it well, and pour therein the said Water, till all be dissolv'd; then mingle the Pearl and Coral together, and that which you have dissolv'd to the Tin-Ice, pour upon the said Pearl and Coral, to cause them to precipitate, and before you mingle them, you must add twice every day Fountain-water, till you perceive no Taste of the Aqua-fortis, and then you shall use it with Peach-Flowers, distilling each apart; and when you use them, take a little quantity of each, and so Compound them.'

Recipes for the teeth were also included, as this one *To whiten the Teeth:*

'Take red Coral, Cuttle-bone, both reduced to a fine Powder, Pearls, Crabs-claws calcin'd, burnt Harts-horn, of each one dram; Salt of Worm-wood a Scruple; make them into a Powder.'

Among other fascinating items in the book are A *remarkable Receipt made of a man's Skull* and *How to make a great deal of Cream*.

In the year preceding publication of the Lémery book, Fra Angiolo Paladini, a skin specialist at the famed Convent of Santa Maria Novella in Florence, had compounded three new cosmetic aids—an almond paste, a lily water, and a cosmetic vinegar—which became very popular with the ladies of the Tuscan court.

The Ladies Dictionary also included a number of recipes. There were, for example, suggestions for the *Body Lean and how to make it Plump and Fat*, as well as the reverse. For *Brows that have their Hair growing too thick or irregular*, the reader is advised to 'take Ivy, Gum, Emmets-Eggs, or Pincent Colophonie, Leeches burnt, half an ounce, grind and mingle them with the Blood of a Frog and annoint the superfluous Hair, and it will come off.'

To remedy the defect of *Brows falling too low over the eyes*, one should take 'a little Mastick, together with the Juice of Colworts, and going to Bed, put the Brow up into its place, and in the form of a Plaister apply the Mastick to it all Night, and in so doing three or four Nights, it will keep in its proper place.'

The instructions for *Brows that have lost their Hair* are intriguing: 'Take Wasps or Bees, burn them to Ashes, and mix the Ashes with Honey, and laying it to the Hair, 'twill quickly come again.'

Finally, *Brows reddish or white are made black by this means*: 'Take what quantity you please of Red Filberds, calcine them in an earthen Vessel, mix it with Goats-grease, and annoint the Brow with it, and if the Skin be soil'd, wash it off with warm water, and in often using, the Hair, 'twill become of a **very** curious Black.'

Passing over *Books, Directions to Ladies about Reading them* ('It is not necessary to read many Books, but to read the best'), we come to *Ceruse*, which is described as 'white-lead, often used by Chyrurgeons in Ointments and Plaister. It is with Painters a principal white Colour; and hath been and still is much used by Women in Painting their Faces.'

In a lengthy discussion of the *Course of Life*, a few remarks are included about the artifices of beauty:

'We are constrained to disallow the practice of some Ladies, who to allay the petty Exorbitancies of too flaming a Colour, expose in the Evening, wherein Dews and Damps fall, their Faces and Naked Breasts to Cynthias moistening Rays, as if the Moon (because pale herself) would make them so, or by spitting in their Faces, scour off the Crimson dye.—Certainly Beauty never consents, that Laundress should whiten her Livery who uses no other Soap than her own Foggy Excrements; such practices, however, since they occasion rheums, Cattarhs,

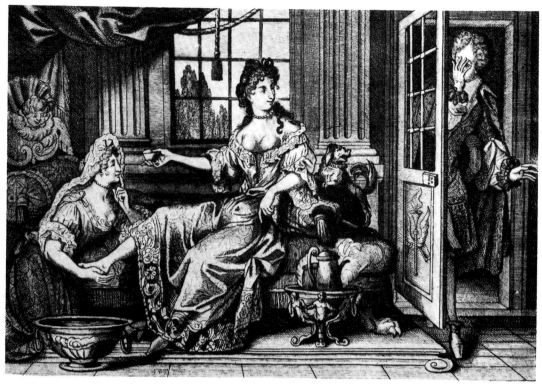

FIG. 118: Undressed for the bath. The visitor is covering his face, not because of the bare bosom, which was customary, but because of the bare calf, which was considered indecent. French engraving, late seventeenth century.

and Distillations, may by those Defects make the Face White and Pallid, but rather diminish than add anything to Beauty, so that we find an Air too dry and parching does Wrinkle and Chap the Skin, so that Art must be called in to work it over with a Beautiful Embroidery.'

Ladies were also advised, when out of doors, to 'make Choice of a Seat some what raised, if it be not too much exposed to the ill conveniences of Foggs and Mists; let it be sheltered round with pleasant Woods and Groves, which may fence you from the blew impressions of a pinching Boreas, and in the Summer secure you so that Sol with his Amorous beams may not kiss away your Beauty.'

In case a lady's beauty did somehow get kissed away by Amorous beams, there was no appropriate recipe. But for ladies who were habitually red-faced, the author suggested first, that they cut down on their drinking, and second, that they prepare a wash from the following recipe:

'Take of Rosewater, a pint, put it into a Glass and steep an ounce of Camphire in it, an ounce of Sulpher beaten to a powder, Myrrh and Frankincense, half an ounce each, set it in the Sun or some warm place, and after ten days end, wash your Face with the Water, and in often doing it your Colour will be restored.'

Freckles, the reader was assured, could be removed by a concoction of oil of tartar, honey, and the sap from a fig tree. But the seventeenth-century woman, like all others before and after, was eventually faced with the eternal problem:

'Fortunes Envy, or Fate, often so orders it that the smiling Glories of Beauties spring are too severely nipt with an early Autum, when sharp scythed Time cuts those flowry Graces down & shrouds them in the furrows of a wrinckled Face: Now to make your Verdant Features flourish in spite of Envy or Accidental decay, and smooth your Face for a new Plantation of Roses and Lillies. — Take our following directions, Bitter Almonds two ounces, Lilly roots dryed and powder'd an ounce, Oyl of Roses an ounce, Virgins Wax half an ounce, make them into an Oyntment over a gentle fire, and anoint the Face with it.' Alternative recipes were provided.

Low foreheads, the reader was told firmly, must be 'raised to a decent height'. In order to do this, the lady was instructed to spread 'Mastick' over the part of the hair which caused the forehead to be too low, to bind it with a fillet over night, then the following morning to 'take it off very quick'. Presumably she could then look under H for headache remedies. A special recipe was included for preventing the hair thus removed from growing back.

For the lady with sufficient patience and determination there was an extraordinary recipe for a concoction that was guaranteed to make the face 'white as Alabaster' and to beautify even a disfigured one:

'Take the most tender and Transparent Talque you can get, slit it into thin slices, put them into a Glass-Viol for ten or twelve days with the Juice of Limmons: During the Frost in Winter, make a Bag of the thickest Cloath you can get, put the steep'd Talque into it, with some hard Flints, being then closely tyed, rub it together with the Flints till the Talque become powder, put it then into a glaz'd Earthen Pot with a narrow mouth, stop the Vessel, and see it be carefully bound about with strong Wire, then put into a Reverbatory twelve hours, then by degrees, take it from the Fire, and being cool, powder it finer with as much speed as may be (to prevent the Airs having too much power over it), put it then into a bag with a book at the bottom to hang a Vessel upon to receive the Liquor, hang the bag then with the Vessel so placed in a Well about a fathom above the Water, till the Humidity begins to drop, then take it out and put it in a damp place, where the wind has no force, and suffer it to hang till all the moisture be drained away; the liquor so received is the water of Talque, and by the same means you may make the Oyl if you put what remains in the bag into a Retort, by degrees giving fire to it, till you have drawn all the Oyl forth, and this is so Excellent a Beautifier that Queens and Princesses may add Splendor to their Perfection by using it.'

A little further on the author (the friendly one) once again defends the ladies against the Christian fathers who 'would make weak people believe that every touch of Colouring added to the Cheeks is a semblance of Hell fire; and their

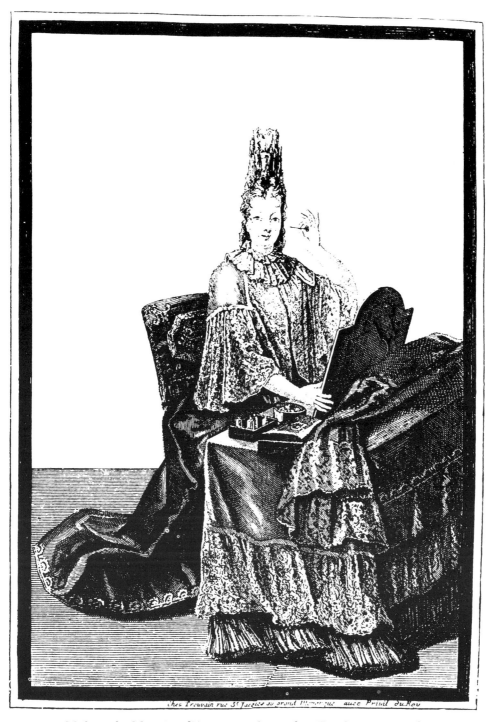

FIG. 119: Madame la Marquise d'Angeau at her toilet. French engraving, late seventeenth century.

curled hair, dangling never so little, an Emblem of the Never dying Worm. Medusa's head is not pictur'd more terrible, with all her Snaky Tresses than they would represent every Ladys, though never so modest and virtuous, whose Hair, Complexion, or Tiring is not naturally her own. But these things ought not to discourage modest Ladys from using such Arts and Adornments as may keep up, repair, or add lusture to their beauty. . . . And since there can be no harm, but good, in beautifying the Face, we see no reason but it may and ought to be used to Good Ends and Purposes. Though Nature is the Elder, Art is the Youngers Sister and may very well assist her where she is wanting or deficient.'

Reluctantly skipping over *Green-Sickness in Virgins*, we go on to patches. The author (the one who hates anything unnatural) never misses an opportunity to lash out at what he disapproves of. Under the heading of *Spots in any part of the body, to remove them*, he says:

'Spots are as great blemishes to beauty in either sex, as in pretious stones, much debasing the worth or value of either; we have seen Faces from whose Features Beauty her selfe might have drawn Patterns, had not Nature studied too much neatness, play'd the Curtezan, and spoiled that which was Lovely and Charming before by over Patching; yet many Ladies never conclude themselves Venus's in beauty unless they have some Artificial Mole, tho such clouded Stars more Eclipse than Increase their Native Lusture.'

After that fairly mild outburst, he does go on to discuss natural spots and how to get rid of them.

Attacking patches, like attacking painting, was, as we have seen, conventional and expected, and ladies who patched doubtless paid no attention at all. But a defense of patches was something out of the ordinary and must have warmed their hearts. The entry headed *Patches defended, in opposition to what is said against it in this book, by another hand* was presumably written by the author who earlier defended painting:

'Painting now not much in use, being almost justled out by Washes, is not the only thing that is censured and objected against; but if a Lady happens to have a Wart or Pimple on her Face, they would not, by their Good wills, have her put a black patch on it, and if she do's, they point at it as a mark of Pride, though we see nature her selfe has adorned the visage with moles and other marks that resemble them, and in imitation of which we suppose they were first used. . . .

'We commonly see little spotty Clouds over the Face of the Sun, yet he is not ashamed of his attraction. . . . The Moon . . . hath in her pale Visage some very remarkable spots, which rather appear as an Ornament than as a disfigurement or defect and may be said to be her chiefest Glory, seeing she is held in everything but that to be inconstant; yet those she never puts off but perpetually wears them, when a Lady puts on her Mask, which is rarely cavill'd at, but held as the Skreen of modest blushes, as well as the shelter of beauty from the too warm

Kisses of the Sun, or parching of the Northern wind, what can that be termed but one great spot to cover the Face. Suppose she cuts her Patches into Stars. They may improve her serious thoughts by minding her as often as she looks on them, of the place to which she is desirous to go. If into Flys, they Emblem to her the Lightness, Vanity, and short duration of things in this World. Or suppose they be cut into the Form of little Worms, then they may put her upon Meditations of Death and the Grave, where those Insects are to be her Companions. . . . The Peacock is set off by Nature with the spotty Glory of his Train; and it is accounted the Rarest Beauty of the Creatures on whom men set the highest value, to be sprinkled or dapled o're by Natures pencil; yet . . . when any such artificial things are seen in a Ladies Face, what Batteries do the Envious and Censorious raise against her Virtues. . . .'

Lest we come away with too one-sided a picture of the delicate seventeenth-century lady of fashion spending countless hours compounding lotions to give her an alabaster complexion, pasting on taffeta patches to make it seem even whiter, and sitting in the shade to avoid being kissed by the sun, it is perhaps worth noting a few cautions the author felt obliged to list under *Manners*:

' 'Tis not manners as soon as you are at table to bawl out, "I eat none of this, I eat none of that. I care for no Rabit; I love nothing that tasts of Pepper, Nutmeg, Onyons, &c." How hungry soever you be, it is indecent to eat hastily or ravenously, as if you would choak your self. — If you happen to burn your mouth, you must endure it if possible, if not you must convey what you have in your Mouth privately upon your Plate, and give it away to the Footman; for though Civility obliges you to be neat, there is no necessity you should burn out your Guts.'

And that practical bit of advice brings us to the end of the seventeenth century.

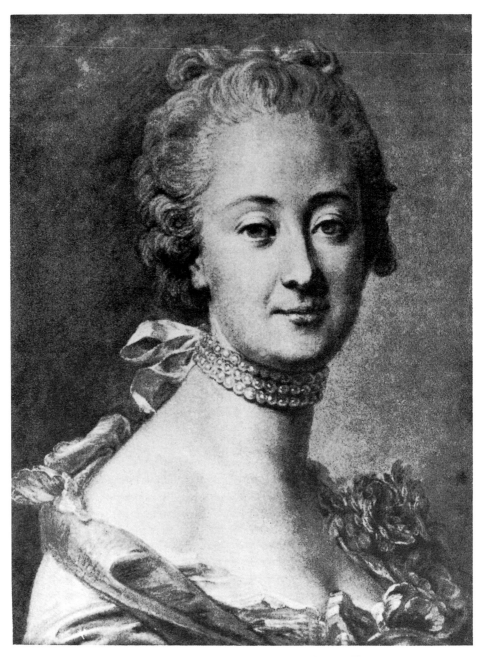

FIG. 120: Portrait of an unknown lady, Paris, 1720. Pastel by Rosalba Carriera.

10 · The Early Eighteenth Century
1700-1737

How capricious were Nature and Art to poor Nell !
She was painting her cheeks at the time her nose fell.

MATTHEW PRIOR

By the beginning of the eighteenth century the voluptuous look of the mid-seventeenth had largely given way to one of painted porcelain, which lasted until the French Revolution. To the lady of fashion some makeup was essential, and as the century progressed, she used more and more of it. Ladies of the French court whitened their faces, pencilled their eyebrows, touched up their veins with blue, and rouged to the limit; only prostitutes, it is said, strived for a natural look. In London, on the other hand, it was the prostitutes who rouged blatantly. Englishwomen of quality made some attempt to imitate nature, though as they grew older, they often grew bolder in a desperate attempt to retain an illusion of youth.

PAINTS AND PAINTING

At the beginning of the century there was published anonymously in London a small book aptly titled *Several Letters Between Two Ladies: Wherein the Lawfulness and Unlawfulness of Artificial Beauty in Point of Conscience are nicely Debated*. It was published, according to the title page, 'for the Satisfaction of the Fair Sex'. It was later assumed, though never conclusively proved, that the author was the Reverend Jeremy Taylor. A handwritten note on the flyleaf of the copy in the British Museum, presumably by the original owner of the book and evidently a scholar of sorts, supports this view. The attitude of the author towards the use of cosmetics—and a somewhat surprising one it is, especially from a man of the cloth—is perhaps indicative of the increasing permissiveness of makeup in the eighteenth century :

' 'Tis my Opinion that Painting the Face is not only lawful, but much to be commended; nay, absolutely necessary, at least if any thing that belongs to Humane kind be so : and this, I hope, I shall be able to prove from several Heads. First, that Woman was made and designed by Heaven for the Pleasure of Man, and if so, certainly 'tis her business and part of her duty to endeavour to contribute to that End for which she was created. . . .

'Improve therefore, ladies, the Beauties Heaven has bestowed upon you, and preserve them as long as you can; for I can see no Reason why the cultivating outward Form should be a Crime since the Improvement of Inward Grace is a Vertue and Duty.'

In the 238-page dialogue, one lady presents the conventional arguments against painting, all of which are demolished (at some length) by her painted opponent.

But lawful or unlawful, moral or immoral, with the debates raging around them, more and more women took to painting. In Tom Brown's satiric *Letters from the Dead to the Living*, first published in 1702, a German doctor and astrologer writes to his friends at Will's Coffee House in Covent Garden:

'If any woman be unwilling to speak to me, they may have the conveniency of speaking to my wife, who is expert in all feminine distempers. She has an excellent cosmetic water to carry off freckles, sun-burn, or pimples; and a curious red-pomatum to plump and colour the lips. She can make red hair as white as a lily; she shapes the eyebrows to a miracle; makes low foreheads as high as you please, has a never-failing remedy for offensive breaths, a famous essence to correct the ill scent of the arm-pits, a rich water that makes the hair curl, a most delicate paste to smooth and whiten the hands; also

A rare secret, that takes away all warts,
From the face, hands, fingers, and privy parts.'

RECIPES FOR BEAUTY

Most of these secrets were to be found in a new version of Lémery's recipe book of 1685, this one called *Curiosa Arcana*, published in 1711. It contained some of the old recipes and many new ones. The one of most interest here is entitled simply *To make the Face Ruddy*, though it turns out not to mean the entire face: 'Take raspings of Brazil and Orcanet dissolv'd in Allum-water, with which wash the Cheeks and Lips.' No other recipes for rouge or face paint of any sort were included. But there was one *To make the Nails Handsome*:

'Take Water of White Horehound, or Sulphur Vine, incorporated with Pitch and Turpentine, with a little Vinegar; or else Myrrh work'd up with Pitch, and a little Juice of Lemons. To take away stagnating Blood from the Nails, use Euphorbium mix'd up with Turkey's Fat; and to remove Proud Flesh use Pouder or Oil of Vitriol.' After compounding some of Monsieur Lémery's recipes, the lady probably *needed* something to make the nails handsome.

There are also useful instructions *To stop the Rottenness of the Teeth* (a grain of salt dissolved in the mouth) and *To make the Body moderately Fat* (which in the eighteenth century evidently required a recipe).

According to the *Spectator*, 'There is not a gentlewoman of a good family in

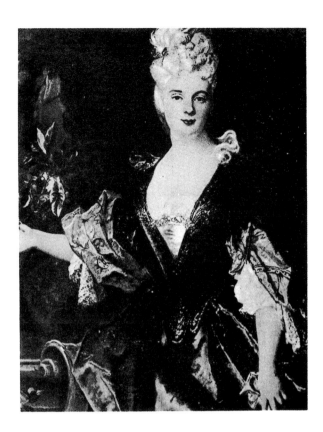

FIG. 121 : Elisabeth de Beauharnais. Portrait
by Nicolas Largillière, early
eighteenth century.

any county of South Britain who has not heard of the virtues of May-dew, or is
not furnished with some receipt or other in favour of the complexion; and I
have known a physician of learning and sense, after eight years' study in the
University and a course of travels into most countries in Europe, owe the first
raising of his fortunes to a cosmetic wash.'

In 1713 a book of recipes entitled *The Queen's Closet Opened* revealed still
more cosmetic secrets. One of the simplest ones, requiring nothing more than
boiling rosemary in white wine, was intended 'To make the Face Fair, and for a
stinking Breath'. Having washed the face with the concoction, one could take
what was left and 'drink thereof' in order to sweeten the breath. No doubt
some bibulous ladies managed to have a considerable amount left over.

The recipe '*For Heat in the Face, Redness, and Shining of the Nose*' was even
simpler and cost nothing. The ladies were instructed to 'take a fair Linnen-cloth,
lay it on the Grass and draw it over till it be wet with Dew : Then wring it out
into a Dish, and wash the Face therewith' as often as they pleased. *May*-dew was
recommended.

Other recipes for the complexion were more complicated but also relied largely
on natural ingredients easily accessible to ladies of the period :

'*A Water of Flowers good for the Complexion of Ladies.* Take the Flowers
of Elder, a Flower-de-Luce, Mallows, and Beans, with the Pulp of Melon, Honey,

and the white of Eggs; and let all be distilled. . . . This water is very effectual to take away wrinkles in the Face, and gives a Vermillion-Tincture to the Skin.

'*Another sort of Water to clear the Face from Freckles.* Take a pound and a half of Strawberries, white Flowers-de-Luce and Beans, of each half a pound; Rocke and Plume-Allum, half an ounce; *Sal Gemmee* and Niter, two Drams: Let all these steep fifteen Days in Malmsey, *Hampshire*-Honey, and white-wine-Vinegar, a quarter of each; and afterwards distill them in a moderate Sand-bath: when you would make use of this Water, dip a fine Rag into it, and apply it to the Part affected, at Night, going to bed; wash it the next Morning, with Nenuphar-water.

'To take away Hair' one was instructed to 'Take the Shells of fifty two Eggs, beat them small and distill them with a good Fire; then with the Water, anoint yourself where you would have the Hair off.' For ladies who had more cats than chickens, the author recommended beating 'hard dry Cats-dung . . . to a Powder' and tempering it with strong vinegar. It was supposed to have the same effect.

To make the Hair grow thick required taking 'three spoonfuls of Honey and a good handful of Vine-sprigs that twist like wire', beating them well, straining their juice into the honey, and using it to anoint the bald places.

Most women made their own perfumes, and the following recipe is included to show how they went about it:

'*To make an excellent Perfume.* Take a quarter of a pound of Rose buds, cut clear from the whites, stamp them very well, adding a good spoonful of Rose-water; and let them stand close stopt all Night: Then take one ounce and a quarter of *Benjamin* beaten fine, and even sifted, (if you please) twenty grains of Civet, and ten grains of Musk, mingle these with the Roses, beating all well together, in order to be made up in little Cakes, and dry'd between Sheets of Paper.'

There is also a recipe for *A water for a weak Brain*, which requires, among other ingredients, 'a Cock that has been chas'd and beaten before it was kill'd'.

Cosmetics were made at home as a matter of both economy and necessity since satisfactory cosmetics were not always readily available in the shops. Items of really fine quality, usually imported, were greatly treasured and were frequently given as gifts. Mary Granville Pendarves, writing to her sister in 1727, mentioned that in a box which was being sent to her she would find, among other things, 'a little Tunbridge jewel box which Mrs Tillier desires you to accept as her fairing; in the first partition there is three cakes of lip salve, in the next a solitary ring which begs the honour of embracing one of your fingers. . . .'

But for women who had enough to do around the house without all of the distilling, straining, grinding, and pounding required for making their own cosmetics and who were willing to make do with commercial products, there were a few available. A bill of 1722 lists powder, pomatum, and a washball for

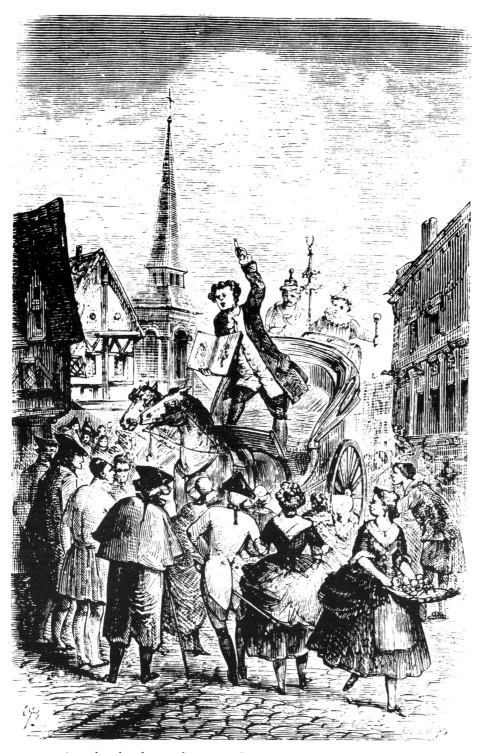

FIG. 122 : A vendor of perfume and cosmetics during the reign of Louis XV.
Nineteenth-century wood engraving.

tenpence, a powder puff, fourpence, and red lead and turmeric, one penny. A two-page advertisement for a remarkable, if unnamed, beauty cream appeared in 1715:

'The only delicate beautifying Cream for Gentlemen and Ladies, for the *Face, Neck,* and *Hands,* which gives such general Satisfaction to all that use it. It surprisingly takes away *Redness, Pimples, Roughness, Worms, Morphew, Scurfs, Sunburn, Freckles, Wrinkles, Pits of the Small Pox,* and other Defilements of the Skin, rendring it delicately fair, plump, smooth, and beautiful, tho' before never so red, rough, discolour'd, wither'd or wrinkled; and no Body can ever discern that you have use any Thing (whereas most other Things too plainly shew themselves), and will in a few Times only Using make even an ordinary coarse Face or Hand look unexpectedly fair; and is as innocent as common *Cream. Young Ladies* use it to preserve their *Bloom,* the *elderly Ladies* and *Gentlemen* to take away *Wrinkles,* (which it wears out) and render their Skin smooth, which, by supplying and plumping up, it performs to Admiration. And as for those Persons who use any thing of a *White,* this is the only Thing to prepare the *Skin* for it, that it may never been seen to lie on.

' 'Tis infinitely beyond any *Almond-Paste,* or *Powder* to clean the *Hands* with, and make them soft, fine, white, and smooth, altho' never so course, red, rough, and chopt before: Nay, even at once only Using, 'twill so recover a red course Hand, as to render it unexpectedly smooth and fine. Now there are a great many very beautiful Ladies who have but indifferent Hands, and would be overjoy'd to make them *white;* this cream will make them so, being so perfect and delicate a Beautifyer, and the Use of it so clean and neat, and has likewise so grateful and pleasant a Scent that nothing can exceed it, and therefore is the only Thing in the World to preserve or regain a fine beautiful Skin and Complexion.

'This cream is in large neat Pots, with the Print of the Sign of *The Necklace for Childrens Teeth* upon each pot, (to distinguish it from the Counterfeits) Price 2s. 6d. which will last a long while: with plain Directions for its Use. And is to be had at the *Crown,* a Milliner's Shop, right against the *King's Arms* Tavern near *Hungerford-Market* in the *Strand.* At Mrs *Garway's* Shop, the Sign of the *King's Arms* at the *Royal-Exchange* Gate next *Cornhill.* At the *Unicorn,* an Apothecary's Shop on St. *Margaret's-Hill* in the *Burrough, Southwark.* At Mr. *Cooper's* the Corner of *Charles-Court.* And of the Authoress, a Gentlewoman up one Pair of Stairs at the Sign of *The Celebrated Anodyne* NECKLACE *for Children's* TEETH, without *Temple-Bar.* Who also sells a curious fine *White* for the Face and Neck, without any hurtful Thing in it, 1s. a Pot. A delicate *Lip Salve,* which will preserve the Lips from *Chopping* all the Winter. A fine Powder for the Teeth. Price 1s.'

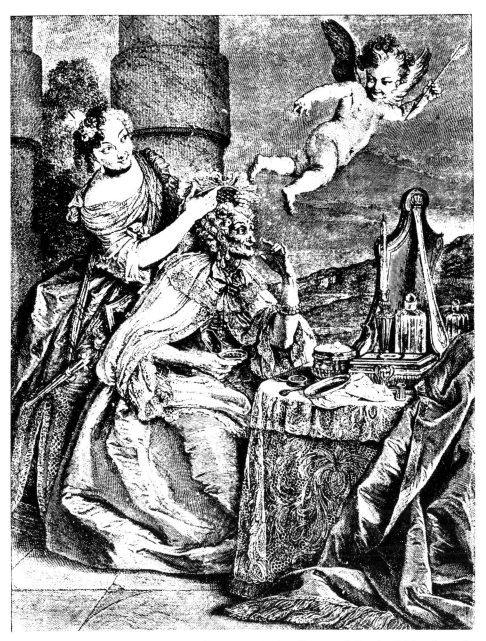

FIG. 123: 'Folly Adorns Withered Old Age with the Charms of Youth.' Mid-eighteenth-century engraving by Coypel. The old lady is holding a patchbox in her hand, and a box of rouge is open on the dressing-table.

APPLYING THE PAINT

In *The Rape of the Lock* Alexander Pope gives us a delightful picture of an eighteenth-century lady at her dressing table:

> And now, unveil'd the Toilet stands display'd;
> Each silver Vase in mystic order laid.
> First rob'd in white the Nymph intense adores,
> With head uncover'd the cosmetic pow'rs.
> A heav'nly Image in the glass appears,
> To that she bends, to that her eyes she rears;
> Th' inferior Priestess at her altar's side,
> Trembling, begins the sacred rites of Pride.
> Unnumber'd treasures ope at once, and here
> The various off-rings of the world appear;
> From each she nicely culls with curious toil
> And decks the Goddess with the glitt'ring spoil.
> This casket India's glowing gems unlocks,
> And all Arabia breathes from yonder box.
> The Tortoise here and Elephant unite
> Transform'd to Combs, the speckl'd and the white.
> Here files of Pins extend their shining rows,
> Puffs, Powders, Patches, Bibles, Billet-doux.
> Now awful Beauty puts on all its arms;
> The fair each moment rises in her charms,
> Repairs her smiles, awakens ev'ry grace
> And calls forth all the wonders of her face;
> Sees by degrees a purer blush arise
> And keener lightnings quicken in her eyes.
> The busy Sylphs surround their darling care,
> These set the head, and those divide the hair,
> Some fold the sleeve, while other plait the gown;
> And Betty's prais'd for labours not her own.

John Gay describes *The Toilette* of Lydia:

> She smooths her brow and frizles forth her hairs,
> And fancies youthful dress gives youthful airs;
> With crimson wool she fixes every grace,
> That not a blush can discompose her face.
> Reclin'd upon her arm she pensive sate,
> And curs'd th' inconstancy of youth too late.

In Wycherly's *Love in a Wood*, published in 1735, Dapperwit, who is trying to arouse Miss Lucy, says to Ranger:

'Pish, give her but leave to gape, rub her Eyes, and put on her Day-Pinner, the long Patch under the left Eye, awaken the Roses on her Cheeks with some Spanish Wool, and warrant her Breath with some Lemon-Peel, Doors fly off the Hinges, and she into my Arms. . . . Beauty's a Coward still without the Help of Art, and may have the Fortune of a Conquest, but cannot keep it: Beauty and Art can no more be asunder than Love and Honour.'

In 1715 J. Bettenham published *The Art of Beauty: A Poem*, a satiric jab at the artifices of the dressing table. In a dedication addressed 'To Belinda', Bettenham says:

'You have distinguished yourself in so remarkable a Manner by your admirable Skill and Knowledge in Cosmeticks, that you are now become, without any Assistance from Nature, one of our most celebrated Oxford Beauties, and no despicable Companion for the tawdriest Gown at the University.'

He then proceeds to dissect the art of artificial beauty step by step, including the gathering and compounding of the ingredients for washes and paints. Finally, after all of the grain has been reaped, the horn ground, the narcissus roots and honey gathered, the gum Arabic procured, and all of the ingredients properly blended, the lady sits at her dressing table and begins her cosmetic ritual:

> The Silver Ceruse first, ye Nymphs, prepare,
> In Native Whiteners exquisitely fair;
> Round this let *Nitre* clasp its Purple Arms,
> And rob itself to give the Ceruse charms,
> Till both in soft Embraces sweetly lost,
> One common, undistinguish'd Colour boast.
> The Rainbow-Flow'r with various Dies succeeds,
> The beauteous Product of *Illyria's* Meads;
> Blend all th' Ingredients on the Marble Stone,
> And crush the diff'ring Colours into one,
> Add balmy Honey, and the Work's compleat,
> The Nymph shall smile, and bless the pleasing Cheat.

THE SPECTATOR

Despite the prevalence of painting, most men disliked it. One Tuesday in the spring of 1711 there appeared in The *Spectator* a classic exchange which editors Addison and Steele said they were publishing not only as a reprimand to ladies for their over-generous use of paint, but as a warning to other men always to examine what they admired.

SIR,

Supposing you to be a Person of general Knowledge, I make my Application to you on a very particular Occasion. I have a great mind to be rid of my Wife, and hope, when you consider my Case, you will be of Opinion I have very just Pretensions to a Divorce. I am a mere Man of the Town and have very little Improvement but what I have got from Plays. I remember in *The Silent Woman* the Learned Dr. Cutberd, or Dr. Otter (I forget which) makes one of the Causes of Separation to be *Error Personae*, when a Man marries a Woman and finds her not to be the same Woman whom he intended to marry, but another. If that be Law, it is, I presume, exactly my Case. For you are to know, Mr. Spectator, that there are Women who do not let their Husbands see their Faces till they are married.

Not to keep you in suspence, I mean plainly that Part of the Sex who paint. They are some of them so exquisitely skilful this Way, that give them but a tolerable Pair of Eyes to set up with, and they will make Bosom, Lips, Cheeks, and Eye-brows, by their own Industry. As for my Dear, never Man was so enamoured as I was of her fair Forehead, Neck, and Arms, as well as the bright Jet of her Hair; but to my great Astonishment I find they were all the Effects of Art: Her Skin is so tarnished with this Practice, that when she first wakes in a Morning, she scarce seems young enough to be the Mother of her whom I carried to Bed the Night before. I shall take the Liberty to part with her by the first Opportunity, unless her Father will make her Portion suitable to her real, not her assumed, Countenance. This I thought fit to let him and her know by your Means.

I am, SIR,

Your most obedient,

humble Servant.

The sympathetic editor then expresses at some length his own opinions on the subject:

'I cannot tell what the Law, or the Parents of the Lady will do for this injured Gentleman, but must allow he has very much Justice on his Side. I have indeed very long observed this Evil and distinguished those of our Women who wear their own, from those in borrowed Complexions, by the *Picts* and the *British*. There does not need any great Discernment to judge which are which. The *British* have a lively animated Aspect; the *Picts*, tho' never so Beautiful, have dead uninformed Countenances . . . the same fixed Insensibility appears upon all Occasions. A *Pict*, tho' she takes all that Pains to invite the Approach of Lovers, is obliged to keep them at a certain Distance; a Sigh in a Languishing

Lover, if fetched too near her, would dissolve a Feature; and a Kiss snatched by a Forward one might transfer the Complexion of the Mistress to the Admirer. It is hard to speak of these false Fair Ones without saying something uncomplaisant, but I would only recommend to them to consider how they like coming into a Room new-painted; they may assure themselves, the near Approach of a Lady who uses this Practice is much more offensive.'

The editor then recounts the case of Will Honeycomb, who fell in love with a vain and ill-natured woman whose beauty, which seemed to increase each day, enslaved him. After she had jilted him and refused to see him, he was reduced to bribing her maid to let him observe her from behind some hangings in her dressing room. 'The *Pict*,' goes the story, 'begins the Face she designed to wear that Day, and I have heard him protest she had worked a full half-hour before he knew her to be the same Woman. As soon as he saw the Dawn of that Complexion, for which he had so long languished, he thought fit to break from his Concealment, repeating that of Chawley:

> Th' adorning Thee with so much Art,
>   Is but a barbarous Skill;
> 'Tis like the Pois'ning of a Dart,
>   Too apt before to kill.

'The *Pict* stood before him in the utmost Confusion, with the prettiest Smirk imaginable on the finished side of her Face, pale as Ashes on the other. Honeycomb seized all her Gally-pots and Washes, and carried off his Handkerchief full of Brushes, Scraps of Spanish Wool, and Phials of Unguents. The Lady went into the Country, the Lover was cured. . . .'

The letter and the editorial comment are followed by an

ADVERTISEMENT

A young Gentlewoman of about nineteen Years of Age (Bred in the Family of a Person of Quality lately deceased) who Paints the finest Flesh-Colour, wants a Place, and is to be heard of at the House of Minheer Grotesque a Dutch Painter in Barbican.

N.B. She is also well-skilled in the Drapery-part, and puts on Hoods and Mixes Ribbons so as to suit the Colours of the Face with great Art and Success.

The original letter may well have been written by the editors as the 'advertisement' surely was.

In France they painted even more. A Turkish ambassador, being asked his opinion of Frenchwomen, replied that he was no judge of painting. Writing of Versailles during the reign of Louis XIV, La Bruyère noted that the women of the district 'hasten the decline of their beauty by the use of artifices which they imagine will increase their charms: they paint their lips, cheeks, eyebrows, and shoulders, and liberally display them as well as their bosom, arms, and ears. . . . If by the fault of nature women became such as they make themselves by art, that is to say, if their complexion suddenly lost all its freshness and looked as fiery and leaden as they make it by the use of rouge and paint, they would be inconsolable. . . . If their wish is to be pleasing to men, if it is for the men's sake that they lay on their white and red paint, I have inquired into the matter, and I can tell them that in the opinion of men, or at least of the great majority, the use of white paint and rouge makes them hideous and disgusting; and that rouge, by itself, both ages and disguises them.'

LADY MARY ON TOUR

In 1716 Lady Mary Wortley Montagu was touring Europe, and in September she wrote to her sister from Vienna. Although she did not mention the ladies' makeup, she did include a description of the hair styles, which she found 'more monstrous and contrary to all common sense and reason than tis possible for you to imagine. They build certain fabricks of Gause on their heads about a yard high consisting of 3 or 4 storys fortify'd with numberless yards of heavy riband. The foundation of this structure is a thing they call a Bourlé, which is exactly of the same shape and kind, but about 4 times as big, as those rolls our prudent milk maids make use of to fix their Pails upon. This machine they cover with their own Hair, which they mix with a great deal of false, it being a particular beauty to have their heads too large to go into a moderate Tub. Their hair is prodigiously powder'd to conceal the mixture, and set out with 3 or 4 row of Bodkins, wonderfully large, that stick 2 or 3 inches from their Hair, made of Diamonds, Pearls, red, green, and yellow stones, that it certainly requires as much art and Experience to carry the Load upright as to dance upon May Day with the Girland. . . . You may easily suppose how much this extrordinary Dresse sets off and improves the natural Uglyness with which God Allmighty has been please'd to endow them all generally. Even the Lovely Empresse her selfe is oblig'd to comply in some degree with these absurd Fashions, which they would not quit for all the World.'

In December Lady Mary wrote to Lady Rich that all the women in Hanover 'have literally rosey cheeks, snowy Foreheads and bosoms, yet Eyebrows, and scarlet lips, to which they generally add Coal black Hair. These perfections never leave them till the hour of their Death and have a very fine Effect by Candlelight, but I could wish they were handsome with a little more variety. They ressemble one another as much as Mrs. Salmon's court of Great Brittain [a wax museum in Fleet Street], and are in as much danger of melting away by too near

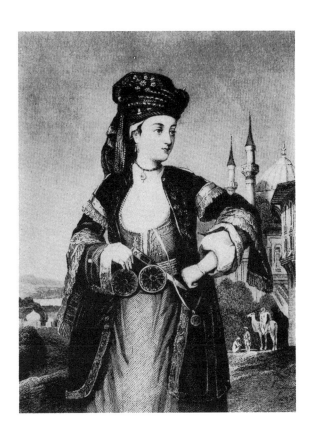

FIG. 124: Lady Mary Wortley Montagu
abroad. Nineteenth-century
engraving.

approaching the Fire, which they for that reason carefully avoid, tho' 'tis now
such excessive cold weather that I believe they suffer extremely by that piece of
selfe denial.'

Writing from Arianopole in 1717, Lady Mary described the Turkish women
as having 'naturally the most beautiful complexions in the World and generally
large black Eyes . . . . They generally shape their Eyebrows, and the Greeks and
Turks have a custom of putting round their Eyes on the inside a black Tincture
that, at a distance or by Candle-light, adds very much to the Blackness of them.
I fancy many of our Ladys would be overjoy'd to know this Secret, but tis too
visible by day. They dye their Nails rose colour; I own I cannot enough accustom
my selfe to this fashion to find any Beauty in it.'

A few weeks later Lady Mary reported her experience with the famous Balm
of Mecca, which was greatly coveted by English ladies:

'As to the Balm of Mecha, I will certainly send you some, but it is not so
easily got as you suppose it, and I cannot in Conscience advise you to make use
of it. I know not how it comes to have such universal Applause. All the Ladys
of my acquaintance at London and Vienna have begg'd me to send Pots of it to
them. I have had a present of a small quantity (which I'll assure you is very
valuable) of the best sort, and with great joy apply'd it to my face, expecting
some wonderfull Effect to my advantage. The next morning the change indeed

was wonderfull; my face was swell'd to a very extraordinary size and all over as red as my Lady's. It remain'd in this lamentable stage 3 days, during which you may be sure I pass'd my time very ill. I believ'd it would never be otherwise, and to add to my Mortification Mr. W reproach'd my indiscretion without ceasing. However, my Face is since in statu quo. Nay, I am told by the Ladys here that tis much mended by the operation, which I confess I cannot perceive in my Looking Glasse. Indeed, if one was to form an opinion of this Balm from their faces, one should think very well of it. They all make use of it and have the loveliest bloom in the world. For my part, I never intend to endure the pain of it again;—let my Complexion take its natural course and decay in its own due time. I have very little Esteem for med'cines of this Nature; but do as you please, Madam, only remember before you use it that your face will not be such as you'l care to shew in the drawing room for some days after.'

A year later she was writing to Lady Rich from Paris of the French ladies, whom she found 'monstrously unnatural in their paint! their Hair cut short and curl'd round their faces, loaded with powder that makes it look like white wool, and on their cheeks to their Chins, unmercifully laid on, a shineing red japan that glistens in a most flameing manner, that they seem to have no ressemblance to Humane faces, and I am apt to believe took the first bit of their dress from a fair sheep newly raddled. 'Tis with pleasure I recollect my dear pritty Country women, and if I was writeing to any body else I should say that these grotesque Dawbers give me still a higher esteem of the natural charms of dear Lady R's auborne hair and the lively colours of her unsully'd Complexion.'

In the spring of 1727 Lady Mary wrote to her sister of the scandalous passion of the sixty-three-year-old Duchess of Cleveland for the twenty-five-year-old Lord Sidney Beauclerk, the exceedingly handsome grandson of Nell Gwynn. Having mentioned the affair, she then describes it in twenty lines of verse:

> The God of Love, enrag'd to see
> The Nymph despise his Flame,
> At Dice and cards mispend her Nights
> And slight a nobler Game;
>
> For the Neglect of offers past
> And Pride in days of yore,
> He kindles up a Fire at last
> That burns her at threescore.
>
> A polish'd white is smoothly spread
> Where whilom wrinkles lay,
> And glowing with an artfull red
> She ogles at the Play.

Along the Mall she softly sails
In White and Silver drest,
Her neck expos'd to eastern Gales,
And Jewells on her breast.

Her children banish'd, Age forgot,
Lord Sidney is her care,
And, what is much a happier lot,
Has hopes to be her Heir.

THE POETS COMPLAIN

Satirizing painted women in verse was commonplace. A manuscript of the early eighteenth century contains several 'Posyes for Trenchers', four lines of which refer to the well-established custom of painting:

Feed and be fatt, heeres painted pears and plumbs
Will never hurt your teethe or spoyle your gums.
And I wishe those girls that painted are,
No other foode than such fine painted fare.

Posies were short epigrams, the shorter the better; and at the end of the sixteenth century, according to Puttenham, they were painted 'upon the back sides of our fruite trenchers of wood' or used 'as devises in rings, and armes, and about such courtly purposes'.

Matthew Prior, at one time Gentleman of the Bedchamber to the King of England, wrote many poems in praise of women and of love. But he also, from time to time, satirized their foibles, as in a poem about *Phillis's Age*:

How old may Phillis be, you ask,
    Whose Beauty thus all Hearts engages?
To Answer is no easie Task:
    For She has really two Ages.

Stiff in Brocard, and pinch'd in Stays,
    Her Patches, Paint, and Jewels on;
All Day let Envy view her Face;
    And Phillis is but Twenty-one.

Paint, Patches, Jewels laid aside,
    At Night Astronomers agree,
The Evening has the Day bely'd;
    And Phillis is some Forty-three.

In *Jinny the Just*, a thirty-five-verse poem printed for the first time in 1907, Matthew Prior again criticized women's painting:

Of such terrible beauty She never cou'd boast
As with absolute Sway o'er all hearts rules the roast
When J —— bawls out to the Chair for a Toast;

But of good Household Features her Person was made,
Nor by Faction cry'd up nor of Censure afraid,
And her beauty was rather for Use than Parade.

Her Blood so well mix't and flesh so well Pasted
That tho her Youth faded her Comliness lasted;
The blew was wore off, but the Plum was well tasted.

Less smooth than her Skin and less white than her breast
Was this pollisht stone beneath which she lyes prest:
Stop, Reader, and Sigh while thou thinkst on the rest.

Although it is seldom mentioned, some ladies of fashion in the early eighteenth century evidently wore false eyebrows. Prior was so delighted with the possibilities for mishaps to false eyebrows that it required four poems to exhaust his invention and his interest:

A REASONABLE AFFLICTION

From her own native France as old Alison past,
She reproach'd English Nell with Neglect or with Malice,
That the Slattern had left in the Hurry and Haste,
Her Lady's Complection and Eye-brows at Calais.

ANOTHER

Her Eye-brow-box one Morning lost,
(The best of Folks are oftenest crost)
Sad Helen thus to Jenny said,
Her careless but afflicted Maid;
Put me to bed then, wretched Jane;
Alas! when shall I rise again?
I can behold no mortal now:
For what's an eye without a brow.

ON THE SAME SUBJECT

In a dark corner of the House
    Poor Helen sits, and sobs and cries;
She will not see her loving Spouse,
    Nor her more dear Picquet-allies;
Unless she finds her Eye-brows,
    She'll e'en weep out her Eyes.

ON THE SAME SUBJECT

Helen was just slipt into bed;
Her Eye-brows on the toilet lay;
    Away the Kitten with them fled,
As fees belonging to her prey.

For this Misfortune careless Jane,
Assure yourself, was loudly rated;
    And Madam getting up again,
With her own hand the Mouse-trap baited.

On little things, as Sages write,
Depends our human joy, or sorrow;
    If we don't catch a Mouse to-night,
Alas! no Eye-brows for to-morrow.

PATCHING

In 1711 the *Spectator* noted that women looked like angels and, the editors added, 'they would be more beautiful than the sun, were it not for the little black spots that break out in their faces, and sometimes rise in very odd figures. I have observed that those little blemishes wear off very soon; but when they disappear in one part of the face they are very apt to break out in another. Insomuch that I have seen a spot in the forehead in the afternoon which was upon the chin in the morning!'

The little blemishes, cut out of silk or velvet or even paper and applied with mastic, continued to wander about the faces of women — and sometimes men — throughout the century. A prominent marquise is reported to have appeared at a party wearing sixteen of them, one in the shape of a tree on which were perched two love birds. Sometimes the patches were cut in the shape of silhouettes of friends or family. At Zwickau in 1705 beauty patches were prohibited by law, but elsewhere they were rampant.

The political significance of patching was pointed out in the summer of 1711 by a correspondent who had observed at the opera two parties of well-dressed women, seated in opposite side-boxes, evidently 'drawn up in a kind of battle-array one against another. After a short survey of them, I found they were patched differently; the faces on one hand being spotted on the right side of the forehead, and those upon the other on the left. I quickly perceived that they cast hostile glances upon one another, and that their patches were placed in those different situations as party-signals to distinguish friends from foes. In the middle boxes, between these two opposite bodies, were several ladies who patched indifferently on both sides of their faces, and seemed to sit there with no intention but to see the opera. Upon inquiry, I found that the body of Amazons on my right hand were Whigs, and those on my left Tories; and that those who had placed themselves in the middle boxes were a neutral party, whose faces had not yet declared themselves.'

An anonymous correspondent to the *Spectator* in January 1712 described a female puppet he had examined at the shop of a French milliner, who assured him that the puppet's complexion reflected the latest fashion in Paris. The correspondent complained about a small patch on its breast, which, he said, he could not suppose was 'placed there with any good design'.

A correspondent to *The Gentleman's Magazine* in 1732, referring to what seemed to him strange customs in hair, beards, and complexions, wrote:

'Our Ladies formerly would not stir out of doors without a Mask; now they wear none. We look on it as ridiculous in the Savage Women to think to set off their Faces with the Figures of Trees, Animals, or Butterflies: Is it less so in our Ladies to cover their Faces with Patches, as if full of flies?'

Patches required patch boxes, called *boites à mouches* by the French. They were usually rectangular, sometimes oval or round, and in appearance often very like snuff boxes, though flatter. Although any small box could be used as a patch box and may often have been, those designed for the purpose were hinged and had a small mirror inside the cover for convenience in applying the patches away from one's dressing table. These boxes, especially the ones now to be found in museums, were often exquisitely made by the finest goldsmiths and silversmiths of the day and sometimes even decorated by famous painters. In the seventeenth century carved wooden boxes were not unusual (Plate 14-G). Miniature portraits often appeared on the boxes (Plate 17-K). Patch boxes for the dressing table were more likely to be of porcelain or enamel (Plates 15-20), often considerably larger than the elegant flat boxes designed to be carried about (Plates 18-H and 20-E, for example). Madame Pompadour used an enamelled patch box in the form of a swan.

Tiny gold boxes designed to hold both rouge and patches (*boites à rouge et à*

PLATE 15 : EIGHTEENTH-CENTURY
COSMETICS CONTAINERS

A 1760's, English. Blue glass scent
   bottle, enamelled and gilded.
   (*Victoria and Albert Museum*)
B 1755, English. Staffordshire salt-
   glaze patch box. (*British Museum*)
C 1760s, English. Patch box matching
   scent bottle in A, above. (*Victoria
   and Albert Museum*)
D 1780, English. Wedgewood per-
   fume bottle. (*British Museum*)
E Patch box, painted enamel on
   copper. About 2 inches in diameter.
   (*Dublin National Museum*)
F 1776, English. Leeds cream-ware
   patch box.
G Mid-century, French. White enam-
   elled pomatum jar with silver
   mountings.
H *c.* 1720–1735, French (St Cloud).
   Pomatum jar in soft-paste porce-
   lain. Design in deep blue on white.
   Style of Bérain. About 2¼ inches
   high. (*Metropolitan Museum of
   Art, New York*)

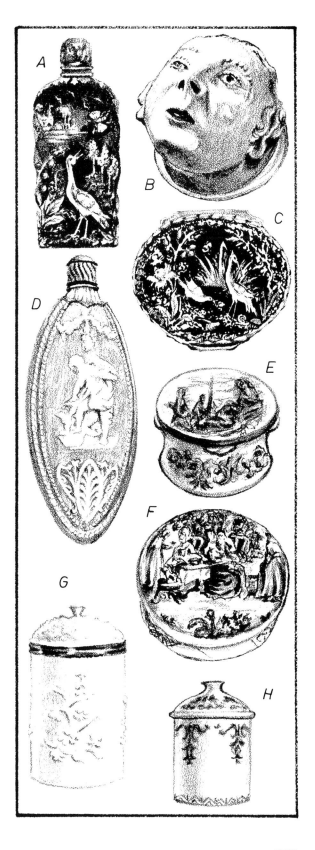

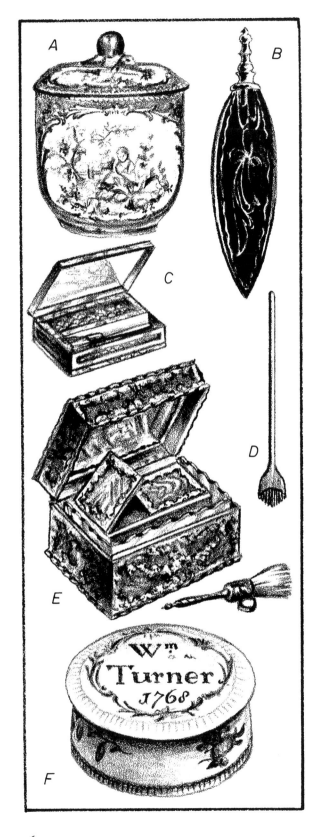

PLATE 16 : EIGHTEENTH-CENTURY
COSMETICS CONTAINERS
AND ACCESSORIES

A   Mid-century, French. Pomatum jar of Sèvres porcelain. (*Metropolitan Museum of Art, New York*)

B   Moroccan. Antimony box of black wood inlaid with design in silver wire. $3\frac{7}{8}$ inches long. (*Dublin National Museum*)

C   1784–89, French. Enamelled gold rouge and patch box. Hinged cover on both top and bottom. About 2 inches long. (*Metropolitan Museum of Art, New York*)

D   Probably *c.* 1770, English. Eyebrow comb used by fops.

E   1747–48, French. Rouge box of chased gold with agate panels. There are 2 inner compartments with gold and agate lids, a compartment for a chased gold brush, and a mirror in the inside of the cover. Size, $2\frac{1}{8} \times 1\frac{5}{8} \times 1\frac{1}{4}$ inches.

F   1768, English. Leeds patch box.

PLATE 17 contd.

K   Oval rouge box. Milk glass with enamelled metal cover, inscribed 'In Remembrance of a Friend'. About $1\frac{1}{2}$ inches in diameter. (*Museum of Art, Edinburgh*)

L   *c.* 1750, French. Ivory and tortoise-shell patch box with painted miniature. About 3 inches in diameter. (*Dublin National Museum*)

PLATE 17 : EIGHTEENTH-CENTURY
COSMETICS CONTAINERS

A First quarter, French (St Cloud). Covered rouge jar of soft-paste porcelain. Gold on white. (*Metropolitan Museum of Art, New York*)

B *c.* 1750, German (Meissen). Patch box with flat back and hinged cover for hanging on the wall. Porcelain with gold. (*Victoria and Albert Museum*)

C English. Patch box of enamelled copper. Printed transfer motto on cover — 'To the fairest and the rarest'. Deep blue enamel box with white top. About ¾ inch in diameter. (*Dublin National Museum*)

D English. Oval patch box of enamelled copper, inscribed 'I give to receive what will not deceive'. Blue-green enamel with white top. (*Dublin National Museum*)

E Chinese. Box for vermilion in soapstone porcelain. Blue on greyish white. (*Victoria and Albert Museum*)

F English. Patch box of enamelled copper. (*Dublin National Museum*)

G English. Patch box of enamelled copper. Orchid enamel, about 1 inch in diameter. (*Dublin National Museum*)

H Japanese, probably eighteenth century. Ivory makeup box with 2 compartments. Shown without outer cover. About 2½ inches long. (*Dublin National Museum*)

I English. Rouge pot of tin-glazed earthenware ('delftware'). The entire bottom section of the pot is solid, leaving only a very shallow depression for the rouge. (*Victoria and Albert Museum*)

J *c.* 1750, French. Gold and agate rouge box. About 2½ x 3 inches. (*Metropolitan Museum of Art, New York*)

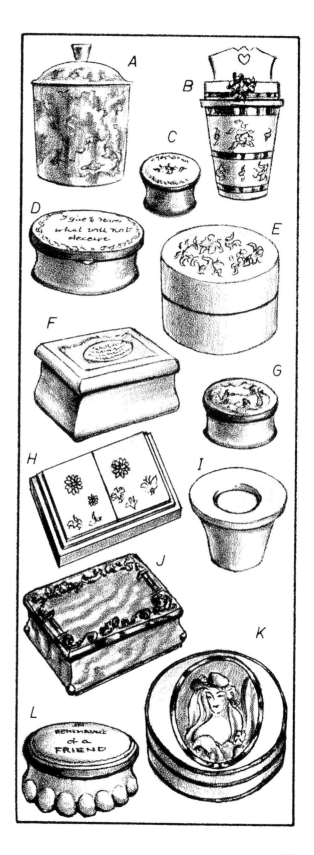

PLATE 18 : EIGHTEENTH-CENTURY
COSMETICS CONTAINERS

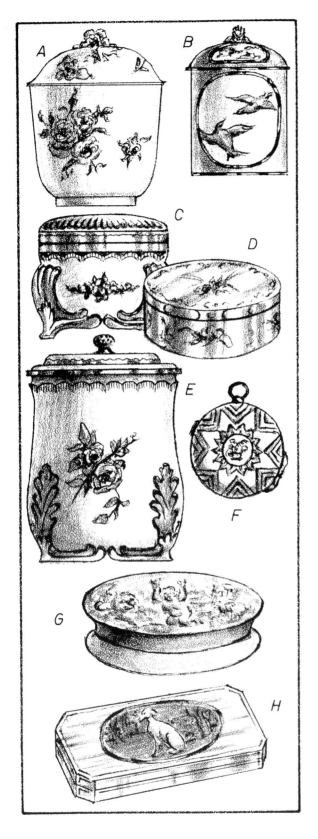

A   *c.* 1750–60, French. Pomatum jar of soft-paste porcelain.

B   1756, French (Sèvres). Pomatum jar of soft-paste porcelain, one of a matching pair. Green with gold edging, rose-coloured flower on cover. (*Metropolitan Museum of Art, New York*)

C   1763, 1764. Patch box of Sèvres porcelain. Part of a toilet service consisting of 2 powder bowls, 2 patch boxes, 2 pomatum pots, clothes brush, and shaving brush. White and apple green, enriched with gold and painted with flowers. About 3 inches in diameter. (*Wallace Collection*)

D   1759, 1760, French. Oval patch box of vari-coloured gold. About 2¾ inches long. (*Metropolitan Museum of Art, New York*)

E   1763, 1764. Pomatum jar of Sèvres porcelain. Part of a toilet service (see C above). About 5 inches high. (*Wallace Collection*)

F   Late eighteenth century, English. Patch box of enamelled copper. (*Dublin National Museum*)

G   *c.* 1797, French. Carved boxwood patch box, inscribed 'Le Lion de France'. About 3 inches in diameter. (*Victoria and Albert Museum*)

H   Late eighteenth century, Paris. Gold patch box with miniature painted on ivory. Signed 'Isabey'. About 4 inches long. (*Metropolitan Museum of Art, New York*)

PLATE 19 : EIGHTEENTH-CENTURY
COSMETICS CONTAINERS
AND ACCESSORIES

A   c. 1755, French (Mennecy). Patch box of soft-paste porcelain. Silver mountings. About 2½ inches long. (*Metropolitan Museum of Art, New York*)

B   1795, English. Mahogany pomatum jar, one of 3 in a dressing table. The bottom rim is attached to the table top, and the jar sits down into it. (*Metropolitan Museum of Art, New York*)

C   1782–83, French. Gold and enamel rouge and patch box. Brush is missing from the front compartment. Box can be opened from either top or bottom. (*Metropolitan Museum of Art, New York*)

D   1773–74, French. Double-lidded patch box of translucent royal blue enamel and gold. There are 2 compartments with enamelled covers and an open compartment for the brush. Mirror is in the cover. Size, $2\frac{3}{16}$ x $1\frac{5}{8}$ x $\frac{7}{8}$ inches. (*Louvre*)

E   1778, French. Gold rouge box decorated with opalescent peach enamel and borders of orange and white. Diameter, 1¾ inches.

F   c. 1750, French. Patch box of Sèvres porcelain. Designed to hang on the wall. Note similarity to patch box shown in Plate 16-B.

G   English. Patch box of Battersea enamel.

H   English. Patch box of Battersea enamel.

I   c. 1790. Ivory patch box with Wedgewood cameo. About 3 inches in diameter. (*Brooklyn Museum*)

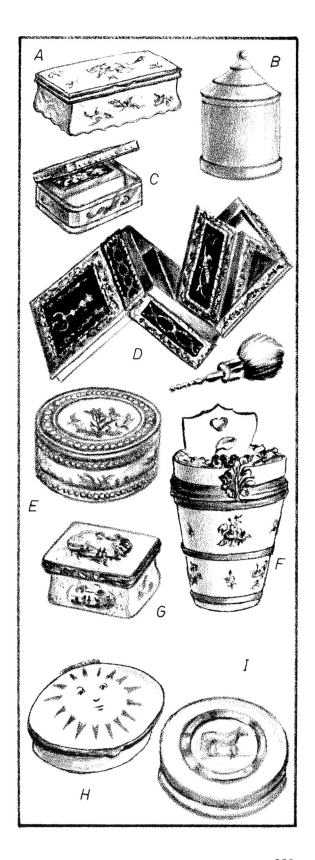

209

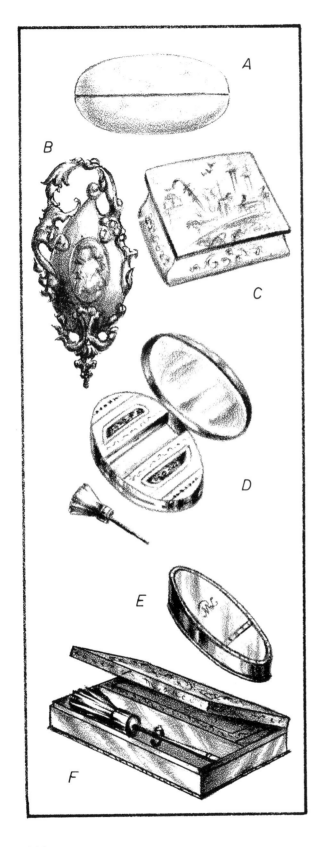

PLATE 20 : EIGHTEENTH-CENTURY
            COSMETICS CONTAINERS
            AND ACCESSORIES

A Chinese, Ch'ing Dynasty. Peach-bloom porcelain rouge box with cover. (*Metropolitan Museum of Art, New York*)

B Early years, French. Scent flask of carved boxwood. (*Victoria and Albert Museum*)

C Mid-century, English. Enamelled patch box. (*Art Institute, Chicago*)

D 1787, Paris. Gold patch box with mirror and rouge brush, decorated with deep blue and white enamel. (*British Museum*)

E 1781–82, London. Silver patch box. A snuff box in the same pattern was deeper and was hinged at the centre. (*Art Institute, Chicago*)

F 1783, Paris. Gold box for rouge and patches. (*Metropolitan Museum of Art, New York*) *mouches*) were popular, and a good many are still to be seen in museums (Plates 16-C, 19-C-D, and 20-D-F). Usually there were two lids, the principal one with a mirror on the inside. This part of the box was divided into two or three compartments, one of them open and containing a tiny round makeup brush with a gold handle. The other compartment or compartments, always covered, could be used for rouge, eyeshadow, or any other cosmetic. The underside of the box, with its own lid, contained a shallow compartment well suited to holding patches.

Criticism of patching continued; and when Massilon, bishop of Clermont, preached against the fashion, more patches than ever were worn and were called *mouches de Massilon*. They were generally considered to make a woman look younger. Madame de Genlis is quoted as remarking to a gentleman whom she had just permitted to watch her apply some patches to her face, 'Well, what do you think of that! Would you not take me for a girl of twenty?'

MEN AND COSMETICS

Many men of the period patched and painted, some obviously, some not. The obvious ones were a favourite subject for satire, as in this first stanza of a song from Thomas Baker's *Hampstead Heath*, published in 1706:

> A wig that's full
> An empty scull,
> A box of burgamot;
> A hat ne'er made
> To fit his head,
> No more than that to plot.
> A hand that's white,
> A ring that's right,
> A word-knot, patch and feather;
> A gracious smile,
> And grounds and oyl,
> Do very well together.

The 'hat ne'er made to fit his head' refers to the custom of carrying the hat under the arm so as not to disarrange the enormous curled and powdered periwig. Tom D'Urfey, in one of his songs mentions

> ... beaus that in boxes
> Lye snuggling their doxies,
> With wigs that hang down to their bums.

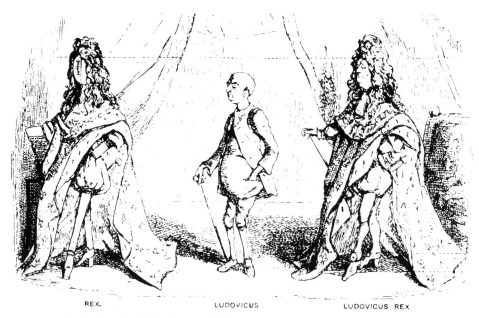

REX.   LUDOVICUS   LUDOVICUS REX

FIG. 125: 'Ludovicus Rex'. Caricature of Louis XIV. From Thackeray's *Paris Sketch-Book*, 1840.

D'Urfey has more to say about fops in a song from his comedy *The Modern Prophets*:

> I hate a fop that at his glass
>   Stands prinking half the day;
> With a sallow, frowsy, olive-colour'd face,
> With a powder'd peruke hanging to his wast,
> Who with ogling imagines to possess.
> And to hew his shape doth cringe and scrape,
>   But nothing has to say.

Book II of Joseph Thurston's *The Toilette*, a criticism of over-emphasis on personal decoration and under-emphasis on natural beauty, pertains to men, with emphasis on hair and dress:

> At Eyes alone our Beaus direct their Art,
> Nor know the nobler Conquest of the Heart;
> With her own Arms a Mistress they pursue,
> Snuff, Powder, Patches, Paste, and Billets doux.
> Man's hardy Mould is in his Habit lost,
> And Beaus assume the Softness of their Toast. . . .

I have beheld a Beau of hapless mind,
To some old Peruque add a Tail behind;
Then, Pleas'd, survey the inconsistent Grace,
And claim Alliance with the Pig-tail Race:
How would our Conoisseurs be pleas'd to see
Debilitated Bob commence Toupet!
Of all Improvements this appears the worst,
For Queues, like Poets, must be born at first.

In Book III Thurston returns to the ladies, mentioning jewelry, dress, and beauty, inner and outer, but, curiously, never a word about makeup. And yet rouge was so much a part of eighteenth-century life that it seemed quite natural to make up the dead to give them a lifelike appearance. Even Cardinal Pamphili was rouged for lying in state in Rome.

11 · The Mid-Eighteenth Century
1737-1770

What makes Clodio, who always was fond of new faces,
So notoriously constant to Fulvia's embraces?
Ask Fulvia the cause — she can tell you the true one,
Who makes her old face every morning a new one.

ANONYMOUS

By this time the clergy had wearied of its ranting against cosmetics, though it had not entirely given in. The Bishop of Amiens, on being asked by a lady for his advice about the wearing of rogue, replied, 'One casuist affirms in one sense, a second casuist in another. I choose, my dear madam, a happy medium; I sanction *rouging*. Paint, dear daughter, paint, since you so wish; but only on one cheek dear lady!' Whereupon the good lady laughed, it is said, till both her cheeks were red.

PAINTED LADIES

In 1740 Horace Walpole wrote from Florence to Henry Seymour Conway about Lady Mary Wortley, who, he said, 'is laughed at by the whole town. Her dress, her avarice, and her impudence must amaze any one that never heard her name. She wears a foul mob that does not cover her greasy black locks, that hang loose, never combed or curled; an old mazarine blue wrapper that gapes open and discovers a canvas petticoat. Her face swelled violently on one side with the remains of a ———— , partly covered with a plaister, and partly with white paint, which for cheapness she has bought so coarse that you would not use it to wash a chimney.' The word omitted by the publisher was probably 'gumma', an indication of siphilis, which Lady Mary is not known to have had.

At another time Walpole described a well-known lady of the day as having 'large fierce black eyes rolling beneath lofty arched eyebrows, two acres of cheeks spread with crimson, an ocean of neck that overflowed and was not distinguishable from the lower part of her body, and no portion of which was restrained by stays'.

But it was not only the men who were critical of women's painting. In one issue of *The Female Spectator*, Eliza Hayward remarked that she did not descend 'so low as to take notice of the curling-irons, the false locks, the eyebrow shapers,

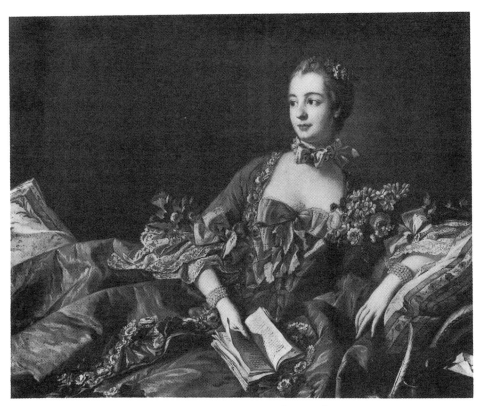

FIG. 126: Madame de Pompadour (1721–64). Painting by Boucher.

the pearl cosmetic, the Italian red, or any of those injudiciously called face-mending stratagems'. It was in 1740 that Mary Granville Pendarvis described Lady Baltimore as looking 'like a *frightened owl*, her locks strutted out and most furiously greased, or rather gummed and powdered'.

There were still high-ranking women who flaunted fashion and refused to paint. Marie-Thérèse of Spain, first wife of the Dauphin Louis (son of Louis XV and father of Louis XVI), objected to painting her face. But upon her arrival in France in 1745, the King made it clear that she would be expected to follow the French fashion, which demanded a chalk-white face, black patches, and flaming red cheeks. And the more the natural charms faded, the more heavily the paint was applied. Madame de Pompadour's final act, after receiving the last rites from her priest, was to rouge her face. Then she closed her eyes and fell asleep, and presently she was dead.

In 1750 Horace Walpole was still reporting on women's cosmetic habits. In a letter to Horace Mann he quoted some verses current at the time. One of them, quoted at the beginning of the chapter, refers to Lady Caroline Petersham and

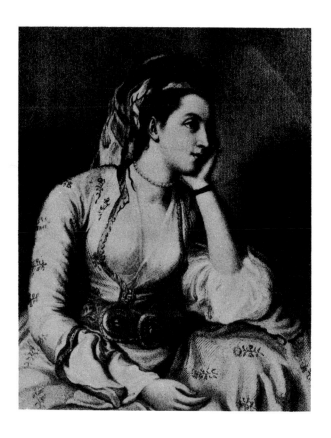

FIG. 127: Maria, Lady Coventry, 1753. One of the famous Gunning sisters, she met an early death as a result of using makeup containing poisonous white lead. Engraving by H. Cook, 1835.

her lover, Harry Vane. Another, entitled *Who is This?*, is about Lady Caroline and her friend Elizabeth Ashe:

> Her face has beauty, we must all confess,
> But beauty on the brink of ugliness:
> Her mouth's a rabbit feeding on a rose;
> With eyes — ten times too good for such a nose!
> Her blooming cheeks — what paint could ever draw 'em?
> That paint, for which no mortal ever saw 'em.
> Air without shape — or royal race divine —
> 'Tis Emily — oh! fie! — 'tis Caroline.

Two months later, in writing to George Montagu, he reported going in the evening to pick up Lady Caroline at her house, where he 'found her and the little Ashe, or the pollard Ashe, as they call her; they had just finished their last layer of red and looked as handsome as crimson could make them'.

Two years later, again writing to Horace Mann, Walpole reported on the return of Lady Caroline and Lady Coventry (Figure 127) from Paris: 'The French would not conceive that Lady Caroline Petersham ever had been handsome, nor that my Lady Coventry has much pretence to be so now. . . . Poor Lady Coventry was under piteous disadvantages; for besides being very silly, ignorant of the world, breeding, speaking no French, and suffered to wear neither red nor powder, she had that perpetual drawback upon her beauty, her lord, who is sillier in a wise way, as ignorant, ill-bred, and speaking very little French himself —just enough to show how ill-bred he is. . . . He is jealous, prude, and scrupulous; at a dinner at Sir John Bland's, before sixteen persons he coursed his wife round the table, on suspecting she had stolen on a little red, seized her, scrubbed it off by force with a napkin, and then told her that since she had deceived him and broke her promise, he would carry her back directly to England.'

Lord Coventry was, however, no more successful than other men throughout history in attempting to dictate women's fashions, singly or en masse. The lady continued to paint, subtly at first, then more boldly, and presumably he adjusted to it.

But men other than her husband found her painting excessive. Lord Chesterfield wrote that 'Lady Coventry adorns herself too much, for I was near her enough to see manifest that she had laid on a great deal of white which she did not want, and which will soon destroy both her natural complexion and her teeth.' And in a very short time it destroyed her as well. At twenty-seven she died of the poisonous paints (some say of consumption), and in the last days of her illness her once-beautiful face had become so ravaged that she kept the curtains of her bed drawn and refused to permit a lamp in the room. Her younger sister (Figure 128) also fell seriously ill from use of the paints, but she survived.

THE USE OF ROUGE

Many men rouged, though not so heavily as the women—at least, not for a while. But in 1768, when English dandies were beginning to paint their cheeks and lips, blacken their eyebrows, and perfume themselves, they were mercilessly satirized by writers and caricaturists, as in the following verse:

> A coxcomb, a fop, a dainty milk-sop
> Who, essenced and dizened from bottom to top,
> Looks just like a doll for a milliner's shop;
> A thing full of prate and pride and conceit,
>   All fashion, no weight,
> Who shrugs and takes snuff, and carries a muff,
> A minnikin, finicking French powder-puff.

Children's rouge often rivalled that of their mothers. When Henrietta, the young daughter of Louis XV, died, her face was painted as heavily as it had been in life. It is said that Marie Leszcynska, queen of Louis XV, though she painted a little on canvas, was the only woman at court who did not paint her face. A pious woman, concerned more with domestic than with social matters and more interested in improving her mind than her appearance, the Queen simply had no wish to display herself or to participate in what seemed to her the frivolous and fruitless activities of the court. In the painted eighteenth century, this seemed eccentric, to say the least. By this time the painting had been going on for so long and had become so much an accepted part of life that there was only occasional criticism of it on either moral or aesthetic grounds.

Casanova was of the opinion that the rouge, though excessive, had its attractions and that the charm of the ladies' painted faces lay in the carelessness with which the rogue was applied, without the slightest attempt at naturalness. 'It is put on,' he wrote, 'to please the eye, for it creates the illusion of sensuality, promising fulfillment in orgies of love.'

In David Garrick's *Miss in her Teens* (1747), we find the description of an attentive male friend who seems to enjoy the young lady's toilette without being stimulated to provoke an orgy:

> He speaks like a lady for all the world, and never swears, as Mr. Flesh does, but wears nice white gloves, and tells me what ribands become my complexion, where to stick my patches, who is the best milliner, where they sell the best tea, and which is the best wash for the face and the best paste for the hands; he is always playing with my fan, and showing his teeth; and when ever I speak, he pats me — so — and cries, 'The devil take me, Miss Biddy, but you'll be my perdition — ha, ha, ha !'

Sir Harry Beaumont, in his *Crito: A Dialogue on Beauty* (1752), though far more tolerant than many of his contemporaries, objected strongly to the excessive makeup of the French:

'The Covering each Cheek all over with a burning Sort of red Colour, has long been look'd upon in a neighbouring Country to be . . . necessary to render a fine Lady's Face completely beautiful. . . . The First time I saw the Ladies all rouged in the Front of the Boxes at the Opera in Paris, they seem'd to me to look like a long Bed of high-colour'd full-blown Peonies in a Garden.'

A portrait of Marie de Verrières, painted by Drouais in 1761, shows her very heavily rouged all along the cheekbone, close to the eye, the rouge extending from nose to ear and downwards in a generally triangular pattern over most of the cheek. A French portrait by Nattier, dated 1756, shows the rouge applied in a round pattern on the most prominent part of the cheekbone. In Nattier's portrait of Madame de Pompadour we find a round pattern placed

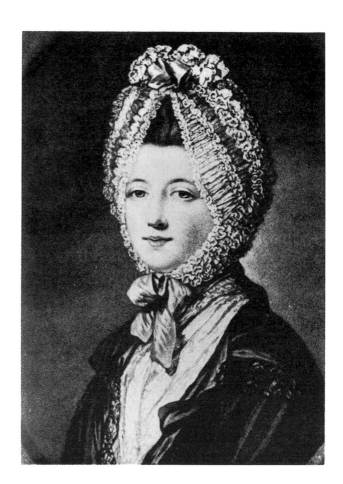

FIG. 128: Elizabeth Gunning, Duchess of Hamilton and later Duchess of Argyll. Like her sister, Lady Coventry, she was noted for her beauty. Engraving by John Finlayson.

slightly lower on the cheek. And in a mid-century French portrait by Van Loo, the rouge is bright pink, in a round pattern, placed low and near the mouth. There are tiny rosebud lips, natural brown eyebrows, and hair powdered grey.

Reports from Abroad

Leopold Mozart, father of the composer, wrote to his wife from Paris in 1763 that he really could not say whether Parisian women were beautiful or not since they were 'painted like Nuremberg dolls, and so disfigured by this repulsive trick that the eyes of an honest German cannot recognize a naturally beautiful woman when he sees her'.

In the summer of 1765 Lady Sarah Bunbury wrote to Lady Susan O'Brien from Paris about the fashions there:

'There are very few handsome women in Paris: the Dss de la Valliere, who is fifty-two, is the handsomest woman I saw, but indeed she is extraordinary.

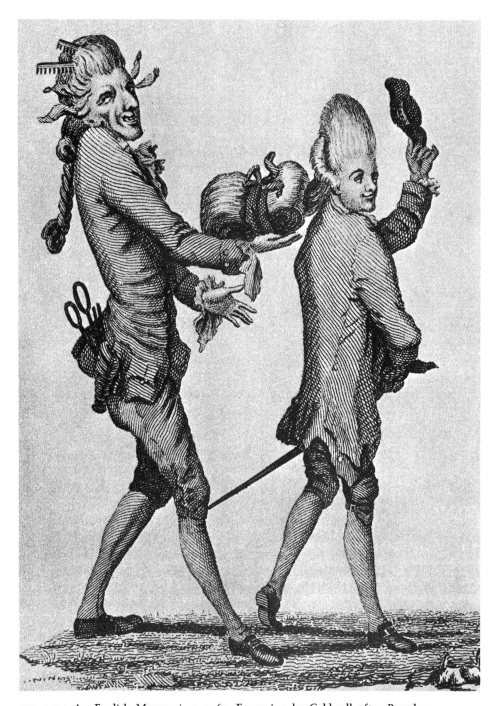

FIG. 129: An English Macaroni, *c.* 1760. Engraving by Caldwell after Brandom.

Her face is now as beautiful as an angel, & really looks only twenty-five; her person is bad, but she hides that with a cloak. The Pss of Monaco is reckoned a great beauty there, here she only would be a very pretty woman; her face is round & flat, but her countenance is meek & sweet, her complection very fine, & her figure the most perfect of any woman in the world, I believe. She is the only lady who don't wear rouge, for all the rest daub themselves so horribly that it's shocking. Madme D'Egmont is the next beauty: she has a pretty Chinese face, is very affected & fashionable & so is made a beauty. The Pss of Chimay, who is my favourite, is not reckoned a beauty; she is quite unaffected & simple in her manner, her figure is like Ly Mary FitzPatrick's but taller, her head is like the Gunnings', her complection good if she did not ruin it, her eyes small & dark, & she has regular, small features.'

Sir Harry considered the two prettiest women he had ever seen to be 'the Duchess of B***, in France, and Mrs. A***, in England; and the very Reason why I should give the Preference to the latter of the Two is that the former is obliged, by the Fashions of the Country where she lives, to heighten the Colour of the Roses which Nature has scattered over her Cheeks, into one great Mass of Vermilion.

'Were a Frenchman, on his first Coming over hither, to see a Set of our greatest Beauties all in a Row, he might probably think them like a Bed of Lilies; or, at least, like a Border of light-colour'd Pinks.' The Prince of Annanaboo expressed the opinion that a celebrated English beauty 'would be the most charming Woman in the World if she was but a Negro'. But it was only the fashionable, upper-class women who were pale, not their servants. 'The honest Rustic,' says Beaumont, 'can think himself happy in his Woman of a good strong Make and sun-burnt frowsy Complexion.'

Richard Chandler described with admirable detail the eye makeup used by contemporary Greek women:

'For colouring the lashes and sockets of the eye, they throw incense of gum laudanum on some coals of fire; the smoke which ascends is intercepted with a plate, in order to collect the soot. This I saw applied. A girl sitting, cross-legged as usual, on a sofa, closing one of her eyes, took the two lashes between the fore-finger and thumb of her left hand, pulled them forward, and then thrusting in, at the external corner, a sort of bodkin or probe which had been immersed in the soot, and withdrawing it, the particles previously adhering to the probe remained within the eye-lashes.'

In addition, they cleansed their skin thoroughly, whitened their teeth, darkened their eyebrows, reddened their lips, and painted their cheeks with *sulama*, which, Van Egmont reported, not only reddened them beautifully, but imparted to the skin 'a remarkable gloss', giving the effect of porcelain. Van Egmont added that the artifice could be easily discovered by chewing on a clove, then breathing on the lady's face, which would immediately turn yellow. He did not say whether this lack of gallantry was customary among men (or jealous women) or whether it was, perhaps, merely experimental on his part. But he did add that because of the mercury content of the paint, the teeth of the user were badly damaged. Greek girls, he reported, sometimes gilded their faces, especially on their wedding day. This was considered to be 'irresistibly charming'.

One of the most highly coloured families in Europe was that of the Duke of Medina. Travellers, it is said, went miles out of their way to see them. When he was young, the Duke wore a lump of vermilion on one temple to match a wen on the other. Later he married such an extravagantly painted woman that the local wits speculated as to whether or not, when their faces were juxtaposed, the colours ran together. And Walpole described Benedetta, the duke's sister, whose colour increased with age, as being painted and peeled like an old summer house, with her chin bristles sprouting through the plaster.

Fashionable ladies, who often spent hours being enamelled and coiffed, would sit in state for an hour or so in order that friends and their servants might see what had been wrought. It is reported that a lady's maid, arriving late at a party, explained that she had gone to see the Duchess of Montrose, who was 'only showed from two to four'.

The elderly Duchess of Bedford was too impatient for all that sitting. Horace Walpole wrote to George Montagu in 1761 of the coronation of George III, reporting the 'Lord Bolinbroke put on rouge upon his wife and the Duchess of Bedford in the Painted Chamber; the Duchess of Queensberry told me of the latter, that she looked like an orange-peach, half red and half yellow'. Two years later he wrote to Horace Mann:

'Did I, or did I not, tell you how much I am diverted with his Serenity of Modena's match with that old, battered, painted, debauched Simonetta? . . . Two-and-twenty years ago she was as much repaired as Lady Mary Wortley, or as her own new spouse. Why, if they were not past approaching them, their faces must run together like a palette of colours, and they would be disputing to which such an eyebrow or such a cheek belonged.'

In describing life in eighteenth-century Venice, Philippe Monnier writes:

'Look well upon this Don Alonso, as he enters, bows, kisses his lady's hand, and . . . settles himself smiling on the edge of an arm-chair. He is a curious character. Adorned, bedizened, smart as a tailor's dummy is this man, made up, as Ugo Foscolo says, entirely of negatives; being neither lover, friend, nor valet, and yet partaking of the functions of all three. . . . He is one of the most familiar figures in eighteenth-century Venice. He is the cicisbeo or *cavaliere sirvente*. . . . The cicisbeo visits her when she is abed or newly risen, at her toilet, in her morning-gown. He receives all her confidences and knows all her secrets. . . . He hunts for the pin to fasten her neckerchief, hands her the mirror when she would dress her hair, hands brush and scent-bottle, manicure-set, hare's foot,

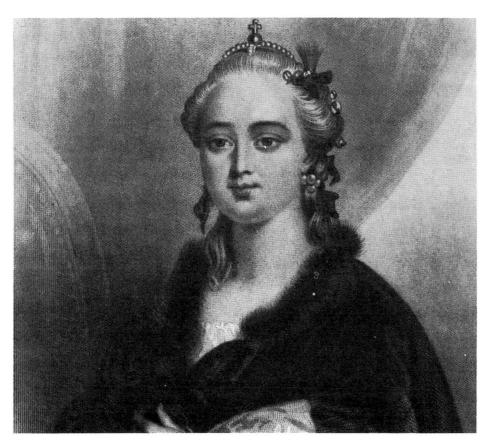

FIG. 130: Catherine the Great (1729–96). Nineteenth-century steel engraving. Note her full face and lips, double chin, large, dark eyes and full, dark brows.

powder-box, and powder-puff. Familiar as a lady's-maid with clasps and buttons, he acts upon a nod or gesture. He moistens the tip of his finger, seizes a beauty-spot, and plants it on the place appropriate; he knows where to put "the man-slayer", "the coquette", the saucy, the passionate, the rakish, the majestic beauty-spots — the last being set in the middle of the forehead.'

In the early autumn of 1764 Mrs James Harris (later Lady Malmesbury), writing to her son, commented that the Spanish Ambassadress was 'very well in her person, and not a disagreeable face, but with rather too much yellow mixed with the red; she appears to be between thirty and forty, and, without joking, would look very agreeable if she added blanc to the rouge instead of gamboge'. It was about this time that kissing on the forehead was introduced since it was the 'only spot on the face where the touch would not risk a confusion of complexions'.

Women of the Middle East had been painting for centuries. Lady Mary herself

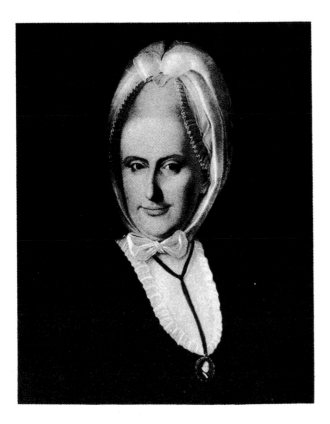

wrote from India about a visiting Moorish lady of high rank, who was 'slim, genteel, and middle-sized; her complexion tawny, as all the Moors are; her eyes as black as possible, large and fine, and painted at the edges, which is what most of the Moors do; her lips painted red, and between every tooth, which were fine and regular, she was painted black, to look like ebony. All her attendants, which were about thirty ladies, were the same; her face was done over like frosted work with leaf gold; the nails of her fingers and feet (for she was bare-footed) were painted red, and likewise the inside of her hands. You will perhaps think this a strange description, but I assure you it is literally true. . . . Her hair was as black as jet, very long and thick, which was combed neatly back, and then braided till it hung a great deal below her waist.'

CITIZEN OF THE WORLD

Oliver Goldsmith's *Citizen of the World*, first published in 1762, contains a letter comparing English and Oriental ideas of beauty and customs in makeup. The letter is purported to be 'from Lien Chi Altangi, to the care of Fipsihi, resident in Moscow; to be forwarded by the Russian caravan to Fum Hoam, First President in the Ceremonial Academy at Pekin, in China:

'When I had just quitted my native country and crossed the Chinese wall, I fancied every deviation from the customs and manner of China was a departing from nature; I smiled at the blue lips and red forheads of the Tonguese; and could hardly contain myself when I saw the Daures dress their heads with horns; the Ostiacks powdered with red earth; and the Calmuck beauties, tricked out of all the finery of Sheep skin, appeared highly ridiculous: but I soon perceived that the ridicule lay not in them but in me; that I falsely condemned others of absurdity, because they happened to differ from a standard originally founded in prejudice or partiality. . . .

'You are not insensible, most reverend Fum Hoam, what numberless trades, even among the Chinese, subsist by the harmless pride of each other. Your nose-borers, feet-swathers, tooth-stainers, eye-brow pluckers, would all want bread, should their neighbours want vanity. These vanities, however, employ much fewer hands in China than in England; and a fine gentleman, or a fine lady, here dressed up to the fashion, seems scarcely to have a single limb that does not suffer some distortions from my art.

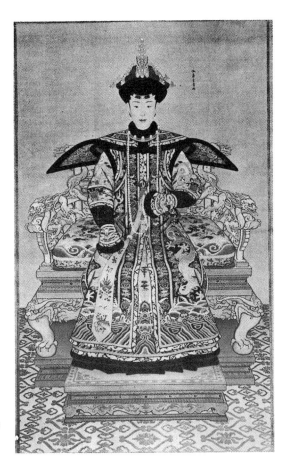

FIG. 132: 'First-rank lady' of Chinese Emperor Ch'ien-lung (1736–1795).

'To make a fine gentleman, several trades are required, but chiefly a barber. . . . To appear wise nothing more is requisite here than for a man to borrow hair from the heads of all his neighbours and clap it like a bush on his own: the distributors of law and physic stick on such quantities that it is almost impossible, even in idea, to distinguish between the head and hair.

'Those whom I have been now describing affect the gravity of the lion: those I am going to describe more resemble the pert vivacity of small animals. The barber, who is still master of the ceremonies, cuts their hair close to the crown; and then, with a composition of meal and hog's lard, plaisters the whole in such a manner as to make it impossible to distinguish whether the patient wears a cap or a plaister: but to make the picture more perfectly striking, conceive the tail of some beast, a greyhound's tail, or a pig's tail, for instance, appended to the back of the head, and reaching down to that place where tails in other animals are generally seen to begin; thus be-tailed and be-powdered, the man of taste fancies he improves in beauty, dresses up his head, features face in smiles, and attempts to look hideously tender. Thus equipped, he is qualified to make love, and hopes for success, more from the powder on the outside of his head than the sentiments within.'

The English ladies he finds 'horridly ugly', in no way resembling the small-footed beauties of China. 'I shall never forget,' he goes on, 'the beauties of my native city of Nangfew. How very broad their faces; how very short their noses; how very little their eyes; how very thin their lips; how very black their teeth; the snow on the tops of the Bao is not fairer than their cheeks; and their eyebrows are small as the line by the pencil of Quamfi. Here a lady with such perfections would be frightful: Dutch and Chinese beauties, indeed, have some resemblance, but English women are entirely different; red cheeks, big eyes, and teeth of the most odious whiteness, are not only seen here, but wished for; and then they have such masculine feet, as actually serve *some* for walking!

'Yet, uncivil as nature has been, they seem resolved to outdo her in unkindness; they use white powder, blue powder, and black powder for their hair and a red powder for the face on some particular occasions.

'They like to have the face of various colours, as among the Tartars of Coreki, frequently sticking on, with spittle, little black patches on every part of it, except on the tip of the nose, which I have never seen with a patch. You'll have a better idea of their manner of placing these spots, when I have finished a map of an English face patched up to the fashion, which shall shortly be sent to increase your curious collection of paintings, medals, and monsters.

'But what surprises more than all the rest is, what I have just now been credibly informed of by one of this country; "Most ladies here (says he) have two faces; one face to sleep in, and another to shew in company: the first is generally reserved for the husband and family at home, the other put on to please strangers abroad; the family face is often indifferent enough, but the

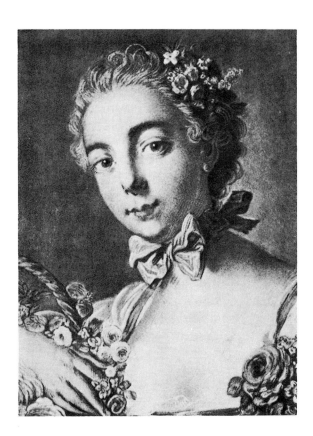

FIG. 133: Girl with flowers. Chalk drawing
by Boucher, c. 1740.

out-door one looks somewhat better: this is always made at the toilet, where
the looking-glass and toad-eater sit in council, and settle the complexion of the
day".

'I cannot ascertain the truth of this remark; however, it is actually certain
that they wear more clothes within doors than without; and I have seen a lady
who seemed to shudder at a breeze in her own apartment, appear half naked
in the streets. Farewell.'

THE FEMININE IDEAL

Sir Harry Beaumont agrees with Felibien, whom he quotes, as to the characteristics of the ideal feminine face:

The head, he says, should be well rounded and small rather than large, 'the
Forehead white, smooth, and open (not with the Hair growing down too deep
upon it); neither flat nor prominent. . . .

'The *Hair*, either bright, black, or brown; not thin, but full and waving. . . .
The Black is particularly useful for setting off the whiteness of the Neck and
Skin. . . .

'The *Eyes*, black, chestnut, or blue; clear, bright, and lively; and rather large
in Proportion than small.

'The *Eyebrows*, well divided, rather full than thin; semicircular, and broader in the Middle than at the ends; of a neat Turn, but not formal.

'The *Cheeks* should not be wide; should have a degree of Plumpness, with the Red and White finely blended together; and should look firm and soft.

'The *Ear* should be rather small than large; well-folded, and with an agreeable Tinge of Red.

'The *Nose* should be . . . of a moderate size, strait, and well-squared; though sometimes a little Rising in the Nose, which is but just perceivable, may give a very graceful Look to it.

'The *Mouth* should be small; and the Lips, not of equal thickness; they should be well-turned, small, rather than gross; soft, even to the Eye; and with a living Red in them. A truly pretty Mouth is like a Rose-bud that is beginning to blow. . . .

'The *Skin* in general should be white, properly tinged with Red; with an apparent Softness, and a Look of thriving Health in it.'

COSMETIC AIDS

In order to approximate these characteristics, in case she did not already have them, the eighteenth-century lady had available a wide variety of cosmetic aids, some of them lethal.

In 1765 Lady Sophia Thomas asked Horace Walpole to have the Earl of Hertford, who was in Paris, send to London twelve bottles of *le Baume de Vie*, prepared by Monsieur Lièvre, apothecary to the King. The following year he wrote to Miss Anne Pitt from Paris that he could find no way of making her room look French 'but by sending it a box of rouge'. Later he sent Lady Hervey and Madame de Boufflers 'a box of pomatums'. The following winter he wrote to Sir Horace Mann that 'that pretty young woman, Lady Fortrose, Lady Harrington's eldest daughter, is at the point of death, killed, like Lady Coventry and others, by white lead, of which nothing could break her'. One of the others was Kitty Fisher, a courtesan who posed for Reynolds.

Le Camus gives us a 'Library of the Toilet' (in *The Art of Preserving Beauty*), in which he lists the various toilet articles and preparations used by ladies of the eighteenth century. It seems worthwhile to include a major part of the list since it gives perhaps the best picture to be found anywhere of what the ladies had to work with:

WATERS

Water of Silverweed, of Cedar, without Equal, of the Queen of Hungary, where the Lemon predominates, wherein the Bergamot abounds, wherein the Cedar is superior, wherein the Amber prevails, of Balm, of Luze, Vulneray, of Roses, Plantain, Jonquil, Violet, Pink, Jasmine, Orange-flower, Bergamot, Yarrow, Scurvy-grass, Myrtle, Angelica, Honey, English, without Odour, Lavender, Simple, of Lavender, distill'd, Red, Barbel, Bean, Lettuce, Eyebright, of the Sultanesses of Cordona, of Portugal, for a Marshall's Lady, of Popouri, of the smaller Lemons, of Brandy, Simple, with Camphire, Perfumed, of Guaiacum, of Strawberries, of Cyprus, of Ambret, of Florentine Orris.

ESSENCES

Essence of Lemons, of Bergamot, of Cedar, of Oranges, of the smaller Lemons, of Jasmine, of Spanish Jasmine, of Nerote, of Pinks, of Gilli-flowers, of Cinnamon, of Ben, of Amber, of Roses, of Lavender, of Aniseed, of Fennel.

SPUNGES

Fine Spunges prepar'd for the Body, for the Teeth, for the Beard.

POMATUMS

Pomatum simple, White, Red, Yellow, of Cucumbers, of Snails, of the four Cold Seeds, for the Chaps of the Lips, with the Flowers of Oranges, with Bergamot, with Lemons, of green Walnuts, with Jasmine, with the lesser Lemons, with Lavender, with Pink, with Violet, with Tuberose, with Jonquil, with Sheep's Trotters, with Cedar, with the Caffias, of Frangipane, with Amber, of Portugal, of Italy, of Rome, of Provence, of the White of Pearls, in a Cane, in a Pot.

OILS

Oil of sweet Almonds, of bitter Almonds, press'd without Fire, of Hazel, of Ben, of Poppies, of Flower-de-Luce, of Roses, of Cinnamon, of Storax, of Tartar *per Deliquium*.

VINEGARS

Vinegar of Roses, of the Four Robbers, of Surat, Roman, of Venus.

PASTES

Paste of sweet Almonds, of bitter Almonds, of dried Almonds, of sweet and bitter Almonds, Liquid, Greasy, Yellow, with Honey, for the Queen, with Soap.

WASH-BALLS

Wash-balls Common, of pure Soap, of odoriferous Soap, Marbled of Provence, of pure Neapolitan Soap, Perfumed, of Bologne, of Frangipane, White, Brown, Light, Heavy, Amber'd, with Lavender, Grey with Lavender, Grey with Amber, Grey with Lemon, Grey with Bergamot, of Neroli, of Amber.

POWDERS

Powder Common, very Fine, purified with Brandy, purified with Spirit of Wine, White, Black, Brown, Fair, Grey, Flesh-colour'd, Rose-colour'd, Cherry-colour'd, for a Marshal's Lady, with Violet, with Orris, with Pink, Orange-flower, of Jonquil, of Tuberose, of Yarrow, of Beans, English, Cyprus, Bright of all Colours.

RED PAINT

Red in a Pot, in Powder, for the Fair, for the Brown, with different Colours, of Paris, of Spain, of Portugal, of Nismes, Carmine, Fire, Rose, of different Colours.

PATCHES

Patches of Velvet, of Sattin, of Taffety, Superfine, Unmatch'd.

VIRGIN'S MILK

White, Red, of Rome.

PAINT

White of Pearls, White of different Kinds.

HEAD-BANDS

For the Wrinkles of the Forehead.

The head-bands were often of linen-lined leather and were worn at night, as were face masks for wrinkles elsewhere. If the report of an English parson is to be credited, the Countess of Thanet's mother, more interested in rejuvenating her husband than herself, killed a man and fed her husband the distilled remains. The parson recorded only the deed, not the results of the treatment. The idea, successful or not, did not catch on, and other women usually let their husbands grow old and continued to use for themselves more prosaic methods for keeping fit — such as wearing chicken-skin gloves during the night to keep the hands soft and white. Some thirty years later, when, it appears, they were no longer in use, a London perfumer explained that these gloves had not been made of chicken skin, as one might suppose, but rather 'of a thin, strong leather, which is dressed with almonds and spermacetti, and from the softening, balmy nature of these gloves, they soften, clear, smooth, and make white, the hands and arms. And why the German ladies gave them the name of chicken gloves is from their innocent, effectual quality.'

THE ART OF PRESERVING BEAUTY

The preceding list of cosmetic aids is taken from a book by Antoine Le Camus entitled *Abdeker: or, the Art of Preserving Beauty*, published in London in 1754. It is written in the form of a story, in which Abdeker, a physician, gives instructions for achieving and maintaining beauty. According to the preface, the book 'is a translation of an Arabian Manuscript, which Diamantes Utaste, Physician to the Turkish Ambassador, brought to Paris in the year 1740'. When the question of painting arises, Abdeker recommends compounding 'four Ounces of the Oil of Ben, an Ounce of Virgin Wax, and two Drams and a half of Magistery of Bismuth', the bismuth being preferable to tin or lead because of its whiteness. The result was Spanish White, which was dissolved in Flower-de-Luce Water before being applied to the face.

As usual in such books, the reader was given several choices. Another recipe for the same purpose, called simply *An Excellent White Paint for the Face*, required that a mixture of hartshorn, rice flour, white lead, cuttle-fish bone, frankincense, mastick, and gum arabic be diluted in rose-water and used for washing the face. Still another recipe for white paint was somewhat more complicated:

'Take any Quantity you please of Sheep's Trotters well chopp'd; break the long Bones in order to get at the Marrow. But that you may effect it with greater Facility, macerate the Bones for a Day or two in Water, which you must change three or four times a Day. Keep the Vessel in a Cellar; and to every Dozen of Sheep's Trotters add half a Dozen Calves-Feet. When you have obtain'd their Marrow, wash it several times, renewing the Water each time. Repeat the Washing till it becomes very white; and also wash the Bones well, after taking out the Marrow, and boil them in clear Water for an Hour or two. Strain through a Linen Cloth; and let the liquid Part that passes through, settle for twelve Hours. Take off with a Silver Spoon the Oil that comes to the Top, and mix it with the Marrow which you have prepared as above. Melt the whole over a gentle Fire, and for every four Ounces add an Ounce of Borax, and the like Quantity of Roch-Alum burnt. When the whole is sufficiently hot, add two

Ounces of the Oil of the four Cold Seeds press'd without the Help of Fire, and a small Quantity of Kid's-Grease. Strain through a Piece of clean Linen, and keep it for Use. Some, instead of Kid's-Grease, use a small Quantity of Wax or Sheep's Tallow; but the Wax dries and chaps the Skin, and the Sheep's Tallow grows reddish, and makes the Face look yellow.'

The frequent references to white paint for the face as enamel or varnish, though they may lead to confusion in the contemporary mind, are not quite so inappropriate as they might seem since a sheen or lustre to the complexion was considered most desirable. Perhaps this was related to the fashionable dull, flat appearance of the powdered hair. Since natural highlights in the hair were practically eliminated, it may have seemed reasonable that they should be emphasized in the face.

Le Camus includes in his book a simple recipe for *Varnish for the Face*:

'Put into a Bottle twelve Ounces of Brandy, an Ounce of Sandarach and half an Ounce of Benjamin. Shake the Bottle often and afterwards let it settle. When you use it, wash your Face beforehand, and it will give it the handsomest lustre imaginable.'

One of Abdeker's favourite recipes requires tartar of white wine, nitre, pewter, rock alum, and brandy. And then there is the intriguing recipe for *Oil of Pearls*:

'Put upon a Plate any Quantity you please of Pearls, and pour over them some good distill'd Vinegar. When the Pearls are dissolved, add a small quantity of Gum Arabic, keep the Solution for Use. Wash your Face before you bathe it with this Solution, which will soon dry of itself. This is one of the best Secrets that have been invented for rendering the Face both white and fair.'

For rouging the cheeks, Abdeker suggests pomatum coloured with alkanet root, a scarlet ribbon dipped in water or brandy, or scarlet wool, which, he says, will give the cheeks 'a very handsome Red'. He also mentions that some women use red lead for the same purpose. Proceeding, then, to the metallic paints, he says:

'Cinnabar is composed of Brimstone and Mercury. When it is reduced to a Subtil Powder in a Marble Mortar, it acquires so lively and so high a Colour that it is called Vermilion. Some ladies mix it with Paint wherewith they rub their Cheeks, which is very dangerous; for by using it frequently they may lose their Teeth, acquire a stinking Breath, and excite a copious salivation.' Despite such warnings, some ladies continued to use the poisonous paints.

The rouges coloured with vegetable dyes were much safer. Abdeker gives *The Secret of a Turk for making an excellent Carmine*:

'Take a Pound of the best rasp'd Brasil Wood, and steep it for three or four days in a sufficient quantity of White-Wine Vinegar. After that boil it for half an Hour; strain it through a strong Piece of Linen, and put it again over the Fire. You must likewise dissolve by itself eight Ounces of Alum in a sufficient Quantity of White-Wine Vinegar. Mix both Liquors together, by stirring them in a Mortar; and there will arise a froth, which is the Carmine. Skim it off, dry it, and keep it for Use. Cochineal or red Sanders may be used instead of Brasil wood.'

Le Camus then includes a recipe for *Another Kind of Red Paint*, using red wine instead of vinegar. It is to be applied by dipping a bit of cotton into it and rubbing it on the cheeks. Still another liquid vegetable rouge is described under the heading *A Kind of Paint that resembles the Natural Red*:

'Take Benjamin, Brasil Wood, Roch-Alum, of each half an Ounce. Macerate the Whole in a Pint of strong Brandy for the Space of twelve Days: shake the Bottle every Day, let it be well cork'd, and keep it for Use. A slight Touch of this Liquor gives such a beautiful Red to the Cheeks that it can hardly be distinguished from the natural: And what renders this Secret the most valuable is, that its use is attended with no ill Consequences. Such Women as dare not paint for fear it should be perceived, may use this composition without any Danger of being suspected.'

For the lady preferring a different type of moist rouge, there was a recipe for *An Oil for Painting the Cheeks Red*:

'Take ten Pounds of sweet Almonds, an Ounce of red Sanders in Powder, and

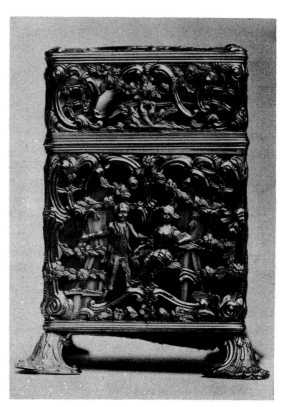

FIG. 134: Box for cosmetics implements. English, eighteenth century.

an Ounce of Cloves. Beat them well together in a Mortar; pour four Ounces of White Wine thereon, and three ounces of Rose-Water. Shake the Vessel every Day for eight days successively; press out the Oil in the same Manner used in making Oil of Sweet Almonds.'

In addition to advising the ladies on whitening and rouging the face, Abdeker provided recipes for keeping the skin in good condition, including an intriguing one for a *Water to Preserve a Fresh Complexion*, requiring calves' feet, melons, cucumbers, freshly laid eggs, pumpkin, lemons, whey, rose-water, silver-weed, plantain water, and borax. Then there was *A Secret to take away Wrinkles, communicated by a Persian to a Grecian of seventy-two Years of Age, who by the Benefit of it did not seem to be above 25*. But this recipe turns out to be the old one with the wine and the fire shovel published by Lémery in the seventeenth century (see p. 178). Like the recipe for Queen of Hungary water, it appeared again and again, even as late as the nineteenth century.

The term *Virgin's Milk* appears from time to time. It could be made, according to Abdeker, 'by pouring a great deal of Water upon the Dissolution of Lead in Vinegar. The Liquor that results from this Operation is as White as Milk.' Abdeker also provided a recipe for *Distill'd Water for giving a beautiful Carnation*, prefacing it by commenting that it could be used by 'such Ladies as have a disagreeable Colour:

'Take two Quarts of Vinegar, three Ounces of Mouth-Glue, two Ounces of Nutmegs, six Ounces of common Honey: Distil with a slow Fire; add to the distill'd Liquor a small Quantity of red Sanders, in order to give it a little Colour. Before using it the Face should be wash'd with Soap-Water; but after using the distill'd Water the Face is not to be wash'd, that it may grow fair and red and look healthy. This Secret was communicated by a Lady that never failed to make use of it, whether she pass'd the Night at Gaming, or whether she was fatigued after a Ball, or after Suppers that are not ended till the first Approach of Aurora.'

Then there is *A Remarkable Secret*:

'Make a Hole in a Lemon, fill it with Sugar-candy, cover it with Leaf-Gold, and over the said Gold apply the Part of the Peel you have cut off; afterwards roast your Lemon under the warm Ashes. When you have a mind to make use of it, squeeze out a little of the Juice through the Hole you have already made, receive the Juice in a clean Cloth, and rub your Face therewith. This Juice is very efficacious for cleansing the Skin and rendering the Complexion bright and fair.'

There are a few additional recipes for cosmetics which may be of interest:

RED POMATUM FOR THE LIPS

Take an Ounce of white Wax and of an Ox's Marrow, three Ounces of white Pomatum, and melt all in a Bath-Heat. Add a Dram of Alkanet, and stir the Mass till it acquires a red Colour.

Others chuse to use the Ointment of Roses, which is thus prepared:

Take Hog's Lard wash'd in Rose-water, red Roses, and pale Roses; beat all in a Mortar, mix them together, and let them macerate for two Days. Then melt the Lard and strain it, and add the same Quantity of Roses as before. Let them macerate in the Fat for two Days, and afterwards let the Mass boil in a Bath-Head. Strain it with Expression, and keep it for Use.

Some are accustom'd to wash their Lips with pure Brandy in order to make them look red.

POMATUM FOR TAKING AWAY POCK-HOLES

Take of Rose-colour'd Pomatum an Ounce, of corrosive Sublimate a Dram; apply it to the Pock-holes with a Partridge-Feather. The Dose of the corrosive Sublimate may be increased according to the Circumstances: But the Administration of this Remedy requires the utmost Precaution, lest it should excite an Inflammation of the Erysipelas.

RECEIPT FOR CHANGING THE TAWNY COLOUR OF THE FACE

One may . . . bruise some Strawberries upon the Face at going to Bed and let them dry thereon during the Night, and the next Morning wash it with Chevril Water. By this means the Skin becomes fresh and fair and acquires a beautiful Lustre. It is one of the best Methods that can be used in such Cases; and the Prescription is not to be found in any Book of Cosmetics.

WATER TO TAKE AWAY THE SPOTS OF THE FACE

Take two Pounds of Bastard Rhubarb and Melon-Seed, ten swallow's Eggs, half an Ounce of Nitre, and two Ounces of white Tartar; distil all in a Glass Alembic, and wash your Face with the distill'd Water.

PATCHES AND PATCHING

The Art of Preserving Beauty also includes a description of Abdeker painting the Sultaness:

'He pulled out a small Box that contain'd Vermilion; he took a Pencil, dipp'd it therein, and dextrously painted the Cheeks of the Sultaness. Fatima consulting her Looking-glass, I do not know myself, cried she: Heavens! What a Prodigy! My Cheeks are as red as Tyrian Purple, and as radiant as a Flame.'

Presumably Fatima was at last as beautiful as paint could make her — until a fly landed near her eye, and it seemed to her that it set off the vermilion. But when she turned her head, the fly flew off. Abdeker was prepared. 'He immediately took a patch of black Taffety, which was cover'd with Gum Arabic, and cut it in the Form of a Lozenge, and applied it to the Spot where the Fly had been placed. . . . At the same Time . . . he cut the Taffety in the Form of a Half-Moon and applied it to her Temples. . . . Whilst she spoke . . . she cut out another Patch, which represented the Full Moon and placed it in the midst of her Forehead, saying, As this nightly Luminary eclipses the Sun, so in like manner do you rule over my Soul, in spite of all the Allurements of Grandeur whereby Mahomet endeavours to captivate my Eyes.

'Abdeker . . . contrived also in his Turn an allegorical symbol that fully expressed all the sentiments of his Acknowledgment. He gave the Figure of a Star to a Patch of Taffety. . . . After making various Experiments upon Patches of all Sizes and Figures, Fatima observed that she should not apply too many of them, and that one or two were enough. Afterwards she establish'd as a general Rule that none of them should ever be put into the small Dimples which the Poets have imagined to be the Habitations of Love and of the Graces. She contrived likewise to give them different Names, according to the different Characters they imprinted on the Face. She call'd the Patch that was at the exterior Angle of the Eye *Killing*, because it contributed to give a sharp and lively Look; and named that which was in the midst of her Forehead *Majestic*, because it gives a noble Air. That placed in the Fold that is form'd in the skin by laughing she nam'd *Jovial*; that in the midst of the Cheek, *Gallant*; and that near the Lips *The Coquet*. This last is also known by the Name of *Prude*, and the *Gallant* by the Name of *Jiltish*. In a Word, each of them had a Name answerable to the Effect it produced.'

There were still occasional complaints about patching from critics and from the general public, but the bite had gone out of them. In the same year that Le Camus' work was published, a distressed contributor to *The World* wrote, 'Though I have seen with patience the cap diminishing to the size of a patch, I have not with the same unconcern observed the patch enlarging itself to the size of a cap. It is with great sorrow that I already see it in possession of that beautiful mass of blue which borders upon the eye. Should it increase on the left side of that exquisite texture, what an eclipse have we to dread! But surely it is to be hoped that the ladies will not give up that place to a plaster which the brightest jewel in the universe would want lustre to supply.'

COSMETICS FOR MEN

In the autumn of 1754 the editors of *The Connoisseur* described the ultra-fashionable men of the time:

'They have their toilettes, too, as well as the ladies, set out with washes, perfumes, and cosmetics, and will spend the whole morning in scenting their linen, dressing their hair, and arching their eyebrows. Their heads (as well as the ladies') have undergone various mutations and have worn as many different kinds of wigs as the block at their barber's. About fifty years ago they buried their heads in a bunch of hair; and the beaux (as Swift says) "lay hid beneath the penthouse of a full-bottomed perriwig". But as they then shewed nothing but the nose, mouth, and eyes, the fine gentlemen of our time not only oblige us with their full faces, but have drawn back the side curls quite to the tip of the ear.'

This description, predictably, brought letters from the readers, one of which, from a Mr W. Manly, was published the following April. Mr Manly closes his letter by saying, 'I am ashamed to tell you that we are indebted to Spanish Wool for many of our masculine ruddy complexions. A pretty fellow lacquers his pale face with as many varnishes as a fine lady. . . . I fear it will be found, upon examination, that most of our pretty fellows who lay on Carmine are painting a rotten post.'

The young editors, who went under the collective name of Mr Town, took the opportunity for further comment:

'The male beauty has his washes, perfumes, and cosmetics and takes as much pains to set a gloss on his complexion as the footman in japanning his shoes. He has his dressing-room and (which is still more ridiculous) his Toilet too, at which he sits as many hours repairing his battered countenance as a decayed toast dressing for a birth-night.'

The collective Mr Town then describes a visit to a young gentleman's dressing room:

'I could not but observe a number of boxes of different sizes, which were all of them Japan, and lay regularly disposed on the table. I had the curiosity to examine the contents of several: in one I found lip-salve, in another a roll of pig-tail, and in another the ladies black sticking plaister; but the last which I opened very much surprised me, as I saw nothing in it but a number of little pills. I likewise remarked, on one part of the table, a tooth-brush and sponge, with a pot of Delescot's opiate; and on the other side, water for the eyes. In the middle stood a bottle of Eau de Luce and a roll of perfumed pomatum. Almond pastes, powder puffs, hair combs, brushes. nippers, and the like, made up the rest of this fantastic equipage. But among many other whimsies, I could not conceive for what use a very small ivory comb could be designed, till the valet informed me that it was a comb for the eyebrows.'

In the eighteenth century the American colonists of the upper classes were following British and French cosmetic practice and still importing their cosmetics from Europe. Every gentleman had his dressing box equipped with shaving necessities, soap, powder puffs, brushes, oil and scent bottles, curling irons, scissors, rouge, if he used it, and often writing materials.

After shaving, followed by the use of a face lotion, he would apply rouge, not always subtly, powder, and sometimes patches. Gilbert Vail mentions among the possessions of Captain Giles Shelley of New York two patch boxes in which he carried 'the fashionable mouches' to wear 'upon his cheekes'.

But for most men the major cosmetic adornment was the wig. John Still, a barber and wigmaker, announced in 1750 his arrival in the New World:

> This is to acquaint the Public that there is lately arrived from London, the Wonder of the World, an Honest Barber and Peruke-maker, who might have worked for the King, if His Majesty would have employed him; it was not for the Want of Money that he came here, for he had enough of that at Home; nor for the Want of Business that he advertised himself; but to acquaint the Gentlemen and Ladies, That such a Person is now in Town, living near Rosemary-Lane, where Gentlemen and Ladies may be supplied with the Goods as follows, viz. Tyes, cuts and bob Perukes; also Ladies' Tate-matongues and Towers after the Manner that is now wore at Court. By their humble and obedient servant, John Still.

A competitor of Mr Still's tried to capture his share of patronage by means of an unconventional advertisement in the *New York Gazette* in 1756:

> Me Givee de advertisement of every Body in New York. . . . Yes, dammee, me advertise for makee de Vig, Cuttee or curlee de Hair, dressee and shavee de Beard of the Gentleman, sellee de Pomates, and de Powdre, so sweet for de Hair, and de Vig, for makee a bon Approach to de Madammoselle. . . . N.B. Me makee all de Bon Taste, Alamode de Paris; and me no chargee above three Hundred per Cent, more dan all de Workmans in Town.

For Dressee de Hair ...	...	...	...	...	...	£0	6	6
For Curlee de Hair ...	...	...	...	...	...	0	4	0
For Cuttee de Hair ...	...	...	...	...	...	0	6	6
For Makee de Bag ...	...	...	...	...	...		10	6
For Makee de Ramille de Halfe de Pistole								
For Makee de Toupee de Halfe de Pistole								
For Von Stick de Pomat ...	...	...	...	...	...	0	2	6
For Von Bottle de Lavender ...	...	...	...	...	...	0	4	0

And so in de Proportion.

Along with the nuisance and expense of keeping his wig or wigs adequately powdered and curled, the eighteenth-century man had to keep his face clean-shaven. Since progress along these lines was painfully slow and the process itself never a particularly enjoyable one, the announcement in 1745 of a proposed

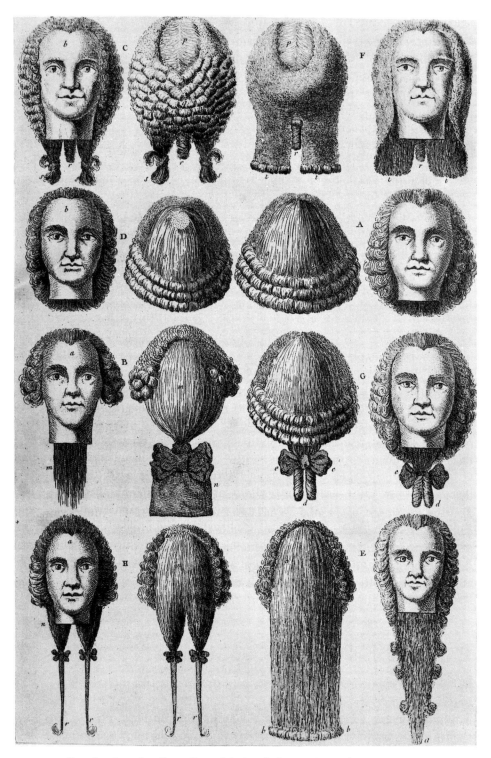

FIG. 135 : French wig styles. From Garsault's *Art du Perruquier*, 1767.

machine for shaving men en masse aroused considerable interest, even hope. An engraving of the invention, published on the twenty-ninth day of November, was captioned, 'A Perspective View and Section of an Engine Propos'd to be Built by Subscription, which will Shave Sixty Men a Minute, also Oyl and Comb and Powder their Wigs'. The shaving engine was 'to be Work'd by a Horse . . . which spurs himself if he does not perform the Task assign'd him'.

In the round, wooden construction, not unlike a merry-go-round, there was, at each station, a complicated system of blades, which 'in their Rotation are Wip'd, Set and Strap'd by Spunges, Hornes and Leathers affixt in proper Places'. There were holes for heads to be stuck through and steps to stand on, with an occasional shelf for the very short. Above the holes there were pegs for hats, and below there were 'Doors to put their Wigs in, on Blocks to be Comb'd, etc.' The oiling and combing, also automatic, was to be accomplished by means of 'a Vertical Wheel with Combs and Spunges'. For those who wanted powder there were 'Cocks which by turning more or less by a Continual Blast will Powder to your likeing'. Behind each patron — on the outside wall of the construction — there were windows alternating with mirrors and under each window 'a Cistern for Water, on the top of which is Casteel-Soap and Brushes for Lathering the Face. Under each Cistern is a Sink to carry off the Foul Water, under the Looking-Glasses are Rowling Towels.'

There was to be one engine built for every five hundred subscribers, each of whom had to pay a guinea a year for the service. One barber expressed the hope that in spite of the possible usefulness of the machine 'in preventing the Continuation of that abominable Custom of Shaving on Sundays . . . Legislation will take in Consideration, and prevent this Machine or Engine from working on Week Days'.

In January subscribers were advised that 'they are desir'd to give their Attendance on Wednesday next at Mr Bridel's, the One-Tun in the Strand, between the Hours of Six and Eight in the evening, to make Choice of a proper Place to erect the same on', and in March there was a request for bids from manufacturers of razors, pointing out that each engine would require 180 dozen blades. From that point on, enthusiasm evidently waned, for there is no record of the construction of even one shaving engine.

THE COLONIAL LADY

Whereas the gentleman made his relatively simple toilet in the morning, usually immediately after breakfast, the Colonial lady often made hers later in the day, depending on her social obligations. Her toilet box contained many more items than her husband's, including a variety of creams, lotions, washes, dyes, and paints. Some of these she may have concocted herself (some of the better homes had 'still rooms' just for this purpose), some she may have purchased from the local pharmacist or female cosmetician, but the most highly prized were those imported from Europe, especially France.

One of these, called 'The Princely Beautifying Lotion', was said to beautify 'the Face, Neck, and Hands to the Utmost Perfection and it is in the greatest Esteem among the Ladies, etc., of the first Quality. No words can sufficiently express its Virtues, for it is not in the nature of paint which puts a false, unnatural gloss to the Skin, but it is a true Remedy, that by its use really adds a Lustre to the most Beautiful by showing the fine features of the face; and it is so safe, not having the least grain of Mercury in it, that it may be taken inwardly; and if smelled too, it is really good against the Vapors, etc., in Ladies, the very Reverse of all the other Remedies of the kind which raise the Vapors.'

Some of the foreign cosmetics were obtained directly through friends or from importers such as Peter Lynch, who was to be found 'near Mr. Rutger's Brewhouse'. He imported cosmetics, hair dyes, and hair powders as early as 1734; and in 1742 a Mrs Redmond, 'opposite the Fort Garden', was importing patches and patch boxes. These were soon joined by other importers and by those who made their own concoctions.

THE COST OF BEAUTY

A bill of 1759 for cosmetic articles purchased by the Duke of Bedford between March and July lists three pounds of perfumed soap, six bottles of lavender water, one bottle of Hungary water, and large quantities of powder (regular and superfine) and pomade (in both rolls and pots). Bills made out to Lady Caroline Russell for about this same time include stick pomade, soft pomade, grey powder, boxed powder, powder by the pound, and a curling iron. Ordinary hair powder was a shilling a pound, stick pomatum a shilling, and fancier pomatums somewhat more.

It is said that Madame de Pompadour spent as much as 500,000 livres (about $100,000 or more than £40,000) for perfume. And in 1770, upon her marriage, Marie-Antoinette was given a gold and enamelled rouge and patch box which cost 1,200 livres.

HAIR

In the winter of 1765–6 Lady Sarah Bunbury wrote to Lady Susan Strangways that she thought the French dress was gradually coming into fashion, 'tho 'tis almost impossible,' she added, 'to make the ladies understand that heads bigger than one's body are ugly; it is growing the fashion to have the heads *moutoné*; I have cut off my hair, & find it very convenient in the country without powder, because my hair curls naturally, but it's horrid troublesome to have it well curled; if it's big it's frightful. I wear it very often with three row of curls behind & the rest smooth with a fruzed *toupé* & a cap, that is, *en paresseuse*. There is nobody but Ly Tavistock, who does not dress French, who is at all genteel, for if they are not French they are so very ill dressed, it's terrible. Almost everybody powders now, & wears a little hoop; hats are vastly left off; the hair down on the forehead belongs to the short waist, & is equally vulgar with poppons, trimmings, beads, garnets, flying caps, & false hair. To be perfectly genteel you must be dress'd thus. Your hair need not be cut off, for 'tis much too pretty, but it must be powdered, curled in very small curls, & altogether be in the style of Ly Tavistock's, *neat*, but it must be high before & give your head the look of a sugar loaf a little. The roots of the hair must be drawn up straight & not fruzed at all for half an inch above the root; you must wear no cap, & only *little little* flowers dab'd in on the left side; the only feather permitted is a black or white sultane perched up on the left side, & your diamond feather against it. . . . The men's dress is exactly what they used to wear latterly; that is 3 or 4 curls high at the sides. Some people wear it cut short before & comed up *en brosse* very high upon the top of the head, it's called *à la greque*, & is very pretty when well done. Mr. Robinson says that everybody now dresses their hair so well that the old Makaronis must be quite plain to distinguish themselves, & indeed it's true, tho' I think this style much prettier than the hair down at the ears in Sr Charles' style. . . . By the way of new married folks, Ld Newnham & Mr Mackenzie are the only people I think; Ly Newnham was a Miss Vernon, she is not pretty but as Ld. N. makes her wear rouge & dresses her very well, she is very tollerable.'

High foreheads were in fashion, and ladies who did not have them naturally, plucked their front hair in order to get them. So important did it seem that mothers sometimes used walnut oil on their children's foreheads to prevent the growth of hair. Bandages impregnated with vinegar and cat's dung were also used with the hope of preventing the growth of hair, and depilatories could be bought from cosmetics shops. Some women then, as now, had facial hair to cope with and used home-made depilatories containing quick-lime to remove it. It is said that the Duke of Newcastle paid £400 to have his wife's facial hair permanently removed, yet in a letter of 1755 Horace Walpole refers to the Duke's retirement, adding that he can now let 'his beard grow as long as his Duchess's'.

BATHING AND PERFUMES

In a letter to Richard West, dated 21 April 1739, Horace Walpole writes that 'even the princesses of the blood are dirty enough to have shares in the banks kept at their houses. We have seen two or three of them; but they are not young, nor remarkable but for wearing their red of a deeper dye than other women, though all use it extravagantly.'

The painting often seemed a practical as well as a decorative function — it helped to cover the marks of smallpox, which was very common at the time, and it also covered the accumulation of dirt. Frequent washing was still considered unhealthy. Louis XIV bathed only once a year — a sort of spring cleaning. For the most part he was content with a little eau de cologne on his hands and face. This may have taken off some of the surface dirt, but it was totally inadequate as a deodorant.

Precepts for proper behaviour, published by a French missionary in 1749, suggested that it was proper to clean the face every morning with a white cloth but unwise to wash with water since that made one susceptible to colds in winter and sunburn in summer. The author considered it unseemly to apply patches to the face or to paint with white or vermilion, which merely served to prove that one did not have natural beauty. And he did not approve of cutting the eyebrows too short.

Like many before him, he warned against blowing one's nose with one's hand or in one's sleeve. Scratching the head in public he considered indecent, and he noted that it was the habit of some women to tap their heads frequently in order to dislodge the vermin in their head-dresses. He suggested using less powder and pomatum, which tended to attract the vermin and to trap them inside the coiffure.

Nor did he approve of cleaning one's teeth with the fingernails, but he found a toothpick or a quill quite acceptable. The gesture of pushing one tooth forward with the thumbnail in order to express dislike or disdain for someone was considered extremely uncivil. And it was no less uncivil to suck drippings from the nose into the mouth. The bathing situation being what it was, perfumes were used in profusion by both men and women, and a lady's lover was expected to wear the same scent that she did. Louis XV insisted on his apartments' being perfumed with a different scent each day. Louis XIV, it is said, did not like heavy perfumes.

The English, though by modern standards hardly meticulous in their personal habits, were considerably cleaner than the French. And there were those who thought highly enough of cleanliness to counsel their children about it. Philip Dormer Stanhope, Earl of Chesterfield, was one of these. He wrote voluminous letters to his son on a variety of subjects, most of them offering fatherly advice, which he obviously expected to be followed.

In November 1750 he advised, 'When you come to Paris . . . let your man learn of the best *friseur* to do your hair well, for that is a very material part of your dres. . . . In your person you must be accurately clean; and your teeth, hands, and nails, should be superlatively so: a dirty mouth has real ill consequences to the owner, for it infallibly causes the decay, as well as the intolerable pain of the teeth; and it is very offensive to his acquaintances, for it will most inevitably stink. I insist therefore, that you wash your teeth the first thing you do every morning, with a soft spunge and warm water, for four or five minutes; and then wash your mouth five or six times. . . . Nothing looks more ordinary, vulgar, and illiberal, than dirty hands and ugly, uneven, and ragged nails. . . . You must keep the ends of them smooth and clean, not tipped with black, as the ordinary people's always are. The ends of your nails should be small segments of circles, which, by a very little care in the cutting, they are very easily brought to; every time that you wipe your hands, rub the skin round your nails backwards, that it may not grow up and shorten your nails too much'.

If teeth were not well cared for in the eighteenth century, and they usually were not, it was not for want of reminders. In 1750 there appeared from time to time in the *London Gazette* an advertisement for 'Mr. Greenough's Tinctures, the one of which perfectly cures the Scurvy in the Gums, fastens and preserves the Teeth, renders them white and beautiful, prevents their decaying, and keeps such as are decayed from becoming worse. The other, for curing the Tooth-Ach, gives ease in a few Minutes, and in a little Time perfectly cures it, even when most violent.' The tinctures, 'too well known to the Nobility and Gentry (and indeed to the World in general) to need any further recommendation', were sold 'only by J. Newbery, at the Bible and Sun, near the Chapter-House in St. Paul's Church-yard' and by 'T. Greenough, Apothecary, near St. Sepulchre's Church'. The price was one shilling a bottle.

12 · The Late Eighteenth Century
1770-1800

If the young men of this age are so silly
as to be allured by a little red paint,
why red paint must be used;
but for married women, mistresses of families,
mothers, for these to be greedy
of the gaze and admiration of the other sex
is disgusting and betrays a frivolity of character
unbecoming the dignity of a matron's situation.

THE GENTLEMAN'S MAGAZINE, 1792

In the latter part of the eighteenth century bright red lips and magenta cheeks on a chalk-white face were fashionable, though the shade of red depended on the quality of rouge the lady was able to obtain. The portrait painters usually represented the colouring with a vermilion tint. A Gainsborough portrait of Mrs Grace Dalrymple Elliott shows her rouge applied rather low, extending from cheekbone to jawbone in a generally triangular pattern. Sir Thomas Lawrence's portrait of Elizabeth Farrer, done a few years later, also shows the rouge low on the cheek but applied in a round pattern.

PAINTS AND PAINTING

The English Parliament, taking note of the spread of painting, expressed its alarm and disapproval by passing a law as unenforceable as it was naïve, stating that 'All women, of whatever age, rank, profession or degree, whether virgins, maids, or widows, that shall from and after this act impose upon, seduce or betray into matrimony any of His Majesty's subjects by the use of scents, paints, cosmetics, washes, artificial teeth, false hair, Spanish wool, iron stays, hoops, high-heeled shoes, or bolstered hips, shall incur the penalty of the law now in force against witchcraft and like misdemeanors, and that the marriage, upon conviction, shall stand null and void.' The ladies, needless to say, continued to paint. In fact, the December 1776 issue of the *Lady's Magazine* contained an amusing essay 'On the modern Fashion of Painting' which seems well worth quoting:

'A Great deal of wit and raillery has been exerted by several polite writers against the predominant fashion among the ladies, of setting off their charms

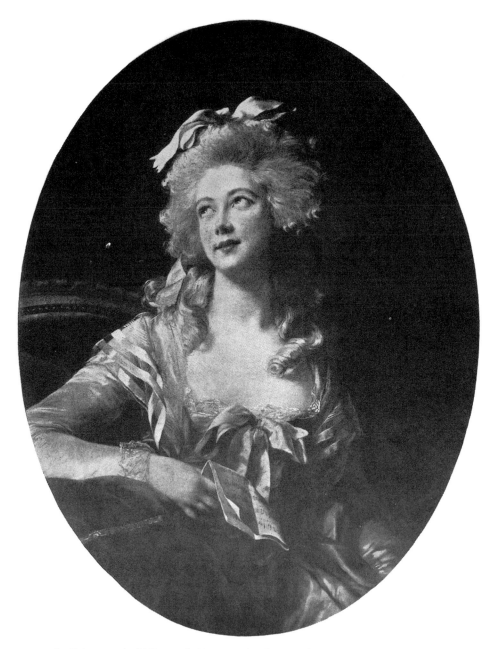

FIG. 136: Princesse de Talleyrand. Painting by Louise Elisabeth Vigée-Lebrun, late eighteenth century.

with the addition of paint.—Our great Shakespeare has put a very severe remark into the mouth of his Hamlet, in the scene with Ophelia:—"Heaven hath given ye one face, and ye make yourselves another."—This thought has been twisted and tortured into a thousand different shapes by every little endeavourer at an epigram for a long time past, and the custom has been frequently censured as a folly imported from our neighbours the French. As the art of giving an artificial tincture to the skin appears to me to admit of many favourable circumstances, I shall employ this essay in vindication of my pretty countrywomen.

'It may seem at first an extreme bold position, if I assert that painting is not an importation of modern refinement, but originally of English growth; and yet, that this is the real state of the case, is sufficiently known to the most superficial dabbler in history.' The correspondent quotes Julius Caesar's description of the early Britons painted blue with woad, which, he adds 'lends them a formidable aspect in battle. This, I think, may serve to obviate the imputation of imitating the French in this particular, which I take to be a point of some consequence, as by this we cannot be charged with the levity of having servilely copied from others. We find that the ladies among the British Picts went entirely naked and painted their bodies all over with the woad above-mentioned.

'This must, undoubtedly, have afforded great scope for fancy, and in those days there must certainly have been many eager rivalships among the fair for pre-eminence in point of taste for painting. As the whole lovely body was ornamented with different figures and sundry various representations, according as imagination suggested, the variety of new fashions must have been extremely entertaining, each fair one being studious to adapt to each different part of the body that degree of colouring, and that form which must have proved most becoming.

'As painting, therefore, was the universal practice among our ancestors, I am strongly inclined to think it laudable in the amiable sex at present. I must, however, take notice, by the way, of one circumstance, in which the modern practice of painting differs from ancient simplicity. I do not find in the account of any historian, that the female British Picts applied the least tincture of the woad to the natural complexion of their faces. For a bloom and a vivacity of colour they trusted to exercise, fresh air, and wholesome diet: but as the fashionable vigils of gaming were unknown in those days, it must be allowed that this is an improvement upon the fashions of our progenitors: and, indeed, it could not be expected that in those rude times so elegant a diversion could be known. For this we are indebted to modern refinement, which has introduced improvements in manners, as well as in arts and sciences.'

In a subsequent issue another correspondent expands on the theme with tongue in cheek:

'When simple nature is left to her own disposal, is she not rude and unpolished? and is it not principally owing to the effects of art that nature is brought nearest to perfection? with what degree of propriety, then, can we discommend those ladies who, to heighten the natural bloom and complexion of their countanance, make use of the finest colours that art can procure?

'To speak then, as far as this custom concerns the preservation of our health, to me it appears that painting cannot be prejudicial when it provides against the openness of the pores and the dangers of the cold. . . . To embellish as many parts of the body as still remain open to the view would be one of the greatest improvements upon the English character for beauty and symmetry of proportion; because the beautiful ivory that so distinguishes the bosom and the neck would shew itself to much greater advantage when placed in opposition to a variety of colours.'

Brushing aside the legal, moral, and aesthetic issues, a book entitled *The Art of Beauty* warned against the popular white paints which, the author said, 'affect the eyes, which swell and inflame, and are rendered painful and watery. They change the texture of the skin, on which they produce pimples and cause rheums; attack the teeth, make them ache, destroy the enamel, and loosen them. They heat the mouth and throat, infecting and corrupting the saliva, and they penetrate through the pores of the skin, acting by degrees, on the spongy substance of the lungs, and inducing diseases. Or, in other cases, if the paint be composed of aluminous or calcareous substances, it stops the pores of the skin, which it tarnishes, and prevents the perspiration, which is, of course, carried to some other part, to the peril of the individual. . . . To the inconveniences we have just enumerated, we add this, of turning the skin black when it is exposed to the contact of sulphureous or phosphoric exhalations. Accordingly, those females who make use of them ought carefully to avoid going too near substances in a state of putrefaction, the vapours of sulphur, and liver of sulphur, and the exhalation of bruised garlic.' But the warning was not new and fell on deaf ears. The ladies continued to enamel.

John Almon described such an enamelled lady in 1777:

> Her hair's like the sea, deck'd with shells, lovers pledges,
> Where hearts are entangled like fishes in sedges;
>
> . . . .
>
> From each new acquaintance, she still exacts garnish;
> Like iv'ry her teeth, and her cheeks are like — varnish.

This was also the year that Lady Sarah Lennox, who very nearly married George III, mentioned in a letter to Lady Susan O'Brien that she had heard that 'Lady Ilehesten appeared at the Opera without powder, dressed in a poking, queer way, with Ly Sefton, & caused great speculation to know who that queer but pretty little vulgar woman could be that Ly Sefton brought with her. Now,

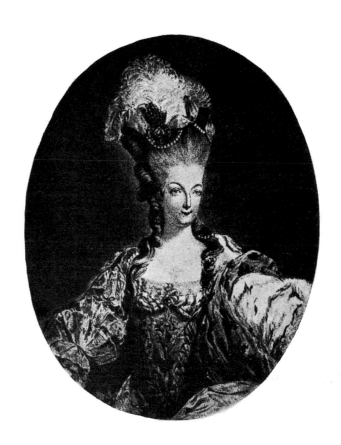

FIG. 137: Marie-Antoinette, consort of
Louis XVI. Engraving by
François Janinet, 1777.

to be sure, it requires nothing but a short examination to find out that the
genteel Ly Sefton is in *nature* a most compleat vulgar; to my certain knowledge
her gentility never went further than her dress, & the "*pretty, vulgar little
woman*" has more true real gentility about her than most people I know, for
her understanding is enlarged, & her mind very far above the common rate. But
such is the world that a little powder & gauze properly disposed secures a proper
respect, & the neglect of it gives a *mauvais ton*, which 'tis sometimes a little
troublesome to overcome.'

Horace Walpole wrote to George Selwyn from Paris in 1775 that 'feathers
are waning, and almost confined to *filles* and foreigners. I found out an
Englishwoman at the Opera last night by her being covered with plumes and
no rouge, which made her look like a whore in a salivation; so well our
countrywomen contrive to display their virtue!'

By 1781 it was estimated that Frenchwomen used two million pots of rouge
a year. Madame Dugazon alone bought six dozen pots (at six francs each) from
Montclar, the perfumer. There were nearly a dozen kinds of rouge available,
liquid and dry, in a variety of shades, including mauve. At this time Friedrich
Nicolai observed that upper class women in Stuttgart rouged much more
naturally than the French.

In four lines J. B. B. Nichols describes The Dressing-Table of Marie-Antoinette:

> This was her table, these her trim outspread
> Brushes and trays and porcelain cups for red;
> Here she sat, while her women tired and curled
> The most unhappy head in all the world.

Even as late as 1783, when *The Young Quaker*, a comedy by George Colman, was first produced, there were those who resisted the fashion of painting. In the epilogue to the play, the character of Dinah assures the audience proudly that though she is now married and will be called Dinah Sadboy for life,

> Still shall my cheek shew Nature's white and red;
> No cap shall rise like steeple from my head;
> Powder, pomatum, ne'er my locks shall deck,
> Nor curls, like sausages, adorn my neck.

But Dinah Sadboy was the exception. Women of fashion continued to paint furiously. Lady Archer was one. Notorious at the gaming tables, she was equally notorious for her excessive use of makeup (see Figures 138 and 139), as implied in an item in the *Morning Post* for 5 January 1789:

> The Lady Archer, whose death was announced in this paper of Saturday, is not the celebrated character whose *cosmetic powers* have been long held in public estimation.

This was followed three days later by another item:

> It is said that the dealers in *Carmine and dead white*, as well as the *Perfumers* in general, have it in contemplation to present an address to Lady Archer, in gratitude for her not having DIED according to a late alarming report.

The eminent painted lady was also the inspiration for the following verse:

> Antient Phyllis has young graces,
> 'Tis a strange thing, but a true one;
>   Shall I tell you how?
> She herself makes her own faces,
> And each morning wears a new one;
>   Where's the wonder now?

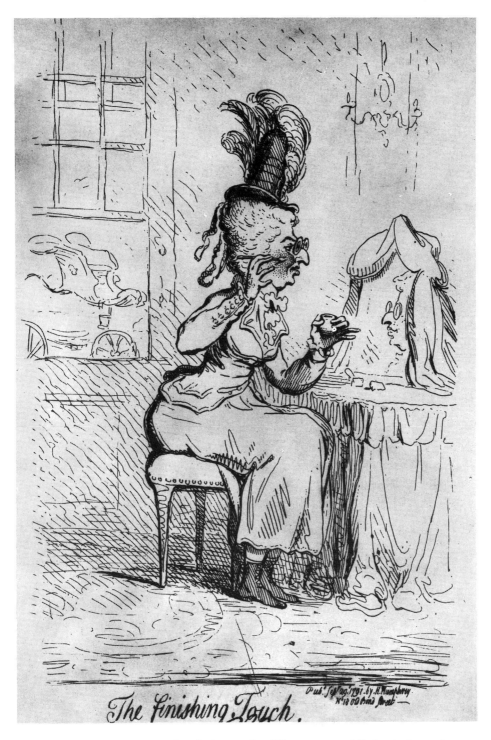

The finishing Touch.

FIG. 138: 'The Finishing Touch'. Caricature by Gillray, 1791, of Lady Archer, who was noted for her excessive use of makeup.

Among the men, fops painted their faces obviously, whereas those others who chose to paint at all, usually did so more or less secretly, with a hope of deception which, more often than not, was unsuccessful. Even today we are aware that the elderly Lord Ogle tried to add youth to his face and sparkle to his eyes with a faint tincture of rose, discreetly applied with full intent to deceive.

One of the best descriptions of the contemporary application of makeup comes from William Barker, of 6 King Street, Holborn, who wrote a short *Treatise on the Principles of Hair-Dressing; in which the Deformities of Modern Hairdressing are pointed out, and an elegant and natural Plan recommended, upon Hogarth's immortal System of Beauty.* Although no date of publication is given, one is led to the conclusion that it must have been written about 1786. Mr Barker, who was understandably distressed by the current hair styles, did not miss the opportunity for a few jibes at the French, whose fashions were so influential in England:

'If it is the ambition of my fair country-women to imitate the French ladies, I sincerely wish they would desist from the pursuit of what is impossible to attain. The French ladies being in general of a dark complexion, are very similar to each other when dressed for public appearance; for the fashion of wearing their rouge is systematical; and that fashion, when it does alter, alters always with a very remarkable variety. From a little below the eye there is sometimes drawn a red streak to the lower temple and another streak in a semicircular form to the other line. If the eye-brows are not naturally dark, they make them so; and unless ladies have very striking personal singularities, it is difficult to distinguish them asunder: their manners too so widely differing from the reserve of the English, renders imitation in that particular as burlesque and ridiculous as in the article of dress. Sometimes the French ladies, like the pallid Italian women of the opera, put on rouge of the highest colour in the form of a perfect circle, without shading it off at all; this is done to give a fire to the eye, which they think adds a spirit to conversation and a force to the art of ogling.' But Mr Barker added that Marie-Antoinette had introduced a more natural application of rouge.

During the reign of Louis XVI a Madame Josse provided ladies of the court with a vegetable rouge said to be as beautiful as natural colouring. There was also a Mlle Martin who supplied rouge in pots of Sèvres porcelain. Madame Tallien took strawberry and raspberry baths and was sponged with milk and perfumes.

Among his other accomplishments — house painter, hypnotist, healer, swindler — Count Cagliostro was a purveyor of cosmetic aids for both men and women. When he and his wife Lorenza (or the Countess Seraphine, as she preferred to be called) opened a shop in London in 1776, he was enormously successful in convincing his patrons, male and female, of the effectiveness of his products,

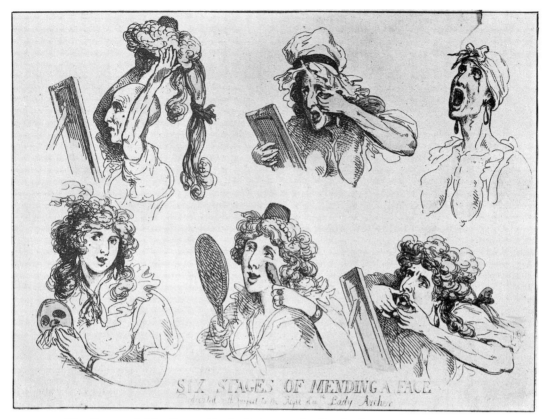

FIG. 139: 'Six Stages of Mending a Face'. Caricature by Rowlandson, 1791. 'Dedicated with Respect to the Right Honble Lady Archer.'

which included love potions, beautifying waters, sexual rejuvenators, and fake lottery tickets. The latter got him sent to prison in England, after which he went to Paris, spent some time in the Bastille, then returned to Sloane Street, Knightsbridge, with more nostrums, which he had some difficulty in promoting in spite of their popularity in Paris.

According to an advertisement of 1774, a rouge called Bloom of Circassia was being imported into New York for the first time. 'It is allowed,' read the advertisement, 'that the Circassians are the most beautiful women in the world. However, they derive not all their charms from nature. A gentleman long resident there in the suite of a person of distinction, well-known for his travels through Greece, became acquainted with the secret of the Liquid Bloom, extracted from a vegetable produce of that country, in general use there with the most esteemed beauties. It differs in all others in two very essential points. First, that it instantly gives a rosy hue to the cheeks, not to be distinguished from the lively and ornamental bloom of rural beauty, nor will it come off by perspiration, or the use of a handkerchief. A moment's trial will prove that it is not to be paralleled.'

The rouge proved to be extremely popular and continued to be used well into the next century. The infuriated early nineteenth-century lady in Figure 156 has knocked over her bottle of Circassian Bloom on to the floor.

A few of the cosmetics in use in the American colonies at the time, as listed by Gilbert Vail, include Apley's Violet Water, Balm of Mecca, Bavarian Red Liquor, Carmine, Ceruse, Chinese Wool, French Red, Italian Red, Imperial Cold Cream, Lady Molyneux's Italian Paste, Royal Cosmetic Beautifying Lotion, Spanish Papers, Spanish Red, Strawberry Cosmetic, and Venetian Paste. This Venetian Paste was 'well-known to the ladies for enamelling the Hands, Neck and Face, of a lovely white; it renders the most rough Skin smooth and soft as Velvet, and entirely eradicates Carbuncles and other Heats of the Face, or Nose and cracking of the Lips at this Season of the Year.' In 1774 it cost six shillings per pot.

PLOCACOSMOS

James Stewart's *Plocacosmos*, a rare and extraordinarily detailed book on hairdressing, published in 1782, contains a section on cosmetics giving precise meanings of terms in use at the time. Many of these had been used for a century or more and continued to be used until the Victorian age. 'Cosmetic,' says Stewart, 'is a term used for any preparation or means employed to beautify and embellish the face and preserve or improve the complexion; as ceruse, and the whole tribe of fucuses, washes, cold creams, lip salves, &c. &c.

'Ceruse is a white calk of lead, used in painting and cosmetics, made by calcining that metal in the vapour of vinegar.

'Ceruse is made of a thin lamina, or plates of lead, made up into rolls, and so placed as to receive and imbibe the fumes of vinegar contained in a vessel, and set over a moderate fire; the lamina are by means thereof concreted into a white crust, which they gather together, and grinding it up with water form into little cakes. Conder shews how to make ceruse of tin and urine. Ceruse makes a beautiful white colour and is much used by the painters both in oil and water colours. It makes the principal ingredient in the fucuses used by ladies for the complexion. Taken inwardly it is a dangerous poison and soon shews its malignity on the outside, spoiling the breath and teeth and hastening wrinkles and the symptoms of old age.

'The best ceruse is that of Venice, but this is rare; that chiefly used is either English or Dutch, both of which have more miol in them than white lead. The latter, however, is the better of the two.

'Fucus is a term used for paints or compositions applied to the face to beautify it and heighten the complexion. Old women make use of fucuses to appear

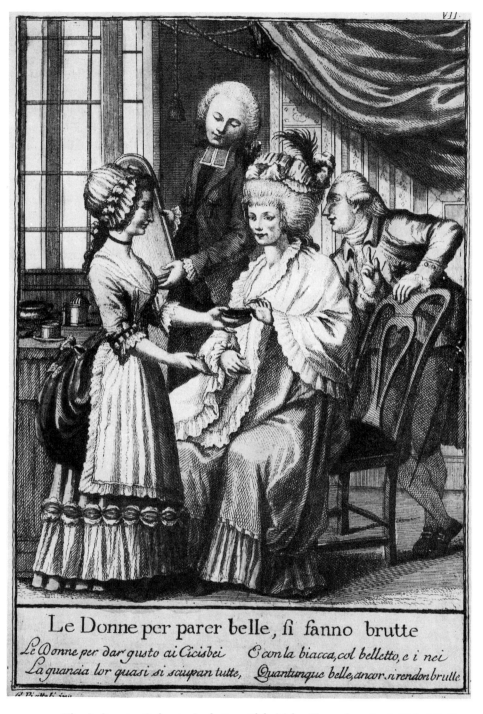

VII.

Le Donne per parer belle, si fanno brutte

Le Donne per dar gusto ai Cicisbei   E con la biacca, col belletto, e i nei
La guancia lor quasi si scuopan tutte,   Quantunque belle, ancor si rendon brutte

FIG. 140: 'The Ladies, in Order to Look Beautiful, Make Themselves Look Ugly.' Italian
engraving by Piattoli, 1786.

young. The fucus made with ceruse is corrosive and pernicious to the skin. The chymists abuse the ladies in selling them oil of bricks as an excellent fucus. Pliny says that the fucus of the Roman dames was a kind of white earth, or chalk, brought from Chios or Sanos, dissolved in water. The *fucus folimanni* is a composition of prepared sublimate, in great repute among the Spaniards of Peru. Of all the fucuses used by the ladies to whiten the complexion and hide the defects thereof, the least pernicious and that used with the greatest safety is the *Spanish White*, which is made of isinglass dissolved in spirits of nitre and precipitated into a very fine powder by means of salt water.'

Stewart, a hairdresser who considered himself also an authority on cosmetics, health, good manners, child rearing, and acting, mentioned that he had in his possession 'at least fifty receipts, all of equal ingenuity and efficacy, as well as utility, and even elegance, as well as an improvement on the manners of this nation; and however enigmatical it may seem, I can with justice say, the more such articles are encouraged in a land, the more flourishing that country must be.'

One of his ingenious, efficacious, and useful recipes was for *Lip Salve or Pomatum for the Lips*:

'Take half a pound of caul of mutton cut into pieces, and melt it in a little saucepan, and pass it through a piece of cloth, and put in another pan four ounces of wax, and when melted mix it with the mutton grease; then put in it balm of oil mixed together, and melt it again in the balneum mariae; when it is almost cold, put in it four drachms of carmine, and stir it till the pomatum be of a rose colour; then grind it well upon marble, and melt it again in the balneum mariae; when it is melted and cold, put some essence of rose in, and the pomatum salve is done.'

PIGEON'S WATER

In the late summer of 1778, a gentleman correspondent, writing to the *Lady's Magazine*, admitted that the fair and delicate complexions for which Danish women were famous, were due in part to a cosmetic wash known as Pigeon's water, the recipe for which was supposed to be secret, but which he obligingly quoted:

'Take of the water of nenuphar or water-lilly, bean water, melon water, cucumber water, and the juice of lemons, of each one ounce; of briony, wild succory, flowers de luce, borage, and bean-flowers, of each an handful; of white pigeons seven or eight, pluck them, and cut the heads and ends of the wings, then mince them very small, and put them, with the other ingredients into an alembic; add also four ounces of double-refined sugar, one drachm of borax, and as much camphire; the crumb of four small white loaves new from the oven, and a pint of good white wine. Let them digest in the alembic seventeen or eighteen days, after which distil the whole and reserve the water for use.

'Before this water is used, they make the skin perfectly clean with the following composition. Take about the fourth part of the crumb of a rye loaf, fresh from the oven, the whites of four fresh eggs, and a pint of vinegar: beat them well together, and strain the whole thro' a linen searse. Many ladies in this country who are full *fifty* years of age, preserve by these means all the freshness and bloom of *twenty-one*.

'This cosmetic I beg leave to recommend to the ladies of Great Britain, instead of those artificial colourings which are now in vogue, and which will inevitably destroy the finest complexion in a short time.'

The letter is signed by William Wimple. It is interesting to note that Mr Wimple's recipe, with only minor variations, appeared in the 1784 edition of *The Toilet of Flora*.

THE TOILET OF FLORA

In London, in 1775 (about the time the firm of Houbigant was established in Paris), women were busy brewing various concoctions for cleansing, softening, painting, and powdering their faces. *The Toilet of Flora* is, as the subtitle accurately states, 'a Collection of the Most Simple and Approved Methods of Preparing Baths, Essences, Pomatums, Powders, Perfumes, and Sweet-scented Waters'. It is an extraordinarily useful book for anyone examining the history of cosmetics; and, since a second edition was published in 1784, it must have proved of some practical value to women of the eighteenth century. The recipes quoted here are from the second edition. We begin with part of the charmingly tactful introduction:

'The chief Intention of this Performance is to point out and explain to the Fair Sex the Methods by which they may preserve and add to their Charms; and by which many natural Blemishes and Imperfections may be remedied or concealed. The same Share of Grace and Attraction is not possessed by all of them; but while the Improvement of their Persons is the indispensable Duty of those who have been little favoured by Nature, it should not be neglected even by the few who have received the largest Proportion of her Gifts. The same Art which will communicate to the former the Power of pleasing, will enable the latter to extend the Empire of their Beauty. It is possible to remove or, at least, to cover the Defects of the one Class, and to give Force and Lustre to the Perfections of the other.'

All books of the period giving hints on beauty contained various recipes for cosmetic washes. One of the more intriguing recipes in this book — for a wash called *Imperial Water* — begins, 'Take five quarts of Brandy'. After the addition of frankincense, mastic, benjamin, gum arabic, cloves, nutmeg, pine-nuts, sweet almonds, and musk, all bruised and distilled, one has, to judge from the book, a very versatile cosmetic: 'This water takes away wrinkles and renders the skin extremely delicate; it also whitens the Teeth and abates the toothache, sweetens the breath, and strengthens the gums. Foreign ladies prize it highly.'

Quite a different sort of lotion, called *The Divine Cordial*, was evidently intended for the patient lady with plenty of time and a large flower garden:

'To make this, take, in the beginning of the month of March, two ounces of the Roots of the true Acorus, Betony, Florentine Orrice-roots, Cyprus, Gentian, and sweet Scabion; an ounce of Cinnamon, and as much Yellow Sanders; two drachms of Mace; an ounce of Juniper-berries; and six drachms of Coriander-seeds; beat these ingredients, in a mortar, to a coarse powder, and add thereto the outer Peel of six fine China Oranges; put them all into a large vessel, with a gallon and a half of Spirit of Wine; shake them well, and then cork the vessel tight till the Season for Flowers. When these are in full vigour, add half a handful of the following: viz. Violets, Hyacinths, Jonquils, Wall Flowers, Red, Damask, White, and Musk Roses, Clove-july-Flowers, Orange Flowers, Jasmine, Tuberoses, Rosemary, Sage, Thyme, Lavender, sweet Marjoram, Broom, Elder, St. John's-wort, Marigold, Chamomile, Lilies of the Valley, Narcissuses, Honeysuckle, Borage, and Bugloss.

'Three seasons are required to procure all these Flowers in perfection; Spring, Summer, and Autumn. Every time you gather any of these Flowers, add them immediately to the infusion, mixing them thoroughly with the other ingredients; and three days after you have put in the last Flowers, put the whole into a glass cucurbit, lute [seal with mud or clay] on the head carefully, place in a water bath over a slow fire . . . and draw off five quarts of Spirit, which will prove of a rare quality. As a medicine, it is far more efficatious than Balm-water; and for its fine scent, one of the best perfumes.'

There was also a recipe *To Remove Worms in the Face*, containing, among other ingredients, melon seeds, egg whites, bread crumbs, and white roses.

It is interesting to note that the sponges ladies used for the face and sometimes for the teeth evidently could not be purchased ready to use but had to be prepared:

'Steep in Water some time the finest and thinnest Sponges you can pick out; wash them well, dry them, and soak them in Brandy a whole day; then squeeze the Brandy out, and dry them again. Lastly, dip them in Orange flower Water, and let them remain in it eleven or twelve hours. When squeezed and thoroughly dried, they are fit for use.'

Since the skin of the fashionable eighteenth-century lady was supposed to have a slight natural shine to complement the hair dulled with powder, the book

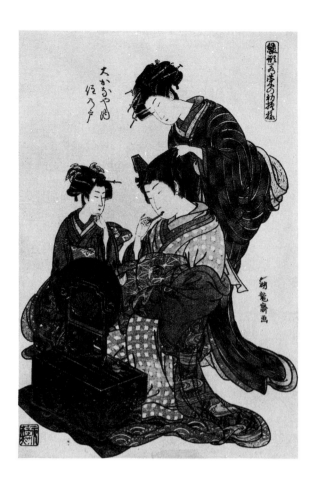

FIG. 141 : Eighteenth-century Japanese courtesans applying makeup. Woodcut
by Korinsai.

contains a recipe for *An Admirable Varnish for the Skin*:

'Take equal parts of Lemon Juice, and Whites of new laid Eggs, beat them
well together in a glazed earthen pan, which put on a slow fire, and keep the
mixture constantly stirring with a wooden spatula, till it has acquired the
consistence of soft butter. Keep it for use, and at the time of applying it, add a
few drops of any Essence you like best. Before the face is rubbed with this
varnish, it will be proper to wash with the distilled Water of rice. This is one of
the best methods of rendering the complexion fair and the skin smooth, soft, and
shining.'

There is in the book a large number of recipes for pomatum, for both skin
and hair. One for *Cucumber Pomatum* requires hog's lard, ripe melons and
cucumbers, verjuice, pippins, and cow's milk. After much melting, washing, and
straining, it is to be kept 'in a gallypot tied over with a bladder'. There are
several recipes for colouring the face, fewer than one would expect in view of the
amount of painting that was done, but probably as many as the limited materials
of the time made possible. One is for *A Distilled Water that tinges the Cheeks a
beautiful Carnation Hue*:

'Take two quarts of white wine Vinegar, three ounces of Isinglass, two
ounces of bruised Nutmegs, and six ounces of Honey: distil with a gentle fire,

259

and add to the distilled Water a small quantity of Red Sanders, in order to colour it. Before the Tincture is used, a Lady should wash herself with Elder-flower Water, and then the cheeks will become of a fine lively vermillion that cannot be distinguished from the natural bloom of youth.'

There are, in addition, recipes for scarlet lip salves, which, like many other recipes in the book, are lifted directly from *The Art of Preserving Beauty* of Le Camus. One recipe for lip salve suggests that the lady add some gold leaf if she wishes.

One way of blackening the eyebrows was to rub them frequently with ripe elderberries. For the brows, lashes, or lids one might use burnt cork, lamp black, burnt ivory shavings, burnt cloves, or even 'the Black of Frankincense, Rosin, and Mastic. This Black,' the reader was assured, 'will not melt nor come off by sweating.' Evidently some blacks did.

Eyebrows were also shaped, professionally or at home, and false eyebrows were still worn occasionally and occasionally lost.

For dyeing the eyebrows black, the ladies (or perhaps the gentlemen) were instructed to wash the brows 'with a decoction of Gall Nuts; then wet them with a pencil or a little brush dipped in a solution of Green Vitriol, in which a little Gum Arabic has been dissolved, and when dry, they will appear of a beautiful black colour'.

To change the Colour of the Hair one was supposed to wash the head with spring water, then dip the comb in oil of tartar, and comb the hair in the sun. The author's guarantee was encouraging: 'Repeat this operation three times a day, and at the end of eight days at the most the hair will turn black'. For scenting the hair, a little oil of benjamin was recommended.

For men who wished *To change Hair or Beard black*, there was a less simple but perhaps quicker method:

'Take Oil of Costus and Myrtle, of each an ounce and a half; mix them well in a leaded mortar; adding liquid Pitch, expressed Juice of Walnut Leaves and Laudanum, of each half an ounce; Gall-nuts, Black-lead, and Frankincense, of each a drachm, and a sufficient quantity of Mucilage of Gum Arabic made with a decoction of Gall Nuts.'

The recipe ends with the curious instruction to 'Rub the head and chin with this mixture after they have been shaved'.

The book also contains a recipe for *A Fluid to die the Hair of a flaxen Colour*. There is, in fact, a wide variety of recipes for doing things to the hair — colouring it, taking it off, keeping it on. One is a *Receipt to thicken the Hair and make it grow on a bald part*:

'Take Roots of a Maiden Vine, Roots of Hemp, and Cores of soft Cabbages, of each two handfuls; dry and burn them; afterwards make a lye with the ashes. The head is to be washed with this lye three days successively, the part having been previously well rubbed with Honey.'

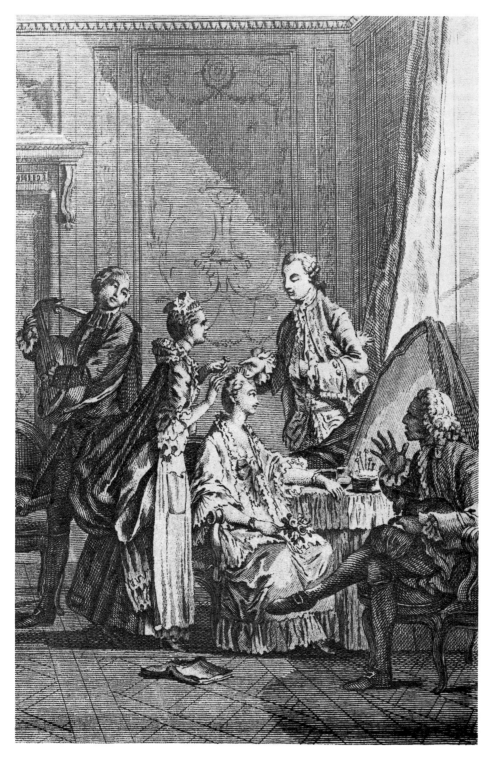

FIG. 142: The Toilette. Engraved in 1777 for the *Lady's Magazine*, it represents a period at least fifteen to twenty years earlier. The engraving depicts the moment when Priscilla's new admirer presents her with a costly egret, which is inexplicably embellished with a diamond the girl's father has lost. The father, at the right, registers astonishment. 'But what,' asks the editor, 'is the moral of this interesting story?'

A *Powder to prevent Baldness* is a marvel of simplicity: 'Powder your head with powdered Parsley Seed, at night, once in three or four months, and the hair will never fall off'. Other recipes for encouraging the growth of hair contain such ingredients as the juice of nettles, wormwood, Southernwood, sage, betony, vervain, dill, mistletoe, hemp, bear's grease, and red wine. Somehow the powdered parsley seed seems the best choice.

There is, in addition, *A powder to nourish the Hair*, which is supposed not only to increase growth of the hair, but to enliven the imagination and improve the memory.

One of the more interesting dentifrices mentioned is *A Coral Stick for the Teeth*:

'Make a stiff Paste with Tooth Powder and a sufficient quantity of Mucilage of Gum Tragacanth: form with this Paste little cylindrical Rollers, the thickness of a large goose quill, and about three inches in length. Dry them in the shade. The method of using this stick is to rub it against the teeth, which become cleaner in proportion as it wastes.'

This is followed by a recipe *For rotten Teeth* and another entitled *An approved Receipt against that troublesome Complaint called The Teeth Set on Edge*. This latter involved chewing purslain, sorrel, almonds, walnuts, or burnt bread. Scrubbing the teeth with gunpowder was said to give them 'an inconceivable whiteness'.

In 1787 Joseph II prohibited the use of white paint because of its harmful effects on the skin and general health and severely taxed the use of rouge.

In the *Lady's Magazine* for February 1793, Dr A. Fothergill, a physician from Bath, in some 'Remarks on Cosmetics', lamented the fact that most cosmetics probably contained lead, mercury, or bismuth:

'Carmine, or harmless rouge (as the ladies are pleased to term it), is a preparation of cochineal in nitrous acid, with some other ingredient, which is kept a profound secret. This favourite composition, which gives the roseate bloom to their countenance, being prepared with a strong mineral acid, is perhaps not altogether so very innocent as they imagine; besides, its excessive dearness renders it an object of adulteration; and vermilion (a preparation of mercury), though an humble imitation, affords a cheap and inviting ingredient to mix with it. To this, in its simple or combined state, they are generally beholden for their roses; while a calx of lead, or what is equally pernicious, the magistery of bismuth, gives the last polish to the lily whiteness which so dazzles our eyes. It is thus our modern Hebes attempt to preserve a perpetual bloom, and to hold wrinkles and old age at defiance. But, alas! these pernicious ingredients, although only used externally, are liable to be imbibed at every pore, and thence convey a slow poison into the system, highly injurious to health: and, what may appear still more formidable, destructive to beauty: —For, dismal to relate, the cold cream, the pomade divine, or, whatever specious titles such compositions may assume, at last betray their trust; and, instead of beauty, produce real deformity.

'This poisonous composition is generally dignified by the pompous title of pearl powder and sold as perfectly innocent; it has, however, proved fatal to some and ruined the health of many others without being even suspected. I am credibly informed that those ladies who are in the habit of enamelling their faces, necks, and bosoms with this white paint generally fall early victims to their own indiscretion; — but particularly so if they chance to undergo the small-pox, even by inoculation. Nor is this to be wondered at, the pustules being unable to penetrate outwardly through the enamelled skin, the virus recedes inwardly and preys on the vital organs.

'The artificial roses soon fade, the angelic whiteness contracts a dingey brown, when the mask falls off, and the spectre stands confessed, particularly on exposure to the sun, a hot fire, or sulphureous vapours. Strange that British ladies, to whom nature has been so bountiful, should distrust their native charms, and have recourse to such wretched substitutes of art! — Is it not truly mortifying that they should thus stoop to adorn, or rather disguise, their persons at the expense of their health?'

In concluding, Dr Fothergill told his readers that there was one simple cosmetic he could recommend with confidence as 'a perfectly safe, cheap, and efficacious substitute for all the pernicious tribe above-mentioned, and which may be freely used without any risk of detection — a cosmetic which boasts the highest antiquity and is perhaps the only true one acknowledged by nature. It is not only innocent, but highly conducive to health. It clears the complexion far beyond the milk of roses; and when accompanied with regular hours and brisk exercise in the open air, diffuses over the countenance more animated bloom than the finest rouge. It is now almost needless to add that this grand secret is no other than *Cold Spring Water*.' This no doubt came as a great disappointment to his readers.

CRITICS OF PAINTING

A letter to the editor of *The Gentleman's Magazine*, dated 27 April 1792, complains about the continued prevalence of painting in England:

'I remember some years ago to have read a pamphlet, published about the time of Charles II, against face-painting. Can you, or any of your readers, inform me where one may be procured? Such a treatise seems now much wanted. Great and little, old and young, paint their faces, nay, "avow the fact, and glory in the deed." Not only her Grace and Lady Betty put on a little rouge when they dress for the drawing-room; but Mrs. and Miss Drivequill must bedaub their

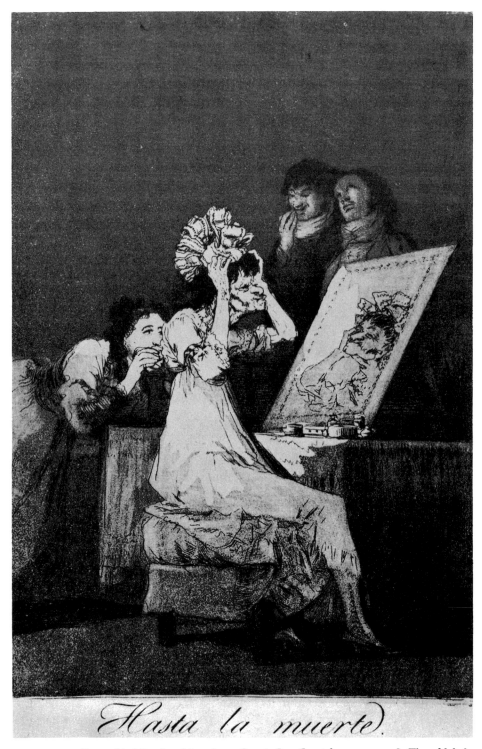

FIG. 143: 'Till Death'. Mixed etching from Goya's *Los Caprichos, c.* 1793–8. The old lady
has her paints in front of her and is evidently completing the ritual of beautification.

cheeks with red paint, or they would appear *quite particular at Mrs. Parch-ment's private party.*

'For the single ladies who follow this practice there is some excuse. . . . Husbands must be had, and if the young men of this age are so silly as to be allured by a little red paint, why red paint must be used; but for married women, mistresses of families, mothers, for these to be greedy of the gaze and admiration of the other sex is disgusting and betrays a frivolity of character unbecoming the dignity of a matron's situation. . . . The ladies sometimes assent that they put on paint to please their husbands. Is it possible that a British husband can desire his wife to make herself a gazing stock for every coxcomb! But if it is for the good man's personal satisfaction that all these pains are taken, let the fair one remember that to be consistent the rouge box must be had recourse to in the morning before breakfast, as well as before dinner, when she sits alone with her husband, as well as when she issues forth to a rout.'

The Gentleman's and London Magazine of 1792 published six *Original Epigrams to a Lady who Painted*, translated from the original French of Breboeuf:

I

Candour said I did my duty,
Cloris, when I prais'd your beauty;
But the Druggist overhearing,
Said it was beyond all bearing,
Her Beauty! Said th' astonish'd wight,
You deprive me of my right;
It shall be hers, I'll grant your will,
When for the pains, she pays my bill.

II

Let low bred cits of their finances boast,
Yours must by far exceed all common cost;
Tho' they oft sport new liveries and new lace,
You ev'ry day can sport a span new face.

III

Transcendent artist! matchless skill is thine,
To do thee justice mocks my weak design;
Since to thy skill, the faint attempt must fail,
Who'rt copy, painter, and original.

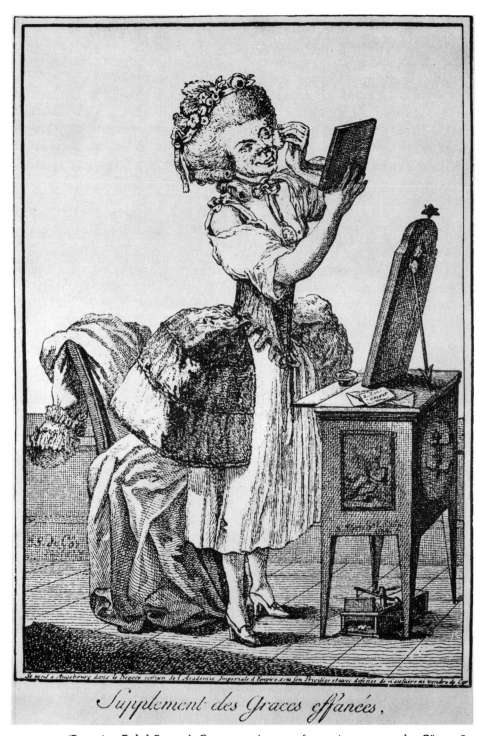

Supplement des Graces effacées.

FIG. 144: 'Restoring Faded Beauty'. German caricature of an aging coquette by Göz, 1784.

IV

Cloris! 'tis just we on your charms bestow
The rose's coral, and the lily's snow;
With such as these they most relation claim,
Their birth, their beauty, and their fall the same;
Like those they flourish with the morning light,
And fade at noon, or disappear at night.

V

Yes, yes, thy mystic hand we all must own,
That takes up youth, or wrinkled age lays down;
Cloris by day with all the virgins glow,
At night her *grandam* in her native snow.

VI

To Cloris still the faithful muse shall give
That well-earn'd praise the modest must receive;
Who young, could captivate each wand'ring heart,
Does still in age preserve her wond'rous art.
Tho' then your aspect fill'd the breast with fight,
You wound us still, but most you wound our sight!
Horror, not love, does now the twain pursue,
Who daring ventures the terrific view;
Yet still by prudence faithfully you steer,
Who cannot love, you justly make to fear.

A long poem entitled *On Female Conduct* appearing later in the year, contained one verse relating specifically to the toilet:

What is your sex's earliest, latest care,
Your heart's supreme ambition? — To be fair:
For this the toilet every thought employs;
Hence all the oils of dress and all the joys;
For this hands, lips, and eyes are put to school,
And each instructive feature has its rule.

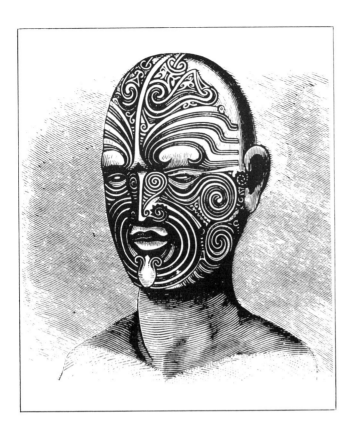

FIG. 145: Tattooed head of a New
Zealand chieftain. Nine-
teenth-century wood
engraving.

THE VOYAGES OF CAPTAIN COOK

On the other side of the world, men and women were also painting. During his
world travels, a good many of which took place in the 1770s, Captain Cook
meticulously recorded his impressions of the natives he met and observed, always
including notations on their hair and the colour, natural and artificial, of their
skin. When he arrived in New Zealand, he noted in his log that 'the native
women paint their faces with red ochre and oil, which is generally so moist as
to make an imprint on anyone who embraces them. Many of our sailors were
thus marked on the nose.' At one time the men drew designs on their faces with
charcoal before going into battle. Later they were tattooed. (See Figure 145.)
Unfortunately, tattooed heads brought such a good price from Europeans that
tattooed men were more in danger of their lives than others.

The Tahitians, Cook reported, used rancid coconut oil on their hair and
tattooed their bodies. 'This is done by inlaying the colour of black under their
skins in such a manner as to be indelible. Some have ill-designed figures of men,
birds, or dogs; the women generally have the figure Z simply on every joint of
their fingers and toes; the men have it likewise, and both have other different
figures, such as circles, crescents, etc., which they have on their arms and legs;

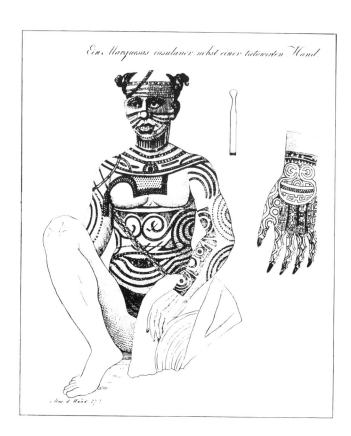

FIG. 146: Tattooed native of the
Marquesas Islands. Early
nineteenth-century engra-
ving. The stick in the
middle is used for
tattooing.

in short, they are so various in the application of these figures that both the
quantity and situation of them seem to depend entirely upon the humour of
each individual, yet all agree in having their buttocks covered with a deep black.
Over this most have arches drawn one over another as high as their short ribs,
which are near a quarter of an inch broad. ...

'The colour they use is lamp black, prepared from the smoke of a kind of oily
nut, used by them instead of candles. The instrument for pricking it under the
skin is made of very thin flat pieces of bone or shell. ... One end is cut into sharp
teeth, and the other fastened to a handle. (See Figure 146.) The teeth are dipped
into black liquor and then drove, by quick, sharp blows struck upon the handle
with a stick for that purpose, into the skin so deep that every stroke is followed
with a small quantity of blood. The part so marked remains sore for some days
before it heals. As this is a painful operation, especially the tattowing their
buttocks, it is performed but once in their lifetimes; it is never done until they
are twelve or fourteen years of age.'

The brown-skinned, black-haired Maoris, especially the older ones, tattooed
their faces with black and occasionally other parts of the body as well, mostly
with spiral designs applied with great precision. These might cover the entire
face, only part of it, or only one side. Women tattooed their lips black, and both

269

sexes painted their faces and bodies, on occasion, with red ochre mixed with fish oil. The Australian aborigines, on the other hand, used a white paint on their faces and bodies, each individual evidently making up his own design.

The copper-skinned native men of the Friendly Isles sometimes coloured their short, dark hair red, white and blue and shaved their beards with sharp shells. The men tattooed their bodies 'from the middle of the thigh to above the hips; the women, only lightly on their arms and fingers'. On Easter Island the men tattooed from head to foot; the women, only slightly. Both used red and white paint, the red being made from tamarick.

In the New Hebrides, Captain Cook found the natives reasonably handsome and 'of a very dark colour, but not black. . . . They make themselves blacker than they really are by painting their faces with a pigment of the colour of black lead. They also use another sort which is red, and a third sort brown, or a colour between red and black. All these, but especially the first, they lay on, with a liberal hand, not only on the face, but on the neck, shoulders, and breast.'

The American Indians on Nootka Sound, Cook reported, always painted their bodies red and their faces black, bright red, or white. The white, said the Captain, 'gives them a ghastly, disgusting aspect. They also strew the brown martial mica upon the paint, which makes it glitter, the ears of many of them are perforated in the lobe, where they make a pretty large hole; and two others higher up on the outer edge. In these holes they hang bits of bone; quills fixed upon a leathern thong; small shells; bunches of woollen tassels; or pieces of thin copper, which our beads could never supplant. The septum of the nose, in many, is also perforated, through which they draw a piece of soft cord; and others wear, at the same place, small thin pieces of iron, brass, or copper, shaped almost like a horseshoe, the narrow opening of which receives the septum, so as that the two points may gently pinch it; and the ornament thus hangs over the upper lip.' On special occasions the face was 'variously painted, having its upper and lower parts of different colours, the strokes appearing like fresh gashes, or . . . besmeared with a kind of tallow, mixed with paint, which is afterward formed into a great variety of regular figures, and appears like carved work'.

In discussing the adornment of women of the East Indies, William Alexander wrote:

'They have a variety of paints to improve the charms of nature, these they mix and lay so artfully upon their cheeks and eyes that it is exceedingly difficult to discover them; they likewise paint the extremities of the nails, but in this instance, departing entirely from nature, they lay on a fine red so thick that on the slightest view it appears to be the work of art. Black moles on the face have long been considered in the East as particularly beautiful. In the songs of their poets and works of their painters, this fancied elegance is seldom forgot; and to supply it when wanting, was probably the cause which first introduced black patches.'

They also used a variety of perfumes, for which they often spent more than they did on clothing and jewelry. Dr Alexander then supplied a few notes on Americans, whom he considered to be 'the least favoured by nature and to have made themselves the least assistance by art. . . . Our European traders judge of the fortune of an American by the trinkets on the crown of his head, at his ears, wrists, fingers, &c.; by the quantity of red paint daubed on his face, and by the finery at the collar of his shirt, if he happens to have one, which is far from being always the case.'

Having warmed to his subject, Dr Alexander added that 'some nations of savages, not contented with such ornaments as are loose and easily detached from the body, have contrived to ornament the body itself by incisions, stainings, and paint. The Chilesian women of the province of Cuyo and the plains on the East side of the Andes paint some part of their faces of a green colour. In several of the islands lately discovered in the Great Southern Ocean, a variety of indelible stains are made in different parts of the body by certain materials which sink into small punctures made in the skin. In Otaheite, this operation is called *tattowing* and reckoned so essentially necessary that none of either sex must be without it, especially the women.

'What they chiefly pride themselves in is long threads of human hair, plaited so as hardly to be thicker than sewing silk, and often a mile or more in length, without a single knot; these they wrap round their heads in a manner that shews they are neither void of taste nor elegance, sticking flowers and springs of evergreen among them, to give them the greater variety. European satirists are apt to declaim against our ladies for spending so much time under the operation of a French hair-dresser, while even these untutored people cannot be supposed to employ much less in twisting so many yards of rope round their heads and giving it the necessary decorations.'

Arabian women, it was reported, stained their nails red and their palms and soles with henna. The eyes were lined and the eyelashes blackened with *kochhel*, a lead ore. Eye makeup was also used by some men. All men wore beards, which in eighteenth-century Europe were completely out of fashion and rarely seen. Older men sometimes dyed their white beards red, but the practice was not well thought of. The Persians blackened their beards, even when they were naturally black, and the custom was said to be catching on among fashionable young Turks.

In 1792 a curious miscellany on female beauty, extracted from Du Halde, appeared in the *Lady's Magazine*:

'The ladies in Japan gild their teeth; and those of the Indies paint them red. The blackest teeth are esteemed the most beautiful in Guzurat, and in some parts of America. In Greenland the women colour their faces with blue and yellow. However fresh the complexion of a Muscovite may be, she would think herself very ugly if she was not plaistered over with paint. . . . In some countries, the mothers break the noses of their children; and in others press the head between two boards that it may become square. The modern Persians have a strong aversion to red hair: the Turks, on the contrary, are warm admirers of these disgusting locks. The Indian beauty is thickly smeared with bear's fat. . . .

'In China, small eyes are admired, and the girls are continually plucking their eye-brows that they may be small and long. The Turkish women dip a gold brush in the tincture of a black drug, which they pass over their eye-brows. It is too visible by day but looks shining by night. They tinge their nails with a rose colour. . . .

'The female head dress is carried, in some countries, to singular extravagance. The Chinese fair carries on her head the figure of a certain bird. This bird is composed of copper or of gold, according to the quality of the person; the wings spread out, fall over the front of the head-dress, and conceal the temples. The tail, long and open, forms a beautiful tuft of feathers. The beak covers the top of the nose; the neck is fastened to the body of the artificial animal by a spring, that it may the more freely play and tremble at the slightest motion.

'The extravagance of the Myanteses is far more ridiculous than the above. They carry on their heads a slight board, rather longer than a foot, and about six inches broad; with this they cover their hair and seal it with wax. They cannot lie down, nor lean, without keeping the neck very straight; and the country being very woody it is not uncommon to find them with their head-dress entangled in the trees. Whenever they comb their hair, they pass an hour by the fire in melting the wax; but this combing is only performed once or twice a year.

'To this curious account . . . we must join that of the inhabitants of the land of Natal. They wear caps, or bonnets, from six to ten inches high, composed of the fat of oxen. They then gradually anoint the head with a purer grease, which, mixing with the hair, fastens these *bonnets* for their lives.'

Japanese women rouged their lips (Figure 147) and whitened their skin (Figure 148).

THEATRICAL MAKEUP

In *A Treatise on the Principles of Hair-Dressing*, William Barker explains that his method of dressing the hair for Mrs Siddons and other theatrical clients 'tends principally to the setting off the features of the face and the hue of the complexion, and that my curling also, as well as powdering hair, are governed not by fashion, but by the formation of the face and neck, the colour of the skin, and the lights, whether natural or artificial, by which the face and neck are to be viewed. The hair, in an artificial light, is only to be considered as a mean to give a fine colour to the complexion by such shade and light as the stage

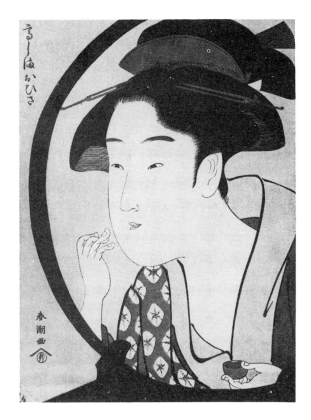

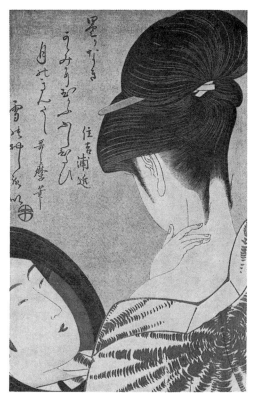

FIG. 147: Japanese lady rouging her lips. Eighteenth-century woodcut.

FIG. 148: Powdering the neck. Japanese woodcut by Utamaro.

affords, which will, in every possible instance, alter the face and natural colour of the complexion. This may be demonstrated by the absolute necessity which stage performers are under of using colour on their faces; and it is evident that young men who perform old characters, by a judicious application of white and red and a few black lines drawn with Indian ink, often wear the appearance on the stage of eighty or ninety and are altogether so much altered that their most intimate friends do not know them.'

Until greasepaint was invented in Germany about the middle of the century, the actor's makeup kit was very limited indeed, including little but a lard-and-white-lead paint, burnt cork, ashes, white chalk, black crayon, and carmine. Considerable reliance was therefore placed on beards and wigs.

Figure 149 shows a Japanese actor having his face painted in the stylized tradition of the Kabuki and Nō theatres. White paint was usually used on the face for both men and women — originally to make the faces more visible in the dark theatres. The actor's brows were blocked out with the white paint and new ones painted on with black above his own. The eyes were lined and the lips painted. For male characters stylized designs were often painted on the face, using both line and colour to represent emotions or character traits. Originally, all parts had been played by women, but on 23 October 1629, the Women's

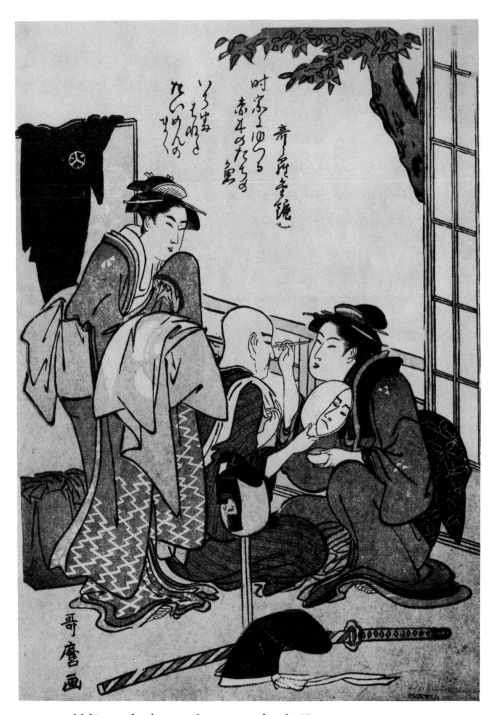

FIG. 149: Making up for the stage. Japanese woodcut by Utamaro.

Kabuki was outlawed, according to Ernst, for both moral and political reasons. For a short time women continued to play women's parts, but after 1630 all parts were played by men, and it was not until 1868 that women were permitted to perform in public at all. The Kabuki theatre is still exclusively male.

Mountains of Hair

Perhaps critics of fashion would have had even more to say about the excessive use of cosmetics if they had not been so busy satirizing the hair styles, which year by year were growing more preposterous. The following song is included here to help round out the picture of the eighteenth-century woman:

THE MOUNTAIN OF HAIR

You maids, wives, and widows of Britain draw near,
I'll sing you a ditty will tickel your ear;
How maids, wives, and widows now fashion their hair,
With fine lappets behind, and mountains of hair.

My lady she goes to the ball and the play,
She rambles all night and she sleeps all the day,
And then in the evening to church does repair,
With her lappets behind, and mountains of hair.

And Miss Sally also, her own serving maid,
Who keeps up the jest to keep up her trade;
She shews her white breast, and her bosom quite bare,
With her fine lappets behind, and mountains of hair.

There's millers', bakers', and shopkeepers' wives,
They'll have their hair dress'd to keep up their pride,
The landlady sits dress'd up in her chair,
Her head she can't move for the weight of her hair.

Then in comes the farmer's wife 'mongst all the rest,
'A barber this minute, my hair must be drest;
And if you don't dress it a yard high, I do swear,
The devil may pay you for dressing my hair.'

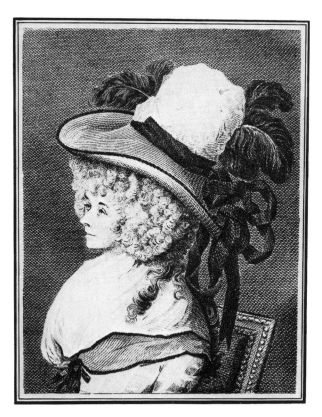

FIG. 150: Engraved portrait of Mrs Hannah
Cowley (1743–1800), dramatist
and poet.

Then in comes the butcher's wife, greasy and fat,
She will have her hair dress'd and what of all that;
A fine leg of mutton, or shoulder, I swear,
She gives to the barber for dressing her hair.

Miss Jenny, they tell me, is breeding a kind,
And Molly is left in the same state, I find,
And when the young babes come into their care,
They'll curse their lappets, and damn their false hair.

Believe me, dear ladies, you're all in the wrong,
I tell you: and that makes an end of the song;
When your hair's finely dress'd, I plainly do see,
You look like an owl in an old Ivy-tree.

In December of the same year Mary Granville Delany wrote from London to
a friend, 'I hear of nothing but balls and high heads — so *enormous* that nobody
can sit upright in their coaches, but *stoop forward* as if they had got the
children's *chollick*. Surely there is an influenza of the *brain*, which must account
for the present vagaries and be some excuse.'

On a Wednesday morning in May 1780 Mrs Delany wrote from London to her friend Mrs Port about a concert the previous night to celebrate the opening of Mrs Walsingham's new house and her daughter's birthday. 'The concert was splendid,' wrote Mrs Delany, 'rows above rows of fine ladies with *towering tops*. Not having been much used to see so many together I must own I could not help considering them with some astonishment and lamenting that so absurd, inconven^t, and unbecoming a fashion should last so long, for though every year has produced some alteration, the *enormity* continues, and one of the most beautiful ornaments of nature, fine hair, is entirely disguised; it appears to me just as ridiculous as if Mr Port was to fell all his fine hanging woods and feathered hills, and instead of all the beautiful hues of various native greens, should plant only *Scotch firrs* and *brambles*!'

Around 1770 the Macaronis, a group of fashionable young men who had travelled in Italy, burst forth in London with their patches and powder, their foppish dress, and their exaggerated clubbed wigs, giving the satirists fresh material for several years, as in this last verse of a song with 'words by Mr. Oakman':

> Five pounds of hair they wear behind,
>   The ladies to delight, O;
> Their senses give unto the wind
>   To make themselves a fright, O;
> This fashion who does e'er pursue
>   I think a simple-tony,
> For he's a fool, say what you will,
>   Who is a Macaroni.

But fool or not, the Macaroni had an enormous effect on fashions for both men and women, as attested by a song called *The Female Macaroni*:

> No ringlets now adorn the face,
>   Dear nature yields to art;
> A lofty head-dress must take place,
>   Absurd in ev'ry part.
> Patch, paint, perfume, immodest stare,
>   You find is all the fashion;
> Alas, I'm sorry for the fair
>   Who thus disgrace the nation.

Only a little later, in 1775, David Garrick was satirizing the ladies' fashions in a musical farce called *May-Day, or the Little Gypsey*:

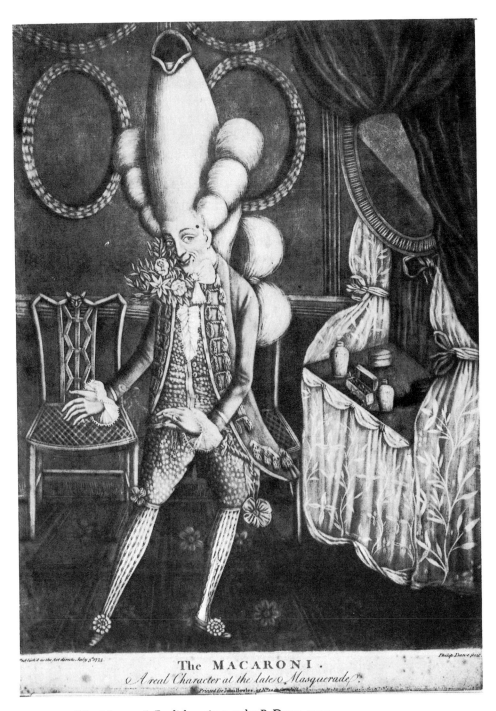

The MACARONI.

A real Character at the late Masquerade.

FIG. 151: 'The Macaroni'. English caricature by P. Dawe, 1773.

> The ladies I vow,
> I cannot tell how,
> Were now white as curd, and now red.
> Law, how you would stare
> At the huge crop of hair,
> 'Tis a hay-cock at top of their head.

Nor did he ignore the men :

> Then the fops are so fine,
> With lank-waisted chine,
> And a skimp bit of a hat,
> Which from sun, wind, or rain,
> Will not shelter their brain,
> Though there's no need to take care of that.

A piece called 'The Modern Belle', published in the *Universal Magazine* in 1776, concentrated on the women :

> Void of talents, sense, and art,
> Dress is now her better part.
> Sing her daub'd with white and red;
> Sing her large terrific head,
> Nor the many things disguise,
> That produce its mighty size;
> And let nothing be forgot,
> Carrots, turnips, and what not;
> Curls and cushions for imprimis,
> Wool and powder for the finish;
> Lace and lappets, many a flag,
> Many a party-colour'd rag,
> Pendent from the head behind,
> Floats and wantons in the wind;
> Many a gem, and many a feather,
> A fine farrago all together,
> By whose wool and wire assistance
> (Formidable at a distance,
> As the elephants of yore
> A fam'd queen to battle bore)
> They with terror and surprise
> Strike the poor beholder's eyes.

> What a quantity of brain
> Must he think such heads contain!

After the travelling Macaronis had disappeared, the stay-at-homes who imitated them and perhaps went to even greater cosmetic and sartorial extremes were known as Jessamies. The *Morning Post* in July 1789 reported 'not a man in the nation, no not even Lord Effingham, who bestows so much time and attention in rendering the external appearance of his head, elegant in the extreme, than the Earl of Scarbourough. It is said that his Lordship keeps six French frizeurs, who have nothing else to do than dress his hair. Lord Effingham keeps only Five!!!'

In his *New Bath Guide* Christopher Anstey satirizes the various fashions of the times, including hairdressing and face-painting. Most of the head-dresses he mentions are illustrated in *Fashions in Hair*. The following lines are from 'A Modern Headdress':

> What base and unjust accusations we find
> Arise from the malice and spleen of mankind!
> One would hope, my dear mother, that scandal would spare,
> The tender, the helpless, and delicate fair;
> But alas! the sweet creatures all find it the case,
> That *Bath* is a very censorious place.
> Would you think that a person I met since I came,
> (I hope you'll excuse my concealing his name)
> A splenetic ill-natured fellow, before
> A room-full of very good company swore,
> That, in spite of appearance, 'twas very well known,
> Their hair and their faces were none of their own:
> And thus without wit, or the least provocation,
> Began an impertinent formal oration:
> 'Shall nature thus lavish her beauties in vain
> 'For art and nonsensical Fashion to stain?
> 'The fair Jezebella what art can adorn,
> 'Whose cheeks are like roses that blush in the morn?
> 'As bright were her locks as in heaven are seen,
> 'Presented for stars by th' Egyptian queen;
> 'But alas! the sweet nymph they no longer must deck,
> 'No more shall they flow o'er her ivory neck;
> 'Those tresses which Venus might take as a favour,
> 'Fall a victim at once to an outlandish shaver;
> 'Her head has he robb'd with as little remorse
> 'As a fox-hunter crops both his dogs and his horse:

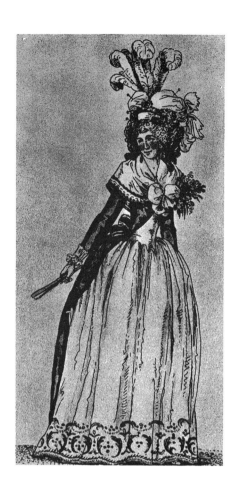

FIG. 152: Fashionably dressed lady of the 1790s. The heavily applied rouge was as fashionable as the feathers. Ink and watercolour sketch from a French fashion journal.

'A wretch that, so far from repenting his theft,
'Makes a boast of tormenting the little that's left:
'And first at her porcupine head he begins
'To fumble and poke with his irons and pins,
'Then fires all his crackers with horrid grimace,
'And puffs his vile *Rocambol* breath in her face,
'Discharging a steam that the devil would choak,
'From paper, pomatum, from powder, and smoke.
'The patient submits, and with due resignation
'Prepares for her fate in the next operation.
'When lo! on a sudden a monster appears,
'A horrible monster, to cover her ears;
'What sign of the zodiac is it he bears?
'Is it *Taurus's tail* or the *tête de mouton*,
'Or the *beard of the goat* that he dares to put on?
' 'Tis a wig *en vergette*, that from Paris was brought,
'*Une tête comme il faut*, that the varlet has bought
'Of a beggar whose head he has shav'd for a groat:

'Now fix'd to her head, does he frizzle and dab it;
'Her foretop's no more — 'tis the skin of a rabbit —
' 'Tis a muff — 'tis a thing that by all is confest
'Is in colour and shape like a chalfinch's nest.

    'O cease, ye fair virgins, such pains to employ,
'The beauties of nature with paint to destroy;
'See Venus lament, see the Loves and the Graces,
'How they pine at the injury done to your faces!
'Ye have eyes, lips, and nose, but your heads are no more
'Than a doll's that is plac'd at a milliner's door.'

    I'm asham'd to repeat what he said in the sequel,
Aspersions so cruel as nothing can equal!
I declare I am shock'd such a fellow should vex
And spread all these lies of the innocent sex,
For whom, while I live, I will make protestation
I've the highest esteem, and profound veneration:
I never so strange an opinion will harbour,
That they buy all the hair they have got of a barber;
Nor ever believe that such beautiful creatures
Can have any delight in abusing their features:
One thing tho' I wonder at much, I confess, is
The appearance they make in their different dresses;
For indeed they look very much like apparitions
When they come in the morning to hear the musicians,
And some I am apt to mistake, at first sight,
For the mothers of those I have seen over night:
It shocks me to see them look paler than ashes,
And as dead in the eye as the busto of Nash is,
Who the ev'ning before were so blooming and plump,
— I'm griev'd to the heart when I go to the pump.

Hairdresser William Barker credited Marie-Antoinette with 'introducing the fashion of wearing a kind of orange coloured powder, which, by an artificial light, looks like what is vulgarly called red hair, but which has a very good effect in an assembly, if the lady's complexion should be bad. On the heads of some fine women, it has quite a contrary effect, as powder of such an hue, even with the assistance of rouge on her cheeks, must give her face a livid cast, and her neck must appear as if painted a dead white.'

For ladies who wished to compound their own hair powders, Stewart gave instructions on how *To Make Powders of Various Colours*:

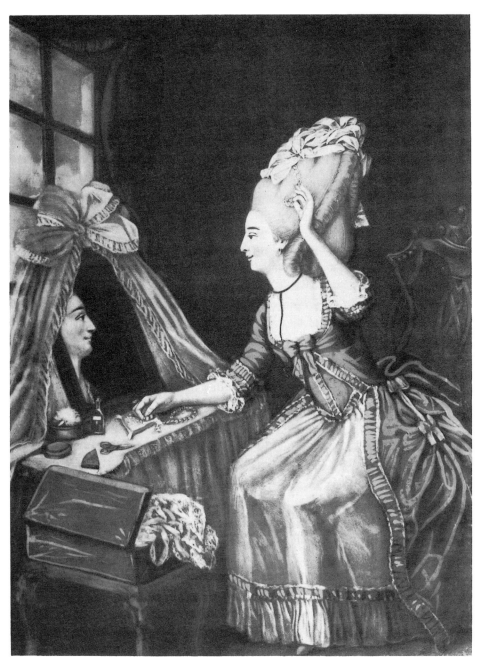

FIG. 153: 'Miss Rattle Dressing for the Pantheon.' English caricature, late 1770s.

'Take a pound of ivory black, in powder, and pass it through a sieve, and a pound of fine powder, which you must put on the fire, in a new saucepan, till is turns very black; then wet it with half an ounce of eau de Mareschalle. After that take of cloves, four drachms; cinnamon, two drachms; ginger, four drachms, dry these three pieces upon a red-hot shovel; after that peel them, and beat them to powder so that they might pass through a sieve; then mix them all together, and the black powder will be done. This is the powder that is called the Poudre à la Mareschalle and that serves to make up all the other kind of coloured powders, except the fair, the rose, and the red. It may be remarked that the Mareschalle cannot be made properly in this country; all made here having a foetid, hot disagreeable smell and hurtful to the hair; while that from Paris is cool, sweet, wholesome and fragrant.'

Various colours of hair powder were used throughout the decade. Although Mr Barker suggested that in general it would be wise to leave the choice of the right one to the hairdresser, provided he was a man of taste, he did offer a few suggestions:

'White powder is regaining its general use and promises to be the universally adopted taste, but the use of white powder in the extreme is an error that a nice distinguishing taste for elegance can never altogether adopt, because the colour of the powder must ever be governed by the prevailing tints of the person's complexion. A brown beauty and a fair beauty should not use the same coloured powder;—the reason must be self-evident. Ladies who take exercise and have the lovely glow of health in their cheeks, however fair and beautiful the complexion may be, should not use white powder alone, as the effect ever must be that the light acting on white without absorbing one ray, the reflected rays cast a shade on the face that discolours the real complexion and gives it the semblance of a dusky brown. On the contrary, a lady who leads a sedentary life and is little exposed to the air will have a rather languid aspect; a very little brown mixed with white powder will therefore give great assistance to such a complexion, enliven the appearance of the eyes and face, and animate the whole form.

'There is a coloured hair (I mean the yellow, vulgarly called red, of a more than common bright tinge) to which a deep brown or chocolate powder gives the happiest cast, infinitely surpassing the grey powder, and saving the trouble and expense of staining the hair by advertised nostrums of a mineral, poisonous, destructive effect, which are generally applied by persons wholly ignorant of the nature and quality of hair. This powder, judiciously applied, has the same happy effect on flaxen and grey hair, with this difference as to the latter, that it must be used in its pure state, not lowered by the least mixture of white. . . .

'There are very few heads of hair which do not require the aid of colouring, as well as enriching. Pomade and powder are the best materials for that purpose I know of and have hitherto been so approved, none better having been yet

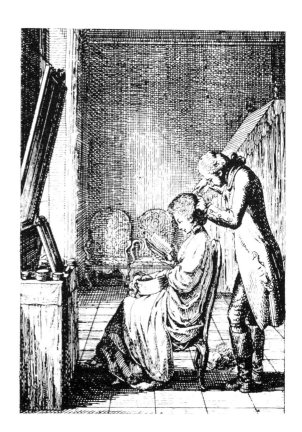

FIG. 154: Woman at her toilet, 1779. Etching
by Chodowiecki.

discovered; but the profusion with which these articles, valuable in themselves,
is too frequently used, is productive of as injurious effects as the inordinate
application of rouge. When ladies, desirous of a florid complexion and out of
humour with Nature for having been rather unkind in that particular, first
begin the use of that imaginary ornament, they apply it with a sparing hand;
but daily habit and the love of admiration tempting them by degrees to enlarge
the portion, those articles, which applied with discretion would tend to embellish,
are laid on in such profusion, and particularly the rouge, that the beholder turns
aside, the eye declining to encounter so glaring an object.'

Various kinds of pomatum or grease were used for making powder adhere to
the hair. One of the earliest references to Bear's Grease for the hair is to be found
in an advertisement in *The Times* for 7 February 1793:

> JUST KILLED, an extraordinary fine Fat Russian Bear, at Ross's Ornamen-
> tal Hair and Perfumery Warehouse, No. 119 Bishopsgate Street (late
> Vickery's), three doors from the London Tavern.
>
> The excellent virtue which the fat of Bears possesses has been exper-
> ienced by thousands of both sexes, and of all Ages, in this Metropolis. To
> those who have used the real Bears' Grease, it is evident no Grease what-
> ever beside, retains its moisture so long upon the head, it being the only
> thing possible to make the Hair grow thick and long, recover it after

illness, prevent it falling off, or turning grey, during life; being the most efficacious remedy for making the Hair grow on Horses' knees when broken or chafed.

It is sold at 1s. per ounce, or 16s. the pound, to be seen cut off the Animal in the presence of the purchaser.

HELP WANTED

Even in the eighteenth century women were pouring out their personal problems to unseen but sympathetic journalists. The following letter was purported to be written in the summer of 1775 to a Mrs Grey, who conducted a column in the *Lady's Magazine* called 'The Matron':

MADAM,

I am young and pretty, I am, of course, much followed by the men; I have also a very extensive acquaintance among my own sex, but I am afraid that the latter are more likely to do me mischief than the former, as they are always advising me to do every thing which the man, whom I prefer, disapproves.

When I first began to be taken notice of, I not only wore what was fashionable, but took particular care also that it should look becoming as well as genteel, and it had so good an effect, that I soon gained a very agreeable lover . . . with whom I think I can be happy, would my female friends let me alone; they are continually teizing me because I do not dress to the very extremity of the fashion and would not let me rest till I braided and bunched out my hair over a load of wool of a preposterous height and size, and placed the poke of my cap quite on the hinder part of my head, till it stuck out almost a quarter of a yard behind my hat, which with the addition of lappets, ribbons, &c. certainly made my head look out of all proportion.

In consequence of this way of dressing my head, Mr. Fairlove (that is the name of my lover) gently hinted that he thought a reduction of my *coëffure* was necessary, as it actually was swelled to a most enormous size. I thought his observation so judicious that I readily began to pull down all that was superfluous behind, and appeared with my head of a decent and becoming size.

All the women now attacked me at once — 'Lord!' cried one, 'what have you done to yourself to day? — I never saw you look so forlorn! — You are an absolute dowdy!' 'Bless me,' said another, 'how you have spoilt your hair! Why, it is quite thin; there is but one curl on a side (when

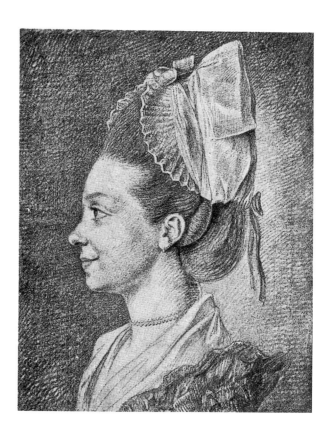

FIG. 155: Portrait of Babette Renelle.
Drawing by Chodowiecki,
c. 1770.

every body wears three at least) and no bag at all. Surely you have studied to make yourself as frightful as possible ! . . .'

Mortified at being thus found fault with by those who had not, I knew, the same pretensions to person as myself, I stuck out my hair and cap still more than ever, resolving not to be outdone by any body. Mr. Fairlove, now lifting up his hands and eyes at the sight of me, expressed the utmost surprise. 'I flattered myself, madam,' said he, 'that what I mentioned with regard to your head dress, had brought you to reason, but I find that I flattered myself too soon. You are more attached to the most preposterous of all fashions than you are to me. . . .' Thus, you see, it is impossible for me to please both my friends and my lover; I must, therefore, give up the one or the other, if you cannot put me into a way to please them all. Without giving general satisfaction, I cannot enjoy that tranquillity which would be most agreeable to me.

I am, madam,

Your very humble servant,

Lucy Weaver.

P.S. I cannot think why my female acquaintances will not let me alone. I never trouble myself about their heads.

PROBLEMS IN CLEANLINESS

In a letter to the editor of the *Lady's Magazine* in the summer of 1775, a 'Lover of Cleanliness' expressed puzzlement over the neglect of cleanliness by women who seemed to be going out of their way to be attractive, yet displayed 'a set of teeth covered with filth. If,' the correspondent concluded, 'that trouble were taken in cleaning the teeth, which is done by making themselves more disagreeable in the use of nauseous perfumes, they could not fail of being much more amiable in the opinion of delicacy.'

Teeth were often poor, even among fairly young people, often being described as yellow, black, jagged, or rotten. False teeth were available but not common. George Washington wore wooden ones, and before he was forty, Lord Hervey had a set made of Egyptian pebble. (Pebble was also used for ground lenses in optical instruments.) Ivory, bone, gold, enamel, and porcelain were also used, often secured with wire, springs, or pure luck, which one could not count on. George Washington's dropped out at least once during a public speech. Such dentures were satirized in three lines from *Excursions to Parnassus*:

> Can i'vry teeth at sixty-one,
> Tho bought of March, be deem'd thy own,
> Display'd in lucid rows?

More than half a century later the anonymous authors of *Habits of Good Society*, reminiscing about the past, touched on the carelessness of their forebears in the matter of personal cleanliness. 'Our great-grandmothers were afraid of cold water,' they wrote, 'and delicately *wiped* their faces with the corner of a towel no larger than a pocket handkerchief. There were those among them who boasted that they had never washed their faces in their whole span of existence, lest it should spoil their complexions, but had only passed a cambric handkerchief over the delicate brow and cheeks, wetted with elderflower water or rose water. I believe the nearest approach to the ablution we now diurnally practise was the bathing their lovely countenances in May-dew, esteemed the finest thing in the morning for the skin by our belles of the last century: so they turned out betimes in high-heeled shoes and *négligés*, trotted down the old avenues of many a patriarchal home to the meadow, and saturating their kerchiefs in May-dew, refreshed with it the cheeks flushed over-night at quadrille or great cassino, and went home contented that a conscientious duty had been performed.'

Princesses, it seems, were no cleaner than anybody else, and sometimes less so. In his diary for Wednesday, 18 February 1795, the first Duke of Malmesbury wrote:

'Argument with the Princess [Caroline of Brunswick] about her toilette. She piques herself on dressing quick; I disapprove this. She maintains her point; I however desire Madame Busche to explain to her that the Prince is very delicate, and that he expects a long and very careful *toilete de propreté*, of which she has no idea. On the contrary, she neglects it sadly and is offensive from this neglect. Madame Busche executes her commission well, and the Princess comes out the next day well washed *all over*.'

Lady Mary Wortley Montagu was notoriously lax in her personal cleanliness. When chided by a friend at the opera because her hands were dirty, she replied, characteristically, 'What would you say if you saw my feet?'

In eighteenth-century France private bathtubs were often found in the better homes, and it became the custom for one to receive visitors, male or female, while in the bath. On these occasions, a pint or two of milk was often added to the water for the sake of modesty rather than for any salutary effect it might have on the skin. This is probably the source of many reports of affluent women bathing luxuriously in milk to preserve their skin, though undoubtedly there were women who followed Poppaea's example and bathed in milk with no visitors on hand at all. Marie-Antoinette, more modest than some of the French-born ladies of the court, bathed in a long flannel robe buttoned up to the neck.

Men who had no bathtubs and liked cold baths, bathed nude in the Seine, occasionally shocking prudish females. The women, who were not permitted the same freedom as the men, could for three sous use enclosed cold baths set up at various points on the river. The men could also use them but had to stay on their own side. Towels were available for one sou. Other baths, some fairly elaborate, were established in boats on the river bank. One which was opened in 1761 near the Pont Royal was forty-one feet long and divided into two levels. This was arranged to accommodate both men and women. The water, pumped from the river, was filtered before it reached the baths. Another bath on the Quai d'Orsay was free to poor people who had proper certification from their doctor or curate. Steam and shower baths were also available at houses in the area.

In 1782, after people had once more become accustomed to bathing from time to time, a doctor of theology, who evidently believed that Godliness did not require *complete* cleanliness, published a manual reviving the notion that water applied to the face was harmful and that one should clean the face each morning by rubbing with a white cloth. Even this was a considerable step forward from the carelessness of Lady Mary Wortley and most of her contemporaries, but meticulous cleanliness would have to wait until the nineteenth century, when Beau Brummell made it fashionable.

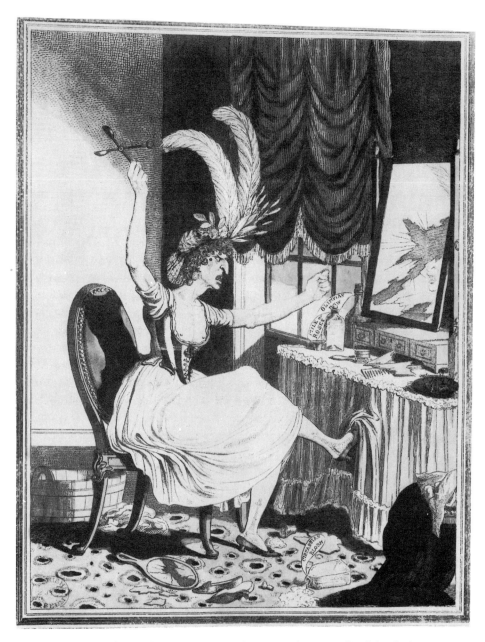

FIG. 156: 'The Looking Glass in Disgrace'. Caricature by Isaac Cruikshank, between 1805 and 1810.

13 · The Early Nineteenth Century
1800-1837

I cannot see any shame in the most ingenuous
female acknowledging that she occasionally rouges.
It is often, like a cheerful smile on the face
of an invalid, put on to give comfort to
an anxious friend.

MIRROR OF THE GRACES

The nineteenth century saw the pendulum swing away from the obvious, highly artificial makeup of the eighteenth century to subtle, natural, deceptive makeup or none at all. At no time in the century was makeup completely abandoned by all women in the Western world, though during the peak of the Victorian influence in England and America, it sometimes *seemed* to be. Most men simply assumed that whatever colour their wives had was natural, and the wives made sure that their husbands' illusions were not shattered. Other women were less naive, but so subtle was the deception that they could seldom be sure. For most of the century obvious makeup was not socially acceptable and was rarely seen.

FROM PAINTED TO PALE

In the early years of the century young and fashionable cheeks were brightly rouged. A portrait by Sir Thomas Lawrence, painted about 1803, shows the rose-coloured rouge applied in a large round pattern. The lips were also rose. But after about 1806 the makeup became more subdued and, when used at all, was often so artfully applied as to escape detection. Even the Empress Joséphine, who devoted considerable time to her makeup, was somewhat secretive about the cosmetics she used.

About this time an unidentified fashion editor, quoted by Lester and Oerke, wrote that the tinting of the face and lips was considered permissible only for those upon the stage. 'Now and then,' wrote the editor, 'a misguided woman tints her cheeks to replace the glow of health and youth. The artificiality of the effect is apparent to everyone and calls attention to that which the person most desires to conceal. It hardly seems likely that a time will ever come again in which rouge will be well-nigh universally employed, but until that time does come, a person could not make a greater mistake than to use it upon the face.'

Yet older women often clung not only to their rouge but to their white enamel as well, as noted disapprovingly in *The Habits of Good Society; A Handbook of Etiquette for Ladies and Gentlemen*, published in London in 1859:

'The celebrated Mrs. Fitzherbert was rouged to the very eyes; those beautiful deep blue eyes of hers. The old Duchess of R——— enamelled, and usually fled from a room when the windows were opened, as the compound, whatever formed of, was apt to dissolve and run down the face. Queen Caroline (of Brunswick) was rouged fearfully; her daughter, noble in form, fair but pale in complexion, disdained the art.'

In the summer of 1817 Lady Granville described Lady Stuart as being 'very agreeable and amiable, and by dint of rouge and an auburn wig looks only not pretty, but nothing worse'. She found Miss Rodney to be 'a very pretty girl, but with rather too much rouge and *naiveté*'.

But with cosmetics, going out of fashion simply meant going underground. Women continued to paint, but they pretended not to. In November 1810 Lady Granville, the former Lady Harriet Cavendish, wrote to her brother that she had grown very thin and pale and that a female friend had strongly recommended rouge. Husbands, she assured Lady Granville, never noticed such things, for if they did, her own husband would be furious with her. 'And,' Lady Granville added, 'the little man would be so, for he is still wondering and exulting over her having left off being pea green.'

With rouge out of fashion, a pale, ethereal look came into vogue. The Psyche look (from Gerard's *Psyche et l'Amour*) was greatly admired and widely imitated, often with the help of face-whitening lotions.

In the French Restoration the classic look disappeared, and ladies tried to look like figures out of the mass book—pale, slender, delicate, spiritual, slightly indisposed, given to attacks of the vapours. They used a ghostly white makeup and quantities of rice powder. Their makeup, if not imitated, was often matched by the dandies, who whitened the backs of their hands and rouged their palms.

In 1811 a Lady of Distinction, in a little book called *Mirror of the Graces*, spoke firmly to women about the use of cosmetics:

'The custom which some ladies have, when warm, of powdering their faces, washing them with cold water, or throwing off their bonnets, that they may cool the faster, are all very destructive habits. Each of them is sufficient . . . to spread a surfeit over the skin and make a once beautiful face hideous for ever.'

She made a strong plea for beautiful complexions—but only real, never artificial, and she refused 'to tolerate that fictitious, that dead beauty which is composed of white paints and enamelling. In the first place, as all applications of this kind are as a mask on the skin, they can never, but at a distant glance, impose for a moment on a discerning eye. But why should I say a *discerning eye*? No eye that is of the commonest apprehension can look on a face bedaubed with white paint, pearl powder, or enamel, and be deceived for a minute into a

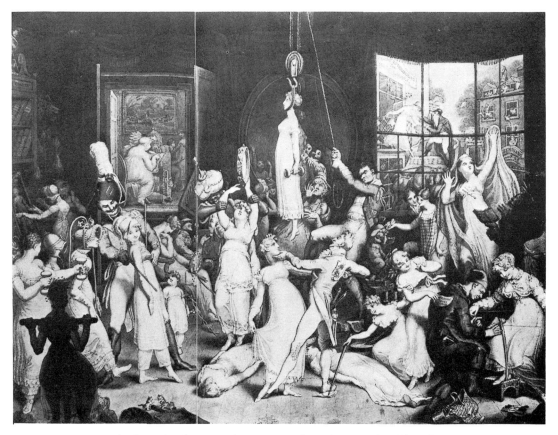

FIG. 157: Beauty school in London, c. 1800. Watercolour drawing by Edward Francis Burney.

belief that so inanimate a "whited wall" is the human skin. . . . Perhaps the painted creature may be admired by an artist, as a well executed picture; but no man will seriously consider her as a handsome woman.

'White painting is, therefore, an ineffectual, as well as a dangerous practice. The proposed end is not obtained; and, as poison lurks under every layer, the constitution wanes in alarming proportion as the supposed charms increase.'

Curiously, she is more permissive about red, which 'leaves three parts of the face and the whole of the neck and arms to their natural hues. . . . A little vegetable rouge tinging the cheek of a delicate woman, who, from ill health or an anxious mind, loses her roses, may be excusable; and so transparent is the texture of such rouge (when unadulterated with lead) that when the blood does mount to the face, it speaks through the slight covering and enhances the fading bloom. But though the occasional use of rouge may be tolerated, yet my fair friends must understand that it is only *tolerated*. Good sense must so preside in its application that its tint on the cheek may always be fainter than what nature's palette would have painted. A violently rouged woman is one of the most disgusting objects to the eye. The excessive red on the face gives a coarse-

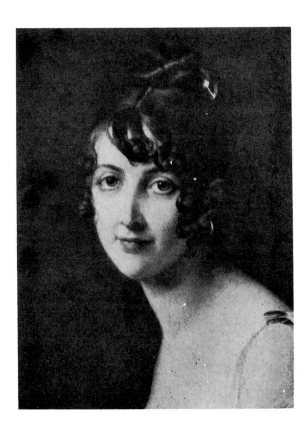

ness to every feature and a general fierceness to the countenance, which transforms the elegant lady of fashion into a vulgar harridan.'

But she does not approve of using rouge deceptively, for it seems to her 'so slight and so innocent an apparel of the face (a kind of decent veil thrown over the cheek, rendered too eloquent of grief by the pallidness of secret sorrow)' that she 'cannot see any shame in the most ingenuous female acknowledging that she occasionally rouges. It is often, like a cheerful smile on the face of an invalid, put on to give comfort to an anxious friend.'

Having admitted the possibility of using rouge and made the necessary excuses for it, our Lady of Distinction then proceeds to explain exactly how it should be applied:

'French women, in general, and those who imitate them, daub it on from the bottom of the side of the face up to the very eye, even till it meets the lower eyelash, and creeps all over the temples. This is a hideous practice. It is obvious that it must produce deformity instead of beauty, and, as I said before, would metamorphose the gentlest-looking fair Herse into a fierce Medusa.

'For brunettes, a slight touch of simple carmine on the cheek, in its dry powder state, is amply sufficient. Taste will teach the hand to soften the colour by due degrees, till it almost imperceptibly blends with the natural hue of the skin. For fairer complexions, letting down the vivid red of the carmine with a mixture of fine hair-powder, till it suits the general appearance of the skin, will have the desired effect.'

But rouge, we are told, is the 'only species of positive art a woman of integrity or of delicacy can permit herself to use with her face. Her motives for imitating the bloom of health may be of the most honourable nature, and she can with candour avow them. On the reverse, nothing but selfish vanity and falsehood of mind could prevail on a woman to enamel her skin with white paints, to lacker her lips with vermilion, to draw the meandering vein through the fictitious alabaster with as fictitious a die. Penciling eyebrows, staining them, &c. are too clumsy tricks of attempted deception for any other emotion to be excited in the mind of the beholder than contempt for the bad taste and wilful blindness which could ever deem them passable for a moment. . . . Let every woman be content to leave her eyes as she found them and to make that use of them which was their design.'

Yet in the back of the book the author does include a recipe for lip salve containing 'a small portion of alcanna root, sufficient to colour it a bright vermilion'.

THE ART OF BEAUTY

Judging from *The Art of Beauty; or, the Best Methods of Improving and preserving the Shape, Carriage, and Complexion*, published in London in 1825, the attitude toward painting was more permissive than it would be later in Victorian days:

'Ought people to use paint? Why not? When a person is young and fresh and handsome, to paint would be perfectly ridiculous; it would be wantonly spoiling the fairest gifts of nature. But, on the contrary, when an antique and venerable dowager covers her brown and shrivelled skin with a thick layer of white paint, heightened with a tint of vermilion, we are sincerely thankful to her; for then we can look at her at least without disgust. And are we not under obligation to her for being at the pains to render herself in reality more ugly than she is, in order that she may appear less so.'

The author then argues strongly in favour of rouge and asks, 'In an age when women blush so little, ought we not to value this innocent artifice, which is capable of now and then exhibiting to us at least the picture of modesty, and which, in the absence of virtue, contrives, at least, to preserve her portrait. . . .

'It is not the present fashion to make so much use of red as was done some years ago; at least, it is applied with more art and taste. With very few exceptions, ladies have absolutely renounced that glaring, fiery red with which our antiquated dames formerly masked their faces.'

It is then suggested that ladies would do well to compound their own rouge

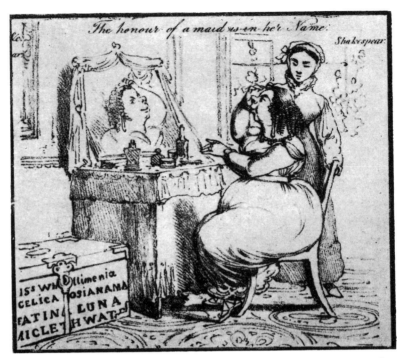

FIG. 159: 'The Honour of a Maid is in Her Name.' English caricature, 1826.

and avoid the risk of the dangerous metallic paints by using harmless vegetable dyes from 'red sandal wood, root of orchanet, cochineal, Brazil wood, and especially the bastard saffron, which yields a very beautiful colour when it is mixed with a sufficient quantity of talc. Some perfumers compose vegetable rouge, for which they take vinegar as the excipient. These reds are liable to injure the beauty of the skin; it is more advisable to mix them with oily or unctuous matter, and to form salves. For this purpose you may employ balm of Mecca, butter of cacao, spermaceti, oil of ben, &c.'

Spanish wool was frequently mentioned in the eighteenth century as a cosmetic for both men and women and was evidently still in use. Of the several sorts, it is stated in the book that 'that which is made here in London is by far the best; that which comes from Spain being of a very dark red colour, whereas the former gives a bright pale red; and, when it is very good, the cakes, which ought to be of the size and thickness of a crown-piece, shine and glisten, between a green and a gold colour.

'This sort of Spanish wool is always best when made in dry and hot summer weather, for then it strikes the finest blooming colour; whereas, what is made in wet winter weather is of a coarse dirty colour, like the wool from Spain. It is, therefore, best always to buy it in the summer season, when, besides having it at the best time, the retailer can likewise have it cheaper; for then the makers can work as fast as they please, whereas, in winter, they must choose and pick their time.'

An interesting variation called 'Spanish papers' is described as being 'of two sorts: they differ in nothing from the above, but the red colour, which in the latter, tinges the wool, is here laid on paper; chiefly for the convenience of carrying in a pocket-book.

'This coloured wool comes from China, in large round loose cakes, of the diameter of three inches. The finest of these give a most lovely agreeable blush to the cheek; but it is seldom possible to pick more than three or four out of a parcel, which have a truly fine colour; for, as the cakes are loose, like carded wool, the voyage by sea, and the exposure to air, even in opening them to show to a friend, carries off their fine colour.'

There were also Chinese boxes of colours, each containing 'Two dozen of papers, and in each paper are three smaller ones, viz. a small black paper for the eyebrows; a paper, of the same size, of a fine green colour, but which when just arrived and fresh, makes a very fine red for the face; and, lastly, a paper containing about half an ounce of white powder (prepared from real pearl), for giving an alabaster colour to some parts of the face and neck.

'These are not commonly to be bought, but the perfumer may easily procure them by commissioning some friend who goes to China to purchase them for him.'

As to the application of the colours, the reader is informed that the red powders 'are best put on by a fine camel-hair pencil. The colours in the dishes, wools, and green papers, are commonly laid on by the tip of the little finger, previously wetted. As all these have some gum used in their composition, they are apt to leave a shining appearance on the cheek, which too plainly shews that artificial beauty has been resorted to.'

THE DUTIES OF A LADY'S MAID

This same year another book was published in London containing much of the same information on cosmetics, word for word. Which book appeared first or who copied whom it would be difficult to say. Perhaps both anonymous authors (or editors) simply lifted the material bodily from an earlier source. In any event, this second book, which is somewhat broader in scope, concerns *The Duties of a Lady's Maid; with Directions for Conduct, and Numerous Receipts for the Toilette.*

The book is divided into two parts—*Duties of Behaviour* and *Duties of Knowledge and Art.* The first part covers such subjects as Religion, Honesty

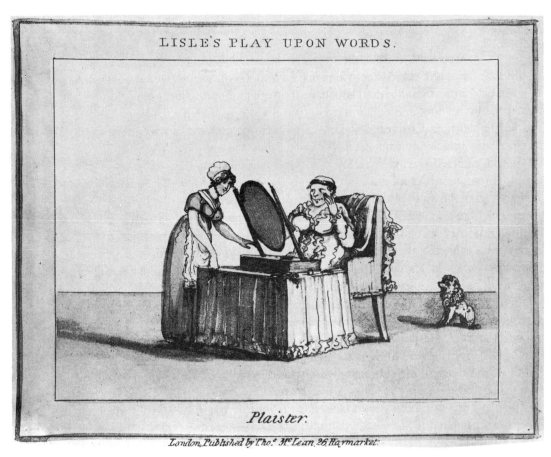

Plaister.

London, Published by Thos. McLean, 26 Haymarket.

FIG. 160: 'Plaister'. English caricature, c. 1825.

and Probity, Diligence and Economy, Attention, Familiarity with Superiors, Good Temper and Civility, Confidence in Keeping Family Secrets, and Vulgar and Correct Speaking. Under the latter heading the aspiring maid is informed that she must say 'A bit *of* paper', not 'a bit paper'; 'the child *cries*', not 'the child *roars*'; and 'she was married *to* him', not 'she was married *on* him'. She will also learn, if she is an apt pupil, that she must always refer to 'bread and cheese', never to 'cheese and bread'. And she will find, still further on, a list of 'vulgar Irish sounds' which she must assiduously avoid.

In the second part of the book the fledgling maid can learn about Taste in Colours of Dress, Artificial Flowers, Stays and Corsets, Padding and Bandaging to Improve the Figure, Display of the Forehead, Taste in Dressing the Hair, and, eventually, Cosmetics and Paints and the Use and Abuse of Soap. The author begins by firmly warning the reader to avoid any cosmetic labelled 'Kalydor' or 'Rowland's Lotion' since they 'are mostly all dangerous repellants, being composed of mercury and other deleterious drugs'.

The first step in beautification is to get rid of unwanted spots or moles, though they sometimes, the author admits, 'give a certain archness to the countenance and expression to the looks and serve as foils to set off the lustre of the skin, and in women of dark complexions they are particularly becoming, for such spots are real patches which they have received from the hand of Nature.' But she (or he) adds that one can have too much of a good thing and removal may be called for. She recommends 'the distilled water of the great blind nettle'.

For removing freckles, when hats and veils have failed to prevent them, the author suggests dipping a bunch of green grapes in water, then sprinkling them with alum and salt, wrapping them in paper, and baking them under hot ashes. The juice is then squeezed out and used for washing the face. There is also an interesting recipe for removing wrinkles:

'Take two ounces of the juice of onions, the same quantity of the white lily, the same of honey, and an ounce of white wax. Put the whole into a new earthen pipkin till the wax is melted; then take the pipkin from the fire, and in order to mix the whole well together, keep stirring it with a wooden spatula till it grows quite cold. You will then have an excellent ointment for removing wrinkles. It must be applied at night when going to bed and not wiped off till morning.'

One of the most coveted cosmetics of the period was the same Balm of Mecca with which Lady Mary Wortley Montagu had such an unpleasant experience in Turkey a century earlier. Imitations sold under that name and manufactured in London and Paris sold for twenty-five to thirty-five shillings an ounce, whereas the real Balm of Mecca cost at least four guineas. One of the more esoteric duties of a lady's maid, and one presumably possessed by few, was to be able to distinguish between the two. This could be done, according to the author, by pouring a drop of balm into water, then spearing the drop with an iron knitting needle. If the entire drop adhered to the needle, the balm was genuine. No special instructions were given for dealing with the irate lady who discovered her four-guinea balm was not genuine. Eastern ladies presumably had no such problem, and the author describes how Egyptian ladies used the balm:

'It is at the bath that they anoint themselves with this balm. They remain in the bath until they are very warm; they then anoint the face and neck, not slightly like the women of the East, but with an ample and copious ablution, rubbing themselves until the skin has absorbed the whole. They then remain in the bath until the skin is perfectly dry, after which they remain for three days with the face and neck impregnated with the balm. On the third they again repair to the bath and go through the same process. This operation they repeat for the space of a month, during which time they take care not to wipe the skin.'

The European ladies were more frugal with the expensive balm and usually diluted it with oil of sweet almonds or virgin's milk. Recipes for various washes are included in the book. One of the more interesting is the Danish pigeon water described in the previous chapter.

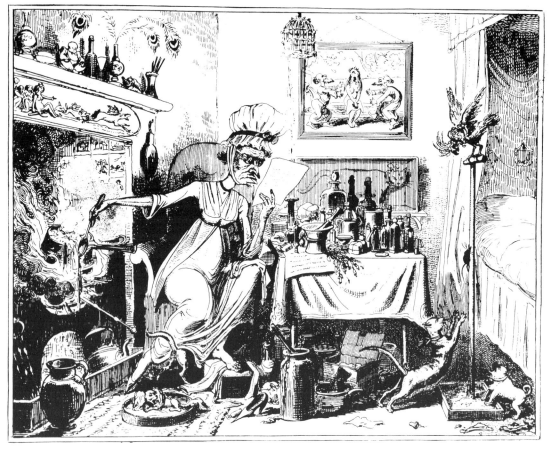

FIG. 161: Mixing a Recipe. English caricature, 1835, of do-it-yourself recipes for cosmetics and home remedies.

In a general summary, the author lists the forms of cosmetics in current use:

'Some are liquid, others mucilaginous, and others have vinegar for their vehicle. Others again resemble pastes and ointments. People should avoid the use of cosmetics with the composition of which they are not acquainted. There are cosmetics which at first produce an astonishing effect and ultimately ruin the skin. . . . Mucilaginous cosmetics possess the property of rendering the skin more supple, softer, and more polished. . . . I cannot say the same of vinegars, which are used by ladies, and are often very pernicious. They evidently give lustre to the skin and brilliancy to its colour and sometimes even remove spots; but they alter the texture of the cutaneous organ, dry it, and produce premature wrinkles. I cannot warn you too strongly against the frequent use of them.'

Pastes and ointments she approves of, but paints, she says, 'cannot give the skin the desired qualities and only instate them in a manner more or less coarse'. But she admits they are quicker and 'for persons too plain or too old, paints afford a convenient resource, a last and only method of disguising either the defects of the complexion or the ravages of time.

'In these observations I allude more particularly to white, for if ever paint were to be proscribed, I should plead for an exception in favour of rouge, which may be rendered extremely innocent and be applied with such art as sometimes to give an expression to the countenance which it would not have without an auxiliary. I therefore think it would be very wrong to include rouge in the same proscription as white. The latter is never becoming, but rouge, on the contrary, almost always looks well.'

Despite her disapproval of white paint, the author gives a recipe for its preparation—one not containing harmful metallic ingredients. The recipe, which requires that Briançon chalk be powdered by rubbing it with a dog's skin, is similar to those in other books.

It can, we are told, 'be used in the same manner as carmine, dipping your finger or a piece of paper, or what is preferable to either, a hare's foot, prepared for the purpose, in ointment, and putting upon it about a grain of this white, which will not be removed even by perspiration. . . . The same ingredients may be used for making rouge.' The discussion of rouge is identical to that in *The Art of Beauty*.

Three recipes are included for darkening the eyebrows and eyelashes:

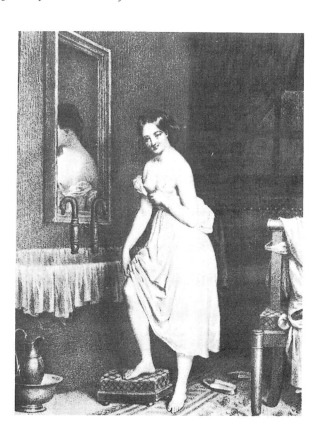

FIG. 162 : Lady about to enter a bathtub.
French engraving, *c.* 1830.

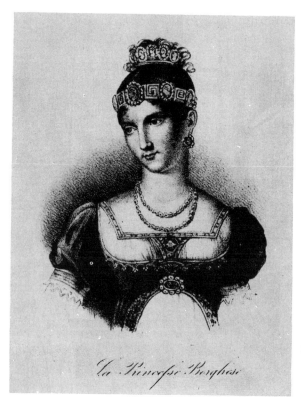

FIG. 163 : Pauline Bonaparte,
later Princess Borghese
(1781–1825).
Lithographed portrait.

'*How to Blacken the Eye-lashes and Eye-brows.* Rub them often with elder-berries. For the same purpose, some make use of burnt cork or clove burned at the candle. Others employ black frankincense, resin, and mastic: this black, it is said, will not come off with perspiration.

'*Wash for Blackening the Eye-brows.* First wash with the decoction of galls; then rub them with a brush dipped in the solution of green vitriol, and let them dry.

'*Black for the Eye-brows.* Take one ounce of pitch, a like quantity of resin and of frankincense, and half an ounce of mastic. Throw them upon live charcoal, over which lay a plate to receive the smoke. A black soot will adhere to the plate; with this soot rub the eye-lashes and eye-brows very delicately. This operation, if now and then repeated, will keep them perfectly black.'

In the same year in which these two books were published, Napoleon's sister, Pauline Bonaparte, the Princess Borghese (Figure 163), died at the age of forty-five. Having been a great beauty and a frivolous and extravagant woman, her final concern when she knew death was near, was to have her most elegant court dress and her jewels put on, her hair dressed, and, like Madame Pompadour, her face powdered and rouged. Then she asked that her face be covered with a cloth so that if her features were distorted at the moment of death, they would not be seen.

HELP FOR WOMEN

Another anonymous work was published in Boston in 1833. It relied heavily on previously published books, but it boasted an extraordinarily informative title page: *The Toilette of Health, Beauty, and Fashion; Embracing the Economy of the Beard, Breath, Complexion, Ears, Eyes, Eye-Brows, Eye-Lashes, Feet, Forehead, Gums, Hair, Head, Hands, Lips, Mouth, Mustachios, Nails of the Toes, Nails of the Fingers, Nose, Skin, Teeth, Tongue, &c. &c., including the Comforts of Dress and the Decorations of the Neck; also the Treatment of the Discolorations of the Skin, Corns — Eruptions — Spots — Pimples, Scorbutic or Spongy Gums, Tainted Breath — Tooth-ache — Carious or Decayed Teeth — Warts — Whitlows, Prevention of Baldness, Grey Hair, etc., with Directions for the Use of Most Safe and Salutary Cosmetics — Perfumes — Essences — Simple Waters — Depilatories, and other Preparations to Remove Superfluous Hair, Tan, Excrescenses, etc. and a Variety of Select Recipes for the Dressing Room of Both Sexes.* Since the technical information in the book seems to have been copied from other books we have already discussed, a single paragraph concerning the current attitude toward cosmetics will suffice:

'Many, indeed, are the authorities that might here be adduced in favor of simple cosmetics, for one good one against them. There are frequent opportunities of observing the astonishing difference which exists between females who bestow constant and judicious care in the preservation of their beauty and those who neglect to cultivate their charms. If a fortunate change of circumstances should enable a young female of limited means, who previously had scarcely attracted any observation, to attend to the minute details of the toilette, in a short time a new beauty may be seen to expand in her. How many rural females, with charms somewhat rustic, and figures rather coarse, have by means of a short residence in town, and the use of the toilette, presented us with a brilliant spectacle of the most pleasing and no less astonishing metamorphosis. The change holds good in both sexes.'

In 1827 Anthony Imbert, a New York painter who had his 'lithographic office' at 79 Murray Street, published a tiny volume entitled *The American Toilet.* Each of the twenty pages consisted of a small lithograph of some object which might be associated with a lady's toilet, such as a mirror, ring, necklace, or perfume bottle. Each lithograph had a hinged section which could be lifted up, revealing a single word — HUMILITY, CONTENTMENT, INNOCENCE, CHEER-

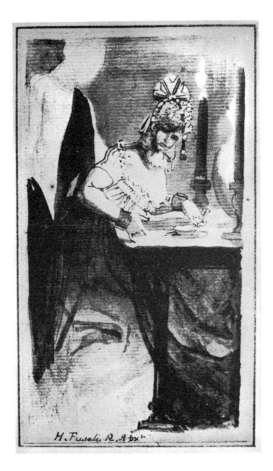

FIG. 164: Woman at her dressing-table. Drawing in pen and ink and watercolour by Henry Fuseli, early nineteenth century.

FULNESS, MODESTY, FIDELITY — and each page, a heading and one or two rhymed couplets at the bottom of the page. The cut-glass covered dish containing CONTENTMENT appeared below the heading *A Wash to Smooth Wrinkles*. The couplet read:

> A daily portion of this essence use,
> Twill smooth the brow, and tranquil joy infuse.

MEEKNESS was *A Necklace of the Purest Pearl*:

> This ornament embellishes the fair,
> And Teaches all the ills of life to bear.

A jar of *Genuine Rouge* contained the word MODESTY:

> Touch with this compound the soft lily cheek
> And the bright glow will best its virtue speak.

The little book was evidently a considerable success for in 1867 a new version, called *The Toilet* and lithographed in colour, appeared with the following notation preceding the title page:

'Many years ago Miss Hannah and Miss Mary Murray of New York, ladies of great wealth and culture, designed *The Toilet*. They cut pictures from papers and pasted them on the leaves of little blank books, and the descriptions were in their own handwriting. It was originated, and sold, for charitable purposes, and the demand for it was so great that at length one thousand dollars was realised from the sale of it and given to the Foreign Missionary Society. In Dr. Spring's Life of Miss Hannah Murray, published by the "Carters", there is a letter to her from Dr. Jonas King, of Greece, dated 1830, approving of their "beautiful Toilet". To show his appreciation, he mentioned that he had presented a copy of it to the Duchess of Broglie, of Paris, a lady eminent for the "adorning" of her heart and mind.'

After 1828 those who preferred to buy their cosmetics could go to Guerlain, which supplied lip pomades for both men and women. The lady in Figure 167 has a jar of lip pomade on her dressing table and a bottle of hair colouring next to her wig box.

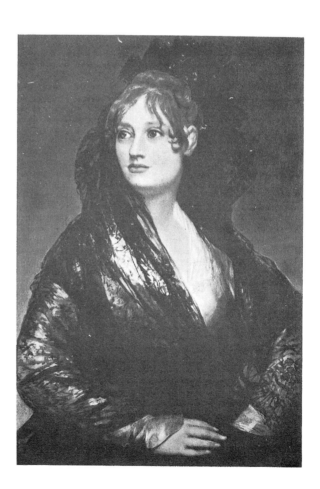

FIG. 165: Doña Isabel Cobos de Porcel.
Portrait by Goya, c. 1806.

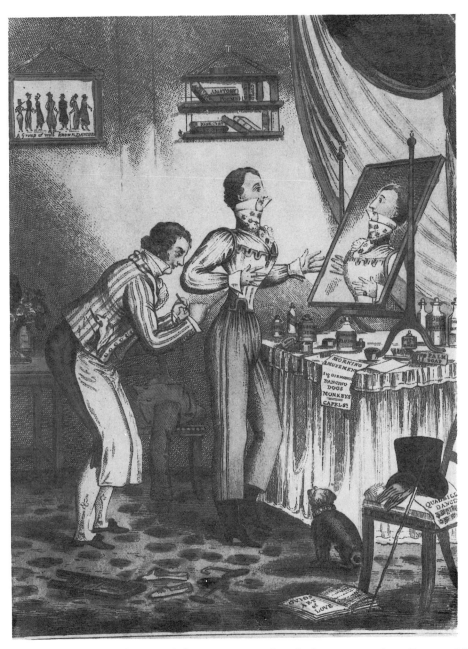

FIG. 166: Dandy's Toilette. English caricature, *c.* 1810. Such cosmetic aids as Russian Oil, Musk, Otto of Roses, Curling Fluid, Palm Soap and a pot of rouge can be seen on the dressing-table.

MAKEUP FOR MEN

Despite a decline in the open use of cosmetics, there were still a few men who hadn't given them up. Jacques Boulenger reports that in 1821 a fop living in a London hotel was overheard asking his valet for 'his corset, his stays, oils, perfumes, all sorts of waters'. When he finally went out, he had the look of a wasp, his neck held in a vast cravat, from which there barely emerged cheeks reddened with makeup and glistening hair, artfully set. Another dandy of the same period is described as 'made up and perfumed like a bouquet of tuberoses'.

HAIR

Tricossian Fluid was still being used in the nineteenth century. An American importer, Mr Overton, encouraged ladies to visit his establishment, 'where may be seen specimens of red or grey hair changed to various beautiful and natural shades of flaxen, brown, or black. As many ladies are compelled from their hair changing grey, at a very early period, to adopt the use of wigs, such ladies are respectfully informed that their own hair may be changed to any shade they choose, in the course of a few hours, by the use of the never failing *Tricosian fluid*, and such is its permanence, that neither the application of powder, pomatum, or even washing, will in the least alter the color. It is easy in application and may be used in any season of the year, without danger of taking cold, being a composition of the richest aromatics, and highly beneficial in nervous headaches, or weakness of the eyes. To convince the nobility, etc., any lady sending a lock of her hair, post paid (sealed with her arms so as to prevent deception), shall have it returned the next day, changed to any color showed at the places of sale. Sold in bottles at one Pound, one Shilling.'

Since there was not enough obvious makeup to satirize, writers turned their attention to hair. Although *Fashions in Hair* contains a considerable amount of nineteenth-century writing on the subject, the following ballad, called *Paper'd-up Hair*, provides an interesting addition:

> Of all the gay fashions that are come in vogue,
> Since wearing the mantle, or bonny red brogue,
> There's none so praiseworthy — you'll find — I declare,
> As the elegant fashion of papering the hair.
>
> The modern dames, both abroad and at home,
> Have got such a fashion of wearing the comb;
> To church or to market, they cannot repair,
> But must take an hour to paper their hair.

When in the evening they change for to walk,
To see their sweethearts, and with them to talk,
An hour or two they must certainly spare,
To fit in their combs, and to paper their hair.

From walking at evening these ladies retire,
They draw up their seats, and chat by the fire,
The tongs then to warm, they ready prepare,
To squeeze up the papers quite tight in their hair.

And when that these ladies give over their talk,
Then up to the looking-glass straight they will walk,
They'll dance, and they'll caper, their arms they will square,
To see if the papers look tight in their hair.

It's the cheapest of curling that ever was found,
You may do it with pipes, white, black, or brown;
For colour of hair, I suppose they don't care,
For they tear up the Bible to paper their hair.

All you young lads that are frisky and trig,
Pray shun the old females that wear a false wig;
To toy with a young one, still make it your care
Whose delight is to trim up, and paper her hair.

Should you meet with a female, whose hair is cut short,
Among other fair ones she is but a sport;
She looks very shabby and out of repair,
When she's wanting the comb, and the paper'd-up hair.

But when they are married, it's just the reverse,
The paper and combs they quickly disperse;
For nursing and cooking is then their whole care,
They may then bid adieu to the paper'd-up hair.

TRAVELS ABROAD

In the nineteenth century the British travelled widely in Europe and the East, and a number of them wrote detailed descriptions of women's cosmetic habits. Sir Robert Ker Porter complained that the beautiful women of Russia enamelled

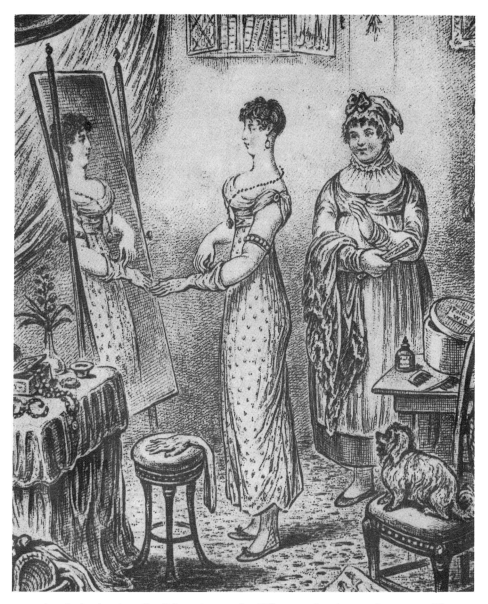

FIG. 167: Lady dressing. English caricature by Gillray, early nineteenth century. There is a rouge pot on the dressing-table and a bottle of hair colouring by her wig box.

their faces so heavily that not a trace of the original texture could be seen, and that the surface was so stiffened by the paint that 'not a line shows a particle of animation excepting the eyes, which are large, dark, liquid, and of a mild lustre,

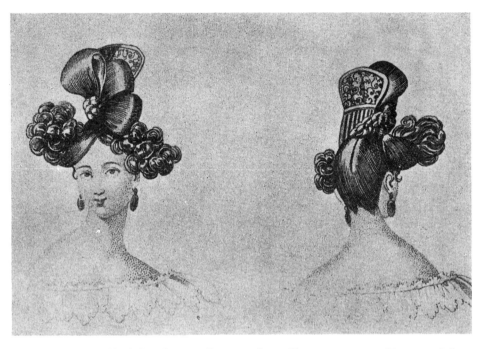

FIG. 168: Fashionable lady of 1831. Drawing from *Theaterzeitung*, a Viennese fashion journal.

rendered in the highest degree lovely by the shade of long black lashes and the regularity of the arched eyebrow.' While in Persia, he visited a royal bath at Tabreez:

'The attendant brings from the cistern, which is warmed from the boiler below, a succession of pails full of water, which he continues to pour over the bather till he is well drenched and heated. The attendant then takes his employer's head upon his knees and rubs in with all his might, a sort of wet paste of henna plant, into the mustachios and beard. In a few minutes this pomade dyes them a bright red. Again he has recourse to the little pail and showers upon his quiescent patient another torrent of warm water. Then, putting on a glove made of soft hair, yet possessing some of the scrubbing-brush qualities, he first takes the limbs, and then the body, rubbing them hard for three quarters of an hour. A third splashing from the pail prepares the operation of the pumice-stone. This he applies to the soles of the feet. The next process seizes the hair of the face, whence the henna is cleansed away, and replaced by another paste, called *rang*, composed of the leaves of the indigo plant. To this succeeds the shampooing, which is done by pinching, pulling, and rubbing, with so much force and pressure as to produce a violent glow over the whole frame. . . . This over, the shampooed body . . . is rubbed all over with a preparation of soap confined in a bag, till he is one mass of lather. When the soap has been washed off with warm water, the bather is led to the cistern and plunged in. After five or six minutes he emerges and has a large, dry, warm sheet thrown over him, in which he makes his escape back to the dressing-room. During the process of the bath many of the Persians dye, not only their hair black, but their nails, feet, and hands, a bright red.'

The Persian ladies regarded the bath as a place of amusement and made appointments to meet friends there, often spending 'seven or eight hours together in the carpeted saloon, telling stories, relating anecdotes, eating sweetmeats, sharing their Kaliouns, and completing their beautiful forms into all the fancied perfections of the East; dying their hair and eye-brows, and curiously staining their bodies with a variety of fantastic devices, not unfrequently with the figures of trees, birds and beasts, sun, moon, and stars.' In Bagdad lower class women often stained 'their bosoms with the figures of circles, half-moons, stars, &c., in a bluish stamp'.

In *Glimpses of Life in Persia*, Lady Sheil wrote that the Persian lady's palms and the tips of her fingers 'were dyed red with a herb called henna, and the edges of the inner part of the eyelids were coloured with antimony. All the Kajars have naturally large arched eyebrows; but, not satisfied with this, the women enlarge them by doubling their real size with great streaks of antimony: her cheeks were well rouged, as is the invariable custom among Persian women of all classes.'

Chinese women used face-packs of tea, oil, and rice-flour at night and rice powder during the day. They rouged their cheeks, lips, nostrils, and even the tip of the tongue with carmine. Another traveller reported that Orientals used *schnouda*, a white cream made of jasmine pomade and benzoin, to give a subtle but transient glow to the cheeks.

Like the Japanese Kabuki and Nō makeups, the makeup for a geisha is traditional, and the geishas of the twentieth century could just as well have posed for the woodcuts of Utamaro. The mask-like makeup begins with a layer of pink and white. In Tokyo the geishas apply the pink first and brush white over it; in Kyoto the procedure is reversed. This foundation is then thoroughly blended with a very wide, flat, short-bristled brush to give a smooth, porcelain-like finish. Rouge is then brushed delicately onto the cheeks, eyelids, and sides of the nose with a soft brush.

After all paint has been cleaned from the brows and lashes, white rice powder is applied with a cotton puff. Wispy sideburns are lightly pencilled on and the eyebrows painted first with red, then black, allowing only a trace of the red to show. Eyes are lined with red, then black, in the same way, using the same finely pointed brush. Lips are painted a bright vermilion, keeping the mouth relatively small. The traditional black wig completes the doll-like makeup.

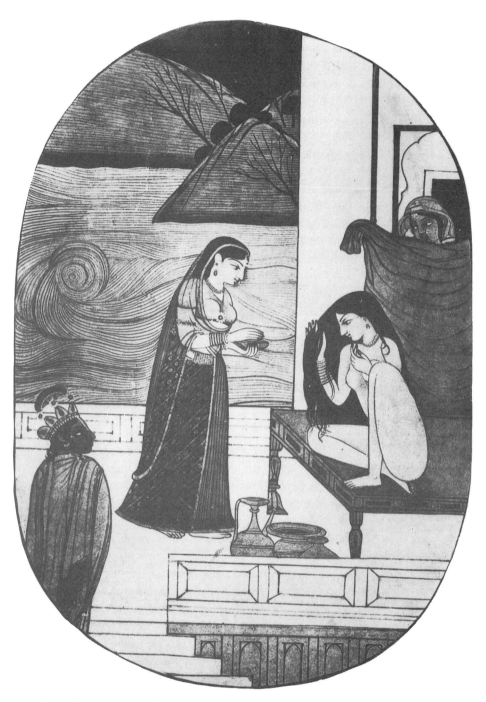

FIG. 169: The toilet of Radha. India, early nineteenth century. The fingertips of both women have been stained with henna.

According to Rimmel, the kohl used for centuries by Arabians for lining their eyes was made, in the nineteenth century and probably for some time previously, by filling a lemon rind with plumbago and burnt copper and placing it on the fire until carbonized. This was then pounded in a mortar 'with coral, sandalwood, pearls, ambergris, the wing of a bat, and part of the body of a chameleon, the whole having been previously burnt to a cinder and moistened with rose-water while hot'.

Arabian complexion powder, called *batikha*, used by the women for whitening the skin, was made of ground cowrie shells, borax, rice, white marble, crystal, eggs, lemons, tomatoes, and helbas (a bitter seed gathered in Egypt) mixed with bean meal, chick-peas, and lentils. This mixture was placed inside a melon, being combined with the melon seeds and pulp. After being thoroughly dried in the sun, it was reduced to a fine powder.

Dye for hair and beards was concocted of fried and salted gall-nuts, burnt copper, cloves, minium, pomegranate flowers, aromatic herbs, litharge, gum arabic, and henna, all pulverized and diluted in the oil used for frying the nuts. This gave a black dye. Henna was used for a reddish tint. They used an almond paste as a substitute for soap, a tooth powder called *souek*, made from the bark of the walnut tree, and a thick turpentine paste as a depilatory.

Rimmel described a toilet bag used in India and often given to the bride by the bridegroom. It contained, among other things, a *pandan* (a box to hold betel), a vial of otto of roses, a *goolabpash* (a bottle to sprinkle rose-water on visitors, whether they wished to be sprinkled or not) a spice box, and a box for *meesee* (a powder of gall-nuts and vitriol for blackening the teeth after marriage), a box for *soorma* to darken the eyelids, another for *kajul* to blacken the eyelashes, a comb, and a mirror. They used a variety of sweet powders and ointments for perfuming their bodies and their clothing and a tooth powder called *Munjun*, composed of burnt almond shells, tobacco ashes, pepper, and salt.

Rimmel reports on the all-day toilet of the son of an American Indian chief named Sa-in-tsa-rish: 'After having greased his whole person with fat to serve as a ground for the paint, and drawn a few streaks on his head and body, he kept looking at himself in a bit of mirror he carried with him and altering the lines until they happened to please him.'

At Aleppo, in Turkey, according to the *Toilette of Health, Beauty, and Fashion* (1833), old men sometimes dyed their beards, and old women dyed their hair with henna, 'which gives them a very whimsical appearance, and many of the men dye their beards black to conceal their age. Few of the women paint except among the Jews, and such as are of the lowest and most debased order; but they generally black their eye brows, or rather make artificial ones, with a certain composition which they call *Hattat*. The practice of late years, however, has considerably declined.'

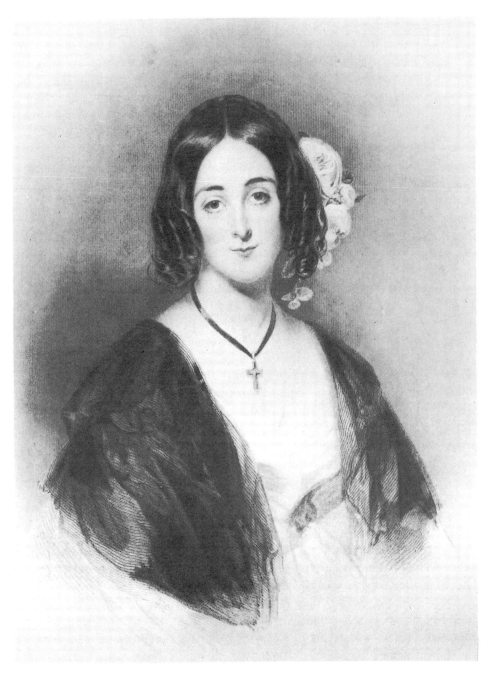

FIG. 170 : The Honourable Mrs Ashley. Steel engraving, London, 1840.

14 · The Early Victorians 1837-1860

Let every woman at once understand
that paint can do nothing
for the mouth and lips.

LOLA MONTEZ

What is commonly thought of as the Victorian influence on makeup — meaning the shift from permissive to deceptive and, more often than not, to none at all — had already begun. A few women still rouged openly and got away with it. In the summer of 1839, early in Victoria's reign, Lady Granville described Mrs Ebrington as 'dressed and rouged like an àltarpiece but still beautiful'. But this was the exception. Most women who rouged did not advertise the fact. Rouge was occasionally seen on elderly gentlemen who clung to the habits of earlier years.

Helpful Hints

Most books and articles of the period confined themselves to discreet, helpful hints on maintaining natural beauty, with or without artifice. Sarah Josepha Hale, editor of *Godey's Lady's Book*, who crusaded tirelessly for the improvement of women, shared with her readers one of her own beauty secrets — the nightly application to her temples of brown paper soaked in cider vinegar. This was worn all night in order to keep the skin around the eyes smooth and free from wrinkles.

An article on cosmetics in *The Penny Magazine* of 1838 approaches the subject diffidently, pointing out that although readers may not approve of cosmetics, some information about their manufacture might 'not be uninstructive'. The writer then lists the two most important objectives of cosmetics — 'to impart a red colour to the cheeks' and 'to whiten the other parts of the skin and neck'. The various rouges in use — dishes, Spanish wool, Chinese boxes — are described, but pure carmine, manufactured from cochineal, is recommended as the most desirable rouge of all.

Elder-flower water and rose-water were the most popular washes of the day; but since they did little or nothing to whiten the skin, white powder was used as well. Pearl powder (made by dissolving seed pearls in acid and precipitating the powder with an alkali) was the most desirable and the most costly. Cheaper pearl powder (prepared from mother-of-pearl or oyster shells) could be obtained, but it had an unnatural sheen. Bismuth powder was considered a good imitation of pearl powder, but unfortunately it turned black on contact with sulphur fumes, causing the wearer considerable distress and embarrassment.

Black for the eyebrows was prepared from lamp-black mixed with a cream or ointment and applied with a camel's hair brush — or pencil, as it was then called. Hence, ladies of the period 'pencilled' their brows. And, in fact, so did some of the men.

The Toilet: A Dressing-Table Companion, published in 1839, provides a remarkably complete view of the toilet accessories with which ladies of the period surrounded themselves. 'The following articles,' the reader is told, 'should be kept on the toilet table, ready for immediate use' :

> A Box of Fumigating Pastilles.
> A Lucifer Box
> A Bottle either of Ede's Highly Concentrated Aromatic Spirits of Vinegar, Preston's Smelling Salts, Spirits of Hartshorn, or of Spirit of Sal-volatile.
> A Dressing Case, with Scissors &c. &c.
> A Pincushion and Pins.
> A Paper of Royal Court Plaster.
> A Paper of prepared Gold-beater's skin.
> Half-pint bottle of Rose Water.
> Half-pint bottle of Ede's Royal Extract of Lavender or any of his other Perfumes, viz :
>> The Hedyosmia; or Persian Essence, combining all the fragrant properties of the Odoriferous Compound; being a powerful and colourless *Esprit* for the handkerchief and Toilet.
>> The Odoriferous Compound; or Persian Sweet Bags. This is a very agreeable perfume for scenting clothes, drawers, writing desks, &c., and an effectual preventive against moth.
>> The Extract of Spring Flowers, which is a delicious perfume of exquisite fragrance, and distilled from the choicest flowers when in bloom.
>> True Verbena Extract is an extremely delicate perfume for the handkerchief and a pleasing appendage to the Toilet.
>> Bouquet d'Arabie; an elegant Essence of the most exquisite fragrance, without the evanescent quality peculiar to many advertised perfumes.
> Reece's Walnut Oil Soap.
> Tooth Powder in a box and Brushes.
> Soft Curl Paper.
> Some Hair Oil or Pomatum, Brushes and Combs, &c.

A Pot of Cold Cream.
A Box of Lip-salve.

With this assortment, the lady was presumably ready for any emergency.

FEMALE BEAUTY

Mrs Alexander Walker, writing in 1840 on *Female Beauty*, found cosmetics unnecessary, dangerous, and distasteful, though she made it clear that they were used. Quoting a Mr Alison, she wrote that 'the aversion which mankind have ever shown to the painting of the countenance has a real foundation in nature. It is a sign which deceives, and, what is worse, which is intended to deceive. It never can harmonize with the general character of the countenance; it never can vary with those unexpected incidents which give us our best insight into human character; and it never can be practised but by those who have no character but that which fashion lends them, or those who wish to affect a character different from their own.' Mrs Walker preferred 'an expressive interesting paleness' to any sort of artificial colouring which, she warned, 'never fails to leave behind a dull withered skin'.

Nonetheless, she had to admit that there were available numerous 'preparations of white to improve the complexion, of black to dye the hair, of blue to define the veins, of red to colour the cheeks, of balsams to give brilliancy to the eyes, of carmine to colour the lips'. As for their manufacture, she wrote:

'Many of the pretended cosmetics sold by general perfumers and by a great number of ignorant persons who call themselves chemists, are composed of acids and spirits; and very frequently they are nothing but vinegar or spirits of wine scented. Even eau de Cologne, so much vaunted and so much used, is nothing else than spirits of wine distilled through a few unimportant aromatic herbs; honey water, Hungary water &c. are made in the same way.'

Like many others, Mrs Walker warned her readers against the dangers of metallic paints, especially those containing lead:

'If lead be once introduced into the animal system, although in a very small quantity, it can never be neutralized by art, and never fails to produce the most deplorable effects. Paralysis, contraction, and convulsion of the limbs, loss of strength, and the most painful colics, are its most ordinary effects. . . .

'Even before these consequences show themselves, the complexion becomes dull and tarnished, and the skin appears faded, wrinkled, and ghastly. As soon as the deluded dupe removes the paint from her face, she sees in her glass a skin so wrinkled and a countenance so ghastly that she redoubles the application of cosmetics till she has finally ruined her complexion and destroyed her health.'

Bismuth and lead, in spite of their well-known effects on the skin, continued to be used in white paints. Since the paints tended to remain powdery on the skin (which was not considered desirable) or else to melt with perspiration and streak the face, it is difficult to understand their popularity. Even more distressing was their tendency to turn black when exposed to sulphurous fumes. White paints made of talc, though less dangerous, were seldom of a natural colour or suitable sheen.

Rouge containing vermilion was labelled by Mrs Walker as 'very dangerous, if any portion of its poisonous substance be absorbed by the pores'. It would, she added, corrode and loosen the teeth.

Vegetable rouge was obtained from various sources — sandalwood, madder, orchanet roots, Brazil wood, and especially from cochineal and the carthamus. 'The rouge from the Carthamus, which' Mrs Walker tells us, 'is called Spanish rouge because it was first prepared in that country, and rose en tasse, or pink saucer, because, as a precipitate, it is known under that name in trade, is now the principal basis of red paints. It is with this precipitate, which may be bought cheap at the grocers, druggists, and colour dealers, that different sorts of rouge are prepared. It is used in powder, in pomade, in crèpons or gauze, and in liquid.'

Mrs Walker's description of the manufacture and application of rouge gives a good picture of what the woman of 1840 had available:

'For rouge in powder, they take talc reduced to an impalpable powder and mix it with the rose en tasse, pounding this mixture carefully with a few drops of olive or ben oil, to make it soft and thick. . . . It is then placed in small gallipots in a very thin layer. The powder is applied to the cheeks by means of a little bag or ball of cambric or muslin.

'A pomade of this red paint is easily obtained by adding . . . precipitate of carthamus to a mixture of white wax and soft pomade. It is spread on the face with the finger and rubbed in till it ceases to feel greazy; it will resist moisture and even a slight touch. This is perhaps the most favourable and the most agreeable form in which rouge can be used.

'Rouge en crèpons are pieces of gauze or silk or crape (whence the name) which are rolled up so as to form a ball, and which have been previously steeped in rouge. These crèpons last a long time; and they are not more objectionable than any other powder.

'Liquid rouge heightens the colour of the skin, has the appearance of the natural complexion, and adheres a long time to the face. The brilliancy, however, thus produced, is afterwards dearly paid for: this vegetable rouge is very injurious to the skin. . . .

'The green red is simply rose en tasse poured whilst still moist, into rouge pots, where, on becoming dry it assumes naturally an olive green tinge, which changes to a lively red when it is moistened with a little fresh water.

'As all these rouges preserve a portion of the juice of the citron employed in manufacturing them from the carthamus, they dry and produce a contraction of the skin which prematurely destroys its freshness. . . .

'The root of the Bugloss is used in the composition of many cosmetics. The rouge, of which it is said to be the base, is vaunted as the best and the least dangerous. It remains several days on the face without fading; water is said to brighten its brilliancy . . . and it is pretended that it does not so seriously injure the skin. From some of these circumstances, it must be a dye and cannot but be hurtful.

'Chinese rouge in leaves, or cochineal rouge, is one of the most beautiful and most expensive. It is extracted from cochineal by means of alcohol diluted with water. The dye being filtered is diluted with a little gum arabic and boiled till there remains very little liquor. What remains, being glutinous, is spread upon paper cut in the shape of large leaves and then dried in the shade. To apply this to the cheeks or lips it is sufficient to detach it with the finger moistened with water.'

Mrs Walker follows this with a recipe (sulphate of iron, distilled water, gum water, and eau de Cologne) for darkening the eyebrows but says there is no safe way of dyeing or darkening the eyelashes. As for milk baths, the author is not encouraging:

'Milk and cream are doubtless preferable to most other applications; but still they are dirty, clog the skin, and injure it in the end. Nature certainly never meant that people should plaster their food over the outside of their Bodies.'

In the 1840s tooth powders were criticized as being harmful to the teeth. Some of them, coloured with lake or carmine, were reported to contain, among their less exotic ingredients, powdered coral, seed pearl, drabs' eyes, terra signillata, pumice-stone, cuttle-fish bone, burnt egg shells, and pulverized porcelain.

Mid-Century Cosmetics

As the Victorian influence became more pervasive, the use of cosmetics became more furtive, particularly in the United States. Despite the example of George Washington, who was perfumed and powdered along with other men of his class, sentiment against any use of cosmetics by men was becoming exceedingly strong — so much so, in fact, that the revelation that Martin Van Buren used such cosmetic aids as Corinthian Oil of Cream, Double Extract of Queen Victoria, and Concentrated Persian Essence, helped to end his political career.

But elsewhere, essential items for a gentleman's toilet, listed in one of the manuals popular in the nineteenth century, included tweezers for removing superfluous hair, a sharp knife for cutting the nails, hair oil, dye for the hair and

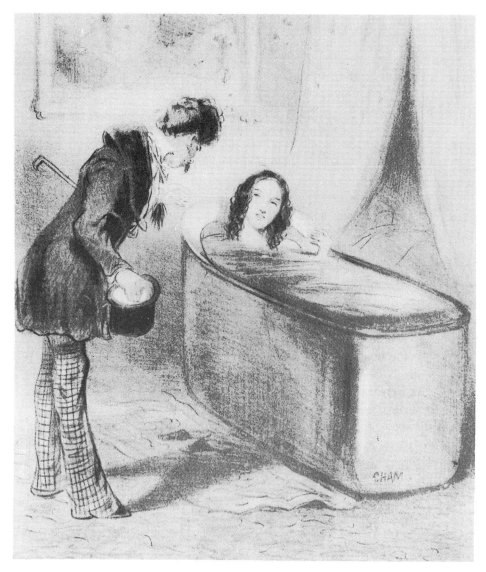

FIG. 171 : In the bath. Lithograph by Cham, Paris, *c.* 1850.

beard, perfumed chalk for sallow complexions, and a little rouge (which was to be used with great care so as to avoid detection).

Cosmetics available in the United States at mid-century included Macassar Oil, Florida Water, Freckle Wash, Indian Hair Dye, Gilman's Liquid Instantaneous Hair Dye, Vinaigre Rouge, Pearl Powder, Otto of Roses, Orange Flower Water, Bear's Oil, Buffalo Oil, Lavender Water, Hair Powder, and a variety of colognes. In 1846 Theron T. Pond began manufacturing Pond's Extract, one of the first widely distributed American cosmetics.

Fashionable ladies in Paris at this time hoped to improve the complexion and avoid wrinkles by sleeping with their faces bound up with thin slices of raw beef. Madame Vestris used her own special anti-wrinkle paste instead. The paste, made by beating together whites of four eggs boiled in rose water, half an ounce of alum, and half an ounce of sweet almonds, was spread on a mask of muslin or silk and worn all night.

WOMEN'S HAIR

In his 'Criticism on Female Beauty', published in *Men, Women, and Books* in 1847, Leigh Hunt stipulated that women's hair should be long, soft, flexible, thick, and of a colour suitable to the skin. For women whose hair grew low on the nape of the neck, he preferred that they wear it in long hanging locks rather than turned up with a comb. He liked ringlets hanging about the forehead and felt they suited almost everybody. 'But,' he added, 'the fashion of parting the hair smoothly and drawing it tight back on either side is becoming to few. It has a look of vanity instead of simplicity. The face must do everything for it, which is asking too much.'

Basing his argument on the fact that if Venus were bald, she would not be Venus, Hunt preferred 'the help of artificial hair to an ungraceful want of it. We do not wish to be deceived. We should like to know that the hair was artificial, or at least that the wearer was above disguising the fact. This would show her worthy of being allowed it. We remember, when abroad, a lady of quality, an Englishwoman, whose beauty was admired by all Florence; but never did it appear to us so admirable as when she observed one day that the ringlets that hung from under her cap were not her own. Here, thought we, it is not artifice that assists beauty; it is truth. . . . Oh, wits of Queen Anne's day, see what it is to live in an age of sentiment, instead of your mere periwigs, and reds and whites! . . . Affectation and pretension spoil everything; sentiment and simplicity warrant it. Above all things, cleanliness. . . . Let a woman keep what hair she has, clean, and she may adorn or increase it as she pleases.

'Oil, for example, is two different things, on clean hair and unclean. On the one it is but an aggravation of the dirt; to the other . . . it may add a reasonable grace. . . . A lover is a little startled when he finds the paper in which a lock of hair has been enclosed, stained and spotted as if it had wrapped a cheesecake. Ladies, when about to give away locks, may as well omit the oil that time and be content with the washing.'

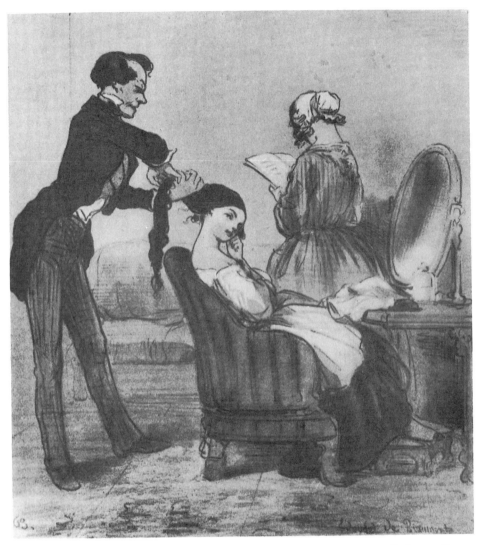

FIG. 172: Actress and hairdresser. Lithograph by Edouard de Beaumont, Paris, *c.* 1859.

TOILET TABLE TALK

In 1856 a small paperback book entitled *Toilet Table Talk*, by S. J. Brown, was published in London. It is of interest chiefly for the formulas it contains for the compounding of various cosmetics. Since there are evidently very few copies of the book in existence, it is probably worthwhile to set down here some of the formulas which differ from those in other books of the period:

ROUGE FOR THE COMPLEXION

Carmine in fine powder, one part; levigated chalk, five parts. Mix.

TURKISH BLOOM

Gum benzoin, one pound; powdered red sanders, one and a half pound; dragon's blood, two and a half ounces; alcohol, one gallon. Digest for fourteen days and filter.

SPANISH LADIES' ROUGE

Take tincture of carmine or cochineal, any quantity, wet some cotton wool with it, and repeat the operation until the wool has sufficient colour.

WINDSOR SOAP

Hand soap, seven pounds; water to soften, then add oil of carraway, two drachms; finely powdered cassia, three ounces. Form into cakes.

HUDSON'S COLD CREAM

Oil of almonds, eight ounces; white wax, one ounce; spermacetti, one ounce. Melt, and when cooling, stir in rose-water, four ounces; orange-flower water, one ounce.

CELEBRATED HONEY ALMOND PASTE

Take honey, one pound; white bitter paste, one pound; expressed oil of bitter almonds, two pounds; yolks of eggs, five. Heat the honey, strain, then add the bitter paste, knead well together, and lastly, add the eggs and oil in alternate portions.

There is also a recipe, presumably for a fairly large family, for *Farina's Eau de Cologne*, requiring, for a start, seventy gallons of alcohol. Other ingredients include sage, thyme, mint, spearmint, calamus aromaticus, angelica root, rose petals, violets, lavender, orange blossoms, wormwood, nutmeg, cloves, cassia, mace, sliced lemons, sliced oranges, and a variety of essences. This was to be macerated for twenty-four hours, then agitated for twelve days, and finally allowed a week's well-deserved rest.

LOLA MONTEZ

One of the most celebrated beauties of all time, adventuress, self-styled Spanish dancer (born in Ireland), mistress of Liszt and Louis I of Bavaria, Lola Montez was hissed off the stage in London, was reduced to poverty in Brussels, single-handedly faced and conquered a hostile mob in Warsaw, very nearly fomented a revolution, became the power behind the throne in Bavaria, and was one of the most celebrated women in Europe before her luck finally ran out. It was in 1858, when she was nearing the end of her short life, that a book of beauty hints bearing her name was published. The book was an unexpected mélange of Victorian prudery, common sense, conventional recipes, and advice listed from other books. The recipes included one from the court of Spain for giving 'a polished whiteness to the neck and arms:

'Infuse wheat-bran, well sifted, for four hours in white wine vinegar; add to it five yolks of eggs and two grains of ambergris, and distill the whole. It should be carefully corked for twelve or fifteen days, when it will be fit for use.'

French and Italian ladies — especially, according to Madame Montez, dancers, musicians, or others engaged in physical exercise — were given to a pre-bed rubdown of a mixture of deer fat, Florence oil, virgin wax, musk, white brandy, and rose water. This was supposed to impart elasticity to the muscles.

Madame Montez (if it was indeed she who actually did the writing) prefaced her book of recipes with a statement that they were in use 'among the fashionable belles of the various capitals of the Old World. I give them as *curiosities*,' she added, 'desiring that they may pass for what they are worth and no more. If, however, a lady wishes to use such helps to beauty, I must advise her, by all means, to become *her own manufacturer* — not only as a matter of *economy* but of *safety* — as many of the patent cosmetics have ruined the finest complexions and induced diseases of the skin and of the nervous system, which have embittered the life and prematurely ended the days of their victims. For a few shillings and with a little pains, any lady can provide herself with a bountiful supply of all such things, composed of materials which at any rate are harmless and which are far superior to the expensive patent compounds which she buys of druggists.'

Madame Montez mentioned an English lawsuit involving a Mr Dickinson, a Mrs Vincent, and a Mr MacDonald, each of whom claimed to have invented a popular cosmetic selling for 7s 6d a pint. As a result of the suit, the lotion was revealed to be compounded of $1\frac{1}{2}$ ounces of bitter almonds and 15 grains of corrosive sublimate to a quart of water. The total cost was twopence for the ingredients and threepence for the bottle — a profit, Madame Montez was quick to point out, of 1,700 per cent.

Further on in her preface, which seemed intended to justify the enhancement of personal beauty, she noted that 'The Baroness de Staël confessed that she

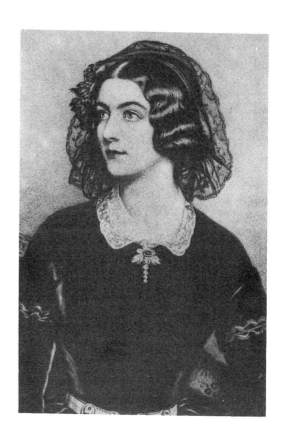

FIG. 173: Lola Montez (1818–61).

would exchange half her knowledge for personal charms, and there is not much doubt that most women of genius to whom nature has denied the talismanic power of beauty, would consider it cheaply bought at that price. And let not man deride her sacrifice and call it *vanity* until he becomes himself so morally purified and intellectually elevated that he would prefer the society of an ugly woman of genius to that of a great and matchless beauty of less intellectual acquirements. All women know that it is *beauty* rather than genius which all generations of men have worshipped in our sex. Can it be wondered at, then, that so much of our attention should be directed to the means of developing and preserving our charms? . . . Preach to the contrary, as you may, there still stands the eternal fact that the world has yet allowed no higher "mission" to women than to be *beautiful*. Taken in the best meaning of that word, it may be fairly questioned if there *is* any higher mission for woman on earth.'

Madame Montez was distressed to report that 'young girls of the present day sometimes eat such things as chalk, slate, and tea-grounds to give themselves a white complexion. I have no doubt,' she added, 'that this is a good way to get a *pale* complexion, for it destroys the health and surely drives out of the face the natural roses of beauty and instead of a bright complexion produces a wan and sickly one.' But neither did she approve of obvious whiting applied to the outside:

'If Satan has ever had any direct agency in inducing woman to spoil or deform her own beauty, it must have been in tempting her to use *paints* and *enamelling*. Nothing so effectually writes *memento mori*! on the cheek of beauty as this ridiculous and culpable practice. Ladies ought to know that it is a sure spoiler of the skin, and good taste ought to teach them that it is a frightful distorter and deformer of the natural beauty of the "human face divine". The greatest charm of beauty is in the *expression* of a lovely face, in those divine flashes of joy and good-nature and love, which beam in the human countenance. But what expression can there be in "a face bedaubed with white paint and enamelled? No flush of pleasure, no thrill of hope, no light of love can shine through the incrusted mould". Her face is as expressionless as that of a painted mummy. And let no woman imagine that the men do not readily detect this poisonous mark upon the skin. Many a time I have seen a gentleman shrink from saluting a brilliant lady, as though it was a death's head he were compelled to kiss. The secret was, that her face and lips were bedaubed with paints. All white paints are not only destructive to the skin, but they are ruinous to the health. I have known paralytic affections and premature death to be traced to their use. But alas! I am afraid that there never was a time when many of the gay and fashionable of my sex did not make themselves both contemptible and ridiculous by this disgusting trick.'

This is a curious foreshadowing of Madame Montez's own premature death from paralysis three years later, though her use of cosmetics is not known to have been a contributing factor.

She also disapproved of the excessive use of powder:

'None but the very finest powder should ever be used, and the lady should be especially careful that sufficient is not left upon the face to be noticeable to the eye of a gentleman. She must be very particular that particles of it are not left visible about the base of the nose and in the hollow of the chin. Ladies sometimes catch up their powder and rub it on in a hurry without even stopping to look in the glass, and go into company with their faces looking as though they just came out of a meal-bag. It is a ridiculous sight, and ladies may be sure it is disgusting to a gentleman. . . .

'But it is proper to remark that what has been said against white paints and enamels does not apply with equal force to the use of *rouge*. Rouging still leaves the neck and arms and more than three-quarters of the face to their natural complexion, and the language of the heart, expressed by the general complexion, is not obstructed. A little vegetable *rouge* tinging the cheek of a beautiful woman, who, from ill health or an anxious mind, loses her roses, may be excusable; and so transparent is the texture of such *rouge* (if unadulterated with lead) that when the blood does mount to the face, it speaks through the slight covering and enhances the fading bloom. But even this allowable artificial aid must be used with the most delicate taste and discretion. The tint on the cheek should always be fainter than what nature's pallet would have painted. A violently rouged woman is a disgusting sight. The excessive red on the face gives a coarseness to every feature and a general fierceness to the countenance, which transforms the elegant lady of fashion into a vulgar harridan. But in no case can even *rouge* be used by ladies who have passed the age of life when roses are natural to the cheek. A *rouged* old woman is a horrible sight — a distortion of nature's harmony!'

If the paragraph above sounds familiar, it is because most of it is lifted verbatim from *Mirror of the Graces*, published seven years before Madame Montez was born. Some twenty years before the publication of her book, her attitude toward rouge had been quite different, for she was then conspicuous for her rouged lips and cheeks at a time when obvious rouging was considered neither fashionable nor proper. And at that time her extraordinary beauty needed little help from cosmetics.

A few pages later Madame Montez warned her readers about eye makeup, which she found 'absurd and ruinous to beauty. . . . There is' she believed, 'almost invariably a lovely harmony between the colour of the eyes and its fringes and the complexion of a woman, which cannot be broken up by art without an insult to nature. The fair complexion is generally accompanied with blue eyes, light hair, and light eyebrows and eye-lashes. . . . But take this fair creature and draw a black line over her softly tinctured eyes, stain their heavy fringes with a sombre hue, and how frightfully have you mutilated nature! . . . If a woman has the misfortune from disease, or otherwise, to have deficient eye-brows, she may delicately supply the want, as far as she can, with artificial pencilling; but in doing this she must scrupulously follow nature and make the colour of her pencilling correspond with her complexion.'

Finally, she described the horror of painted lips:

'Let every woman at once understand that paint can do nothing for the mouth and lips, the advantage gained by the artificial red is a thousand times more than lost by the sure destruction of that delicate charm associated with the idea of "nature's dewey lip". There can be no *dew* on a painted lip. And there is no man who does not shrink back with disgust from the idea of kissing a pair of painted lips.'

Yet her own experience clearly would not provide confirmation of this curiously Victorian warning. But for ladies not in the peak of condition, she was willing to permit them to draw the blood to their cheeks with a wash of tincture of benzoin. She also stressed the importance of white teeth and recommended a tooth powder made of prepared chalk, cassia powder, and orris root.

The year following the publication of this book Madame Montez seems to have undergone a religious conversion, perhaps foreshadowed by the uncharacteristic tone of the book, and she devoted the last two years of her life to helping unfortunate women.

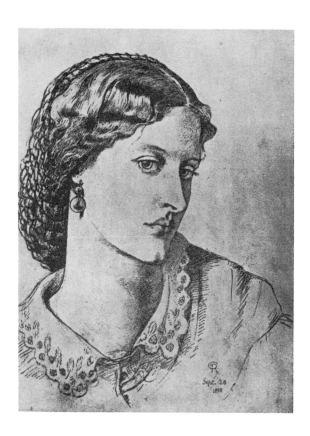

FIG. 174: Portrait of the actress Miss Herbert (Mrs Crabb), by Dante Gabriel Rossetti, 1858.

HABITS OF GOOD SOCIETY

Allowing the female reader only a year to recover from the Montez work, the anonymous authors, one male, one female, of *Habits of Good Society*, published in London in 1859, gave detailed instructions for the personal toilet. This began with bathing, a habit which had evidently fallen into some neglect since the days of Beau Brummel, when it was 'thought proper for a gentleman to change his undergarments three times a day, and the washing bill of a beau comprised seventy shirts, thirty cravats, and pocket-handkerchiefs *à discrétion*. What,' wonders the male author, 'would Brummel say to a college chum of mine who made a tour through Wales with but one flannel shirt in his knapsack?'

The author then describes in four pages how a gentleman should take a bath in a flat metal basin, using a foot-long sponge. One must begin with the stomach and then proceed to the head. From there on, he is on his own. Another five pages take care of the teeth and the nails. Then comes the question of shaving. 'The person who invented razors,' we are told, 'libelled Nature and added a fresh misery to the days of man. . . . As for barbers, they have always been gossips and mischief-makers. . . . Who, in fact, can respect a man whose sole office is to deprive his sex of their distinctive feature? . . . Shaving and fanaticism have always gone together. The custom of the clergy wearing a womanish face is purely Romanist, and I rejoice to see that many a good preacher in the present day is not afraid to follow Cranmer and other fathers of our Church in wearing a goodly beard. . . . It is clear that a Protestant chin ought to be well covered.

'Whatever be said of the clergy, the custom of shaving came to this country like many other ugly personal habits, with the foreign monarchs. As long as we had Plantagents, Tudors, and Stuarts on the throne, we were men as to the outward form. William of Orange was ashamed of that very appendage which it is a disgrace to a Mussulman to be without. Peter the Great had already proved that barber and barbarian are derived from the same root, by laying a tax on all capillary ornaments. . . .

'The beard and the rapier went out together at the beginning of the last century. In the present day many a young shop-boy joins the moustache movement solely with a hope of being mistaken for a captain. Whatever *Punch* may say, the moustache and beard movement is one in the right direction, proving that men are beginning to appreciate beauty and to acknowledge that Nature is the best valet.'

But for those misguided men who persisted in the iniquity of shaving, instructions were given. A case of seven razors, one for each day of the week, was recommended; the common usage of violet powder afterward was not. 'In the first place,' we are informed, 'it is almost always visible and gives an unnatural look to the face. I know a young lady who, being afflicted with a redness in a feature above the chin, is in the habit of powdering it. For a long time I thought her charming, but since I made the discovery I can never look at her without a painful association with the pepper-caster. Violet powder makes the skin rough and enlarges the pores of it sooner or later.'

Having in less than a page disposed of the distasteful subject of shaving, the author returns enthusiastically to beards:

'Beards, moustaches, and whiskers have always been most important additions to the face. Italian conspirators are known by the cut of those they wear; and it is not long since an Englishman with a beard was set down as an artist or a philosopher. In the present day literary men are much given to their growth, and in that respect show at once their taste and their vanity. Let no man be ashamed of his beard if it be well kept and not fantastically cut. The moustache should be kept within limits. The Hungarians wear it so long that they can tie the ends round their heads. The style of the beard should be adopted to suit the face. A broad face should wear a large full one; a long face is improved by a sharp-pointed one. . . . The chief point is to keep the beard well-combed and in neat trim.

'As to whiskers, it is not every man who can achieve a pair of full length. There is certainly a great vanity about them, but it may be generally said that foppishness should be avoided in this as in most other points. Above all, the whiskers should never be curled nor pulled out to an absurd length. Still worse is it to cut them close with the scissors. The moustache should be neat and not too large, and such fopperies as curling the points thereof or twisting them up to the fineness of needles — though patronized by the Emperor of the French — are decidedly a proof of vanity.' The author believed that if a man wore a natural beard and kept it clean and neatly trimmed, he could not go very far wrong.

The hair, he said, should be as simple and as natural as possible, but at the time he found 'nothing unmanly in wearing long hair, though undoubtedly it is inconvenient and a temptation to vanity, while its arrangement would demand an amount of time and attention which is unworthy of a man. But every nation and every age has had a different custom in this respect, and to this day even in Europe the hair is sometimes worn long. The German student is particularly partial to hyacinthine locks curling over a black velvet coat; and the peasant of Brittany looks very handsome, if not always clean, with his love-locks hanging straight down under a broad cavalier hat. . . .

'If we conform to fashion, we should at least make the best of it, and since the main advantage of short hair is its neatness, we should take care to keep ours neat. This should be done first by frequent visits to the barber, for if the hair is to be short at all, it should be very short, and nothing looks more untidy than long, stiff, uncurled masses sticking out over the ears. If it curls naturally, so much the better, but if not, it will be easier to keep in order. The next point is to wash the head every morning, which, when once habitual, is a great preservative against cold. I never have more than one cold per annum, and I attribute this to my use of the morning bath and regular washing of my head. . . .

'As to pomatum, Macassar, and other inventions of the hairdresser, I have only to say that, if used at all, it should be in moderation and never sufficiently to make their scent perceptible in company. Of course the arrangement will be a matter of individual taste, but as the middle of the hair is the natural place for a parting, it is rather a silly prejudice to think a man vain who parts his hair in the centre. He is less blamable than one who is too lazy to part it at all and has always the appearance of having just got up.

'Of wigs and false hair, the subject of satires and sermons since the days of the Roman emperors, I shall say nothing here except that they are a practical falsehood which may sometimes be necessary but is rarely successful. For my part I prefer the snows of life's winter to the best made peruke, and even a bald head to an inferior wig.'

Information on the lady's toilet is equally enlightening as to customs and attitudes of the day. 'In no particular,' the co-author begins, 'has the present generation become more fastidious than in what is requisite for the use of ladies in their own dressing-rooms. Essences, powders, pastes, washes for the hair, washes for the skin, recall the days of one's grandmother, when such appurtenances were thought essential and were essential: for our great-grand-mothers were not rigid in points of personal cleanliness; and it is only

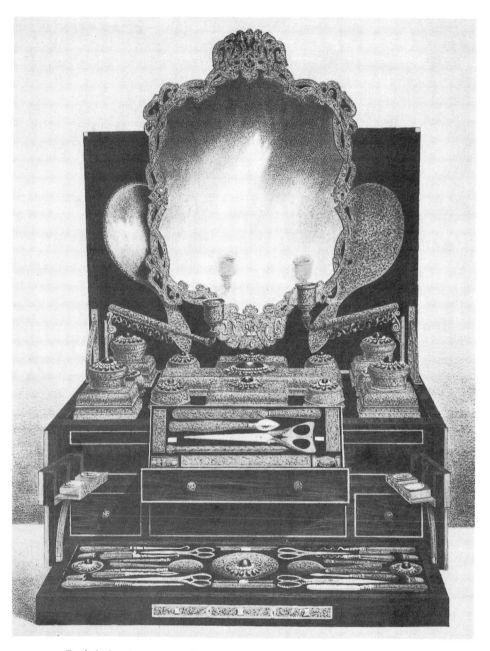

FIG. 175 : English dressing-case, *c.* 1855.

uncleanliness that requires scents to conceal it, and applications to repair its ravages.'

But all the washing in the world will avail nothing if one sleeps too late in the morning. Early rising, we are told firmly, is essential to health. 'No person in good health should remain in bed after seven o'clock, or half-past seven, in the spring and summer; that may, in the present century, when the daughters of England are reproached with self-indulgence, be termed early rising. She may then be down stairs at eight, and without taking a long and fatiguing walk, saunter in the garden a little; or, if in a large town, have time to practice, supposing that the opportunity of going out into the air is denied. By this means, that vigor which is the very soul of comeliness, the absence of hurry and the sense of self-reproach incurred by late rising, and the hunger felt for breakfast, will all conduce to arrest Time, as she hovers over his wholesale subjects, and to beguile him into sparing that process with his scythe by which he furrows the brow of the indolent with wrinkles, whilst he colours the poor victim, at the same time, with his own pet preparation of saffron.'

After throwing open her window for a quarter of an hour and then plunging into a bracing shower, the lady is ready to face her toilet table:

'This, in a lady's as well as in a gentleman's room, should be always neatly set out, and every article placed where it can be most conveniently used. In former times, vast expense used to be bestowed on china, and even on gold and silver toilet-services; then came the war and the national poverty, and those luxurious appliances were let down, if not abandoned. We have now resumed them with a degree of expense that is hardly wise or consistent. The secrets of the toilet were, indeed, no fancied mysteries in former days. Until the first twenty years of this century had passed away, many ladies of *bon ton* thought it necessary, in order to complete their dress, to put a touch of rouge on either cheek. . . . I once knew a lady who was bled from time to time to keep the marble-like whiteness of her complexion; others, to my knowledge, rub their faces with bread-crumbs as one should a drawing. But, worst of all, the use of pearl powder, or of violet powder, has been for the last half century prevalent.

'Independent of all sorts of *art* being unpleasant, no mistake of the fair one is greater than this. She may powder, she may go forth with a notion that the pearly whiteness of her brow, her neck, will be deemed all her own; but there are lights in which the small deception will be visible, and the charm of all colouring is gone when it proves to be artificial. We tremble to think what is underneath.'

She also objects to the unwholesomeness of pearl powder, which, she tells us, interferes with perspiration, 'dries up the cuticle, and invites, as it were, age to settle. Where pearl powder has been made an article of habitual use, wrinkles soon require additional layers to fill it up, just as worn out roads have ruts and must be repaired; but the macadamising process cannot be applied to wrinkles.

'Still more fatal is the use of cosmetics; its extravagance, in the first place, is an evil; but I treat not of the moral question, but of its physical effects. Some women spend as much on essences and sweet waters as would enable them to take a journey, and thus do more for their looks than all that a bureau full of cosmetics could insure.'

She insists on the softest possible water, preferably rain-water, filtered, which is to be 'dashed freely over the face several times, and the process be pursued in the middle of the day, as well as in the morning and at dinner-time; it is true,' she adds, that 'the face may, without that, be *clean* all day, but it will not be *fresh*. The Turkish towels now used so much are excellent for wiping. . . . The body, on the other hand, should be dried with a coarse huckaback, an article unknown in France, but excellent for promoting quick circulation in the frame after bathing. To complete, then, the toilet so far as the person is concerned; with few or no cosmetics, with nothing but the use of soap (the old brown Windsor being still, in spite of all modern inventions, far the best for the skin), to have the water brought in fresh in the morning, as that in the room is seldom, except in winter, really cool, these are the simple preservatives of the skin. . . . Banish . . . every essence, cosmetic, or sweet-water from your toilet; and remember that . . . fresh air . . . and pure water are the best and only cosmetics that can be used without prejudice.'

The remainder of the book covers such intriguing subjects as 'Walking and Driving with Ladies', 'Various ways of Shaking Hands', 'Helping a Lady to Mount', and 'Whom to Invite to Dinner and Whom not'.

PUBLIC BATHS

In the 18 December 1858 issue of the *Illustrated London News*, an article extolling the virtues of the new Metropolitan Baths (Figure 176) states flatly that 'We are not a bathing people. Baths with us are the luxury of the few rather than the necessity of the many. Is it that we are too busy, or too indolent, or that the opportunities are not afforded us of enjoying at a moderate cost this means of ablution?'

In many of the Eastern countries, by contrast, bathing, especially among the upper classes, was general—even in as cold a country as Russia, where high-temperature steam baths were followed by standing naked in the open air to cool oneself. This, to the English mind, seemed excessively rigorous.

But the desirability of more frequent bathing was recognized by a few 'sanitary reformers and professors of social science', who were largely responsible for several 'liberally conducted baths for the working classes'. For the upper classes there were only a few inconvenient and expensive establishments with

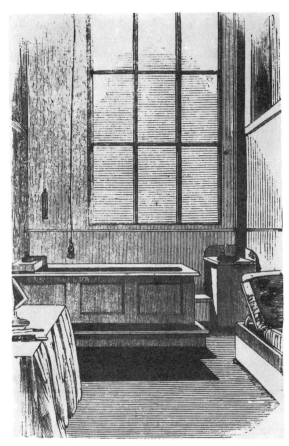

FIG.176: Ladies' bath at the Metropolitan Baths in London,
1858.

'small, ill-lighted closets . . . a scanty supply of water . . . chilly, damp towels,
and truculent attendants', who proportioned 'their civilities to the probable
liberality of the bather.'

But, the writer added with relief, '*nous avons changé tout cela*, which means,
or ought to mean, that a company has established . . . and placed under the
effective management of Mr. H. Mahomet, son of the celebrated Brighton
régisseur des bains, a luxuriously-appointed system of baths, yclept the
Metropolitan. Whether you are healthy or ailing, robust as a Norfolk fox hunter,
or dyspeptic as a London habitué, here you refresh your mind, renovate your
energies, soothe your excitable temperament, dispel your hypochondriac fancies,
or render hardier and more active the already hardy and active frame. You may
subject yourself to medicated vapours, deliciously and subtly fragrant, which
will insensibly purify your blood and invigorate your system, or bring down
upon any offending limb the *thud* of the douche; or be kneaded — we mean
shampooed — with Indian oils; or try experiments with a warm shower or a cold

shower, Russian or Turkish, Vichy, Barège, or Harrogate. You may be sulphurised, and steamed, and iodised. Hot air or hot water, medicated vapour, or medicated fragrance of healthful rosemary, which the patient inhales with intense complacency, until the attendant cries, "Hold, enough!" when he may, if he chooses, plunge into the cold bath in the corner, like a Russian into the Neva, and afterwards rise a renovated and rejuvenated man.'

The estimable Mr Mahomet tended to the needs of the men and Mrs Mahomet to those of the ladies, the sexes being provided with separate entrances to the building at the corner of Jermyn and Bury Streets.

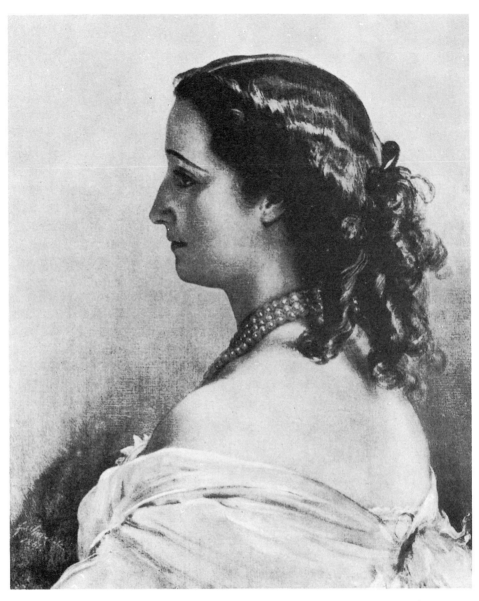

FIG. 177: Empress Eugénie, wife of Napoleon III. Portrait by Winterhalter, 1861.

15 · The Mid-Victorians 1860-1880

If women, prompted by no other motive
than that of pleasing men, paint their faces,
I solemnly declare to them, in the name of the masculine sex,
that they are going a false route
and will only render themselves horrible.

THE ART OF PLEASING

Deceptiveness in makeup seems to be fundamentally unnatural to women, and even the smothering blanket of Victorianism had proved to be only a mild deterrent for the more venturesome. In the 1860s hair powdering was being revived and other cosmetics were being used increasingly. But, predictably, this trend was met with firm resistance, which would last into the next century. Although most women were still discreet, not to say secretive, about their painting, men were beginning to notice cosmetics in the shop windows, if not on the faces. An article in *Chambers's Journal* in 1862 suggests that the disillusioned man 'will not care to press the sweets of coral lips, for fear of soiling his own with carmine pomade, and will value the "network" of veins at the price set upon it by the retailer. Beauty to him will no longer be even skin deep.'

THE GIRL OF THE PERIOD

Mrs Lynn Linton, writing somewhat despairingly in the *Saturday Review of Literature*, described 'The Girl of the Period' as 'a creature who dyes her hair and paints her face as the first articles of her personal religion — a creature whose sole idea of life is fun; whose sole aim is unbounded luxury; and whose dress is the chief object of such thought and intellect as she possesses.' But, she cautioned, 'All men whose opinion is worth having prefer the simple and genuine girl of the past, with her tender little ways and pretty bashful modesties, to this loud and rampant modernization, with her false red hair and painted skin, talking slang as glibly as a man, and by preference leading the conversation to doubtful subjects.'

Mrs Linton's Girl of the Period sounds very much like the French *demi-mondaine*, who whitened her face, rouged her cheeks and her lips excessively, lined her eyes with black, and even wore false eyelashes. Few women of the period went so far; yet, according to *Chambers's Journal*, 'Late disclosures in the Bankruptcy Court prove that enamelled faces are common to women as well as watches, and that the ladies of the present day are quite as ready as their great-grandmothers to sail under false colours, and more cunning in laying them on. Nor is it surprising that these living lies should fail to keep faith with the instrument of deception, while we own we have no sympathy to spare for the bankrupt mistress of such an art, for we would have such debts considered as debts contracted for an immoral purpose....

'Women who know not what exercise is, who shudder at soap, and have an instinctive horror of cold water may well get their white and red from the shop. But Englishwomen, to whom such health-giving agents are familiar friends, need have no recourse to less legitimate means of improving that beauty with which they are so liberally endowed by nature herself. Let the enamellers of faces seek customers elsewhere for their dishonest wares, which the wisest of mankind has emphatically condemned as "neither handsome enough to please, nor wholesome enough to use"!'

MADAME RACHEL

The 'late disclosures at the bankruptcy court' refer, at least in part, to the testimony of the celebrated Madame Rachel, who stated that she was sometimes paid as much as twenty guineas for enamelling a lady's face. But the disclosures and the adverse publicity evidently did not deter women from pouring their husbands' money into her ample pockets. Three years later we find William and Robert Chambers again writing about Madame Rachel, their rapier sharper and more delicately pointed this time. They begin by quoting an advertisement, which they find 'unique in its way — confident in assertion, trenchant in denunciation, and yet with a certain airy grace about it not commonly found united with such intensity:

> MADAME RACHEL takes this opportunity to state that the secret of her beautiful and delicate art of ENAMELLING has descended from generation to generation of her family — therefore all other persons presuming to style themselves enamellers commit a gross fraud on the public at large, which has been proved beyond a doubt.

'This I like, for it shews the lady to be a person of spirit; but it does not tell me all that I want to know. If I wish to be made beautiful — I cautiously abstain from saying "to get enamelled" — what steps am I to take? I learn from another advertisement in another place, that "the following articles are those for which Madame Rachel has the greatest demand":

> Alabaster Powder, Royal Arabian Soap, Alabaster Liquid, Circassian Bloom, Circassian Preparation for the Eyes, Liquid Arab Bloom, Arab Bloom and

Arab Bloom Powder, Magnetic Rock Dew Water from Sahara, Magnetic Cream, Circassian and Arabian Oils for the Hair, Medicated and Preservative Balm, Enamel Powder for the Teeth, Blanchinette Enamel Wash, Albanian Powder, Albanian Cream Powder, Armenian Powder, Pure Extracts of the Lilies, Pure Extracts of the China Rose, Alabaster Cream, Favourite of the Harem's Pearl White, Sultana's Cream, Choicest Perfumes of Arabia, Armenian Liquid for Removing Wrinkles, Circassian Beauty Wash.

'Here is a great choice of beautifying materials, but I cannot help observing that our old friend Mr Barber's Circassian Cream appears among them, although in another guise, suspiciously often. Why should so much that is good for our appearance come from Circassia, and all the rest from Arabia, Albania, and Armenia? Observe, I throw no doubt upon the fact, but only inquire, from simple curiosity, why should there not be a Putney Bloom, a Turham Green Preservative Balm, or even a Camden Town Preparation for the Chin? Why, in the name of native produce and British industry, should I not grow Medicated Balm in a box outside my window, like Mignonette?

'Nay, supposing that the superiority of these far-fetched elixirs is admitted, how am I to apply them, and how often, and how long? Is there no literary work that undertakes to show me in detail how — not I, but somebody who is Beautiful to begin with, is to render him (or her) self *Beautiful for Ever*? There is. A little book with that very title is vended at Madam R.'s magic establishment, which professes — or suggests that it professes — to supply this information; and I have bought it, although it cost me half-a-crown. Two-and-sixpence for a pamphlet of four-and-twenty pages of largish print would be rather dear, if it only treated of politics or polemics; but for the secret of Eternal Youth, it is by no means a high figure.

'The third page (for there is no first or second) is devoted to Women generally; the fourth is dedicated to the Queen; the fifth is occupied with the Princess Royal and the Princess Alice; the sixth speaks very highly of the Princess of Wales; the seventh commends Miss Nightingale, and casually alludes to Jessie Maclean, the heroine of Lucknow; the eighth commemorates the virtues of Grace Darling and of some poor ballet-girl whose clothes caught fire at a theatre; the ninth and three following pages resume the general eulogy upon womankind; and the thirteenth and fourteenth are wholly taken up with a quotation from the *Illustrated London News*. We have only ten pages, therefore, for our money, devoted to the Secret of Eternal Youth. The fifteenth and sixteenth pages themselves do not even at once enter upon this desirable subject, but are mainly occupied with certain wrongs which the great Enameller has suffered at the hands of justice in connection with the beautifying of a lady's complexion. "Let it not, however," says she, "be for a moment supposed that we would presume to act the part of censors. . . . The act of injustice of the one has been amply compensated for by the generosity of others; and we trust we may be pardoned when we apply to ourselves the royal and sacred motto, God and my right."

'This is affecting, but it does not help me, so far as I can see, to be Beautiful for Ever. This, nevertheless, may be owing to my own obtuseness, for the pamphleteer proceeds: "If we do not tire the patience of our gentle readers, we will *further* explain our process, as shewn in the treatment of women and children." In page seventeen, we get a hint of the matter in hand for the first time. "It is principally accomplished by the use of the Arabian Bath, composed of pure extracts of the liquid of flowers, choice and rare herbs, and other preparations equally harmless and efficacious." Page eighteen, however, relapses into the general eulogy of womankind. Page nineteen is devoted to the denunciation of rival establishments: "The author, who had the honour of supplying and arranging the elegant cabinet toilet to the Sultana, the jewels of which were supplied by Emanuel of Hanover Square; who has been especially appointed by the Empress Eugenie and the Court of France as sole importer of Arabian perfumes and toilet requisites — fac-similes of which were presented in golden vases to the Empress Eugenie by the ladies of Paris, under the name of the Senses of Peace; whose talents have been appreciated by the crowned heads of Europe, the aristocracy and the nobility, as the greatest restorer and preserver in the world of female grace and loveliness — the author begs leave to suggest to her fair readers that they cannot be too careful in avoiding the dangerous cosmetics vended by unprincipled persons, who are regardless of the injurious effects to the complexion."

'At page twenty we learn at last the reason why the great Enameller surveys from such a pinnacle all other professors of the same calling. "Having, at an enormous expense, completed the purchase and sole right of the Magnetic Rock Dew Water of Sahara, which possesses the extraordinary property of increasing the vital energies — restores the colour of gray hair — gives the appearance of youth to persons far advanced in years, and removes wrinkles, defects, and blemishes, from whatever cause they may arise, she trusts that the resources at her command will be a sufficient guarantee to her fair readers, should they deem her too presumptuous in extolling her beautiful art."

'This is so far satisfactory: but with respect to the virtues of the Magnetic Rock Dew Water of Sahara, we have absolutely no evidence whatever, except the before-mentioned "Extract of Illustrated London News." Thereby we learn that in the interior of the Great Desert is a magnetic rock, wherefrom a water distils, sparingly, in the form of dew, which appears to have extraordinary properties, since it restores the colour of gray hair, and gives the appearance of youth to persons of considerable antiquity. This precious liquid, we are told, "is brought to Morocco on swift dromedaries for the use of the Court" — or rather, it used to be so, before Madame Rachel deprived them of the luxury, by

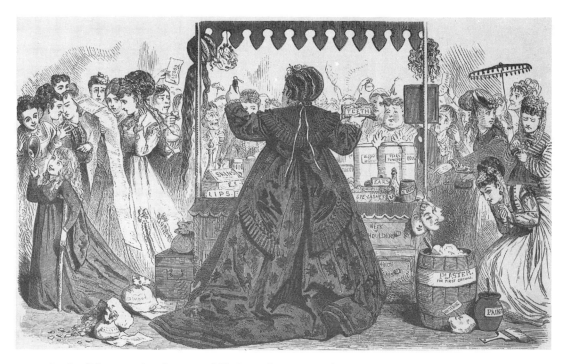

FIG. 178: English cosmetics shop, *c.* 1868. It is the one run by Madame Rachel, who gave her name to a shade of face powder and was occasionally on the wrong side of the law.

purchasing the monopoly of it. "If," says she, "the respectability of this excellent newspaper is not a sufficient guarantee" — although we do not ourselves see how that publication is pledged to the assertion — "if further proofs be needed, the ambassadors from the Court of Morocco can testify to the Magnetic Rock's existence." I venture to think, however, that this is not quite the point. In vain I seek through the remainder of this expensive pamphlet for plain directions how to make one's self Beautiful for Ever. The last four pages are occupied with nothing particular, except that, at the very end, there appears this intimation: "*In our next*, we will endeavour to explain our theory, with advice, and every necessary instruction, concerning the restoration and preservation of female loveliness, with recipes for the same."

'In our *next*? Why, until this dread and disappointing moment, there has not been a hint that the purchase of *another* half-crown pamphlet was expected of us. Upon the title-page is nothing to inform us that this admirable volume is only the first of a series! The date, too, is 1863 — surely between it and 1865 is a longer interval than usual to elapse in the publication of a periodical! It may be that a second work has appeared, unknown to the present writer. It may be that the Secret of Eternal Youth has been meanwhile confided to tens of thousands — but if it has, it has been better kept than most secrets, for I have never heard a whisper of it.

'I have nothing whatever to say against Enamelling, although I understand the process takes more time than a man of business like myself can spare for it. Still less do I object to the Arabian Bath, which Madame Rachel informs us — I have no doubt with truth — is very superior to the Turkish; while my disposition is much too reverent to question for a moment the virtues of the Magnetic Rock Dew Water of Sahara. On the contrary, I do most earnestly hope that the results of these respective elixers are more satisfactory than the literature of which they are the subject. Otherwise, if the Magnetic Rock Dew Water of Sahara costs the the same price as this pamphlet — that is, if it be retailed at half-a-crown a bottle, and I understand that it is quite that price — I shall consider it dear.'

Good Society

In *Good Society*, a book on manners by an unidentified countess, published in 1869, ladies are advised, above all things, never to 'attempt to change the colour of the hair by means of fashionable dyes and fluids. Colour so obtained cannot harmonize naturally with the skin, eyes, and eyebrows that Nature has given. Practices of this kind are simply and strictly immodest. They evince a senseless desire for fashion, and an equally senseless eagerness to attract. Auricomus hair-dyes, like painted lips and cheeks, and pencilled eyebrows and complexions purchased from Madame Rachel, are disgraceful to the wearers. With regard to the art of obtaining a good complexion, we venture to affirm that Madame Rachel is no wiser than ourselves.'

The countess, evidently a woman of strong opinions, also has a few about the gentleman's toilet, which should always begin with a bracing bath and the vigorous application of a flesh brush. Men were advised to remain without clothing 'for some little time' after bathing. The teeth should then be brushed and the nails cleaned and trimmed. 'Long nails,' decreed the countess, 'are an abomination.'

She advised men not to shave, but at the same time, the beard 'should be carefully and frequently washed, well trimmed, and well combed, and the hair and whiskers kept scrupulously clean by the help of clean stiff hair-brushes and soap and warm water. The style of the beard should be adapted to the form of the face, but any affectation in the cut of beard and whiskers is very objectionable, and augurs unmitigated vanity in the wearer. Long hair is never indulged in except by painters and fiddlers. The moustache should be worn neat and not over large. A moustache like that worn by the King of Italy, or a needle-point moustache, *à l'Empereur*, cannot be worn in England with impunity.'

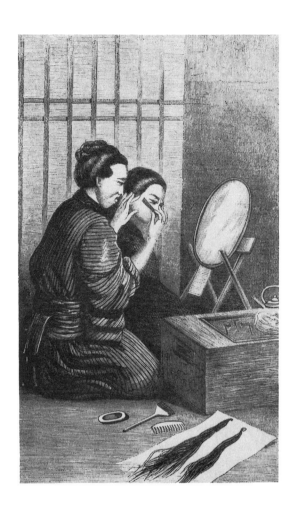

FIG. 179: Japanese ladies shaving, mid-nineteenth century.

The countess did not mention the possibility of women's shaving (see Figure 179).

AIDS TO BEAUTY

In the March 1863 issue of *Cornhill Magazine*, aids to beauty are discussed at some length from both a practical and a moral standpoint. 'If Nature has been niggardly to us,' asks the writer, 'shall we not repair her stinginess by the generosity of Art? Shall we, in candid contentment, display our imperfect complexions, our discrepant teeth, our scanty or objectionable hair, our bulging or unsymmetrical shapes? Shall we not rather seek to hide their defects and so arrange the facts of Nature that we may present a more agreeable aspect even at the expense of perfect sincerity?'

This sounds reasonable enough, remarkably so for a Victorian journalist. But we are very quickly deflated (or gratified, as the case may be) by being informed that there are two methods of hiding defects, 'the Real and the Artificial. In the Real, no deceit is practiced; the best chance is given to Nature to produce an agreeable effect, and nothing is fictitious. In the Artificial there always enters an element of deceit, more or less transparent. Defects are boldly denied, or huddled out of sight, and qualities which have no real existence are assumed.' There we have it — any artifice is deceitful. There's no way we can decently make ourselves prettier without going in for things like exercise and fresh air and plenty of sleep. But wait — there is still hope. The author goes on to say that there are two kinds of artificial aids, and one of them is acceptable, even desirable. Our mind strays to the rouge pot, but our optimism is premature. Only those artificial aids which serve to 'withdraw disagreeable details from observation' (false teeth and glass eyes, for instance) are to be tolerated. Cosmetics are quite another matter.

'Fortunes are made by cosmetics,' we are told bluntly, and we are no doubt expected to react with dismay, if not outrage. 'Large sums, we know, are paid to artists to "enamel" the skins of ladies, bestowing the radiance of health where nature or disease has set a very different sign. Dear Madam, it is all a fiction! Cosmetics are impositions. The credulity of vanity, supported by blank ignorance, may induce you to spend time and money on such appliances to create a "complexion"; but if you knew how your skin was constructed . . . you would as soon think of remedying its defects by the use of cosmetics as of rendering hieroglyphics legible by whitewashing a monument. . . . Resorting to the Artificial methods incurs two serious risks — the risk of injury to health, and the risk of being found out and despised.'

The article then repeats the familiar and sensible warnings about the dangers of enamelling and points out that successful deceit is almost impossible since light falling on the enamelled skin from the side will betray one's guilty secret. Finally, we come to rouge and pearl-powder:

'Rouge is needful on the stage, so long as the present system of lighting the stage continues. . . . Pearl-powder is generally used by foreign actresses and not unfrequently used by English actresses. . . . Both rouge and pearl-powder are much oftener used in drawing-rooms than is suspected — rouge is even used by men — but the moderation with which they are employed causes them to escape general notice, and, at the same time, mitigates their evil effects. . . .

'There are the plain facts. If, therefore, Nature has bestowed on you a brilliant complexion, you have simply to keep yourself in health. If Nature has bestowed on you a skin obstinately brown, or obtrusively spotty, you must resign yourself to the inevitable, and only hope to mitigate the defect, first, by keeping yourself in health, and secondly, by the judicious choice and distribution of colour in costume. In cosmetics there is no help!'

Three months later, in another article on cosmetics, the magazine made it clear that patches, though out of date, had not entirely disappeared: 'The "beauty-spot" still used by humble belles in out-of-the-way districts, is the last relic of the old, often dying, but never entirely dead fashion'. Seven years later writers were complaining that despite violent newspaper attacks against it, the fashion of patching continued.

The use of cosmetics was also revived to some extent in the United States in the 1860s. The Empress Eugénie, it is believed, introduced mascara for the first time, and Charles Meyer, a German teenager, well trained in wigmaking, introduced Leichner's theatrical makeup—the first greasepaint to be made in America. Of greater general influence, perhaps, was the discovery, in 1866, that face powder made from zinc oxide would not discolour, as other face powders did, would not harm the skin, and was considerably less expensive to manufacture. The result was a great boom in the sale and use of face powder, not only in America but in Europe as well.

A correspondent in the *Athenaeum* of November 1865 expressed his outrage against the use of white paints on children. 'Is it possible,' he asked, 'that any woman can be silly enough to paint her children's faces with the pigments that were bought to make her own face "beautiful for ever"? Our eyes seem to report the disgusting fact. What are we coming to? Except in the most debased days of Rome, and those equally vile years when the Grand Monarque ruled France, we do not know that this practice has obtained upon the earth. Whatever a woman may be foolish enough to do with her own countenance in this fashion, she is personally responsible for and may be willing to bear the ridicule which her folly brings with it. A painted child is nothing less than loathsome!'

In his advice to women on *The Art of Pleasing*, published in translation in 1874, Ernest Feydeau expresses firmly negative opinions about painting:

'If women, prompted by no other motive than that of pleasing men, paint their faces, I solemnly declare to them, in the name of the masculine sex, that they are going a false route and will only render themselves horrible. A light touch might be tolerated on a pale complexion: it serves wonderfully to show the brilliance of the eyes and lights up the face with a look of animation; but a coating of white trashy powder, a common mixture of dangerous drugs, smeared from the neck to the roots of the hair, is simply repugnant, if not disgusting. . . . Nature is much more intelligent herself than all the perfumers, hair-dressers, druggists, chemists, and manufacturers of cosmetics, and—question of health apart—gives invariably to each one of us the complexion we deserve to have. That is to say, the one that best harmonizes with our features, the color of our hair and eyes. With a great effort of imagination, I have at last understood that a human being could not be absolutely satisfied with the face Nature had given. But this I cannot conceive, that a creature who has not the slightest idea of ameliorating her disposition, which might perhaps be far easier done, has the absurd predilection of changing her face. All she can do, the only end—even aided by science and art, at the expense of intelligence, patience, and lots of money — obtained is, to make herself uglier than ever.'

Feydeau then becomes more specific:

'One meets often, too often, in the public streets, unfortunate young women that simple-minded people might think afflicted by some terrible disease, who, in the eyes of sensible people, are simply victims of some caprice of bad taste. These women, these unfortunate ones, are not, perhaps, extraordinarily beautiful, nor are they ugly. The greater part of them might be called passably good-looking; a few of them might be called charming. Unfortunately, that does not satisfy their ambition. Nature has given them black, or brown, or blonde hair, complexions to match, youthful repose, eyes sufficiently large to see with, and even to "chain hearts." In an hour of folly they cut off their hair and substitute for it an abominable yellow wig, paint their eyelids and lashes, soil their eyebrows with powdered charcoal, cover their face with flour, paint their lips and gums with red paste of a bad odor, and thus fearfully daubed, resembling the wax dolls one sees in toy-shops, they dare promenade in the sun and brave the bright light of a theatre. And all this to please. They never imagine that they make people tremble. . . . Out of one hundred young women you meet, fifty are made up as I have just described. I know not what ails female youth, but seeing what they do, one would believe they took an interest in the definite triumph of ugliness. . . .

'What renders the Parisian ladies of the third Republic superior to the dames of the Roman Empire is, the latter were simply ridiculous enough to seek means to remedy the inevitable ravages of Nature, by only using cosmetics when they were old and decrepit, while the French ladies have not the patience and the courage to wait so long, but in their youth of bloom and beauty they seek to embellish themselves at the cost of spoiling their charms.'

In Paris and other sophisticated centres of fashion, there were elegant salons where women could have their faces painted by professionals. A pamphlet issued by a Parisian exhibitor at the Centennial Exhibition lists the variety of cosmetics available at his salon:

'Besides being arranged according to their consistency, color, and shade, our fards (paints) are classed according to the purpose intended and the effect of light in the following manner: – white and rose fards with every shade for the complexion; fards for indoors; fards for out-of-doors; fards for daylight; fards for gaslight; fards for court and ball; fards for the eyes; fards for the lips; *réaseau d'azur* to match the veins; hair-dyes and hair-powders; nail-powders; appliances for the application of fards; sanitary compositions to remove fards and to maintain health and freshness of the skin.' For those who wished to paint themselves, a *boîte de jouvence* was available.

Several books were published during this period describing the cosmetics used, frequently their composition, and even their manufacture. Arnold J.

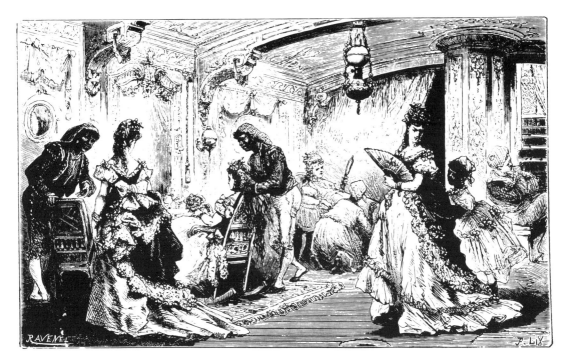

FIG. 180: Beauty salon aboard the *Cincinnati*, 1875.

Cooley was able to list, and in most cases give formulas for, about two hundred cosmetics for the skin, including a wide variety of enamels, rouges, and lip salves, most of them presumably in current use. Drs Brinton and Napheys published a book on *Personal Beauty* in 1870, and four years later came the publication, in English translation, of a book by Dr Pierre Cazenave entitled *Female Beauty; or, the Art of Human Decoration*. The following information, based largely on these three books, covers most of the commonly used cosmetics of the period.

ROUGE

Drs Brinton and Napheys seem to suspect that at the very mention of rouge many women 'will throw up their hands in horror. They associate it, innocent lambs, only with the bedaubed creatures who pace the pavements at night, with Jezebels "who paint themselves" and with actresses who stand before the foot lights, reddened up to the eyes.' Yet Cooley tells us that it is 'extensively employed by ladies to brighten the complexion and gives the seeming bloom of health to the pallid or sallow cheek'. He believed rouge, of all cosmetics, to be the one least injurious to the skin. Cochineal, a small insect found in Brazil, and safflower were the safest sources of red pigment for rouge — carmine being derived from cochineal and carthamine (also called rouge végétale), from safflower. Vermilion, derived from a mercury compound, was cheaper, frequently used, but considered harmful.

Rose en tasse. Rouge in pomade form was usually put up in pots or tiny saucer-like dishes of milk glass or China and applied with the fingers. Containers for rouge pomade are shown in Plate 17-I and Figures 166 and 167.

Rouge en crepons were 'pieces of silk or cotton gauze, twisted into the shape of a plug and imbued with the colouring matter (carthamine)'. They were moistened with alcohol or wine and rubbed gently on the cheeks or lips.

Tampons au rouge were crepons mounted in wooden or ivory handles and applied in the same way.

Rouge en feuilles is described as 'a very elegant preparation . . . usually prepared by depositing a thin layer of the finest carmine on thick paper'. For application, the coating of rouge was taken up from the paper on a moist woollen cloth of soft sponge and rubbed gently on the skin. The effect was said to be 'altogether satisfactory'.

Rose powder was a fine grade of rice meal tinted with carmine and perfumed, often with oil of roses. It could be applied with a powder puff, a camel's hair brush, or a hare's foot.

Enamel powder was a similar form of rouge made from bismuth and French chalk, then coloured and scented. It was applied in the same way.

Damask Rose Drops, according to advertisements, would 'give instant. permanent colour and beauty to the cheeks, lips, and complexion and would 'impart the radiant bloom of youth and defy the closest observer'. They were available in pocket cases for three shillings and sixpence.

Schnouda, sometimes known as Sympathetic Blush, was a colourless liquid which turned to a natural rose colour after it had come in contact with the skin. It was said to be a mixture of cold cream and alloxan, 'the source of which,' remarked Drs Napheys and Brinton mysteriously, 'we hesitate to explain'. Nor were they sure that it was harmless.

Chinese Card Rouge was a colourless liquid made by dissolving pure rouge in a solution of carbonate of soda. As with schnouda, the acid of the skin caused it to turn rose coloured.

Bloom of Roses was used 'to give an artificial bloom to the complexion, the liquid being applied with a camel's-hair brush or the tip of the finger and, when nearly dry, toned off with the corner of a soft napkin'. One recipe called for soft water, lemon juice, sulphuric acid, dried red rose leaves, gum arabic, and esprit de rose, all of which required much stirring, straining, squeezing, dissolving, settling, filtering, and decanting.

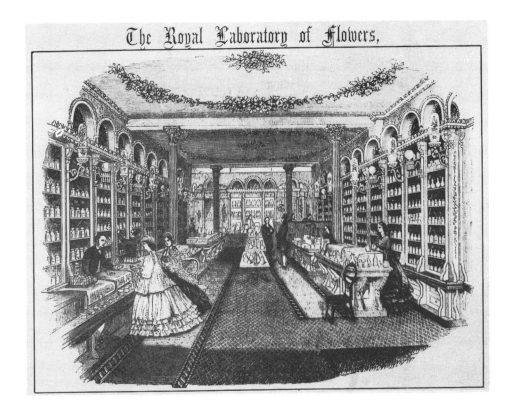

FIG. 181 : Perfume and cosmetics shop of Piesse and Lubin, New Bond Street, London, 1865. 'Manufacturers of Toilet Powders, Odorous Vinegars, Dentifrices, Pomatums, Scented Oils, Perfumed Soap, Cold Cream, Glycerine Jelly, Ivy Paste, Perfumes for the Handkerchief, Scented Waters, Fruit Syrups.'

Peruvian Lip Salve. The best quality lip salve available in the shops could be duplicated at home by combining spermaceti ointment, alkanet root, balsam of Peru, and oil of cloves with the usual heating and straining and pouring into suitable pots or boxes. French, German, and Italian lip salves were also listed.

Rose Lip Salve. This could be purchased in the shops or made at home with equal parts of melted lard and rose leaves coloured with a little alkanet root. Dr Cazenave's recipe called for oil of roses, spermaceti, white wax, alkanet root, and essence of rose. The instructions were to 'put the wax, spermacetti, the oil à la rose, and alkanet root in a bowl or earthen pot. When dissolved, pound the root fine, and let them remain four or five hours so as to extract the color, strain through a fine muslin rag, and add the essence of rose.' He seemed to consider its purpose to be primarily to soften, not to colour.

Dr Cazenave advised using the simple vegetable rouges rather than 'those numberless ones sold under attractive names, about which nothing is known. One of these, which has a wide popularity, is a solution of carmine in rose-water with the addition of a strong caustic ammonia, which latter cannot fail but injure the skin in time. Above all things, beware of *cheap* rouges, and those called "theatre rouges," nearly all of which are coarse colors which give a tawdry and meretricious air to the user and besides that are generally made of vermilion.'

The manufacture of rouge, safe or unsafe, presented technical problems which almost no one but the French had really succeeded in solving. The story is told of a London manufacturer who, in despair, paid a firm in Lyons 30,000 francs for the secret of their process. On being shown through the plant, he found their methods identical to his own. He returned home, tried again, and failed again. On his second visit to Lyons he was asked the state of the weather during his recent attempt. He hadn't the faintest idea. He was then told that the French manufactured their rouge only on the fairest days of their generally favourable climate. The English manufacturer, poorer by 30,000 francs, returned dejectedly to the dampness and fog surrounding his London plant.

Dr Robert Tomes was a champion of natural beauty, and though he recognized the importance of a certain fullness and shapliness of the female lips, he cautioned that 'there is no art potent enough to give the beauty of symmetry which Nature may have refused to the lips. If they become unnaturally pale, more or less rouge mixed with beeswax will give them a deceitful and temporary gloss of nature. To this daubing our fashionable dames are constantly obliged to resort, for their exhausting lives of dissipation impoverish and decolorize the blood, and the effect is apparent at once in the blanched lip. A frequent usage, however, of the lip salve, as it is ingeniously called, but which is merely a red pigment in disguise, so inflames, thickens, roughens, and gives such a peculiar tint to the mouth, that it has the look of the shriveled, purplish one of a sick negress.'

POWDERS

These were the most commonly used means of whitening the skin. Starch was sometimes used, but its effect was not, according to Cooley, 'sufficiently marked to meet the wishes of the majority of those vain enough to employ cosmetics of the kind. The American ladies, who have a passion for painting their necks white, use finely-powdered light carbonate of magnesia. . . . Ladies of the haut ton, however, are not content with the effect of these simple powders and usually employ metallic compounds which possess greater whiteness and brilliancy to revive their faded complexions.'

Drs Brinton and Napheys recommended powdered French chalk or *craie de Briançon* for whitening the face. This was actually not chalk but finely powdered soapstone from Briançon, a small village in the French Alps. The doctors

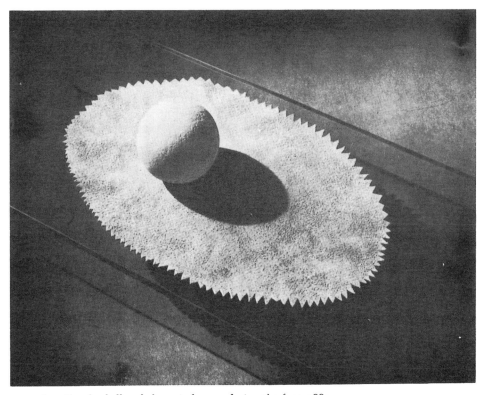

FIG. 182: Powder ball and chamois for powdering the face, 1880.

assured their readers that the powder was harmless, very adhesive, and would not lose its colour. Because of the difficulty of obtaining the French variety, they had examined American quarries and found a suitable substitute in North Carolina. It was, they said, ground and sold 'for various purposes' by a firm in Cincinnati.

Venetian chalk, actually a form of talc, they found inferior to the French powder, both in colour and in adhesive power. They also endorsed the mixing of precipitated carbonate of zinc with French chalk. Finely powdered carbonate of magnesia (also inferior to the French powder) was used by some women.

The doctors, having endorsed the pure products used for face powder, then sharply cautioned their readers about adulterated ones:

'All these powders have the objection that the hue they produce is not a very decided and brilliant one. Therefore the *cosmetiqueur*, with daring hands, has invaded the domain of pharmacy, and laying hold of some of its most potent and dangerous drugs has carried them to his shop to sell to the first chance-comer. This is unwise, and many a tolerable complexion has been wizened into a piece of parchment, many a woman has poisoned her constitution, by ignorantly using these perilous stuffs.'

As for the bismuth used in pearl powder, Brinton and Napheys, contrary to the opinion of many physicians, doubted that it was injurious to the skin or to general health, but they did point out one distressing disadvantage, which had plagued women for more than two centuries.

'It has, indeed, in common with *all* the metallic substances used for this purpose, one serious drawback. They are all changed by sulphurous gases into dark gray sulphurets, and as luck will have it, our coal fires and gas-pipes are constantly ready, whenever the opportunity is allowed them, to fill the apartment with just such gases. The consequence is that on not a few occasions, ladies who at the outset of the evening displayed complexions which made their rivals ready to tear their hair with envy, have come to grief in the most unexpected manner and been obliged to retire in confusion, with their faces of a dirty ash color, owing to some stupid servant mismanaging the furnace and allowing the gas to escape.'

Embarrassing as this might be, it still, in the opinion of the authors, was not a health hazard. But other substances were. Compounds of lead and mercury, which women had been warned against for centuries, were still in use, and once again women were told that if they used them, it was at the risk of their health and beauty and even of their lives. Moreover, these dangerous paints gave a hue so brilliant as to be clearly unnatural. Therefore, concluded the authors, 'from a cosmetic as well as a hygienic point of view, they must be condemned, for the perfection of art is to achieve an absolute resemblance to nature at her best, not to surpass her, nor fall behind her'.

The English version of Dr Cazenave's book, mentioned previously, appeared in 1874, the year the first Hind's Honey and Almond Cream was marketed. As one might expect, the emphasis was on maintaining good health rather than on covering up deficiencies. For protecting and preserving the complexion in general, Dr Cazenave recommended pure rice powder, pulverized starch, a mixture of starch and sub-nitrate of bismuth, or what he called Rose Powder — a compound of rice powder (2 pounds), lake carmine (4 drachms), essence of rose (18 grains), and essence of santal. It was to be spread on the face with a hare's foot or a tuft of down. He also recommended avoiding cold air, water on the face, rich foods, stimulating drinks (unless one was too pale), sitting too close to the fire or in the sun, any expression of strong emotion, and anything which might disturb the mind.

FACE ENAMEL

Cooley warns that 'the unnatural and injurious practice of painting the skin appears recently to have acquired a prevalence in the fashionable world, worthy of the most effeminate days of the most effeminate nations. Formerly, in these realms, the use of face-paints and face-blanches was chiefly confined to the courtesans and ladies of the demi-monde and to actors and actresses, in whom it is necessary to counteract the effects of the artificial lights to which they are exposed. But the case is different now.'

Brinton and Napheys indicated that there had been a rash of wildly exaggerated newspaper reports about ladies who enamelled their faces. One was that the celebrated actress, Madame Vestris, had to sit for hours by the fire to allow her enamel to dry. Another report had it that some New York belles were in the habit of going to Paris annually to have their faces enamelled for the year. One optimistic makeup artist actually advertised in the newspapers for clients to be made up 'to last a day or a year'.

All this, the doctors assured their readers, arose from ignorance. 'The so-called method of "enamelling" is simply painting the face, and for this purpose the artists always prefer the poisonous salts of lead, as they yield much more striking effects. Practice often gives these persons a decided skill in their speciality, but their customers pay for it doubly, first in money and then in health.

'The skin is usually prepared by an alkaline wash, wrinkles and depressions are filled in with a yielding paste, and the colors are laid on to the requisite extent, first the white and then the red.

'No such procedure can give a durable covering to the face, and no one should submit herself to the hands of the ignorant and unscrupulous parties who choose this for a business. The simple and harmless means which we have explained will suffice, if skilfully used, to conceal the ravages of years to any proper extent.'

EYEBROW COLOURING

During this period, according to Dr Cazenave, 'the eyebrows, to be handsome, should be well-furnished with hair, moderately thick, curved, and form a line in the shape of an arch. The head should have more hair than the tail, and the numerous short hairs should lie in and out. The two eyebrows should never meet, and though one often sees them perfectly united, it is at the present day looked upon as a deformity.' Caring for the eyebrows, he says, requires only a soft toothbrush dipped in water with a little cologne. He does, however, give two recipes for darkening the brows:

TO RENDER THEM BLACK

Gall Nuts..................................1 ounce
Oil...3 ounces
Mix with Ammoniac Salt...........1 drachm
Add a little vinegar.

This was to be applied before going to bed and allowed to remain on all night. In the morning the brows were to be washed with tepid water.

TO RENDER THEM BROWN

Lead Filings..............................1 ounce
Iron Dust.................................1 ounce
Vinegar....................................1 pint
Boil all together to reduce to half the original
quantity. Shake it well when cool, and wash
the brows.

Dr Robert Tomes told his readers that eyebrows and lashes were best not interfered with at all except for occasionally rubbing or brushing with a fine cloth or a soft brush.

VEIN COLOURING

But the ladies were not satisfied with whitening and reddening their faces. They also wished to emphasize the blue of the veins. With the demand, Brinton and Napheys pointed out, came the supply :

'It has been done. The elegant world can now provide itself with little jars which contain finely-powdered French or Venetian chalk, made into a paste with gum-water, colored to the proper tint with Prussian blue, and accompanied with little leather pencils, all manufactured on purpose to portray with anatomical fidelity the direction and hue of the veins. The effect, says Professor Hirzel, who talks on this subject with the gusto of a conoisseur, "when the work is artistically performed, is good and natural".'

COMPLEXION AIDS AND WASHES

Various washes for the complexion, often concocted from lemons, cucumbers, or horseradish, were popular. A tablespoon of benzoin in a glass of water, with or without a little glycerine, gave 'virgin's milk', which was highly esteemed for the complexion. These were all harmless and sometimes helpful. But there were other washes available in the stores containing corrosive sublimate, prussic acid, and arsenic. Cold cream, usually made of white wax, spermaceti, oil of almonds, and rose water, was widely used. Physicians were not sure if continued application would injure the skin; but since they looked upon it only as a medication for chapped skin, the question did not seem urgent. Rice powder and powdered arrowroot starch were commonly used to remove shine from the skin but not to whiten it.

For greasy skin inclined to pimples, Dr Cazenave suggested washing with elder water, weak tea, distilled linden water, milk of almonds, or virgin's milk. For a rough or dry skin he recommended a pomade made of oil of bitter almonds, fresh butter, lard, and mutton suet. He also recommended a paste to be applied before going to bed and removed in the morning with cervil water. Following are two recipes for such a paste:

MASK FOR THE FACE

Barley Flour, sifted......................3 ounces
Honey.........................1 ounce, 1 scruple
White of Egg...........................1 scruple
> Mix as a paste.

ANOTHER

White Wax...............................1 ounce
Sweet Almond Oil......................2 ounces
Goat's Grease............................1 ounce
Powdered Starch......................2 scruples

Dr Cazenave also had something for wrinkles, but he made no extravagant promises for it:

BALM TO DIMINISH WRINKLES

Benzoin Water..........................1 drachm
White Honey............................1 ounce
Alcohol......................................1 gill

The reader was instructed to let this macerate for eight days, then to bathe the forehead lightly. For roughness and wrinkles the doctor also recommended a lotion made of turpentine and water. But more interesting, perhaps, was a *Pomade to Conceal Wrinkles*:

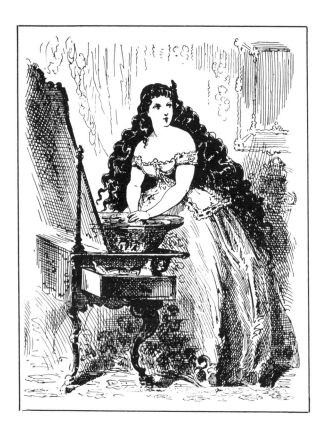

FIG. 183 : Lady at her toilet, 1864. From an advertisement for Perfumerie Anglaise de Rimmel in Paris. The illustration is captioned, 'It is to the products of Rimmel that the suave English ladies owe the golden glint of their silken hair and the diaphanous whiteness of their skin.'

Essence of Turpentine................2 drachms
Mastic....................................1 drachm
Fresh butter.............................2 ounces
Mix and use lightly.

Almond Balls. These were used to soften the skin and prevent chapping and chilblains. They were made by melting together 'in a glazed earthenware pipkin' spermaceti, white wax, oil of almonds, and oil of mace. The hot mixture was poured into egg cups or special moulds to cool. A cheaper recipe substituted suet for the spermaceti and cloves for the mace.

Pommade de Ninon de l'Enclos. A variety of pomades for skin and hair could be obtained. This one was a mixture of oil of almonds, hog's lard, spermaceti, and expressed juice of house-leek. Cooley noted that it was *said* to be very softening, cooling, and refreshing.

Cherry-Laurel Shaving Wash. This was an after-shave lotion made from cherry-laurel water, rectified spirit, glycerine, and distilled water.

Lotion of Cyanide of Potassium. This pleasant-tasting, poisonous compound, containing cyanide of potassium and emulsion of bitter almonds, was also used after shaving, especially to counteract itching or other irritations. The reader was advised to label it POISON, not to swallow it, to keep only a small amount on the dressing table, and to use it on only a small area at a time. Other than that, added Mr Cooley reassuringly, it was perfectly safe.

SOAPS AND DENTIFRICES

Dr Tomes advised readers to throw all of their cosmetic washes into the fire and 'betake themselves to soap', preferably Windsor. He cautioned that cosmetic washes would hide but not remove the dirt and were apt to 'mottle the complexion with brown and yellow spots, like the eyes of grease in an ill-made soup'. United Services Soap Tablets, at fourpence and sixpence each were available, according to advertisements, for those who wanted 'Soft, Delicate, and White Skin with a delightful and lasting fragrance'.

Shaving Paste. This was a mixture of Naples soap, powdered curd-soap, honey, essence of ambergris, oil of cassia, and oil of nutmeg beaten to a smooth paste with rose water and put into covered pots. Alternative recipes were supplied. The paste was applied with the fingers and lathered with a wet brush.

For the teeth Dr Cazenave recommended a half gill each of brandy and alcohol and eighteen grains of oil of mint, well mixed. With another recipe containing brandy, soap, and tincture of pyrethrum, he suggested using a toothbrush.

COURT PLASTER

At this time court plaster was used only to protect cuts or irritations and it was therefore desirable that it should be as inconspicuous as possible. But it is the same material that was used for the black patches of the seventeenth and eighteenth centuries. The preparation is interesting. For Liston's version of the recipe, 1 ounce of isinglass and $2\frac{1}{2}$ ounces of water are kept covered 'in a hot place until the isinglass has swollen and absorbed all the water and become quite soft'. This mixture had then to be beaten, squeezed through muslin, and mixed with alcohol. When this was thoroughly mixed, four coats were applied with a brush 'to the surface of oiled-silk stretched out and nailed on a board'. At this point scent could be added if desired.

Cooley adds that 'the common court-plaster of the shops is generally silk or sarcenet coated with isinglass-size, without the addition of any spirit, with merely a finishing coat of tincture of benzoin or of other aromatic to give it an agreeable odour. Chequered silk or satin is now frequently employed as the basis of the plaster; and, in the fashionable world, flesh-coloured court plaster appears to be the most esteemed. Waterproof court-plaster is simply the common plaster which has been lightly brushed over, on its exposed surface, with pale quick-drying oil. . . . Transparent court-plaster is usually that which is spread on oiled silk. The finest quality of court-plaster of the Paris and London (West-end) houses is now prepared on gold-beater's skin, one side of which is coated with the isinglass solution . . . and the other side with pale quick-drying oil. . . . A flesh tint is sometimes given to this oil . . . by means of a little dragon's blood and annotta in appropriate proportions'. Cooley then noted that gold-beater's skin, with no preparation at all, provided the best transparent court plaster available.

In spite of the considerable increase in the use of cosmetics, conservative Victorianism still kept most women from using makeup openly. Mary Haweis, a parson's wife, seemed unaffected by the current tendency toward artificial beauty. Yet in 1878, in *The Art of Beauty*, she did go so far as to suggest that beetle-browed ladies might do well to take a tip from ladies of centuries past and pluck their eyebrows with the aid of 'tweezers and courage'. But the suggestion had no noticeable effect, and it took another half century for eyebrow plucking to become widespread. If Mrs Haweis had lived to see it, she would surely have regretted her suggestion.

Curiously, for a book on female beauty, there are no hints on makeup, no suggestion that such artifices might be worth a try in emergencies. And yet, in a chapter on what she refers to as *invisible* girls, Mrs Haweis describes a number who could do with some emergency measures — the *Nonentity* ('The prettiness of mere youth lasts a year or two, during which, if poor, the nonentity is idle and ultimately starves'); the *Ill-educated Girl* ('The maiden can never be more than a laughing-stock, who believes that Alexander the Great conquered Britain and that Newton invented electricity'); the *Discouraged Girl* ('Apathy drags its slow length along their minds like a worm which dieth not'); the *Shy Girl* ('Silence which forbids the utterance of thought not seldom destroys the capacity for thought'); the *Stupid Girl* ('She is the most hopeless of the Invisibles . . . yet she may perhaps be of use in hemming dusters and doing what she is told'); the *Plain Girl* ('Do not some people admire a cast in the eye, a slight goitre, even a limp?').

For the plain girl Mrs Haweis offers the most hope of all -— not through makeup but by grace of the artists of the period. 'Morris, Burne Jones, and others,' she points out, 'have made certain types of face and figure once literally hated, actually the fashion. Red hair — once, to say a woman had red hair was social assassination — is the rage. A pallid face with a protruding upper lip is highly esteemed. Green eyes, a squint, square eyebrows, whitey-brown complexions are not left out in the cold. In fact, the pink-cheeked dolls are nowhere; they are said to have no character — and a pretty little hand is occasionally voted characterless too. Now is the time for plain women. Only dress after the prae-Raphaelite style, and you will be astonished to find that so far from being an ugly duck you are a full fledged swan!

'Thus, if pretty, you can do as you like: you can't be spoilt except by time. If plain you cannot do as you like: you must adopt quaintness of action and of garb; but time is powerless to spoil you, and in the long run you have actually the advantage. Whilst your pretty sisters are fretting over their lost bloom, you flourish ever in your soberer hues; the losses of age are more easily replaced in *you* than in *them*, and the probability is that you are more popular.'

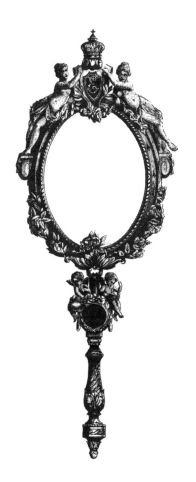 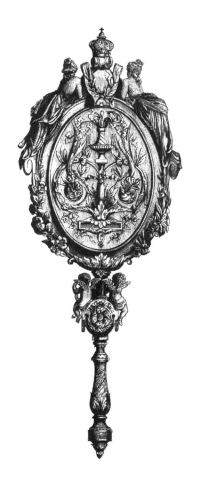

FIG. 184a: Front of hand mirror of carved pear-wood. Paris, 1860s.

FIG. 184b: Back of hand mirror on left.

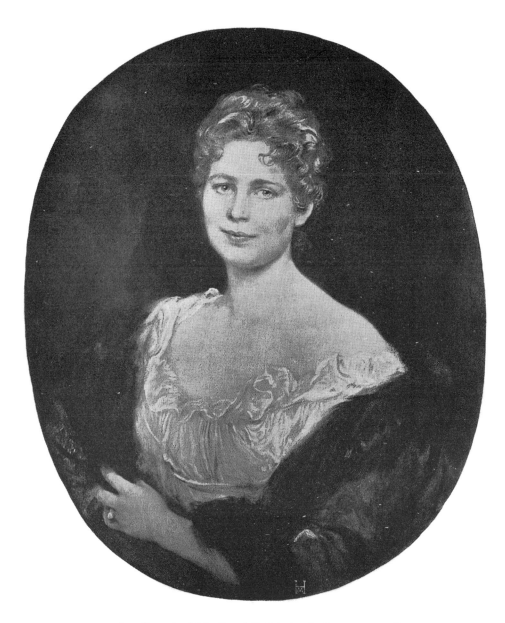

FIG. 185 : Portrait of Mrs C., 1898. Painting by F. A. von Kaulbach.

16 · The Late Victorians 1880-1900

The ladies of St. James's!
  They're painted to the eyes;
Their white it stays for ever,
  Their red it never dies:
But Phyllida, my Phyllida!
  Her colour comes and goes;
It trembles to a lily,—
  It wavers to a rose.

HENRY AUSTIN DOBSON

Women were still divided into those who painted and those who didn't. Among those who did, there were those who admitted they did and those who pretended they didn't. Non-painting was relative, however, for there were few women who did not use cosmetics of some sort, even if only the touch of a moistened red ribbon on their cheeks.

THE PAINTED FACE

According to 'a Professional Beauty', in a book called *Beauty and How to Keep It*, published in 1889, women were rapidly freeing themselves from Victorian attitudes towards makeup:

'The use of rouge and pearl powder seems to have become more fashionable now than it has been for many years, whether it is the result of the severe winters we have or the late hours we keep, I do not know. I have seen girls who are certainly not more than seventeen or eighteen with their faces painted and very badly done into the bargain. It would be so much better to try to correct the faults of the face with a little care and art without covering the *whole* of it with a *mask* of paint. I have seen some hideous specimens lately of painted women who think they are objects of beauty, instead of which they have made themselves objects of ridicule.'

But for those who did paint, she advised them always to have plenty of light in the room before making up the face, 'otherwise the consequence will be disastrous, you will appear with one cheek red, the other pale, one eyebrow high, the other low. For those who can possibly do without, I say, Do not begin to paint the face, it never looks pretty and always gives a hard unnatural expression.'

In *The Truth about Beauty*, published about 1892, Annie Wolf encouraged her readers with the thought that a well-appointed toilet table combined with a certain amount of mental application was 'sufficient to transform a plain woman into a Fra Angelico seraph. There is,' continued Miss Wolf, 'a conventional type of fictitious beauty to be avoided, whose cramped figure, gaudy apparel, and liberal use of paints, dyes and washes constitute her the model of a distinctive class. Concealed from view, all day, under plasters and poultices, like the famous Night Blooming Cereus, she exhales the fragrance of beauty only during the few short, dark hours. From the rims of her *bekolbed* eyes, to the tips of her tomato-stained fingers, she is artificial. No doubt she is as wise as a serpent in recipes for balms, rouge, and dyes, and in the mysteries of puff and plumper. She is neither rare nor inaccessible, and her skilful tactics and meretricious methods are open secrets.'

Instead, the author recommended 'plain living and high thinking' based on 'excellence of blood, bearing, and brains', along with temperance, purity, and exercise.

MY LADY'S DRESSING ROOM

In a book by Baroness Blanche A. Staffe, entitled *My Lady's Dressing Room*, translated (or 'adapted', as the title page has it) by Harriet Hubbard Ayer, the approach seems clear enough when the author proclaims to her readers exactly what they presumably want to hear — that it is right to hide their imperfections. 'There is no falsehood in it; we do not expect our dearest foes to expose their weaknesses. A woman who is indifferent regarding her own appearance cannot hope to preserve the admiration of her husband. On these points a man loves to be deceived, and he is right. What is life, what is love, without illusion?'

If the 1890s lady was led by this introduction to expect the indiscriminate use of makeup to be encouraged or even condoned she was to be disappointed. But suppose we examine first the setting in which the French lady of fashion prepared herself to meet the world:

'The dressing room of a fashionable woman should be as tasteful and comfortable as her social position and fortune permit: simply comfortable if she cannot afford luxury, but supplied at least with all things necessary and useful to a careful toilet. . . . The titled ladies of the eighteenth century, who enjoyed only limited opportunities for their ablutions, had their dressing rooms painted by Watteau, Boucher, Fragonard, etc., and it was here that they received their friends while they were being powdered, painted, and patched. We are too practical to expose delicate and exquisite works of art in this way to the steam and dampness of a room where both cold and hot water are used abundantly.

'The walls of some dressing rooms are covered with tiles in blue, pink, or sea-green. This produces a light, pleasant effect, but is somewhat cold to the

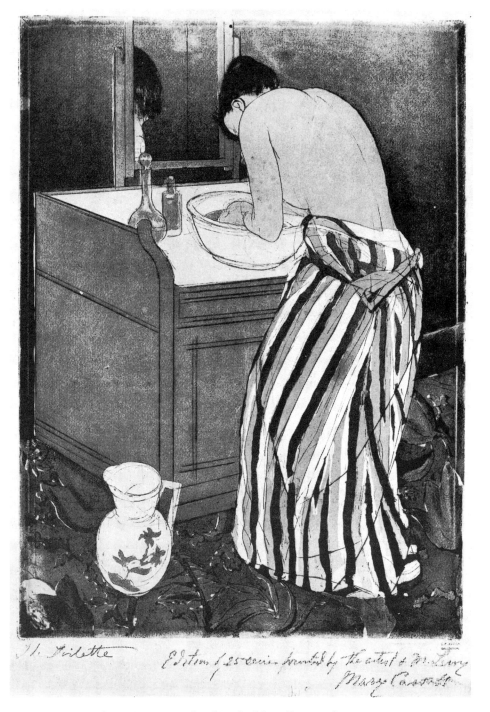

FIG. 186: The Toilette. Aquatint and etching by Mary Cassatt, 1891.

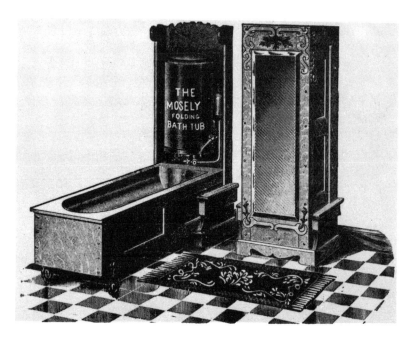

FIG. 187: The Mosely folding bath tub, 1893. The tub was zinc-lined, and
the cabinet was available in three finishes, all with a full-length
bevelled plate-glass mirror. In some models the heater was
replaced by storage shelves.

eye. Generally draperies are preferred. These should be of neutral or delicate
tints, in order not to conflict with the colors of the toilet. Frequently light or
bright silks are covered with thin muslin in order to soften their tone and at
the same time preserve their texture. . . . I prefer a dressing room in which the
principal colour is a pale blue or pink or yellow, with draperies of figured
muslin . . . held back by knots of ribbon. . . .

'From the ceiling should hang a chandelier to be lighted for evening toilets,
its candles securely forced into bobêches of colored crystal as a protection against
dripping wax. This dressing room must be well lighted. The windows, of
unpolished glass, may be ornamented with pretty designs and draped in silk
and muslin, bordered with lace.'

There should be two dressing tables, facing each other, different in dimensions,
but identical in form. The larger was to serve for 'the minor ablutions. It is
provided with a water pitcher and bowl of porcelain, crystal, or silver, selected
with the taste which distinguishes us these days. The dressing table is draped
like the walls. Above it fasten a little shelf on which to place perfumes, smelling
salts, dentifrices, elixers, etc., etc. Beside the bowl, place a soap dish, a box for
brushes, etc., etc.'

The smaller dressing table was to be surmounted by an adjustable mirror framed in silk and muslin with decorations matching the larger. This one, for dressing the hair, was to be supplied with 'all needful accessories, beautiful brushes and combs marked with the crest of their owner, delicate perfumes, creams, and lotions, powder boxes, powder puffs, manicure set, etc., etc.' The Baroness specified projecting bracket lights for each side of this table.

'The fireplace should be at the end of the room, facing the windows. On it place a porcelain clock and one or two vases of fresh flowers. At one side of the fireplace is a couch in blue or some other light color, brocaded with white, and here and there an ottoman and easy-chairs covered in subdued tints.'

The dressing room also contained two wardrobes, one of them with three mirrored doors. 'The wardrobe,' the baroness informs us, 'is no longer used in artistic bedrooms'. The second wardrobe, with floral decorations, was used for keeping supplies of bran, starch, powder, pastes, soaps, and the usual etceteras. The author points out that jugs, pails, and bath gowns must be invisible.

In giving suggestions for a simpler dressing room for less affluent ladies, she suggests concealing the frame of an ordinary mirror with a drapery. 'This is easily arranged by means of hidden tacks. Secure a very simple wardrobe, which you can greatly improve by painting and varnishing. Conceal the water jugs and pails under the valance of the table.' The zinc tub, she suggests, can be hidden under a drapery projecting from the wall. Another possibility, which she did not mention, was the Mosley Folding Bath Tub, illustrated in Figure 187.

HARRIET HUBBARD AYER

Harriet Hubbard Ayer, on the other hand, was unabashedly in favour of cosmetics whenever and wherever they were needed. Writing in 1899 (in her own book this time), she found herself 'a bit amused when anathemas are hurtled at the present use of cosmetics, particularly when a hopelessly soured and pitilessly unattractive female or a blatant, tobacco-smoking, spirituously-odorous male addresses me on the subject. I read from time to time of the untold millions we women are spending annually for our paints and powders and of all the good we might do were we not so given over to vanity and deceit. I have been assured by men who should know, if experience go for anything, that no good woman at any time of the world ever painted her face. I have had Jezebel thrown at me with a pertinent verse of Scripture attached, and with such spite that one would think I personally am accountable for that most trying woman and had given her the formulas for the paints and eye darkeners she adorned herself with before going out to the capture of King Jehu. . . .

'I am not an advocate of indiscriminate painting of the face, of hair dyeing or bleaching, because all are usually unpleasant and perceptibly artificial and unbecoming in their results, but I certainly think a woman should be her own judge in the matter, and the subject is one she is entirely competent to study for herself without masculine interference or dictation. Moreover, I never **knew** a woman who, if she chose, could not deceive the keenest eye of man on **this point**. It is always another woman who first tells a man that her sister uses artificial color or stains her hair.

'There are times in a woman's life when, if she be wise, she will attempt to repair the damage of years and care. When a wife sees a haggard-looking ghost of herself reflected from her mirror, when perhaps she is painfully conscious that the eyes she loves best are turning from her faded beauty to a less worthy object, then I think she is not only justified in delicately simulating, by every aid known to cosmetic art, the charms she has lost, but she is stupid not to do so. It is the plain, unadorned, weary, and too natural woman whose husband invariably falls a victim to the wiles of a Delilah or succumbs to the artificial charms of a Jezebel. The very man who will almost fall in a fit at the sight of toilet powder in his wife's dressing room, will break her heart and waste his substance in the worship of a peroxide or regenerator Titian-red blonde.'

THE ART OF BEAUTY

The last years of the century seemed to be flooded with publications for women. In an anonymously written book on the *Art of Beauty*, the author begins by advising her readers not 'to commence a practice which at first is often really unnecessary, but which often and so soon becomes imperative'. Surprisingly, she states that 'there has not for several centuries been a period when cosmetics were more used than at the present time'. Interpreting 'cosmetics' in its broadest sense, the statement may be less extravagant than it appears on the surface. Certainly, far more women used artificial aids to beauty than would admit it publicly — or privately, for that matter.

It was, our author tells us, becoming 'almost a passion' with some women and was being used by increasing numbers. 'A chemist,' she writes, 'only the other day remarked to me how much the practice had grown of late. "Quite young girls come in now," he said, "and ask for powder and even rouge and eyebrow pencils, without the least embarrassment." Scarcely anything, to my mind, is more revolting than a "made-up" child. And yet at most watering-places nowadays girls of thirteen or fourteen with artificial complexions are far too common. Too visible make-up also is very objectionable. A little good powder, and the use of a few other innocent cosmetics, provided that they are not so palpably applied as to attract undue attention, is, however, quite permissible. . . . I am not, of course, for one instant advocating the indiscriminate use of the almost innumerable preparations which are offered for our beautifying. There are, however, a few cosmetics which are perfectly harmless and innocuous, and, indeed, may be safely relied upon as real beautifiers.'

EVE'S GLOSSARY

Writing in 1897, by which time greater tolerance might have been expected, Margaret Cunliffe-Owen (the Marquise de Fontenoy) showed very little. She begins her chapter on cosmetics in *Eve's Glossary* with an almost audible sigh of resignation:

'It is very much against my inclinations to write about a practice of which I thoroughly disapprove. But, as a great many society women have adopted the custom of "making up", or, to speak more plainly, of painting their faces, I consider it my duty to point out to them how they can do so without endangering forever the beauty of their skin, not to mention their health, which . . . may suffer seriously from the use of poisonous paints, powders, and cosmetics.

'I caution my readers in the most earnest way to pause before they begin to "make up", if they are not yet in the habit of so doing; and if they have, to stop short. I have heard actresses, whose profession obliges them to have recourse to *maquillage*, loudly deplore its effects on their complexion; and it is therefore a mystery to me why women of the world who have no need to do so insist upon plastering their skin with all sorts of pastes and powders, which to begin with, deceive nobody, and which, I may safely add, give any woman an appearance of doubtful respectability.'

Miss Cunliffe-Owen then proceeds with a clear conscience to instruct her readers how to make up. Having done so, she launches into a blanket condemnation of what she has just told us how to do, at the same time clearly delineating the end-of-the-century conservative attitude towards makeup:

'Alas! from the earliest ages woman's besetting sin (or one of them) has been the love of paint. But at least for a good many generations it has been tacitly acknowledged that paint and self-respect somehow could not go in double-harness. . . . As women are credited with desiring to please the opposite sex, it would seemingly follow that the latter must admire what is commonly called "paint"; otherwise we should not be afflicted with the hideous caricatures of nature which are so painfully evident at every gathering of society. This is an egregious mistake, for I have always found that men jeer at painted women . . . and seriously object to *maquillage* where their wives, sisters, or daughters are concerned. How could it be otherwise? Do those who redden their cheeks with rouge, darken their eyes, and cover their complexions with chalk, verily believe that they call back the semblance of youth promised them by cosmetic concoctions? Or by constant contemplation of their own artificiality have they become blind to the spectacle they present to the world? . . . No one who has any idea of modern social life can deny that the use of all the adventitious aids to the toilet which have been condemned since the days of Jezebel —paint, powder, enamel, hair-dye, and every other kind of "beautifier"—is enormously on the increase in society. They seem to have attractions for all ages. . . . The competition for admiration has become so keen that public attention must be arrested at all costs . . . and poor, tender little rosebuds . . . bedaub their clear, fresh, young skins with red, white, and blue—very patriotic colors to be sure, but which look far more in place on the silken folds of Uncle Sam's flag than on the cheeks of his daughters.

'Making up, except when it is done in a very discreet and thoroughly artistic fashion, stamps the most honest woman at least as "fast", and this ought certainly to be sufficient to deter the fair sex from indulgence in so unladylike a practice. A painted, or worse, an enamelled face loses its individual expression; for the artificial complexion constrains one to avoid any passing emotion. Tears would destroy it, smiles or hearty laughter would crack it, and as to blushes— if *fin-de-siècle* women still blush—these delicate waves of color, so becoming to the feminine countenance, are invisible under a thick crust of *blanc de perle* and rouge.'

Miss Cunliffe-Owen, suggesting a suitable decor for a simple dressing room, seemed to be concerned more about decor than about light:

'Have the walls and ceiling covered with pale-green, pale-pink, pale-lemon, or pale-blue Pompadour cretonne—according to your complexion. Cream-hued lace window-curtains underlie those of cretonne, and the floor should be spread with a thick Aubusson carpet harmonizing in color with the hangings. The lounge, chairs, and arm-chairs can be of Japanese bamboo or of pitch-pine, upholstered in cretonne, and a large three-leaved mirror should be placed in a light corner. A long table should be provided for the basin and ewer, the dishes where sponges, toilet-brushes, etc., are contained, and the *flacons* of perfume.

'On another table, surmounted by a mirror, can be put the numerous pieces of the dressing-case, and also a large duchesse-pin cushion made of lace over silk. The newest brushes, boxes, etc., are tortoise-shell inlaid with gold and silver, or ivory inlaid with silver, which is extremely pretty, but somewhat costly. A great many women continue to use the beautiful repoussé silver-backed brushes, with combs in silver frames, heart-shaped trinket boxes, hairpin boxes, hat and clothes-brushes, buttonhook, bottles, tray, etc., and they are likely to remain in vogue for years to come. The tub and its accompanying linoleum cloth are stored away behind a curtain when not in use, and consequently do not detract from the dainty appearance of the room.'

In the same year that Margaret Cunliffe-Owen was writing disapprovingly of makeup, the Sears, Roebuck catalogue, a reliable barometer of what Americans were buying, offered a wide variety of cosmetics, which, the copywriter boasted, could not 'be equalled by any other house either in this country or in Europe, on account of their good and harmless quality and the magical effects produced. They are prepared by a specialist who has made a life study of the science of improving and beautifying the skin, hair, and teeth.' Then, for those women who, along with Miss Cunliffe-Owen, were still resisting cosmetics, there was an additional bit of persuasion: 'It is in the nature of the human family from the savage to the most civilized to use the best means obtainable, by which they can render themselves more pleasing and attractive to others. It is a duty and a pleasure we owe to one another. It is almost criminal to go about with a repulsive complexion, etc., when the means to render yourself attractive are so easily obtainable.' But all writers did not agree on the means.

CARE OF THE SKIN

According to the 'Professional Beauty' who wrote *Beauty and How to Keep it*, hot water is fatal to the skin since it relaxes the tissues and encourages wrinkles. 'To keep the face smooth and soft . . . it ought to be rubbed, on going to bed, with some soothing emollient such as Crème Simon, Cream of Cucumber, or Nadine Cream . . . applied with a fine towel and well rubbed into the skin.' This was to be left on all night, then washed off first thing in the morning with rose water, orange-flower water, or Rowlands' Kalydor. She did not approve of using cold cream or glycerine, which, she warned, encouraged hairs to grow and made the skin yellow. 'There is another way,' she added, 'of keeping the freshness of the skin, but it may not meet in the approbation of my readers, this is, to lay a piece of fresh raw veal on each cheek on going to bed, the veal to be kept in place by bandages of linen. I know that no cosmétique of any kind is equal to this, and it certainly gives the skin a most lovely soft and velvety appearance.'

In addition to thorough washing and proper rest and avoidance of frowning, raising the eyebrows, or laughing excessively, Baroness Staffe suggests face creams and gives her favourite recipe:

'Toward the end of May take a pound of the very freshest, purest butter. Place it in a white basin and expose it to the sun, where it will be well protected from dust, etc. When the butter has melted, pour over it some plantain water, mix well by means of a wooden spatula, and let the sun absorb the water. Pour in more plantain water and repeat five or six times during the day. Continue until the butter has become as white as snow. The last few days add a little orange-flower and rose water. Cover the face at night with this salve, and carefully wipe off in the morning. This is a good and old recipe of the time of the beautiful Gabrielle.'

For impatient ladies who were so unfortunate as to run across the book for the first time after the May deadline, there were other recipes. One of them had the considerable advantage of 'not whitening the coats of partners in a dance'.

Margaret Cunliffe-Owen, on the other hand, leaned towards plain soap and water, and for the first time in history there was a wide variety of soaps available. It might, Miss Cunliffe-Owen thought, be called the Soap Age:

'There are soaps warranted to wage war against and vanquish roughness, redness, and pimples; there are others guaranteed to fortify the most delicate cuticles against wind and weather, and to make shaving even the most stubbly of chins a positive delight; there is even one which defies the wrinkles of old age, another which renders the teeth pearly white and threatens ruin to the dentists. There are others which insure you a charmed life against infectious disorders; another brings about such a state of perfection that it can only be dedicated to the goddess of beauty herself; and another is of such prodigious strength that it can only be likened to a giant. There are even some whose powers are so soothing, and withal so expeditious, as to render the humble home a haven of rest on washing days!'

Annie Wolf permitted a few simple creams and ointments but did not recommend soap. She found bran water preferable, but she considered almond meal, available from the local chemist, even more beneficial. Night masks of suet, raw beef, and wet cotton were 'only to be thought of in exceptional cases'.

For a beautiful complexion Sears, Roebuck offered Lavender Lotion at seventy-five cents a bottle. Almond Nut Cream ('clears the skin from wrinkles, tan, freckles, etc., rendering it soft and white') at fifty cents, Secret de Ninon (for removing freckles) at seventy-five cents, Witch Hazel Toilet Cream ('an elegant preparation for the skin when it is chapped and rough') at twenty-five cents, and Camphorated Cold Cream (for the same purpose) at fifteen cents. For internal use there were Arsenic Complexion Wafers—an excellent medicine for giving to the complexion a clearness and brilliancy not obtainable by external applications, at the same time they improve the general health, causing the figure to grow plump and round'. They were available in the forty-cent and the seventy-five cent size.

For the woman who preferred to brew her own cosmetics from the many available recipes, there were funnels, mortars, measuring glasses, scales and weights, cold cream jars, ointment pots, turned wood boxes, tin ointment boxes, and a variety of bottles. Powder puffs were available for twenty cents and celluloid puff boxes for forty-five cents. There were, in addition, a variety of perfumes, colognes, toilet waters, and depilatories. The listing of these was preceded by a few paragraphs of advice from 'the world renowned Doctor Erasmus Wilson', who warned the buyer that 'a bad complexion will immediately place its possessor in an unfavorable light and blind the eye to every other good quality, either of features or intellect. Not only this, but in many cases will stamp its victims as being vulgar and common and make it impossible for them to rise above these impressions. . . . Anybody with the proper kind of pride should shrink from placing herself in such a position as to require her friends and those whom she is thrown in contact with the necessity of apologizing, even to themselves, for her bad complexion . . . love and admiration are the two great wants in every woman's nature, and beauty alone can aid them in being loved and admired'. In *My Lady's Dressing Room*, the translation of Baroness Staffe's book, emphasis is always on taste and good sense in taking care of oneself. The author recommends bathing the face in warm water with a flat facial sponge and drying the skin carefully with a soft linen cloth. 'Women of leisure,' she adds, 'prefer to wash their faces at bed time.' She also recommends not using soap too frequently and not at all in hot weather, and she prefers lemon juice and strawberry juice to soap for cleansing the skin. She also finds a walk in the rain more useful than a Turkish bath.

Presumably she would not have been greatly impressed by the portable Turkish bath available in New York for three dollars from the Home Turkish Bath Co. For those who wished to avoid the publicity and 'other disagreeable features' of public Turkish baths, the home bath, according to the advertisement, had much to offer: 'Appliances that mitigate and assuage the asperities of a climate, alternating from the torrid heat of midsummer to the Arctic rigors of midwinter, are obtainable, and if only properly brought to the attention of those who would derive benefit therefrom, would go far toward producing that state of health and comfort, in the vain search for which so many thousands desert home and country.' To men the manufacturer guaranteed a clear brain and a strong body and to women, health, strength, and 'the lovely complexion promised, but never given, by cosmetics'. This would seem to be clearly a bargain at only three dollars.

Like all women and all writers on beauty, the baroness is concerned with the aging skin. Some women, she says, apply hot towels before going to bed, others wash in cold water, still others use both hot and cold. 'Lady Londerry, an English beauty,' she tells us, 'retains her youthful charms, which defy the ravages of time, at the cost of infinite pains. Every tenth day she spends in bed sleeping until she awakens naturally, then takes a warm bath, returns to her bed, where a light breakfast is served, tries to sleep again, and if she does not succeed, remains quietly there doing nothing, almost without thinking, in her

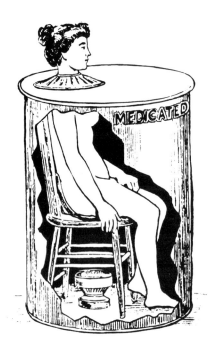

FIG. 188: Portable Turkish bath for home use,
c. 1900.

darkened room. At six in the evening she arises, dines in her dressing room, and remains near the fire inactive until ten o'clock, when she returns to her bed. . . . Occasionally her maid reads to her a light, unexciting romance.'

For the lady lacking a taste for unexciting novels, there were available other beauty books, most of which confined themselves to improving women. But the anonymous authors of *Beauty: Its Attainment and Preservation*, published in 1896, suggest in the first chapter that the problem is not entirely one-sided. 'The effort to be lovely,' they tell their readers, 'should not necessarily be confined to womankind. There is a broad field for improvement in this direction among the opposite sex, and many a woman would be vastly helped in her endeavors to please if "her lord and master" . . . were to administer to his own irritable or otherwise diseased disposition, the wholesome correctives of repression and self-sacrifice and the genial tonics of cheerfulness, kindness, and courtesy.' But that was the extent of their suggestions for the beautification of men. Any advice about artificial improvements in their appearance, beyond cleanliness, neatness, and general health, would have been unwelcome.

In other parts of the book there are such intriguing headings as 'How to Acquire Flesh', 'Cunningly Applied Perfumes', 'A Habit to be Broken', 'The Renovation of Flannels', 'Disadvantages of Colored Underwear', 'A Merry Walk' and 'How to Make a Toilet Table'. According to the authors, evidently a shrewd lot, the first step in making a toilet table is to find a co-operative male relative and tell him what you want.

It was entirely possible, of course, though the authors did not say so, that having constructed a splendidly elegant toilet table, the male relative might then decide to keep it for himself. Margaret Cunliffe-Owen, whose dislike of painted women was exceeded only by her utter contempt for painted men, complained that makeup was 'by no means restricted to the weaker members of society in these decadent and degenerate days, for some of the co-called young "exquisites" which one meets in New York and sometimes also on the Continent are guilty of improving — as they believe — their complexions by *maquillage*. A weak-kneed, miserable, vain specimen of humanity is this sad creature, who has literally no redeeming points that I can discover, but who yet gives himself all the airs of one to whom the universe ought to do homage. He is to be seen at first nights waddling to his seat with a gait which he imagines to be graceful, but which is in reality painfully absurd. His thin, high-pitched voice is heard at private views, pronouncing a languid and final decision upon the merits of the works of art exhibited. He stands against the walls of ballrooms, — unable to dance because nobody asks him, and he could hardly be so manly as to invite anybody, — with poised head and rounded eyes, intent upon his artistic pose, and anxious that every gaze should be upon him. Nor is that all; for, as I have said above, it is an absolute fact that a large number of young men get themselves up. Old beaux I leave entirely out of the question. The rouge pot and the powder puff find a place on the toilet-table of the former. Their eyebrows are darkened; their hair is often crimped or curled and sometimes even dyed, and their figures are trained and artificially improved. . . .

'Many of the toilet shops in London, Paris, and New York would have to put up their shutters if deprived of their male customers. Paint, powder, perfumes, dyes, creams for the complexion, and washes for the hair and moustache are among the more innocent of the purchases of these dandies. Manicure sets to trim their dainty finger-nails, irons for waving and curling that exquisite moustache, which, by the bye, must be dyed to the latest tint of reddish brown, scented sachets to fasten inside their coats, perfumed cachous wherewith to sweeten their breath, — all these and many other items of toilet trickery form part of the indispensable "get up" of our modern ultra society man. Alas! where are the knights of old to whom the weaker sex used to look up! *Mais où sont les neiges d'antan!* Is this to be tolerated? and ought not we, women of sense and heart, to deride these young monsters into abandoning so reprehensible and degrading a custom, and lead the way ourselves in a great measure by discarding all *maquillage*, and by trying, instead, to improve our appearance simply with the aid of daily ablutions, exercise, healthy living, and by the use of such cosmetics as are derived from Nature's rich stock, and which I have described so many times in these chapters?'

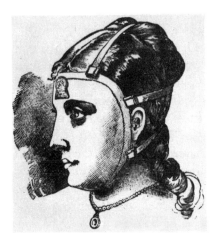

FIG. 189: Madame Rowley's Toilet Mask. From an advertisement of 1889. The mask or 'face glove' was to be worn three times a week.

For women, perhaps more than for men, hands were an important part of skin care. 'It might possibly interest my readers,' wrote the beauty editor of *Vogue* in 1898, 'to know how our great mondaines succeed in preserving, to the most advanced age, unwrinkled and delicate hands, white and velvety, and also endowed with that exquisite pinkish tinge of the palm and finger-nail which is considered as the perfection of la beauté de la main. To begin with, outside of their bath, they never use soap to cleanse their hands during the course of the day, but replace this generally strongly alkaline substance by oatmeal or almond paste, and at night they wear loose white kid gloves which are usually bought at leading parfumeurs, but which can also be prepared at the home if expense entailed seems too great.' Fortunately, the editor happened to have the formula at hand:

'Beat the yolks of two fresh eggs briskly, mixing therewith all the time, and very gradually, two soup-spoonfuls of sweet almond oil, two soup-spoonfuls of rose-water, and one soup-spoonful of tincture of benzoin. When these diverse ingredients have become thoroughly amalgamated, take a pair of white kid, or untanned leather gloves and turning them inside out, dip them carefully in the preparation. Before they become dry, turn them right-side-out again, blowing into the fingers, so as to prevent their sticking, and put them on every night when going to bed. A pair thus prepared ought to last a fortnight. In the morning after removing the gloves, and after having taken one's bath, the fingers and palms as well as the back of the hand should be rubbed very carefully with cologne and then some ordinary zinc ointment should be applied slightly over the nails, for it polishes them and renders them far more transparent and dainty to look at than the various rouges sold for that purpose and which are sometimes extremely injurious.'

According to an 1889 advertisement by the Toilet Mask Company, Madame Rowley's Toilet Mask (or Face Glove) 'Is the *only natural beautifier* for *bleaching* and *preserving* the *skin* and *removing complexional imperfections*. It is *soft* and *flexible* in form, and can be *easily applied* and *worn* without *discomfort* or *inconvenience*. The *Mask* is patented, has been introduced ten years, and is the only *genuine article* of the kind. It is *recommended* by *eminent physicians* and *scientific men* as a *substitute for injurious cosmetics*.'

The mask (or face glove), used by 'famous society ladies, actresses, belles, etc.', was guaranteed to be harmless, inexpensive, and to prevent and remove wrinkles. It would, the reader was assured, save 'hundreds of dollars uselessly expended for cosmetics, powders, lotions, etc., etc.' The illustration accompanying the advertisement is reproduced in Figure 189.

WHITEWASHES AND POWDERS

With makeup still hovering in a sort of no man's land between the deceptive and the permissive, how much paint was used was beginning to be less important than how much could be seen. Harriet Hubbard Ayer warned that 'a sweet and modest woman should be careful to an extreme degree in using artificial expedients during the daytime. The manifestly made-up woman is too atrocious a blot on the landscape to even discuss. At night, for the home-dinner, as well as for opera and ball, the artificial light makes it possible for a woman literally to put on her war paint.'

Whitewashes were still used and still criticized. Annie Wolf called them 'a vulgar pretense. Besides rendering the face dry and chalky and destroying the velvet bloom that is a skin's chief beauty, [they make] an unpleasant impression. If the woman who resorts to them,' warned Miss Wolf, 'is doubted in the male mind and leered upon by masculine eyes and dealt lightly with by masculine tongues, she has only herself to blame and but one gospel to learn by heart; that the worldly and speculative man judges women as he does mines — by surface indications. Cosmetics and enamels are the adjuncts of those misguided women who imitate unwittingly the depraved sisterhood, just as a little child ignorantly repeats profane jargon dropped from a foreign tongue. Creams and lotions should be applied to the skin as salves and ointments are applied to a wound. Disease of whatever nature, wherever located, calls for healing treatment, and in this light only should cosmetics be used. A rough, coarse, and pimply face is quite as disgusting as an open wound or a virulent abscess; but for a lady to appear in the drawing-room, her face covered with a thick coating of cosmetic to conceal defects, is equally as vulgar as for her to leave her chamber with a poultice or plaster spread out in view.'

The authors of *Beauty: Its Attainment and Preservation*, who seem to agree generally with this point of view, begin their discussion of cosmetics with a stern warning that 'the white ingredients of most lotions are highly injurious to the skin and that seen upon the face they also call into question, even though silently, the moral status of the mind. . . . In addition to this . . . the drugs renowned as cosmetics for the skin are the most deadly poisons in the whole catalogue of chemical products. Caustic potash, corrosive sublimate, prussic acid, and arsenic are all used by unscrupulous dealers; and she will be a very wise woman who always endeavors to satisfy herself as to the harmlessness of a cosmetic before she begins to use it.' And yet the authors include, for bleaching the face, a recipe containing cologne, glycerine, and corrosive sublimate. The recipe, they assure the reader, 'will improve any complexion and it is harmless'.

French chalk is recommended for whitening the complexion, and the authors suggest 'a very nice way' to use it: 'Wrap a pellet of the chalk in coarse linen and crush it in water, grinding it well with the fingers. Wash the face quickly with the squeezed pellet, and the wet powder oozing through the linen will leave a fine pure deposit of the chalk upon the skin. Dab the face lightly with a dampened handkerchief to even the deposit, and remove any surplus from the nostrils and brows. It is said that chalk used in this way shows less than when applied dry and is cooling besides.'

There were tinted washes as well as white ones, usually prepared by simply adding a bit of rouge or gamboge to the white wash. A 'truly marvellous' effect, Joseph Begy tells us (in his *Handbook of Toilet Preparations*), can be obtained with a recipe which he calls *Maiden Blush* — a mixture of precipitated chalk, drop chalk, bismuth, borax, carmine, glycerine, bay rum, water, and extracts of vanilla, white rose, jasmine, and musk. It is to be applied to the face, arms, and neck, and 'is not easily detected on account of the natural hue it imparts to the skin'.

For 'an elegant creamy white' skin there is *Snow-Drop Cream*, containing similar ingredients with different fragrances and without the carmine. For a pinker complexion one can blend it with a liquid rouge. It is, says Mr Begy, 'one of the finest combinations I ever put together'. An even more intriguing complexion cosmetic is *The Arabian*, a darker mixture containing both rum and brandy and a little Ylang Ylang.

Mr Begy recommends applying all liquid cosmetics with a soft sponge, allowing them to dry, then rubbing them with a chamois. The results, he assures his readers, will be charming. The advantage of his recipes, he tells the ladies, is that 'you will be in a position to dispense with the preparations that are sold at such exorbitant prices, and in their place you can have yours made from my recipes at considerable less expense and with the assurance of guaranteed excellence . . . securing for yourselves beauty, health, contentment, comfort, and happiness.'

Some of the whitewashes and enamels certainly seemed to provide little comfort. 'The enamelled woman,' wrote Annie Wolf, 'must neither smile nor weep for fear of cracking the ghastly mask. Her porcelain face is cold and expressionless, and her complexion livid in the daytime. And whitewashes! They are even more fatal to the complexion than carmine. In the name of reason and good taste, I proscribe them in the dressing room. A resemblance to Pierrot, the clown, is certainly undesirable.'

Enamelling was not recommended in *The Art of Preserving Beauty* because it clogged the pores of the skin. In addition, it necessitated 'perfect repose of the features so that the emotions, whether happy or sorrowful, must be repressed, thus giving a monotonous, semi-melancholy expression to the face, which cannot prove attractive and, owing to the cause, often occasions sarcastic criticism.' The authors, surely having persuaded any sensible woman not to enamel, then proceed to tell her how to do it:

'In enamelling the face, the skin is first prepared by an alkaline wash, after which all wrinkles and depressions are filled with a yielding paste. Then the face is simply painted, and artists in this line generally prefer to use the poisonous salts of lead for the purpose, as they produce more striking effects than any other pigment. After the white layer is applied, the red tinting is done.'

These familiar instructions were lifted almost verbatim from a previously published book.

Instead of an enamel, Harriet Hubbard Ayer suggested a liquid whitener containing water (boiled and strained), alcohol, zinc oxide, bichloride of mercury, and glycerine. To avoid streaking, the liquid was to be applied with a soft sponge and wiped off with a chamois while still damp. She warned that this was not to be done by the woman herself since there was danger 'of missing ever so small a section of the skin, and this,' she added ominously, 'is fatal'.

Margaret Cunliffe-Owen, having spoken out strongly against making up, then points out that in doing it, one should 'carefully cleanse the skin before and after . . . with very pure white vaseline, which in some measure prevents painting from becoming too irritating. Wipe the face off with antiseptic gauze or tufts of medicated cotton-wool. Under no circumstances should *blanc* of any kind be applied, for not only does it make one look like a *Pierrot*, but this preparation almost invariably contains nitrate of silver or acetate of lead, and even mercury. I hope, therefore, that the good sense of my readers will impel them to taboo this execrable and deleterious paste, which can be advantageously replaced by a light application of a cream which is much used in Oriental harems, acting as a purifier upon the skin rather than injuring it, and which is prepared as follows:

BEAUME DES SULTANES

Incorporate in 4 ounces of sweet almond oil
   320 grains melted white virgin wax
   320 grains whale white
   100 grains finely powdered benzoin
   60 grains tincture of ambergris
   320 grains pulverized rice feculae
   15 grains pure carmine

'Heat and stir thoroughly to mix together; pour into a china jar and allow to cool. This cream must be spread with extreme care and gently rubbed into the skin, taking care not to put any on the eyebrows or in the immediate neighborhood of the eyes. When this is done, dip a swan's-down puff or hare's foot made of eiderdown, in some *Veloutine Rachel* powder, or, if you are very fair, in pink Veloutine. White powder ought never to be used, for a snow-white complexion . . . would be simply ghostly and appalling. Excellent face powder can be prepared at home with very little trouble, the advantage being that one can be certain that the ingredients are absolutely pure.'

Miss Cunliffe-Owen then recommends the flesh-coloured face powder called *Poudre d'Amour*. 'This powder is sprinkled on the face, shoulders, and arms after the *Beaume des Sultanes* has been applied. and wiped off with flakes of cotton or antiseptic gauze. Brush off the surplus with a swan's-down puff, and the skin is now ready for rouging.'

For applying powder generally she preferred a chamois to a puff since the chamois could be used to wipe off the excess powder and keep one's secret from being detected. For those who were 'enamoured of the puff', she suggested a long-haired soft brush for removing the excess. As for the application of powder in public, even in a 'conveyance' before mixed company, Miss Cunliffe-Owen found it disgusting. And this, she said, was being done more and more. A little touching up in the ladies' room, safe from the view of men, she found not only permissible but often desirable.

Chemist Joseph Begy suggests that powder be applied with a chamois, cotton flannel, or a puff, and he cautions the reader that all cosmetic preparations 'must be put on even — not more on one place than on another'. Warning against too generous an application of powder, Baroness Staffe considers 'a face powdered like a clown's' to be ridiculous, unbecoming, and vulgar. 'Powder on the face,' she says, 'should be imperceptible, and if used with discretion is not to be condemned.' Since many of her readers presumably lacked experience in the use of cosmetics, she felt it necessary to caution them not to powder the eyes, eyebrows, and lips.

The Professional Beauty who wrote *Beauty and How to Keep It* agreed on the importance of a light application of powder. 'Some women,' she said, 'have an idea that the thicker it is put on the better it looks! Not at all; this is a great mistake. Powder should be put on the face so lightly and delicately that no one is aware of its presence.' She added that there were three shades available — 'pink, yellow (or Rachel), and white. The first should be used by women of a delicate pink and white complexion, the second by sallow or colourless skins, and the last *never*, it always shows, and is most unbecoming.'

She did not advise the use of home-made powders — 'they are always heavy and rarely succeed in giving the desired effect'. She also considered home-made perfumes a mistake.

Baroness Staffe, on the other hand, advised not buying commercially prepared powders and included the following recipe:

'Fill a new earthen jar with six quarts of water and one kilogramme of rice. Let it soak for twenty-four hours, then bottle. During three consecutive days, put in six more quarts of water each day. Let the rice drip on a new hair sieve which must be used only for this purpose. Then expose to the air, protected from dust, on a towel which has been washed in lye. As soon as it is dry, it must be ground very fine in a clean and covered marble mortar. Lastly, sift through a fine white cloth into the jar. Tie the cloth around the mouth of the jar with a tape, and let it sag in order not to lose any of the powder. The jar should have a tight cover. It is best not to perfume this powder.

'When the powder gives out and cannot be immediately replaced, use, instead, the flour of oatmeal, which can be taken up in small quantities on the puff.'

Reckoning the consumption of face powder in tons, Margaret Cunliffe-Owen warned that it was composed of 'various starches and other ingredients of the nature of which there is some reluctance to speak, because it is not pleasant, perhaps, to be told that potatoes, nuts, French chalk, and ground talc may enter into the composition of these skin-coolers. The public,' she added, 'often displays an extraordinary disregard of its own health in the use of injurious mixtures; and if she does not feel inclined to prepare them herself, the only safe thing for a woman to do is to buy her powders and cosmetics of the best manufacturers, whose reputation is a guarantee that they will not permit adulteration.'

Curiously, Miss Cunliffe-Owen found hair powder quite another matter, and in reporting that French women were beginning to wear their hair powdered, she said that she considered it 'an excellent idea, for not only is powder very good for the hair, but the effect is extremely becoming to both old and young'. She added that 'Patches naturally accompany powder and certainly give much piquancy to the countenance. It is not generally known that these little velvety, artificial beauty-spots, looking so frivolous and tantalizing, were once a symbol of religion.'

In addition to rice powder, with or without impurities, there was Joseph Begy's Violet Powder, which contained arrow-root, orris-root, lycopodium, oil of cinnamon, oil of lavender, and extracts of violet and musk. It was to be applied with a puff and rubbed with a soft cloth to even it. Mr Begy assured his readers it could be used 'with charming results upon the neck and arms'. Talcum powder (powdered magnesium silicate), first manufactured in the United States in the 1890s, was one of the few cosmetic items considered thoroughly respectable.

Sears, Roebuck's Water of Youth, 'a simple preparation much used by a famous French beauty of the last century', was supposed to give the skin 'a youthful fresh softness with a perfect tint'. They also listed miscellaneous powders and creams—Pozzoni's Complexion Powder, Pear's Fuller's Earth, Tetlow's Swan's Down, La Blanche Powder, Elsie Toilet Cream, Vaseline Camphor Ice, Blush of Roses, Couleray's Blanc de Pearl, Champluis Liquid Pearl, Elgin Phantom Powder, Gourad's Oriental Cream, Hagau's Magnolia Balm, Strong's Arnica Jelly, Cold Cream of Roses, and a number of preparations by Harriet Hubbard Ayer.

ROUGE

Rouge was still in a state of dubious respectability. Many women used it, but most of them preferred not to advertise the fact. Margaret Cunliffe-Owen did not 'wish to speak against the use of rouge and pearl powder, but merely to point out to those who use them that they must be used with extreme care and not abused! . . . When rouge is used it ought to be of the very best quality and of the palest rose tint. The common and cheaper kinds will ruin the skin in a very short time as they are composed of inferior carmine. An easy way of painting the face is to put on a layer of cold cream, after which rub in a very little carmine powder, leave it on for a few minutes then gently rub it off with a small piece of cotton wool, this will leave quite enough carmine on the face to give a good colour. The worst of using rouge is that one never knows when to stop; women begin by putting on a little and adding more and more until the whole face is covered with it.'

Baroness Staffe *did* wish to speak out against rouge and tried to induce her readers 'to give up the deplorable and disfiguring habit of painting themselves, a habit which as seriously detracts from matronly dignity, as it compromises beauty and youth'. But for those who persisted, in spite of her advice, she suggested 'where to place the paint on the cheek, according to the usage of the eighteenth century'. Harriet Hubbard Ayer faithfully translated the instructions (given in this book in Chapter 12), then dismissed them in a peremptory footnote, referring to them as 'the opera-bouffe method and . . . not to be recommended'.

Rouge was available in three forms—liquid, cream, and dry. *Liquid rouge* had considerable popularity and was, in fact, preferred by the anonymous authors of *The Attainment and Preservation of Beauty*. It was applied with a soft camel's hair brush, and the effect was supposed to be unusually natural. Commercial preparations were available in tiny bottles, but for women who preferred to make their own, there were recipes in the beauty books.

Joseph Begy suggests a mixture of carmine, ammonia, glycerine, and rose water. It is to be applied with a soft sponge. 'Some ladies,' says Mr Begy, 'love to blend their white complexion preparations on the face in this manner. The white preparation should be put on in the usual way; nicely evened, allowed to dry, then apply a small quantity of the liquid rouge in the center of the cheek; this will produce a very handsome effect; and the blooming complexion so much admired.'

A recipe for a rouge guaranteed to be harmless appeared in *The Art of Beauty* under the name of *mousse de fraises*. It could, the reader was told, easily be made at home during the strawberry season or at any time when the berries could be obtained from hothouses:

'Take three quarts of strawberries, put them in a wide-mouthed thick glass bottle together with a pint of distilled water. Place the bottle in a large saucepan of water on a slow fire and let it boil for two hours. Strain through an extra fine hair-sieve and set aside. When absolutely cool, add : –

> 4 drops attar of roses
> 2 drops attar of neroli
> 12 ounces deodorized spirit
> 15 grains pure carmine, and
> 30 grains best Russian isinglass which has been previously melted.

Keep in a glass jar in a cool place. Both these liquid rouges are applied with a fine sponge.'

For squeamish ladies who could not bring themselves to use anything artificial, the anonymous author of *The Art of Beauty* suggested a little beetroot juice, applied as follows:

'The face should first be carefully and gently sponged in tepid soft water (using no soap), to which it is advisable to add a few drops of Eau de Lubin; or best of all, half-a-dozen drops of Oil of Eau de Cologne. The skin should be thoroughly dried with a soft towel. Next the face should be damped with a fairly strong solution of alum-water, leaving it on to dry; then, after some minutes, use a good powder, putting it on with a piece of clean chamois leather instead of with an ordinary puff, rubbing the powder well into the skin. This being done, a rather thick camel-hair brush should be dipped into the beetroot juice.

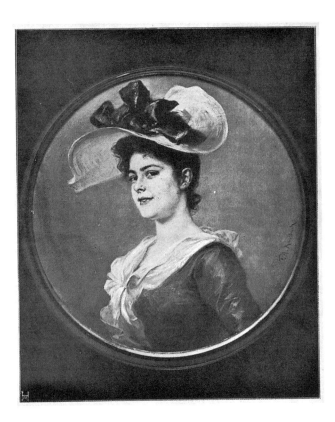

FIG. 190: Portrait of Miss L., 1895.
Painting by F. A. von Kaulbach.

Paint the cheek as desired; then, when quite dry, go over it again with the leather to tone down the colouring.'

Dry rouge was also popular. Margaret Cunliffe-Owen recommends a mixture of carmine and cochineal — 'A piece of fine silk flannel is dipped into the powder, and the cheeks, ears, nostrils, and chin delicately touched therewith, the hand moving with a rotary motion, care being taken not to produce any streaks of color. When only a slight tinge of pink is desired and no grease or powder has been previously applied — this slight heightening of color just suiting women who have a naturally pale, clear skin, and who merely wish to brighten up their face a bit.' Another book recommends a chamois instead of flannel. But the author of *The Art of Beauty* insists that the only safe way to apply dry rouge 'is first to put on a thin layer of cold cream, after which rub in the rouge in powder, leaving it on for a few minutes. Then gently rub it off with a pad of cotton wool. Sufficient colour will remain on the face.' Rouge papers, moistened with a damp sponge or cloth and rubbed on to the face, were recommended in still another book.

Cream rouge was sold in pots or jars and *crépons*, described as 'small pieces of gauze, either silk or cotton, twisted into small balls and colored with carthamine'. These were sometimes mounted on wooden or ivory handles. They were moistened with alcohol and rubbed gently over the cheeks or lips.

Lip rouge was considered less generally acceptable than cheek rouge. Annie Wolf, who did not approve of either one, found red lips 'inharmonious with certain temperaments. All attempts to make the color brilliant will only succeed for a moment and injure the skin. Therefore, do not have recourse to rubbing with alcoholic mixtures, or to cosmetics; you will lose far more than you gain in the end. . . . Alcohol, vinegars, and red paint destroy the delicate skin, which is so much appreciated in a kiss. How often children say to ladies who kiss them: "Your lips prick me" because the skin is rough.

'Many women bite their lips just before entering a drawing-room. Besides the fact that the color thus produced lasts but a moment, frequent biting makes the lips tender and predisposes them to chapping. . . . Do not pass the tongue over the lips. It is contrary to the law of good breeding, and the moisture is injurious.'

Baroness Staffe indicated that lips could be improved by rubbing them with scent and cold cream. Nothing in the way of artificial colouring was even suggested. Harriet Hubbard Ayer more realistically recommended 'a faint addition to the color of the lips, stolen from a stick of French grenadine'.

Sears, Rosebuck's rouge, selling for fifty cents, was described as 'a harmless preparation for giving color to the cheeks and lips . . . a perfectly natural pretty color'. Dorin's Rouge de Theatre could be bought for eighteen cents. Rouge Oriental ('for ladies who are troubled with pallor') cost a dollar.

EYES AND EYEBROWS

Margaret Cunliffe-Owen advised carefully plucking the brows if they were too heavy. However, in the late Victorian period, obviously plucked or very thin brows were not in fashion. In fact, Miss Cunliffe-Owen suggested rubbing too-thin brows three times a day with an infusion of white wine and mint leaves. *The Art of Beauty* recommended small brushes for keeping the eyebrows in order and well arched in order 'to give to the face an air of serenity'. Moderately thick brows were thought to be 'an improvement to the eyes'.

Another writer suggested brushing the brows with oil before going to bed. And she warned the reader never to use a pencil or chalk for the eyebrows since it made the hair fall out. To darken the colour, she suggested holding a small blending stump in the smoke of a candle, rubbing it on a piece of white paper to smooth down the black, then passing it gently over the eyebrows until they had become the shade one wanted. 'Bear in mind,' she warned, 'that this is a very delicate operation and should be done with a steady hand, as nothing looks more horrible than to see the large black band very badly outlined, which passes with some women for eyebrows'. Eyelashes, she told her readers, were to be trimmed and oiled and nothing more.

For colouring the brows and lashes another author mentioned pencils, dyes, diluted India ink, and an interesting cosmetic called frankincense-black, made of frankincense, resin, pitch, and gum mastic. The ingredients were to be mixed and dropped on red-hot coals, the resultant smoke being collected in a large funnel, on the inside of which a black powder would be deposited. This was to be mixed with fresh elderberry juice or cologne and applied with a fine camel's hair brush.

As an alternative, a china or porcelain dish could be held over the flame of a candle or a lamp in order to collect carbon. The carbon would then be applied with a sharpened match stick or even a hairpin. But the results were likely to be lacking in subtlety. A stain for the eyebrows or the hair could be made by boiling walnut bark in water for an hour, adding a lump of alum, then steeping the bark for a week in cologne. The resultant stain was applied with a brush.

For colouring the brows Margaret Cunliffe-Owen gave a recipe for a 'very safe tincture', compounded of red claret, coarse grey salt, sulphate of iron, oxide of copper, gall-nuts, and fine white salt. After being boiled, it was to be strained, poured into a stone bottle, and applied to the brows and lashes with a camel's hair brush, avoiding contact with the skin. After fifteen minutes the tincture was to be washed off.

As for blackening the brows and lashes, the author's attitude was predictable. She mentioned that after thousands of years, kohl was still (in 1897) being used by some women, then added:

'Now kohl in itself is not a harmful substance, but still I cannot recommend it to my readers excepting when they are about to appear on the scene of some amateur theatre; for . . . I do not approve of any kind of paint for the face.'

It is interesting to note that to the conservative woman of the period, dyes were more acceptable than paint. Yet Baroness Staffe who had a horror of dyeing, considered the use of a solution of Chinese ink and rose water 'perfectly harmless'. It was, she said, 'one of the secrets of the harem'. Somehow, in the Victorian era, that seemed to make it acceptable.

Also from the East there was a powder called *Mesdjem*, which was supposed to improve the growth of the eyelashes. It was referred to in the Koran as Ex-Medi and was used by the women of Ammon in 3000 B.C. It was available in 1897 from Parisian perfumers.

Eyebrow pencils — available in black, dark brown, and blonde — were accepted by some, rejected by others. Annie Wolf considered them 'too *voyant*', too easily detected. She preferred a little brilliantine or coconut oil to darken the brows somewhat and for ladies who did not like their brows to meet, a little judicious plucking she found permissible. For temporarily darkening the brows for very special occasions and then only in the evening, a little lamp black might be applied very carefully with a camel's hair brush.

VEINS AND BOSOMS

Blue tint for the veins was listed in *Beauty: Its Attainment and Preservation* as 'another necessity to an artistic make-up of the face. The ingredients of one variety are French or Venetian chalk made into a paste with gum-Arabic water and tinted to the proper depth with Prussian-blue. The mixture comes in little jars accompanied by small leather pencils made expressly for the purpose.' The authors add, in a curiously detached way, as if to deny all first-hand knowledge or responsibility, that 'it is said that if the work is well done, the effect is very natural'. They also suggest a grease pencil with which the veins can be drawn on, then softened by rubbing. Their discussion of accenting veins with blue is strongly reminiscent of a similar discussion by Drs Brinton and Napheys twenty-six years earlier.

Annie Wolf warned that outlining the veins should be attempted only by the experienced. 'The practice of shading and accentuating the bosom,' she wrote primly, 'though often indulged in, is to my mind neither necessary nor a nice one, and therefore I shall not refer to it.'

HAIR

Cosmetics for the hair were accepted more readily than were those for the face. Sears, Roebuck listed Olive Wax Pomatum 'for fixing and lying the hair, whiskers, and mustaches'. It was 'highly perfumed, each stick wrapped in tin-foil'. The price was ten cents. For the man who wanted something less expensive there was French Cosmetique in a round stick, wrapped in foil, in black, pink, or white, for five cents. For forty cents the gentleman could obtain a bottle of Old Reliable Hair and Whisker Dye — 'In use since 1860; will change the color of the hair to a light or dark brown or black in a few hours without doing any injury to it'. For the man or woman who wanted to become a blonde, there was a preparation called Blonde Hair, which was guaranteed to be harmless, cleansing, and strengthening.

Hair goods for both men and women were plentiful. Ladies wigs 'having a graceful and natural appearance not found in wigs of other manufacture' could be bought for as little as ten dollars. A parted puff bang ('made for the fine trade') cost three dollars, and a curled Parisian bang ('a little gem') was only $1.25. Alice waves ranged from three to ten dollars, depending on the quality. A man's weft toupee sold for $5.50 and a hand-ventilated one for ten dollars. Full wigs ranged from eight to twenty-one dollars. Instructions on measuring for a wig were included, the proper measurements being diagrammed on a male head with long sideburns and an extraordinarily thin neck. Moustaches on wire were ten cents (or seventy-five cents a dozen); ventilated ones cost twice as much. Imperials and goatees were ten cents; whiskers, seventy-five cents. Full beards on wire could be bought for eighty cents. Ventilated ones cost $1.75. All the facial hair was available only in medium or dark shades. For the theatrically inclined, there were minstrel wigs for seventy-five cents and eight shades of greasepaint for seventy cents. (See Figure 191.)

FIN DE SIÈCLE

According to the U.S. Census of 1849, there were thirty-nine cosmetics establishments in the country producing $355 worth of cosmetics at a cost of $164. By the end of the century the number of establishments had risen to 262, producing cosmetics valued at $1,222 (about £500) a year. Since many cosmetics were imported, this does not represent the total value of the cosmetics used, but it does set the pattern for the extraordinary development of a major twentieth-century industry.

In an article called 'Powder and Paint', published in *Living Age* in December 1899, I. A. Taylor takes a retrospective look at the nineteenth century:

'A complete alteration has taken place, as every one is aware, within the last hundred years, in the manner of regarding the use of powder and paint — of the employment, that is, of artificial means of embellishment; and it is an alteration which is not at first sight altogether explicable.

'A change of opinion is not satisfactorily explained by the pleasing but improbable hypothesis that it is due to a rapid increase of wisdom since the days when an opposite view obtained; and, if the practice in question be as reprehensible or as repugnant to the taste of the majority as it is now generally felt to be, it would seem to follow that it was no less objectionable in early days. And yet public opinion, as distinguished from the opinion of a comparatively narrow circle, has undergone a curious and significant transformation, by which paint, from a simple extension of the art of dress, frankly employed and frankly acknowledged, has come to be viewed with dislike and even with suspicion by all those outside the limits of the class amongst which it is in use. . . .

'That it is fast gaining ground is apparent; but . . . it will scarcely be denied, even by those who themselves hold no intolerant views that the supplementing of Nature, which in the days of our great-grandmothers was accepted as mere matter of course, is regarded at the present time by the majority of unsophisticated Englishmen with a mixture of contempt and aversion, which, difficult as it might be to explain, is on that account none the less genuine. . . .

'To deal . . . with the motives to which the use of paint is due, it is clear that they have undergone a radical change since the days when ladies produced their

Nursing Bottles, Etc.,—Continued.

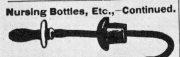

25784 Nursing Bottle Fittings. Rubber nipple and tubing, wood stopper and glass tube.
Each..................$0.05

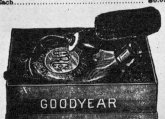

25785 Nursing Bottle. Extra good quality, fittings made of the very best rubber, contains brushes etc., for cleaning. Each..................$0.20

Sponges.

25790 Very Fine, "Small Eye" Sponge. For surgical and nursery use. Each.. $0.06
25792 Small Size Toilet Sponge, for toilet use or can be used in shaving. Each 5½c
25794 Medium Size Sheeps' Wool Sponges, tough and durable. Each.......... 9c
25795 Large Toilet Sponge, suitable for the bath. Each..15c
25796 Large Size Sheeps' Wool Sponges. A very durable sponge. Each..................22c
25798 Cleaning Sponges. When wet they are about 15 to 24 inches in circumference. Suitable for carriage, wood work. etc. Each..................8c

Chamois Skins.

We are headquarters for chamois skins; buy them in large quantities and sell them for less than a retail druggist or dealer can buy them for. Chamois are very useful and should be in every household. Chamois skins are used as follows: Ladies use them for toilet purposes, for cleaning glass, woodwork of all kinds, carriages, silverware or any metal; lining pockets and for chest protectors.
25799 Our Very Fine Toilet Chamois, for applying powder, etc., to the face. Size about 5x6 inches. Each..................$0.05
25801

Style.	A	B	C	D	E	F
Size (inches)	9x8½	12x9	14x11	20x16	26x23	33x25
Each,	.05	.10	.16	.32	.52	.70
1 doz. for	.52	.95	1.60	3.50	5.50	7.50

NOTE.—If a chamois about size 14x11 inches is wanted, order as follows: No. 25801.....style C.

Shaving Sets.

25801½ A Very Special Offer. We have just purchased a very large quantity of Shaving Sets, like cut, at less than one-third the regular wholesale prices. We can thus offer them at a great deal less than the merchant buys them for—probably for ½ what the retailer pays. Set consists of one Sears 1865 warranted razor, "The Clean Shaver," regular retail price $1.25, one fine razor strop, leather handle, patent swivel end, one good shaving cup, one fine shaving brush and one cake of shaving soap. Price of entire set...75c
Retail Price.

Sears' Razor	$1.25
Razor Strop	.40
Shaving Cup	.20
Shaving Brush	.20
Shaving Soap	.10
	$2.15

Our price 75c for the entire set.

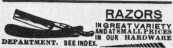

RAZORS
IN GREAT VARIETY AND AT SMALL PRICES IN OUR HARDWARE DEPARTMENT. SEE INDEX.

Human Hair Goods.

Allow about 5 cents postage on hair goods.
Please do not forget to inclose a good-sized sample of the exact shade wanted, and cut it out as near to the roots as possible.
The prices quoted of waves, bangs and switches are for ordinary shades only, and on the basis of a 3-inch parting in the center. Gray and extra shades on larger foundations will cost additional.
There is a great diversity in the styles of hair dressing, according to the tastes of individuals, but none is more in demand than curly bangs, and when used in connection with a nice switch the hair can always be made to look nice, and suitable for any occasion.
There are a great many kinds and styles of "pieces" for the hair, designated by different names. We cannot show or describe them all in our limited space, but if there is any hair work, not here shown, which you may want, please send a description picture of it, and we will guarantee to produce the article for you at the shortest notice.
Any of the goods sent C. O. D., subject to examination, on receipt of $1.00, balance and express charges payable at express office.
Three per cent. discount for cash in full with order.

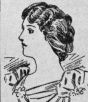

Our $3.00 Puff Bang.

25820 Puff Bang. Parted in the latest style, made for fine trade, on ventilated foundation, with hair lace part.
See cut.
Each $3.00

Parisian Bang.

25822 Parisian Bang. Ladies who do not require large heavy front will find this a little gem; light and fluffy, ventilated foundation.
Each........ .$1.25

Alice Wave.

25823 Alice Wave, invisible hair lace; foundation natural, curly hair; 3 inch part, 12 inches from side to side. Each..................$3.00
Better qualities, $4, $5, $6, $8, and $10.

Ladies' Wigs.

25824 These wigs are all ventilated on a delicate open mesh foundation. They are perfect in fit, having a graceful and natural appearance not found in wigs of other manufacture. Each.
Short hair, cotton foundation..................$10.00
Short hair, silk foundation..................12.00
Hair, 18 inches long..................15.00
Hair, 24 inches long..................18.00
This is only for ordinary shades; light and half gray are worth 25 per cent. more; if very gray, 50 per cent. more.

Men's Wigs.

24825 Men's Toupee, weft foundation. Price each $5.50
25826 Men's Toupee, ventilated foundation. Each $10.00
25827 Toupee Paste, for keeping the same in place. Per stick..................$0.50
25828 Men's Full Wigs, for street wear, weft seam with crown cotton foundation. Price each..................$8.00
25829 Men's Wigs, silk foundation, vegetable net seam. Price each..................$12.00
25830 Men's Wigs, silk foundation, gauze net seam. Price each..................$15.00
25831 Men's Wigs, silk foundation, hair lace. Price each..................$21.00
Extra shades will be charged according to color.
25833 Minstrel Wigs, or plain black negro wigs. Each..................$0.75
25835 Grease Paint, for make-up purposes; eight colors in a box. Per box..................$0.70
We can furnish any kind of a wig for ladies or gentlemen for masquerade, stage or character purposes.

HAIR DYES
HAIR INVIGORATORS . . . . . .
AND A GREAT VARIETY OF TOILET PREPARATIONS IN DRUG DEPARTMENT. PAGES 26 TO 35—WHICH SEE.

How to Measure a Wig.

Directions for measuring the head for a wig to insure a good fit, and mention number of inches.

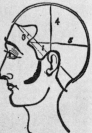

No. 1. The circumference of the head.
No. 2. Forehead to nape of the neck.
No. 3. Ear to ear, across the forehead.
No. 4. Ear to ear, over the top.
No. 5. Temple to temple, around the back.
To Measure for a Toupee.
Cut a piece of paper the exact size and shape of the bald spot, also the measure around the head, and mention which side the parting is on.

Extraordinary Values in Human Hair Switches.

No. 25836 Short Stem Hair Switches, in all ordinary and medium shades; extra shades will cost from 25 to 50 per cent. extra.

Weight. About.	Length. About.	Price. Each.
2 ounces...20 inches....		$0.65
2 ounces...20 inches....		0.90
2 ounces...22 inches....		1.25
2 ounces...22 inches....		1.50
3 ounces...24 inches....		2.25
3½ ounces...24 inches....		3.25

Note—The above 65c. switch has long stem.
French Hair Switches can be made to order from $5.00 to $10.00 each.
No. 25837. Gray Hair Switches, fine quality, short stem. Be sure to send sample of hair.

Weight.	Length.	Each
2 ounces...18 inches....		$1.75
2½ ounces...22 inches....		2.50
3 ounces...24 inches....		4.00
3 ounces...24 inches....		5.45

Note.—The above prices are for medium shades of gray. Where extra white is ordered it will cost ½ or 50 per cent. more.

Full Beards.

25838 On wire..................$0.90
25839 Ventilated..................1.75

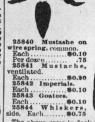
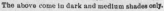

25840 Mustache on wire spring, common.
Each..................$0.10
Per dozen..................75
25841 Mustache, ventilated.
Each..................$0.20
25842 Imperials.
Each..................$0.10
25843 Goatees.
Each..................$0.10
25844 Whiskers, side. Each..................$0.75
The above come in dark and medium shades only.

The Imperial Hair Regenerator.

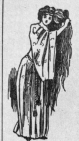

25845 No matter how gray your hair is, or how Bleached or how spoiled by dyes, makes it beautiful, natural, healthy. Restores gray hair to color of youth. Gives the hair new life.
PRICE PER BOTTLE $1.25.

IF WE DON'T PLEASE YOU, IT ISN'T BECAUSE WE DON'T TRY. OUR BEST EFFORTS ARE PUT FORTH TO GIVE YOU PERFECTLY SATISFACTORY SERVICE. WHEN YOU FIND ANYTHING WRONG WITH AN ORDER NOTIFY US AT ONCE, AND WE WILL CHEERFULLY RECTIFY ANY ERROR.

FIG. 191 : Page from the 1897 catalogue of Sears, Roebuck & Co., Chicago.

paint boxes at the theatre and applied it openly, with no desire or expectation that it should remain undetected. In the present day the practice — except, indeed, amongst those whose object seems to be to advertise themselves and their opinions — is mostly carried on in the endeavor to impose upon the world. And to be engaged in a constant effort to deceive, however intrinsically harmless the deception, is apt to have an unfavorable effect upon the character, while it is also productive of the uneasy and anxious frame of mind inseparable from a fear of detection. A habit of concealment is never conducive to happiness, and, while it may also almost be asserted that it will be unsuccessful in the long run, it is equally certain that the world has little mercy upon those it has found out.'

A DEFENCE OF COSMETICS

There seems no better way to bring the nineteenth century to a close and to prepare for the twentieth than to quote liberally from Max Beerbohm's delightful *Defence of Cosmetics*, written in 1894 and published in 1896. Here, then, is Beerbohm's defence:

'For behold! The Victorian era comes to its end. . . . The old signs are here and the portents to warn the seer of life that we are ripe for a new epoch of artifice. Are not men rattling the dice-box and ladies dipping their fingers in the rouge-pot? . . . No longer is a lady of fashion blamed if, to escape the outrageous persecution of time, she fly for sanctuary to the toilet-table; and if a damosel, prying in her mirror, be sure that with brush and pigment she can trick herself into more charm, we are not angry. Indeed, why should we ever have been? Surely it is laudable, this wish to make fair the ugly and overtop fairness, and no wonder that within the last five years the trade of the makers of cosmetics has increased immoderately — twenty-fold, so one of these makers has said to me. We need but walk down any modish street and peer into the little broughams that flit past, or (in Thackeray's phrase) under the bonnet of any woman we meet, to see over how wide a kingdom rouge reigns.

'And now that the use of pigments is becoming general, and most women are not so young as they are painted . . . the old prejudice is a-dying. We need not pry into the secret of its birth. Rather is this a time of jolliness and glad indulgence. For the era of rouge is upon us, and as only in an elaborate era can man, by the tangled accrescency of his own pleasures and emotions, reach that refinement which is his highest excellence, and by making himself, so to say, independent of Nature, come nearest to God, so only in an elaborate era is woman perfect. Artifice is the strength of the world, and in that same mask of paint and powder, shadowed with vermeil tint and most trimly pencilled, is woman's strength. . . .

' "After all," as a pretty girl once said to me, "women are a sex by themselves, so to speak," and the sharper the line between their worldly functions and ours, the better. . . . And, truly, of all the good things that will happen with the full revival of cosmetics, one of the best is that surface will finally be severed from soul. That damnable confusion will be solved by the extinguishing of a prejudice which, as I suggest, itself created. Too long has the face been degraded from its rank as a thing of beauty to a mere vulgar index of character and emotion. . . . And the use of cosmetics, the masking of the face, will change this. We shall gaze at a woman merely because she is beautiful, not stare into her face anxiously, as into the face of a barometer. . . .

'Indeed the revival of cosmetics must needs be so splendid an influence, conjuring boons innumerable, that one inclines almost to mutter against that inexorable law by which Artifice must perish from time to time. That such branches of painting as the staining of glass or the illuminating of manuscripts should fall into disuse seems, in comparison, so likely; these were esoteric arts; they died with the monastic spirit. But personal appearance is art's very basis. The painting of the face is the first kind of painting men can have known. To make beautiful things — is it not an impulse laid upon few? But to make oneself beautiful is an universal instinct. Strange that the resultant art could ever perish! So various in its materials from stimmis, psimythium, and fuligo to bismuth and arsenic, so simple in that its ground and its subject matter are one, so marvellous in that its very subject matter becomes lowly when an artist has selected it! To deny that "making up" is an art, on the pretext that the finished work of its exponents depends for beauty and excellence upon the ground chosen for the work, is absurd. At the touch of a true artist, the plainest face turns comely . . . and, as Ovid would seem to suggest, by pigments any tone may be set aglow on a woman's cheek, from enamel the features take away form. Insomuch that surely the advocates of soup-kitchens and free-libraries and other devices for giving people what Providence did not mean them to receive should send out pamphlets in the praise of self-embellishment. For it will place Beauty within easy reach of many who could not otherwise hope to attain it. . . .

'Ah! Such are the lures of the toilet that none will for long hold aloof from them. Cosmetics are not going to be a mere prosaic remedy for age or plainness, but all ladies and all young girls will come to love them. Does not a certain blithe Marquise, whose *lettres intimes* from the court of Louis Seize are less read than their wit deserves, tells us how she was scandalized to see *"même les toutes jeunes demoiselles émaillées comme ma tabatière"*? So it shall be with us. Surely the common prejudice against painting the lily can but be based on mere ground of economy . . . and who that has ever seen — as I have — a lily really well painted could grudge the artist so fair a ground for his skill? Scarcely do you believe through how many nice metamorphoses a lily may be passed by him. In

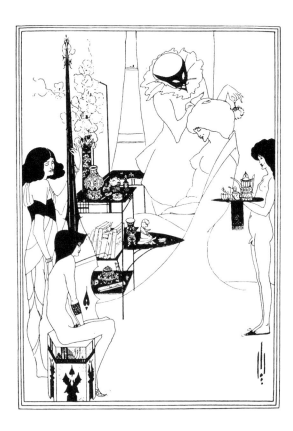

FIG. 192 : Toilet of Salome. One of Aubrey Beardsley's illustrations to Oscar Wilde's *Salome*, 1894.

like manner, we all know the young girl, with her simpleness, her wayward ignorance. And a very charming ideal must she have been, and a very natural one, when a young girl even sat on the throne. But no nation can keep its ideal for ever. . . . What writer of plays . . . ever dreams of making the young girl the centre of his theme? Rather he seeks inspiration from the tried and tired woman of the world, in all her intricate maturity, whilst, by way of comic relief, he sends the young girl flitting in and out with a tennis-racket. . . . The season of the unsophisticated is gone by, and the young girl's final extinction beneath the rising tides of cosmetics will leave no gap in life and will rob art of nothing. . . .

'When your mistress has wearied you with one expression, then it will need but a few touches of that pencil, a backward sweep of that brush, and lo, you will be revelling in another. For though, of course, the painting of the face is, in manner, most like the painting of canvas, in outcome, it is rather akin to the art of music — lasting, like music's echo, not for very long. So that, no doubt, of the many little appurtenances of the Reformed Toilet Table, not the least vital will be a list of the emotions that become its owner, with recipes for simulating them. According to the colour she will her hair to be for the time — black or yellow or, peradventure, burnished red — she will blush for you, sneer for you, laugh or languish for you. The good combinations of line and colour are nearly numberless, and by their means poor restless woman will be able to realize her needs in all their shades and lights and dappledoms, to live many lives and masquerade through many movements of joy. No monotony will be. And for us men matrimony will have lost its sting. . . .

'But that in the world of women they will not neglect this art, so ripping in itself, in its results so wonderfully beneficent, I am sure indeed. Much, I have said, is already done for its revival. The spirit of the age has made straight the path of its professors. Fashion has made Jezebel surrender her monopoly of the rouge-pot. As yet, the great art of self-embellishment is for us but in its infancy. But if Englishwomen can bring it to the flower of an excellence so supreme as never yet has it known, then, though Old England lose her martial and commercial supremacy, we patriots will have the satisfaction of knowing that she has been advanced at one bound to a place in the councils of aesthetic Europe.'

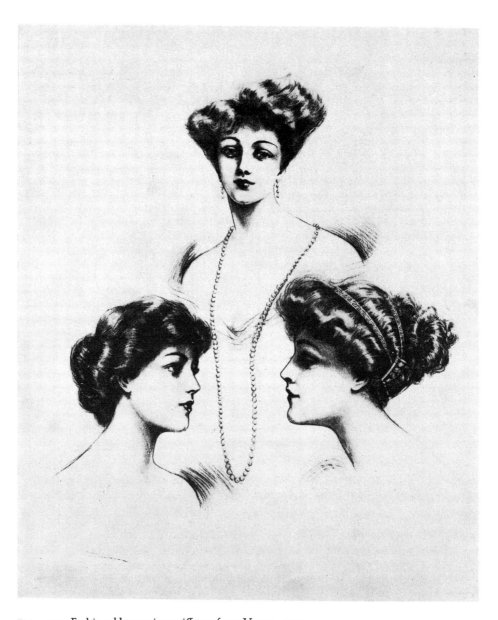

FIG. 193 : Fashionable evening coiffures from *Vogue*, 1909.

17 · The Twentieth Century 1900-1910

At times, the temptation to improve one's appearance,
even if only temporarily, becomes too strong to resist.

VOGUE

In the twentieth century the cosmetics cycle returned to the completely free and open use of makeup. Perhaps for the first time since the ancient Egyptians, the unlimited use of cosmetics came to be universally accepted, both socially and morally. Eventually, even wildly excessive or ridiculous makeup, though it might occasionally be greeted with mild dismay, would more often be looked upon with amused tolerance.

This change, which had barely begun, could be observed in the ambivalence of attitudes towards makeup. In addition to those who remained firmly opposed and those who could see no harm in it, there were others who disapproved in principle but accepted it in practice, and still others who felt it was acceptable only so long as it remained undetected.

THE WOMAN BEAUTIFUL

At the turn of the century Brentano's in New York published a book by Ella Adelia Fletcher entitled *The Woman Beautiful*. This comprehensive volume of 535 pages covers, among other things, physical culture, sleep, correct breathing, the choice of perfumes, and the evolution of taste and includes hundreds of 'Cosmetic and Therapeutic Formulae' for all visible and some invisible parts of the body and a variety of unfortunate conditions. It also provides us today with a detailed picture of the beautiful and not-so-beautiful woman of 1900.

Like most writers on beauty in the nineteenth century, Miss Fletcher seems comfortably Victorian. Her opening chapter, with its highly moralistic and idealistic tone, echoes any number of books which preceded it:

'Assuming that it is not only the natural desire of woman but also her duty to please, in order to succeed, she must train herself to a critical nicety of judgment in choosing her means to accomplish this end. Her grave mistakes are in supposing that imitations, shams, or subterfuges can ever, even transiently, take the place of real charms or genuine emotions. As it will be my endeavor to prove, Beauty is more than skin deep, and such flagrant artifices as paints, rouges, and dyes, made only more conspicuous by combination with Fashion's most daring devices for attracting attention, can no more imitate it than a fragment of window-glass can imitate the diamond's lustre and purity. Every base substitute is sure to result in disastrous failure.'

Creams and lotions did not share the general condemnation of cosmetics designed to colour the skin. And there were plenty of skin creams and lotions available commercially. Unfortunately, one could never be sure what was in them. The only solution to the problem was to compound one's own cosmetics, which the author admitted was troublesome; but, she added, 'the satisfaction of knowing what you are using is immense, and it is dainty work which any girl who has time for it will feel well repaid for doing. She will, moreover, find it a great economy to prepare these cosmetics herself; thus often being able to use them much more freely.' She then outlined the procedure:

'In making all cold creams the manner of manipulation is the same. The fats and oils are put in a *bain-marie* — a double boiler — and warmed by gentle heat till they can be smoothly mingled or creamed. Wanting a *bain-marie*, an earthen bowl placed in a basin of boiling water answers every purpose. The difficult part, that which requires most patience and skill, is uniting the other substances, perfumed waters, aromatic or astringent tinctures, etc., with the fatty base. The perfumed water is poured in very slowly in a fine stream, or even drop by drop, while the mixture is steadily stirred or beaten with a silver spoon or fork. All tinctures or extracts are added last of all, in the same way. Some people use an egg-beater with perfect success.'

One of Miss Fletcher's more exotic recipes was for *Cream of Pond Lilies*, which she especially recommended for oily skins:

Orange-flower water, triple	6 ounces
Deodorized alcohol	$1\frac{1}{2}$ ounces
Bitter almonds, blanched	1 ounce
White wax	1 drachm
Spermaceti	1 drachm
Oil of benne	1 drachm
Shaving cream	1 drachm
Oil of bergamot	12 drops
Oil of cloves	6 drops
Oil of neroli, bigarade	6 drops
Borax	$\frac{1}{5}$ ounce

The author considered it necessary to explain to her readers that shaving cream was 'a saponaceous paste, found ready prepared at most chemists'. Her Cucumber Lotion also contained shaving cream, blanched almonds, oil of benne, and deodorized alcohol blended with the 'expressed juice of cucumbers'. This was recommended as an 'excellent cosmetic with which to massage face and throat, whitening the skin and also toning relaxed tissues'. The preparation of

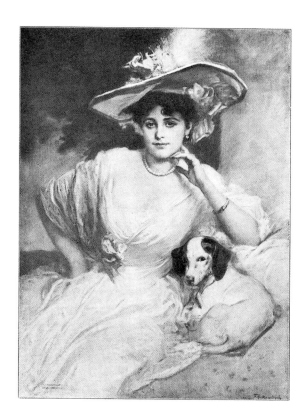

FIG. 194: Portrait of the German actress Tilly Waldegg, 1904. Painting by F. A. von Kaulbach. Heavy eyebrows were still in fashion.

Cucumber Milk must have seemed like just another canning day to the busy housewife:

    Oil of sweet almonds ....4 ounces
    Fresh cucumber juice ....10 ounces
    Essence of cucumbers ....3 ounces
    White Castile soap (powdered) ......¼ ounce
    Tincture of benzoin ....⅔ drachm

'The juice of the cucumbers is obtained by boiling them in a very little water. Slice them very thin, skin and all, and let them cook slowly till soft and mushy; strain through a fine sieve, and then through a cloth. Make the essence by putting an ounce and a half of the juice into the same quantity of high-proof alcohol. Put the essence with the soap in a large jar or bottle — the larger the better, as the mixture requires much shaking. After a few hours, when the soap is dissolved, add the cucumber juice; shake till thoroughly mixed; then pour out into an earthen bowl and add the oil and benzoin, stirring constantly till you have a creamy liquid. Be sure that the cucumber juice is strong, for it is the natural arsenic in the cucumber which imparts its wonderfully whitening power. Put the emulsion in small bottles; keep tightly corked and in the dark; and always shake before using. It is so quickly absorbed by the skin that it is very pleasant to use.'

This must surely have sent a good many ladies rushing to their chemist's and their kitchens. Face powder, another cosmetic which conservative ladies found acceptable, could also be made in one's own kitchen, no doubt at a considerable saving. Freshly gathered flowers—roses and violets were the favourites at the time—were to be buried in a mixture of finely powdered starch and orris-root and renewed once every day for a week. The flowers were then discarded, leaving a pleasantly perfumed powder. For a talcum powder which was 'commended as harmless' the reader was instructed to put 'four ounces of talcum powder in a glass jar, and pour over it eight ounces of distilled vinegar. Let it stand for a fortnight, shaking it daily; then filter it through coarse brown paper, and wash the powder in distilled water—filtering it again—till no taste of the vinegar remains. Mix the powder, together with fifteen grammes of spermaceti finely comminuted, and three grains of carmine, with sufficient violet-water to make a paste. Put in open-mouthed jars and cover with fine linen to protect from dust while it dries.'

One of the more complex recipes for face powder includes cornstarch or rice powder, zinc oxide, drop chalk, white clay, orris root, French chalk, carmine, and the oils of lavender, cloves, cedrat, and rose geranium. After a good deal of being sifted through silk bolting cloth and being tossed about and shut up tightly for a few days, and then being sifted again, it was ready to help beautify milady.

Like other Victorian female writers before her, Miss Fletcher felt that it was necessary, between groups of recipes, to reiterate her firm opposition to painting the face:

'I believe the day is not far distant when artificial make-up, the *maquillage* of the French, will be left to the stage and a certain class of women who announce their "calling" by its use. Could respectable women but grasp the thought in all its clearness, that to strangers their own social position appears more than dubious when they join the "painted and bedizened" sisterhood, they would not hesitate long about risking such misjudgment, but fling the paint and rouge pots far away, and devote themselves sedulously to the recovery of a naturally beautiful skin. . . .

'Always, the beauties of Oriental harems have been devoted to cosmetic arts, but while they have frankly adopted certain artificial methods of enhancing their attractions, they have always had too much regard for the preservation of their beauty to jeopardize it by coating their skins with the deleterious enamels and paints which their Occidental sisters have used. They make an effective *rouge* from the petals of damask roses macerated in white-wine vinegar. Bright crimson silk dipped in spirits of wine and rubbed upon the cheeks, chin, and ears is said to be a safe and harmless rouge that defies detection. That, however, depends upon the hand that applies it. It requires all the skill of a portrait-painter—a deft touch with the fingers and a skillful eye—to make up so that you impose upon even the most indifferent eye. And any make-up which is not discreetly and artistically managed is vulgar in the extreme.

'Of course, I know that there is a large class of incorrigibles who cannot be won over to see the lasting advantage of Nature's method of making a beautiful, translucent skin; and, therefore, I will point out the methods of attempting an imitation of her work which are least harmful. I have already shown that there are times and occasions when it is an advantage to protect the skin. And, further than this, it is always a woman's duty to look her best, sometimes to appear well when she is ill; and it is a harmless subterfuge if, to accomplish this pleasing deception, the pallid countenance for a few hours takes on the blush of health and strength. This can be done by adding just a soupçon of rouge after the Sultana Balm and *Poudre d'Amour*, or by using the *Moyen-âge Invigorant*.'

Having tactfully got round to the possibility of using artificial colour under certain very special circumstances, the author then plunges boldly ahead:

'Genuine rouge is said to be the least injurious of all the substances employed in *maquillage*. It is obtained from a plant, the saf-flower,—*carthamous tinctorious*,—grown in Spain, Egypt, and the Levant; but it is so expensive that its use is quite restricted. Carmine, which comes next, has a most exquisite color, but its constant and long-continued use dries and yellow the skin, much as bismuth does. It is prepared from cochineal, the operation requiring much dexterity and patience, and its success depending upon atmospheric conditions. The test of its purity is that it is entirely soluble in liquor of ammonia.'

Both materials were used in the form of powder, pomade, and liquid. Once again Miss Fletcher warned against the use of vermilion, derived from sulphate of mercury, and an active poison. More and more, women were beginning to think, or at least writers were trying to make them think, in terms of choosing the best available colour for their complexion:

'Some cheeks have a wine-like purplish glow; others a transparent saffron tinge, like yellowish-pink porcelain; others still have clear, pale carmine; others a faint brown that is as much richer than the snow and carmine of the pure blonde as a tinted crystal is finer than a colorless one; but the rarest of all is that suffused tint like apple-blossoms. Therefore, to approach the cunning of Nature's endless variety, it is necessary to modify the tint of rouge by adding a trace of indigo for the deep rose-crimson, or a little pale yellow for soft tints, and the merest soupçon of brown for the creamy rich *brune* complexion. After you have obtained the exact tinge, it is necessary to prepare three shades of it, by adding a little of all the ingredients but the colors to different proportions. Talcum powder is the usual dilutant in a simple mixture.'

The author preferred pomades and liquid rouge to the dry, but she gave recipes for all of them. Many of the recipes were taken from earlier books. *Devoux French Rouge* was a powder made by mixing carmine, oil of almonds, and French chalk and sifting the mixture through silk bolting cloth. *Bloom of Roses* contained ammonia, carmine, rose water, and extract of rose. *Carmine Paste*, which was a little more trouble to make, contained carmine, oil of sweet almonds, extract of rose, and white wax, all of which had to macerate for eight days before it was beaten to a smooth paste. It was especially recommended for evening use — Miss Fletcher did not explain why. *Rouge au Naturel*, she reported, 'is said to defy detection when applied lightly to the cheeks'. Evidently she had not tried it herself. She then added a few instructions for applying rouge:

'It is necessary, however, the moment the first touch of artificial color is given to the face to bring up the adjacent features to harmonize with one another. A startlingly white nose cuts the face in two; so a touch of rouge, deftly blended, is needed on the nostrils; if the nose be large, a very little on the sides will lessen its prominence. The chin, and the lobes and edges of the ears, too, must be touched with rouge; very delicately, and in a rotary motion which will make streaks impossible and leave no edges. The pure extract of China rose-lead, in powder, is said to give a very delicate and lovely tint.'

At the turn of the century ladies were still painting their veins blue. Miss Fletcher, surprisingly, accepted this as a matter of course, giving two recipes, the first for a paint in stick form, which she said was used 'to mark blue veins which a coating of balms or paints has concealed'. She also explained that it required some dexterity to apply in a natural manner. The technique was to 'breathe upon one of the sticks and rub it on the inside of a white glove, then trace the vein with the kid'. It could, she said, be done more deftly with a Japanese brush.

She did not recommend any of the pastes or masks intended for night wear, and she also advised her readers to 'look with a large measure of skeptical tolerance on the absurd directions and warnings which, from time to time, are spread broadcast as to certain methods of doing things. . . . Of this sort is the grave caution not to bend the face over the wash-bowl while bathing it because of the serious tendency to cause the muscles to droop.'

HAIR IN 1901

The *Boston Globe*, in the spring of 1901, described four classic ways of wearing one's hair, each relating to a particular type of gown and hat. To dress one's hair out of harmony with one's gown was 'to commit a grievous anachronism. For instance,' explained the *Globe*, 'if one is wearing an evening dress cut frankly on the pattern that prevailed in the '60s, and adorned with bell-mouthed sleeves of lace, a pompadour headdress or psyche knot would be as shocking as a folding bed in a Louis XVI boudoir. The proper arrangement with the aforementioned type of gown, would be a coiffure pinned rather low upon the back of the head and a straight-around coronet of blossoms and delicate green foliage. On the other hand, for the proper adjustment of a squash hat and the framing of an oval face, the hair must be rolled forward to almost obscure the face. This is technically and properly called the romney wave and is most becoming to youngish faces. . . . Handsome young matrons and the very stately girls affect with their ball and dinner dresses the coiffure de l'opera. For this a dash of hair powder is called into service; silver, gold, or pure white are equally popular and effective, and, when the whole silky suit is softly drawn up to a small knot on the top of the head, a couple of tall black feathers, springing from a rose of gold or silver tissue, is set a trifle to one side of it. . . .

'In Paris, whence we get our hair powders and the romney and opera coiffure, it is not the fashion to wear hair ornaments. The American woman is, however, growing amazingly independent of the Paris fashions, and she wears Sunday coquettish trifles in her admirably arranged head. Big balls of gold threaded and plaited black tulle, from which a black and gold aigrette springs, is one of her favorite ornaments. A flight of blue and black spangled gauze butterflies hovering on wires among a constellation of wired brilliants is another captivating device. Three tiny white ostrich tips dusted with gold powder and springing from a jeweled hairpin tip quivers and glitters over many heads at the opera houses and on ballroom floors.'

Along with the gauze butterflies and quivering ostrich tips, there were doubtless a good many discreetly rouged cheeks and painted veins and perhaps even a few rose-tinted lips. Lip salve was still the least respectable of the available cosmetics. Eyeshadow was not even discussed.

REQUISITES FOR BEAUTY CARE

From time to time unidentified countesses and baronesses have been moved to write books on beauty. The new century had barely got under way before such a book appeared, published in Boston. According to the author (this one a countess), cleanliness is the first requisite in beauty care; but not being satisfied with the available soaps, she recommends that one take '8 oz. 29 grains of "Nice" soap and olive oil soap, cut into small pieces, and place in a little vase of silver or nickel, with a little rose water, some orange-flower water, and 30 grains of boracic acid. When dissolved, pass through a sieve and allow to cool. Again let it dissolve, and add more rose water and orange-flower water, and perfume with your favourite scent'.

She also suggests a second preparation — 'a delicious paste for the skin' — which she prefers to the first. This recipe requires, first of all mixing sweet almond oil with berganistes, essence of bitter almonds, and spirits of cochlearia. You must then crush Savon de Nice in a mortar, 'mix it well with honey, and pour in slowly the perfumed oil as if you were making a sauce mayonnaise; beat it for some time and preserve in pots'. She informs her readers that a good soap can also be made with fruit or glycerine.

As for the dressing room, 'the sanctuary where the idol adorns, before offering herself to the admiration of all', the countess suggests that it be as light as possible. 'We have seen dressing rooms so dark,' she says, 'that they had to be lighted by gas or electricity. But, besides the expense of this lighting . . . this artificial light can be the cause of considerable injury to beauty. . . . And this . . . becomes more serious to those women — too numerous, alas! — who have recourse to rouge and touching up, and who, in a word, enamel themselves. The light from gas or electricity that causes one to enamel too much or too little, in fact, to "make up" badly, can expose one to very disagreeable misadventures.' Having titillated us with the possibility of some interesting tales, the countess drops the matter abruptly and goes on to discuss the contents of a well-arranged dressing room, which, she tells us, 'may be divided into two divisions: one, a table holding a wash-hand basin, a jug, soap dishes, rice powder, and bottles, etc., which serve for the toilet of the face, shoulders, arms; the other the combs, brushes, and all the articles necessary to hairdressing.

'Other toilet accessories, and those which apply to the hands, should be arranged tidily on a little table covered with a cloth of silk or guipure. The toilet set should be as elegant as possible — it is generally made of cut glass. The wash-hand basin and jug should be of fair dimensions, and, if means permit, of silver, or old brass, or china of a simple pattern. Avoid letting marble come in contact with hot water. Place the receptacles which contain the hot water on little round pieces of wood or basket-work. . . .

'An ideal installation in a dressing-room, and what one finds in nearly all well-built, modern houses, is water laid on by a tap immediately over the basin, and emptying under the piece of furniture. This appliance, which has the immense advantage of allowing a free and unlimited flow of water, should be sought by every woman. One can easily arrange hangings to conceal the pipes which serve to carry away the water.'

We then come to the skin, which should be pink and white if possible. To avoid sunburn, we are told, 'there is a very simple method . . . and that is never to go out in the sun or night dew or when the moon is bright, for that tans as quickly as the sun, without covering the face with a fine white, or better still, cream-coloured veil, first putting a little glycerine on the face, and then passing a powder puff lightly over it'.

The author then deals with various skin problems, including freckles (which 'are very very disagreeable to those who are afflicted with them'), and suggests methods of skin care. Finally, on page 90, we come to makeup, about which the countess is admirably specific:

'At this period enamelling is more employed than ever, and yet it does not bear a good reputation. Why? Simply from women abusing it or doing it badly, without taking care to suit it to the various circumstances which call for it. . . . Therefore, if you enamel yourself . . . enamel with discretion and only in the case of necessity.'

As for rouging, the countess quotes the eighteenth-century method as a possibility but recommends instead the nineteenth-century method of applying 'a light coating of cold cream and a cloud of powder, then a little rouge, decreasing in light and shade on the projecting parts and softening them. Then apply the powder again, a second time, very carefully. The red and white thus mix into each other and give the impression of generous blood circulating under a fine skin.'

By using a minimum of white, buying only the best quality rouges and creams, and never leaving makeup on overnight, 'the hurtful influence of enamelling' can, the author promises, be delayed; but, she warns, 'it always ends by making itself felt in lining and yellowing the skin, in rendering it soft and flabby. The best advice one can give on this matter will be that of total abstinence. But alas! this advice, like many others, will, we fear, be very seldom followed.'

For the eyes, the countess recommends plenty of rest, a balanced diet, and practice in front of a mirror to achieve a 'sweet expression'. If one wishes, one may 'rub gently on the lids, with a small brush, a decoction of concentrated walnut leaves. This decoction gives them a beautiful bistre tint which makes the expression extremely langorous.'

The eyebrows, at the beginning of the century, were to be 'thick and well pencilled. The shape of the eyebrows should be a perfect arch, framing the orbit of the eye. When the eyebrows are too straight, they give to the face an astonished air, and when they meet at the root of the nose, they give a hard and fixed expression; it was characteristic, so it is said, of the Fallen Angel and the Wandering Jew, that their eyebrows grew straight across the brow. It is also said that this peculiarity denotes a jealous nature. However that may be, there is a very simple and inoffensive method employed by the Orientals for altering the shape of the eyebrows, lengthening, or blackening them. They trace the shape by means of a pencil steeped in a solution of Chinese ink and rose water.'

The lips, we are told, 'should be of a pretty red strawberry colour', but the colour should be achieved through health, not cosmetics, 'because these substances nearly always produce disastrous effects. In fact, the texture of the lips is very sensitive and can hardly stand painting, and the productions destined to redden the lips only succeed in making the skin hard and wrinkled, and robbing it of all delicacy and pliancy. Other women, without having recourse to painting, have noticed that caustic liquids have the properties of reddening the lips, and they use a quantity of vinegar and alcohol, of which the disadvantages are the same as those of painting.

'And lastly there is a third habit, also as bad and useless as the other two, and that is to bite the lips in order to render them red. The only result of this practice is to predispose them to chaps. There is only one way of reddening the lips without damaging their health, and that is to use some pomade of cucumbers *à la rose*, a very simple production, inoffensive and cheap, and which every chemist can make.'

The rest of the book is devoted to care of the teeth, nose, hair, and the body in general. In the final lines of the last chapter, which is on 'Coquetry', we are told that for women, 'universal knowledge is useless compared with the art of pleasing'.

It is reported that at this time there was in Bond Street a Mrs Pomeroy, who was said to have (perhaps by her own count) ten thousand satisfied clients for her somewhat strenuous beauty services. To remedy skimpy eyelashes, she simply removed a few hairs from the head and sewed them onto the lids. The perenially pale or sallow she sent to a London tattoo-artist, who provided a permanent blush.

THE ART OF BEING BEAUTIFUL

In 1902 a little book entitled *The Art of Being Beautiful* was published anonymously in London. It was written in the form of a dialogue between a young girl and a society beauty, an unidentified Baroness. The tone is one of commonsense throughout; and, like other books of the period, the emphasis is on beauty through health rather than paint:

'A fine complexion may be looked upon as indicative of a sound mind and a sound body. Extreme pallor is at times indicative, not of delicacy, but merely of want of sunshine. The rays of the sun act upon the human being as upon the plant, they bring out the body and brightness of its hue. . . . Open-air life at mid-day is the only cure for delicacy and the only means of acquiring a robustness that is of itself a large fraction of beauty. . . . No woman, while youth and health are hers, should need to paint. She has still the power to acquire a complexion by other means. . . . Have you noticed how many years are added to a young face by the use of paint? That is because the cosmetics hide that inimitable down which is the most exquisite sign of juvenility. You have seen the bloom on the peach! Well, most of our skins have this bloom until it is dried by exposure to fire or wind or worn off by the use of inferior soaps. For this reason you will understand that while middle age might gain, youth would but lose by the use of pigments. . . .

'I have no prejudices against paint. I merely point out how difficult it is to imitate Nature and how insolently daring it is of women to attempt, without a fraction of knowledge of colour, to daily present the public with daubs which are intended to represent the human complexion. . . . But of this we will talk again, for I now expect my dressmaker, who is bringing me a tea-gown of Venetian silk — a lovely gown of dead rose that will not fight my complexion.'

In their next dialogue the Baroness again approaches the question of cosmetics. And by pointing out to her young friend what she should avoid, she makes it clear what many women at the turn of the century were doing. The girl once again asks hopefully about powder, which was generally considered to be a fairly inoffensive cosmetic. The Baroness remains firm :

'Remember that with opaque powder people often do away with the exquisite transparency of blue veins, with the gentle greys and violets that give tone and depth to the eyelids. They rob Peter to pay Paul, as it were. Then, discontented, they go from bad to worse. Be the iris brown, blue, or grey, the tyro bedaubs it with some jetty cosmetic. This generally — by over-strengthening the outline of the eyelids — renders the expression fixed and glassy, and removes the soft, silvery tones which give so gentle a furriness to the eyelashes. I have seen some quite gentle people make themselves appear absolutely ferocious in this way ! Finally, often as not, come finishing daubs of rose; these either impart to the cheeks the indigestible colour of corn-flour impregnated with cochineal, or the vivid geranium scarlet that is seldom seen save on consumptive patients or clowns. . . . Here in England I observe that fair women and dark, the sallow and the florid, the old and the young, all paint — when they do paint — so as to make themselves pink and white and black, like dolls. For a woman to try and knock more than ten years off her age is an arrogance for which she is punished by every glance of the passers-by. When she tries as a brunette to make herself into a blonde by the use of unlimited white chalk, she also makes herself grotesque — as unpleasing as a fly that has dropped into a honey-pot; when, as a blonde, she adorns herself with black eyebrows, like croquet hoops, frankly she becomes alarming, if not detestable.

'Now the *belle Française* . . . merely endeavours to make her own self more acceptable to the eye. If she be a brunette, the powder she deals with is of a delicately saffron hue, slightly warmed with rose, and then — in emergency — to lashes and lids she imparts a delicately sepia touch. She never covers up blue veins. Indeed, she knows so well the value of them that she is apt to err by trying to accentuate them. As a last resource, but only on rare occasions, she uses just a speck or two of carnation (in specks and not in blotches !) to warm the perhaps sickly tint of the cheek bones.'

AVAILABLE COSMETICS

A technical book on cosmetics, written by Dr Theodor Koller and published for the first time in English in 1902, subsequently in 1911, revealed the composition of a great number of popular cosmetic preparations of the period. Here are a few of them:

Crème de Beauté — 'an emulsion of sweet and bitter almonds; of course, without any action at all'.

Blanc de Perles — 'a beautifying wash, consists of scented water containing a little alcohol, and showing a dense white sediment of calomel and lead carbonate'.

Bismuth Powder — 'for beautifying the skin, contains no bismuth, but consists of chalk and clay'.

Vienna Face Water — composed of about 12–13 parts of commercial (plumbiferous) zinc oxide, $1\frac{1}{2}$–2 parts of bismuth oxychloride, and 86–87 parts water, with a few drops of glycerin, rose water, and carbolic acid. It may be injurious.'

Grolich's Face Ointment — 'a white precipitate ointment mixed with bismuth white and scented with rose oil. May be injurious to health'.

Rosy Cheeks without Rouge — 'consists of powdered siliceous sponge. Under the microscope the preparation exhibits numerous siliceous needles, which penetrate the skin, producing mechanical irritation, and thus reddening the face'.

Rouge de Theatre — 'an American preparation for beautifying the skin, consists of talc, chalk, starch, and a little carmine to produce a red colour'.

Grecian Water — 'a cosmetic, consists of 189 parts of scented water with $7\frac{1}{2}$ parts of white precipitate, and may be poisonous'.

Lengiel's Birch Balsam — 'a beautifier and specific against wrinkles, pockmarks, freckles, etc., consists of 5 parts sodium silicate (waterglass), 2 of potash, 1 of soap, 5 of gum arabic and 10 of glycerin, in 400 parts of water; but no trace of birch sap. Any soap will work the same miracle without costing 4s. per bottle, like this preparation'.

Crème Lefebvre — 'a remedy for freckles, is a yellow ointment composed of fat and wax, with a little sublimate. May be poisonous'.

Vogue reported, in 1903, on a new liquid preparation to be used as a substitute for powder. It gave a dull finish and left 'a soft peach look. . . . Women who do not like to use powder will find this a good substitute, it having the additional attraction of being unnoticeable'. It was priced at one dollar a bottle. In the same issue J. Touzeau Saunders of Oxford Street advertised The Bloom of Ninon — 'not a Toilet Powder, but *par excellence* a Complexion powder. It has been for fifty years the standard preparation in England, whose women are noted for their clear and brilliant complexions. Like most imported

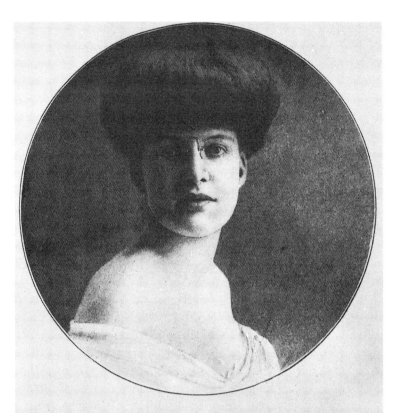

"I was troubled with dandruff, itching scalp and falling hair. Under the use of Crani-Tonic Hair Food, the dandruff disappeared, the itching of the scalp has ceased, the hair has stopped falling out and is growing thick and glossy."

(MISS) AGNES C. FITZPATRICK.

No. 470 W. 150th St., New York City.
April 4, 1903.

An Introduction Offer!

50,000 MAMMOTH TRIPLE SIZE BOTTLES

Crani=Tonic Hair=Food

TO BE DISTRIBUTED

$5 WORTH FOR $1

VOGUE has many thousands of readers, all of whom would find pleasure and benefit in the use of Crani-Tonic Hair-Food if they but knew how delightfully refreshing and beneficial its use is to all who suffer from dandruff, itching scalp, falling hair. We have therefore empowered the Chief Chemist attached to our Laboratories to Give to all who Call, or send to every reader of VOGUE, as an INTRODUCTION, a Large Two-Pound Mammoth Size, $3.00 bottle of Crani-Tonic Hair-Food with Two Cakes of Crani-Tonic Shampoo Soap (regular price 50 cents a cake) and one Tube of Zema-Cream (regular price $1.00), and "Hair Care" and "Hair Education" Books illustrated,) making $5.00 WORTH of the Greatest Hair and Scalp Products in the World, ALL FOR $1.00. Post Office and Express Money Orders, Checks and Drafts are Safer than Currency or Stamps. Any of these can be sent.

$5 WORTH FOR $1

CRANI-TONIC HAIR FOOD is absolutely pure and non-alcoholic, contains no grease, no vulgar perfume, sediment, dye matter or dangerous drugs. It is clean, clear as crystal, delightful to use and certain in its results.

Sold by Dealers in Four Sizes for 50 cts., $1, $2, and $5 the Bottle.

Sent to Any Point on Order, EXPRESS PREPAID.
The $5.00 Bottle is Physician's Size and Holds One Half Gallon.

CRANI-TONIC HAIR-FOOD CO.
526 WEST BROADWAY, NEW YORK

Incorporated May 6, 1899, under the Laws of New York State.

57 HOLBORN VIADUCT, LONDON, E. C.   5 RUE DE LA PAIX, PARIS.

FIG. 195 : Advertisement from *Vogue,* c. 1903.

Toilet Articles, it is sold nearer cost of production than domestic articles of less merit, and retails at 29 cents a box.'

For the lady who not only did not object to powder but liked a little colour in her cheeks as well, the Dr J. Parker Pray Company of New York could supply her with Rosaline — 'The marvelous natural healthy coloring it imparts to the cheeks and lips has made it wonderfully popular with fashionable women. The closest scrutiny fails to detect it, nor can it be displaced by perspiration or bathing.' If the lady was worried about wrinkles, the B. & P. Company of Cleveland was prepared to send her a box of Wrinkle Eradicators and Frowners — 'the greatest aids to beauty ever placed on a woman's toilet table'.

For those women who favoured powder papers, Zeno's Java Powder Book seemed made to order. 'This style of carrying face powder has come to stay,' announced the advertisement. 'We may find improvement on this article, as we have improved on the others, but up to the present time there is nothing in the market that can be compared to Papier Java. We have a cheaper article similar to that offered by some dealers, but we cannot recommend it to women of fastidious taste.

'Papier Java comes in beautiful satin covered booklets in cerise, royal purple, deep red, green, olive, blue, pink, and in fact every color one may desire. The powder is lain on the most delicate rice paper and comes in several tints of white, cream, and pink. Powder applied from these leaflets has the advantage of other forms in that it does not soil the corsage when being applied.'

A subsequent issue of *Vogue* carried an advertisement for Papier Poudré Books, 'The Genuine Made only by the Papier Poudré, 23 Somerset St., London. . . . The genuine are thinly and evenly spread on specially prepared perfumed paper. *Beware of cheap and blotchy imitations* on stiff, hard paper; *they are worthless.*' (See Plate 21-G.)

Vogue, supporting its advertisers, expressed its opinion that nothing could be more convenient or satisfactory than papers of powder. 'A new kind has lately been placed on sale,' the beauty editor informed her readers, 'and they are priced but 25 cents, though they are quite gorgeous affairs of satin lettered with gold. The size is the same as that with which we are familiar as no possible improvement was possible, but the powder is of another make, and I am told is entirely harmless to the most sensitive skin and very fine in quality. A delicate breath of perfume emanates from these little booklets, and the prepared sheets within may be applied without the aid of a looking glass so light is the trace of powder they leave on the skin. If one does not wish to carry the whole book, a few leaves may be detached and tucked within the pocketbook.'

As an alternative, *Vogue* suggested 'a dainty little bag of chamois skin, flat in shape and sparingly perforated on the inner side which is protected by a flap of chamois when not in use. Ribbons tie around the sachet, and the whole makes the smallest kind of a parcel with which one can be burdened. Taffeta in several

PLATE 21 : TWENTIETH CENTURY
1900–1913

A Time of Queen Alexandra. Ointment jar.

B 1904. Silver hand mirror.

C 1913. 'La Petite Victoria' — small, fitted vanity case in lavender, green, or blue leather with card case, pencil, and brass-topped bottles for powder, perfume, and lipstick. Price, $12.50.

D 1907. Magda Toilet Cream — a cucumber cream at 50 cents a pot or 25 cents a tube. Made in London, Boston, Montreal, Sydney, Frankfort, and Johannesburg.

E 1907. Pompeian Massage Cream.

F 1913. Monogrammed ivory mirror, box, nail file, and buffer from a French toilet set.

G 1903. Papier Poudré — book of papers impregnated with face powder.

H 1913. Vanity box in gold plate with mirror in top. Price, $3.50.

I 1904. Silver mirror in chrysanthemum pattern.

J 1903. Polpasta Polishing Paste — 'gives a brilliant polish . . . is a cure for hard nails and callous cuticle'. Price, 25 cents.

K 1909. Olein Daylight Powder.

L 1913. Rite Auto Vanity Case — 'The Newest Viennese Novelty'. Puff is filled with powder. Price, 50 cents.

M 1913. Men's blue or green leather toilet case, lined with pale blue or green satin, containing after-shave lotion, talcum, soap, shaving stick, and toilet water. Price, $10.

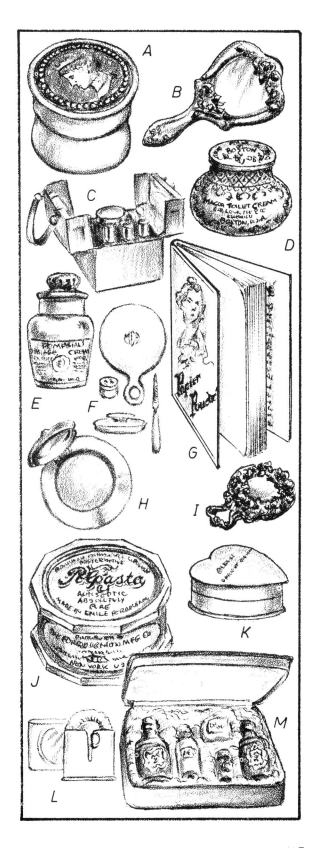

different colors is made into a cover and may match the color of the frock to be worn if desired.'

In August *Vogue* carried an advertisement for a 60-day treatment of Dr Campbell's Safe Arsenic Complexion Wafers and Fould's Medicated Arsenic Soap for one dollar. The treatment was supposed to get rid of pimples, freckles, wrinkles, blackheads, redness of the face or nose, or a muddy, sallow skin.

'The nut brown maid,' warned *Vogue's* beauty expert, 'may be the picture of health, but unfortunately tan and sunburn are anything but poetical in real life, being, on the contrary, often a great detriment to comfort as well as personal appearance. The freshly distilled juice of cucumbers is justly considered one of the most purifying and healing of remedies for this, as well as redness of the skin or chapping.'

In the same column *Vogue* recommended a liquid rouge which was said to be impervious even to sea bathing. 'The reason for this,' *Vogue* explained, 'is a slight admixture of glycerine which also gives the advantage of being able to shade the color gradually into the natural tint of the skin at the edges and thus obviate any crudeness of effect.' It was priced at fifty cents a bottle.

Vogue found another liquid rouge equally attractive. 'I understand,' wrote the editor, 'that its beautiful color is derived from the crushed leaves of crimson roses it being therefore strictly vegetable in substance. The depths of shade can be regulated; when applied lightly only the merest soupçon of color is left upon the cheeks, but if rubbed well in, a much more vivid hue is attainable. If properly applied it is absolutely undetectable, will not rub off and can be delicately shaded at the edges as the liquid is thin and can easily spread out so that it merges imperceptibly into the natural tint of the complexion.

'Red pencils for the lips of exceedingly fine quality sell for $2.50. The use of cosmetics to enhance the color of the lips has become very prevalent of late years. The manner of application is very simple as the pencil has merely to be passed slightly over the moistened lips. Black pencils for the eyebrows and eyelashes are to be had in the best and finest quality for $2. These preparations may seem a little expensive at the first glance, but they are each of exceptional value and the exclusive importation of a small French house well-known among the modish women of Paris.'

Vogue also recommended a new preparation 'for softening and whitening the arms and neck. It is claimed that it leaves the skin very smooth and flexible, the degree of whiteness being easily regulated by diluting with a little rose water. It should be spread on the skin with a fine sponge and not wiped off until all is dry. The tints are white, rose, rachelle, and chair, the price $2.40 for a large bottle.'

In 1903 it was also possible to buy a pneumatic bust.

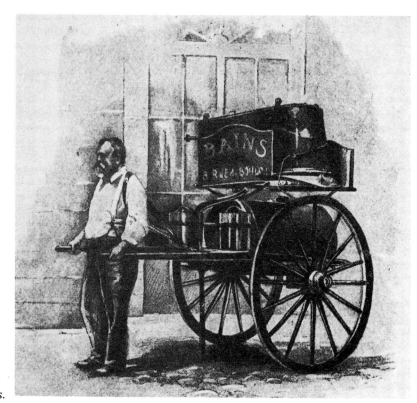

FIG. 196: Old-fashioned Parisian bath wagon, still in use in 1904. Such wagons were also found in other European cities.

DABROOKS' BATH-FUME

Anticipating by some years radio and television commercials, the Michigan Drug Company in 1903 was promoting its products with dramatic dialogue printed in full-page advertisements in women's periodicals. The following exchange, along with an appropriate photograph, appeared in *Vogue*:

Mr. CALVERT — Good morning, Mrs Raymond, what can I do for you to-day?

Mrs. RAYMOND — I want to get six boxes of *Dabrooks' Bath-Fume* to give away to some of my lady friends for a Christmas present.

Mr. CALVERT — I am sorry, Mrs. Raymond, but I do not keep it. I have got something else just as good, that will serve the same purpose, and it retails for half the money.

Mrs. RAYMOND — Yes, I tried some of it, and regret to state that it is of no value. I would rather have *Dabrooks' Bath-Fume* if I had to pay five times the money for it. Why don't you keep it? I buy most of my drugs of you, but it necessitates my going to another drug store to get what I want.

Mr. CALVERT — Yes, I know I have lost some customers by not handling *Dabrooks' Bath-Fume*. I have had a number of calls for that article; also for their *Dabrooks' Locust Blossoms Perfume* and *Dabrooks' Parisian Roses Perfume*. I understand my neighbor across the road is selling a great deal of Dabrooks' goods, and I guess I will have to put the goods in stock.

Mrs. RAYMOND — Well, I will step over to the other drug store and get this *Dabrooks' Bath-Fume* to-day, but when you get the stock in let me know, as I prefer to buy of you. I know you will have a call for it, because lots of my neighbors are using this article for the bath, and think that it is superior to anything in the market.

Mr. CALVERT (as Mrs. Raymond goes out of the store) — This *Dabrooks' Bath-Fume* and *Dabrooks' Perfumes* must be mighty good articles, because I hear the same story nearly every day from customers that come into the store. They seem to be building up a business on *quality* and *reputation*. I think I will send them a nice mail order to-day. I have got to carry the goods that my customers want, and I wish to satisfy them.

THE WINTER OF 1903

In the early winter *Vogue* described the latest fashion in silver dresser sets as having 'lost all pretense of simplicity, being now designed in such heavy, massive fashion that the array of mirrors and brushes seems almost too weighty for the fair hands of the prospective owner. . . . Shapes have lost their accustomed form and follow all sorts of dainty caprice in the matter of outline. Flowers overlap edges with disregard of all set rules, and irregularity of outline gives many an unexpected but welcome change from long familiar standards. One of the most beautiful of inexpensive sets is of this delightful variety, with roses and leaves in a dark gray finish on a background of lighter shade. The flowers are raised two inches from the surface and faithfully carried out in every detail with billows and waves of the silver sweeping into a scroll edge of entirely new shape.'

Although few respectable women of 1903 would openly admit to using rouge, *Vogue*, by recommending undetectable rouges, made it clear that a good many of them did — or wanted to. In December the beauty columnist suggested that the vogue for wearing grey fur, (mole skin, squirrel and chinchilla) had increased the use of rouge. 'Squirrel skin especially,' she pointed out, 'seems to absorb any faint touch of pink in the cheeks and needs a high color to be worn with advantage. For these reasons it may not be uninteresting to hear that a new liquid rouge has lately been imported from France which has many desirable qualities and is as impossible to detect as any artificial coloring matter one can hope to find. If applied with any degree of skill and common sense, it should be able to defy detection even in day time, and may be used in the evening without a single qualm of fear. It is absolutely natural in tint, and being the product of a small and most exclusive house is to be relied upon as being what is claimed.

I am told that the red in rose leaves is the only coloring matter used, and certainly this sounds poetic enough to counteract that unpleasant name of rouge, which, I am sure, all women must dislike.

'Thin in substance, and apparently without a heavy ingredient of any kind, it spreads easily and lightly, sinking at once into the skin and giving a tint which may be varied in depth by the amount of liquid applied. It does not wash off easily and is non-removable in any other way. Price $2.50 a flacon. Absorbent cotton is a good means for application and it is surprising how long a bottle will last, as the size is about two and a half ounces. If desirable a drop on the end of the stopper gives the lips a pinker tone and leaves no greasy look in the wake, as do so many salves for the same purpose.'

Hints from Vogue

The following year *Vogue* was still approaching the problem of rouging with considerable delicacy, being both open-minded and faintly disapproving at the same time. If rouge was to be applied at all, 'it should be approached,' *Vogue* insisted, 'as a work of art, so that there are no traces of its beginning or leaving off'. A foundation cream was recommended, and the lady was advised to have a good light. The actual application of the rouge was passed over quickly. A thin coating of powder was to be applied all over, 'beginning at the forehead and covering the throat; with a second piece of chamois this must be rubbed gently into the skin, touching lightly so that only the superfluous powder is removed. Before leaving one's room, the tips of the fingers may be passed over the face and neck, so that any stray particles not already fastened to the skin are removed. . . . All this description sounds rather artificial, and indeed it may be, but these hints for the woman who employs cosmetics are given so that the results shall have as natural an appearance as possible. It is always to be regretted when artificial means are called in to aid nature, but it cannot be denied that much of this is done in these days.'

The next month the same beauty editor was called upon once again to recommend a cosmetic. There were, it seemed, occasions when ordinary measures were insufficient to cope with deficiencies in the complexion. 'At times,' sighed the editor, 'the temptation to improve one's appearance, even if only temporarily, becomes too strong to resist.' Having firmly established her moral principles and confessed to human weakness at the same time, thus making it possible for all of her readers to identify with her, she plunged ahead with the business of the day, recommending an illusion cream which cunningly concealed defects of the complexion 'under a coating so delicate that it is imperceptible except in results. No suggestion of an enamel is given, but it is a heavy flesh-tinted liquid, that sinks into the pores and leaves an even, white finish which hides most minor

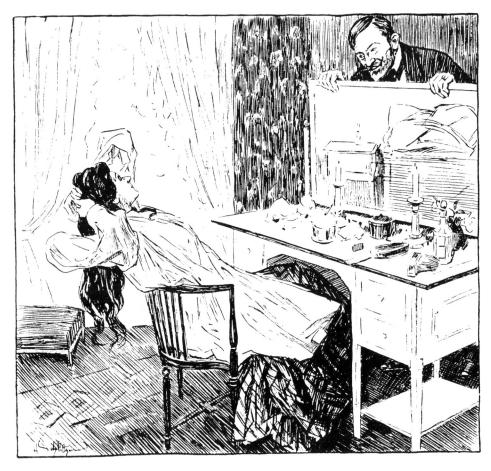

FIG. 197: Miffed. German cartoon by Hermann Schlittgen, *c.* 1905. The husband is criticizing the wife for her use of cosmetics. She asks if he has ever seen her without them.

defects.' Then with no hesitation at all she recommended a perfumed lip salve which cost twenty-five cents and was 'put up daintily in an aluminum case. This is an adjunct of the toilet which almost all women appreciate; it gives the lips a rich, healthy appearance and prevents their chapping or becoming rough.'

Despite serious moral reservations about the use of makeup, most women and a good many men had little objection to colouring their hair, provided it could be done unobtrusively. A steel and nickel comb containing black, brown, or golden dye was simple to use for either hair or moustaches and brought about a gradual change in colour. A single three-dollar comb was supposed to last for a year. *Vogue* endorsed it enthusiastically.

They also recommended use of 'a crayon to deepen the shade of the eyelashes'. It was said to be 'very adherent and bright in color'. Five shades were available

—black, brown, chestnut, blonde, and blue. According to the directions, the crayon was supposed to be warmed before use for better spreading. The cosmetic crayon, along with an eyebrow brush and a cork pencil were packaged in a case and sold for $1.67.

An advertisement for Dream Eyebrow and Eyelash Cream guaranteed that it would darken the brows and lashes and stimulate their growth — '*not a dye*, but a delicate pure cream which if applied faithfully for a week or two will show surprising results'. It was to be had 'in dainty jars' for fifty cents. The same company made Dream Violet Talcum Powder ('in attractive pink and blue silk bags') and Dream Cream for the Complexion ('Removes moth spots, pimples, sunburn'). The advertisement was illustrated with a portrait of the Dream Cream Girl.

About the same time an advertisement by a Madam Julian for the removal of superfluous hair ('no electricity, blue ointment, poison, or pain') showed two identical drawings of young ladies, both with tiny moustaches and incipient goatees.

Almond meal was a popular substitute for soap in the early part of the century. 'As a skin bleacher it is unexcelled,' wrote *Vogue's* beauty editor, 'the softening, refining and soothing qualities are equally worthy of praise and appreciation.'

The New York manufacturers of Liquiderma, a liquid rouge, advertised that 'Unlike powdered or other rouges it does not clog the pores. . . . It will impart a natural ruddy color and its use cannot be detected by one's most intimate enemy'. It sold for fifty cents a bottle. It was to be applied with absorbent cotton and the cheeks then rubbed with a cloth and dusted with powder. This was to be done before retiring. In the morning the face was washed as usual. *Vogue* pronounced the colour extremely natural but warned that it must be used sparingly, one drop being sufficient for both cheeks. It could also be used on the lips.

'You cannot afford to have *wrinkles, sagging cheeks, puffy eyes, unsightly scowls, unshapely ears, noses, lips, chins, thin face* and *scrawny necks, unhealthy complexions,*' warned the advertisement, 'when you can safely and simply, with Dr. Nelden's assistance, be rid of these humiliating disfigurements.' All this was to be done 'Absolutely Without Pain', with 'No Detention Indoors', and with 'Charges Moderate' by A. L. Nelden, M.D., who billed himself as the 'Great Plastic Surgeon'.

In December *Vogue* was enthusiastic about some new 'downy powder puffs with dainty button handles of sterling silver. The patterns are the latest to be found in modern art and usually finished in that soft French gray which is so vastly pretty.' In addition, there were some even newer puffs with long slim silver handles — more chic, decided *Vogue*, but less convenient.

It was in this same year that a Monsieur Coty, trying to sell a new perfume called La Rose Jaqueminot to a Paris department store and being refused permission even to open the bottle, managed on his way out to smash it, enchanting the store full of customers with the delightful scent and launching himself in business.

Tous les Secrets de la Femme

In her *Tous les Secrets de la Femme*, published in 1907, the Baroness d'Orchamps suggests a novel method for achieving naturally red lips:

'Soak the lips for at least five minutes in a glass of warm water. Dry them, then smear them with camphorated pommade. After a quarter of an hour, dry them again with a soft cloth and put on some glycerine. Unless you are seriously anemic, your lips will become as red as carmine.' To this is added a warning: 'Do not misuse this procedure, however, for the glycerine decreases little by little the elasticity of the lips.'

But then the Baroness adds that 'a light sucking of the lips, a little bite, will give to them in an instant a crimson bloom'. As for makeup, it is quite useless, she says. 'Even a slightly trained eye will not be fooled. Paints and salves have the disadvantage of preventing direct contact of the air on the mucuous membranes, which then rapidly turn pale which makes one wish for the natural pink, so diminished from its former bloom.'

She is equally firm about the eyes. 'We can,' she tells us, 'voluntarily accentuate the power of our eyes. We can even use certain artifices to increase the intensity of the look.' But, she concludes, even 'if the artifices, the pencil marks, and the makeup can occasionally correct lack-lustre eyes, they will never increase the beauty, no matter how perfectly they may be done'.

At this time cakes of pressed powder were available in round cardboard or aluminum boxes with puff and mirror for twenty-nine cents. Dr T. Felix Gouraud's Oriental Cream or Magical Beautifier was advertised as 'the least harmful of all the skin preparations'. Pompeian Massage Cream, recommended for men as well as women, was guaranteed to open and clean out the pores, 'restoring free excretion and skin breathing, taking out blackheads, sallowness, and muddiness, animating the blood circulation, and flexing the muscles'.

Mme Leclaire and Harriet Hubbard Ayer

In February the beauty editor of *Vogue* described with extravagant enthusiasm her fifteen-minute beauty treatment at a certain Fifth Avenue salon decorated in Louis XV style, presided over by a sixty-three-year-old beauty, and featuring a secret beauty treatment lost during the horrors of the French Revolution and now rediscovered. Predictably, a March issue of *Vogue* contained a full-page advertisement for Madame Leclaire's Fifth Avenue salon, with pictures of the Louis XV salon and boudoir. Madame Leclaire, now turned sixty-three and possessing 'the velvety, peach-like skin of a baby', was, according to the advertisement, 'a beauty specialist of supreme knowledge and understanding' and was 'prepared to maintain her position with unrivalled authority and power'. She had evidently come a long way since her days in the Austrian convent of the Sacre Coeur, where she whiled away her leisure hours 'aiding in the various manipulations of the chemists'. Her method, which was designed to impart permanent beauty, was described in the advertisement:

'The patron is received in a dainty Louis XV salon, in harmony of pale blue and white, and a charming living proof of MME. LECLAIRE's wonderful skill ushers the visitor into the presence of the famous expert. She herself invariably performs the process. A deep brown substance is spread evenly over the face and remains on for five minutes; by that time a sharp, tingling sensation is experienced, which seems to draw every fibre of the epidermis and imbibes the mysterious substance.

'This application is then entirely removed, and a demulcent and soothing preparation of yellowish tint, resembling honey, replaces it; this remains upon the face for several minutes and imparts a soothing and pleasing sensation, counteracting the effects of the preceding layer. It seems to enter and give fresh life to the skin, effacing lines and hollows, and obliterates in one application any defects which were previously noticeable. The dreaded crow's feet are effectively erased and a youthful bloom imparted. . . .

'After the astringents have been entirely removed, a complexion powder, known only to MME. LECLAIRE, is dusted lightly over the cheeks, and the seance is ended.'

The lady who could not get to New York for her rejuvenation could purchase Mme. Leclaire's cold cream, beauty cream (pink or white), and face powder for five dollars apiece. The pages of subsequent issues of *Vogue* give no clue as to the eventual fate of Mme. Leclaire.

'There has always been a demand on the part of the friends and admirers of Harriet Hubbard Ayer,' began another advertisement in 1907, 'for the famous toilet preparations which she personally prepared and kept for her private use and for her personal friends. These secret formulas have been carefully guarded, and it is with the greatest pleasure and self-congratulation that now for the first time Harriet Hubbard Ayer's friends and admirers, as well as the general public, can obtain these famous toilet preparations.'

The preparations the world had been waiting for included Face Cream ('the most marvelously beautifying skin preparation ever compounded'), Face Powder ('the finest powder ever manufactured'), La Belle Coquette ('a vegetable color-

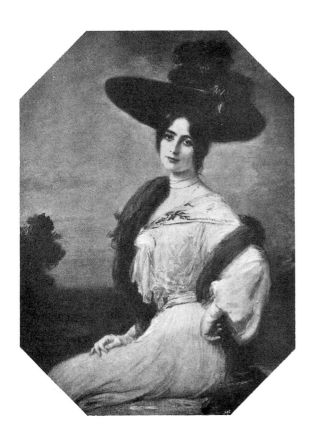

FIG. 198: Portrait of the French actress Cléo de Mérode. Painting by F. A. von Kaulbach, c. 1905.

ing matter which gives a perfectly imperceptible and absolutely natural coloring to the skin'), Wrinkle Eradicator ('the only absolute remedy that has ever been discovered'), and The Genuine Complexion Brush ('the original invention of Harriet Hubbard Ayer and imitated everywhere').

Vogue elaborated on the use of the wrinkle eradicator, which involved stretching the skin smooth and applying a thin layer of the wrinkle paste, which then dried into a firm, transparent film. Vogue agreed with Mrs Ayer that it could be worn during the day without detection (the ultimate criterion for any acceptable makeup in 1907) and that it was helpful. Vogue was equally enthusiastic about La Belle Coquette:

'The most dainty of her sex should be satisfied with the pretty little Limoges bon-bon boxes in which the newest of rouges is housed. The contents are equally satisfactory, and it would be well-nigh impossible to find anything more natural in effect, or a rouge which admits of greater possibilities in shading down the tone at the edges into the white of the skin. It is cream-like in quality but very thin and spreads with marvelous ease, the coloring matter being purely vegetable and of wonderful tint. The shade can be deepened where effective and tapered off in the most natural way, so with even a very moderate degree of skill the effect is really unusually good.'

Madame Leclaire took a different approach from that of Mrs Ayer, inviting women to come to her in confidence 'to have a little chat'. Paint, powder, and paste she considered the 'agents of destruction'. After her own complexion had been 'abominably ruined', she consecrated herself entirely to medical studies and then devoted herself 'to exhaustive researches in order to discover the beneficent secrets of certain fruits and certain mixtures known to the ancients and used by women of former centuries. . . . I do not pretend to be the only one who knows this secret,' she added. 'One of the Queens of Europe is also in possession of it, and her complexion is as universally famous as her name. Can you guess of whom I speak?' Presumably this would immediately bring to mind Marie of Roumania. 'I have a task to perform,' concluded Madame Leclaire bravely, 'and I am giving myself up to it entirely.'

COSMETICS, 1907

In July *Vogue* reported on a rouge 'whose color is so perfect that years were spent by one of the greatest French chemists in bringing it to its present impeccable tint'. This perfect rouge was incredibly priced at $6.90 and came in a china box decorated with cupids.

Liquid nail polishes were so new in 1907 that *Vogue* felt it necessary to explain to its readers that the liquid was 'applied with a brush in a light coating at the bottom of the nail, the fingers being held with a downward incline so that the liquid may spread over the whole surface of the nail. It takes but a few seconds to dry and is followed by a brisk rubbing with a chamois polisher. This produces a wonderful brilliance and will last for several days. The liquid neither stains the polisher or grinds off the surface of the nails.' But for the woman who was not ready for anything so revolutionary, there was a new French polishing powder in cake form, which was rubbed onto the palm of one hand, then applied from there to the nails of the other. *Vogue* said the polish lasted a long time and gave the nails 'a beautiful look of transparency'. Nothing was said about what it did to the palms.

There were other relatively new preparations for the nails as well — a rouge pencil and a paste 'in a small china box', both used for polishing, and a fine white powder 'in a wee box' with a tiny bone spatula for removing stains.

For the woman who could afford it, there was available in 1907 a fitted mahogany dressing table, with silver brushes, combs, glass boxes with silver tops, bottles, hand mirror, nail buffer, button-hook, nail scissors, and file. It was a simple, polished mahogany table when closed, but when the top was raised to a vertical position, side shelves would spring out automatically. The top contained an adjustable mirror, and there were seven cubbyholes at the back with assorted bottles and boxes. *Vogue* noted that one of the bottles was flask-shaped and might 'be utilized as such or for other purposes'. The working area was covered with a glass tray, no doubt to protect the mahogany finish when the flask was in use.

In December *Vogue* reported enthusiastically on a French treatment for complexion ills, available in a home kit of twenty-five applications for $48.75 (about £20). Each treatment required fifteen to twenty minutes and involved mixing a fine white powder with a lotion, resulting in a paste, which was then heated and applied in a thick mask over the face and throat. The paste was moistened with still another preparation while it was on the face. 'The result when all this is removed,' *Vogue* reassured its readers, 'will be a skin made delicate in texture, satiny of finish, clear of tone and wonderfully brightened, with the fresh pink of youth in the cheeks, lines smoothed away where not deep and made much fainter in even the most chronic conditions.'

'Rouge is a cosmetic which I usually have hesitation in recommending,' wrote the beauty editor of *Vogue* just before Christmas, 'but every now and then I come across a production which shows few if any of the usual defects. A word of warning is often necessary to emphasize the unattractiveness of artificial coloring matter when too strongly laid on; the first principle to observe is that it must be unsuspected in order to make the result satisfactory or refined. With some preparations it is difficult to tone the shade into that of the cheeks, although this is one of the very first requisites in a good rouge.' The new rouge was very shadable, 'entirely harmless', made from pure cold cream, and faintly perfumed. It was sold in small china boxes and cost a dollar.

END OF A DECADE

The revised edition of *My Lady Beautiful or the Perfection of Womanhood* by Alice M. Long appeared in 1908. Some of the chapter headings are provocative, if not irresistible—The Sunshine Laboratory; Nature's Roses for the Cheeks; Mrs. Sunshine, the Woman Beautiful; How to Drink Water; The Sweetest Face Imaginable; The Lung Bath; Pearls and Diamonds of Speech; Prescriptions from the Sunshine Dispensary. For the face the author recommends the best vegetable soaps (not too often), pure olive oil (once a week), a teaspoonful of milk and salt (once a month), along with regular exercise, a balanced diet, and happy thoughts. Throughout the 108 pages, the possibility of using makeup is never mentioned.

From the March 7 issue of *The Queen*, one learns of various afflictions of its readers: 'G.S.' had vein marks, 'Julia' suffered from eczema, 'G.P.'s hair was fading, 'Elsie Marguerite' had thin arms, and 'A Dandy' was dissatisfied with the appearance of his or her face. Electricity, medicated waters, hair dye, and face creams were prescribed. By an interesting coincidence, as this issue went to press, 'a fairy play' had just been presented 'by the girls of Glendower House School in aid of the Guild of Brave Poor Things'.

Various fruits and nuts have for centuries been used for the complexion. In 1909 Harriet Hubbard Ayer asked, 'Can you imagine anything more delightful for the complexion than ripe luscious strawberries combined with pure oil of almonds? Ripe strawberries, you know, are Nature's own bleach and tonic for the skin, and the vegetable oil extracted from Persian almonds is an incomparable skin food.' Mrs Ayer called her combination Creme Delicias. For her Lotion Delicias, she combined her abundant supply of fresh, ripe strawberries with crushed rose leaves, toilet vinegar, astringent tonic, and invigorant. 'Isn't that a delightful combination?' asked Mrs Ayer.

With the increasing number of uses being found for electricity, it is hardly surprising that in 1909 an advertisement headed WHY NOT BE BEAUTIFUL should feature a photograph of a smiling, attractive young woman plugged into an electric socket. 'Women who know the value and power of beauty,' the advertisement read, 'will not permit their cheeks to become colorless, haggard, and wrinkled, with dark circles under the eye, crow's feet, etc. . . . There is no occasion for women having wrinkles or crow's feet before sixty if she will use THE DAVIS ELECTRIC MEDICAL BATTERY, the greatest and latest invention for administering Electricity into the human system. It causes rich red blood to go leaping, bounding, and tingling through the body, stimulating vigorous blood circulation — nature's beauty food. Destroys old age microbes — endorsed by leading physicians. Recommended especially for Rheumatism, Paralysis, Chronic Headaches, Nervousness, Worn Out Systems, Insomnia, etc. Nothing like it.'

18 · The Twentieth Century 1910-1920

It is not necessarily vanity that brings out
the powder-puff, but a courteous regard
for the esthetic sensibilities of others.

RICHARD LE GALLIENNE

Early in the century of the beauty shop, Mrs Elizabeth Hubbard published a little pamphlet of *Helpful Advice to Women who would be Beautiful*. The advice seemed designed to emphasize the advisability of paying a visit to Mrs Hubbard's Fifth Avenue salon, where one could obtain a Grecian Muscle-Strapping Treatment of the Face and Neck, Grecian Muscle Oil, Grecian Daphne Skin-Tonic, Grecian Cream of Velvet, Grecian Snowflake Cream, Grecian Lotos Beauty Cream, Grecian Japonica Lotion, Grecian Freckle Cream, Grecian Lilium Hand-Cream, Grecian Eye-Bandelettes, Grecian Beauty Sachets, Grecian Wrinkle Plasters, and approximately three dozen additional Grecian preparations.

For the woman who chose to paint, there was Grecian Rose Bloom (a liquid rouge), Grecian Lip-Pencil (for a 'rosy, healthy looking mouth'), Grecian Enamel (for whitening the neck and arms), Grecian Face Enamel (in a 'youthful flesh tint of pale ivory-pink'), Grecian Eyelash and Eyebrow Ointment ('it darkens them without staining the flesh'), Grecian Eyelash Cosmetique (applied with a small brush), and, for variety, an Oriental Grease Rouge, put up in small jars suitable for carrying in the purse.

Mrs Hubbard was also prepared to supply a Grecian Forehead Strap, a Grecian Combination Throat and Chin Strap, a Grecian Nasal Clamp, Grecian Rubber Gloves, and Grecian Masks made of kid or rubber. Treatments were available at the salon ($2 for a 'muscle-strapping treatment') or at one's home or hotel ($3 for the same treatment). There were also do-it-yourself home-treatment kits for $4, or the same thing in a 'Japaned Beauty Box' designed for travelling, for $30.

Having decided she needed help in selling her Grecian products, Mrs Hubbard took Florence Nightingale Graham, a determined and energetic Canadian woman, into the firm. After a brief and stormy partnership, Mrs Graham borrowed six thousand dollars from a cousin, chose the name of Elizabeth Arden, and launched one of the most successful careers in the history of the cosmetics business. She spent most of the six thousand on furnishing a four-room salon and paid it all back in four months. In 1929 she refused an offer of fifteen million dollars for the company.

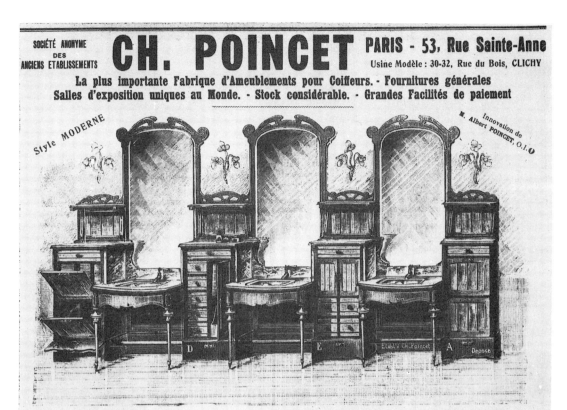

FIG. 199: Furnishings for hairdressers' shops. French advertisement, 1913.

BEAUTY PARLOURS

Beauty parlours in the early twentieth century were no better than their owners, as a former employee of one of them made clear in the pages of the *Delineator*:

'The proprietor of the beauty parlor where I started to learn beauty culture proved to be a man who had absolutely no knowledge of anatomy, physiology, medical therapeutics, or chemistry. He had simply invested money . . . in a "parlor", which an interior decorator had beautified with white enamel paint, soft gray-green hangings, gleaming mirrors, and artistic electroliers. Outwardly it shrieked sanitation; behind the curtains it reeked with germs. . . . Prices were arranged on a sliding scale, regulated wholly by the experience and worldly knowledge of patrons. The hairdressers were men, English and French. Most of them were inveterate gamblers, and their morals and conversation were such that when I saw young, unchaperoned girls enter their curtained booths for a loose wave or a Marcel, I trembled and wondered why their mothers took such risks.'

The anonymous author reported that operators frequently suggested brightening the hair a little. Having been given permission to do that, they would proceed with a full bleach job. 'When at last the chemically treated mass is dry, Madam almost faints. . . . It is copper-toned, brass-hued, or the regulation peroxide blond, according to the daring of the operator.' Now that Madam's faded complexion no longer matches her hair, she is turned over to the makeup specialist for a touch of rouge, eyebrow pencil, lip salve, and powder. 'And so,' concludes the author sadly, 'the wholesome normal woman who came into the shop for a shampoo and a loose wave fares forth a slave to make-up.'

LETTERS TO THE EDITOR

Letters to newspapers' beauty editors in the early years of the new century revealed nothing very new or surprising. Women with freckles wanted to get rid of them; women with straight hair wanted it curly; women with short eyelashes wanted long ones. One woman wanted to get rid of her husband's double chin; another wanted to know how to make her daughter's nose stop growing; still another wanted to know how not to become any taller, and she wanted to know it by the following Sunday. Women unhappy with their looks and susceptible to advertising wore wrinkle plasters, chin straps, face masks, and forehead bands and massaged their faces with Japanese wooden balls. Many of them wrote, often in desperation, always with implicit faith, to the beauty editors.

'I am so worried about my cheeks,' wrote one young lady, 'as I look like a ghost, and have you something that will brighten their color? I do not like to use rouge. I am going to be maid of honor on the seventeenth of this month and I want to make an impression on the man I am going to stand up with, so please help me.' A young man wanted to know how to make his hair grow 'gradually darker into a black'. In addition, his eyebrows were too thin and he wanted them heavier; also, they were light, and he wanted them dark. Not only that, but his hair was of two different colours. 'You can imagine how I feel,' he wrote to the editor.

The most touching letters of all were from girls whose problems stemmed from the social conditions of the day and seemed almost beyond the help of any beauty editor. Here are three of them:

> I am twenty-three years old and three years married. I used to be pretty, but now I ain't pretty at all. I got wrinkles like I was fifty, and I ain't round and pink at all. I do washing, ironing, and scrubbing, also bring up my coal and wood. It is four flights. Do you think that can have anything

to do with my not being pretty any more? My husband still loves me, but I am afraid he won't after a while if I go on getting more wrinkles. He said yesterday I ain't so pretty as I used to be, and it's awful to know he found it out already.

I don't look healthy, I am yellow. Some say it is because I work in a tailor shop, that I sit all day, but I can't help myself; I can't succeed at no other trade, as I am handy at a needle so thought maybe you could give me something to make me not so yellow.

Can you tell me something to wear in my cheeks to fill them out? I am a white goods maker, and I get so tired I think it makes my cheeks so hollow. If you could tell me something to wear at night to make them grow out round. I read a piece: it said it was every girl's duty to be as pretty as she could, but how is she going to do it when she works so hard?

BEAUTY IN 1911

In January, V. Darsy in New York advertised a leather case of cosmetics for motoring:

'It is always very important to take care of the skin if one wishes to look young and fresh even in advanced years, but especially so when speeding over the country in an automobile. We have gotten up the most perfect Motor Box, containing every possible requisite the fair motorist may need to protect her skin against the coarsening influences of sun, wind, and dust.

'The box is made of black leather and leather lined with secure compartments for every bottle and jar. There are Darsy's creams, soap, powder, rouge, etc., and Sonya Rejuvenating Milk and Rejuvenator. An empty space is big enough to hold a purse, a veil, etc.'

The box also contained eye wash and an eye cup for removing cinders from the eye. The price was twenty dollars.

In the same month there was an advertisement for the Davenport Sanitary Pocket Tooth Brush — 'Practical, Artistic, Economical . . . Highly Ornamental for the Dressing Table' — and on the following page, one for the Secret of Beauty, which did not 'rub off like dry powder' and imparted 'a delicate velvet-like softness to the skin without leaving the slightest trace that would suggest its use'. It was supposed not to 'paint, bleach, dry, or contract the skin'.

For fourteen years a Mrs Adair had been selling toilet preparations in New York, but as will happen in the business world, a competitor had evidently tried to take advantage of Mrs Adair. An advertisement for her Ganesh Toilet

Preparations and Facial Treatments proclaimed in bold-faced type that 'FALSE RUMORS have been circulated to the effect that Mrs. Adair will discontinue her New York branch. THESE RUMORS ARE ABSOLUTELY UNFOUNDED and are circulated with malicious intent. THE MARVELOUS GROWTH of Mrs. Adair's business has never been greater than at the present time. It continues to record increases irrespective of seasons and conditions. *There are no similar preparations or treatments*, neither has Mrs. Adair any pupils in New York other than those working for her at her Salon at 21 West 38th Street'. But somewhere in New York there must have been those, covetous of Mrs Adair's business, who claimed otherwise.

Like most beauties and beauty authorities of her period, Lillian Russell relied largely on exercise, diet, and rest to keep young and attractive. But she did recommend a good cold cream:

'I think that made of almond-oil is the best — the best, that is, except the one that I am some day going to have manufactured myself, if I ever get around to it! The most important ingredient is mutton-tallow, such as your mother used to grease your nose with, except that it is five times refined and is redolent with the odor of violets. It is the tallow with which the manufacturers of French perfumes extract the scent from flowers. . . . As to the almond cream . . . let it remain on the face and the neck as long as you can and then remove it with gauze. Sterilized gauze, which I buy in lengths of twenty-five yards, is all that ever touches my face. Never a towel, never anything rough! As for the rest, I advise you to wash your face in hot water and with soap once a day. You should steam it, I think, if you do not take turkish baths. . . . I should do nothing further except to dust a little powder over my face and throat.'

In 1911 Ingram's Milkweed Cream was being advertised in the *Delineator*. The advertisement, showing five opened jars of Milkweed Cream with a beautiful lady's head protruding from the mouth of each ('There is Beauty in Every Jar') promised 'unusual and quick-acting therapeutic properties. It tones, softens, and whitens the skin — soothes and stimulates the youthful glow in the face of woman'. The cream, continued the advertisement, was 'universally used by the famous beauties of the stage' and 'publicly praised and recommended by them'. It sold for fifty cents a jar. Velveola, 'the Milkweed Cream Face Powder, smooth, finely pulverized and exquisitely scented', cost twenty-five cents. For fifty cents one could buy a wooden box of Pozzoni's Complexion Powder — 'The Greatest Beautifier of them All . . . the only complexion powder that really clings'. Hinds Honey and Almond Cream, at fifty cents a bottle or twenty-five cents a tube, was recommended for both men and women.

Elsewhere in this issue the reader was urged to write for hair to be sent on approval. Straight switches were to be had for as little as ninety-five cents. Men's and ladies' wigs were fifty dollars.

In this same year a little book of coloured drawings of boxes and jars and

jewelry, all with parts to be lifted to reveal a one-word virtue, and all accompanied by a few lines of verse, was published in Philadelphia. This version of
the book, called *My Lady's Toilette*, is remarkably like *The American Toilet*,
published in 1827, and *The Toilet*, published in 1867, both discussed in previous
chapters. The 1911 book is described as 'a series of illustrations, designed and
executed more than a century ago by Catharine Shephard, of Virginia, and
presented by her to her favorite niece. The original which is a treasured heir-
loom, is yellowed with age, and the ink somewhat faded, but the water colors
are still bright and indicate considerable talent and artistic ability, in spite of
somewhat obvious mistakes in perspective.'

A yellow dish labelled *Genuine Rouge* is accompanied by a rhyming couplet:

> Touch with this compound the soft likely cheek
> And the bright glow will best its virtues speak.

Lifting the cover of the dish reveals the word 'Modesty'. Beneath a box of
Fine Lip Salve, one is cautioned to

> Use daily for your lips this precious dye,
> They redden & breathe sweeter melody.

The word inside the box is 'Cheerfulness'.

NEW PRODUCTS, 1912

In January 1912 *Vogue* announced a new liquid face powder, 'not sticky like
so many powders of this variety' and 'medicated so that one can reasonably
believe it pure'. The powder came in natural, flesh, and brunette and was used
primarily for whitening the neck and arms, though it could be used on the face
if one wished. The price was one dollar, postpaid.

Vogue warned about the dangers of impure face creams, some of which,
they said, contained white lead. But they highly recommended a cream scented
with orange blossoms which was freshly made for each purchaser and delivered
within thirty-six hours for one dollar a jar. Besides cleansing the skin, it would,
Vogue assured its readers, eliminate lines and wrinkles.

Other preparations were made 'entirely from the fruits and nuts which are
most nourishing to the skin'. *Vogue* recommended leaving a little of the almond
cream on over night and in the morning a face bath of cold water containing
ten drops of astringent lotion. Then a little violet face powder (white, rose, or
brunette) to give the skin 'a soft transparency rather than the heavy, chalky
look that some powders do', and the lady was ready to face the world once
more.

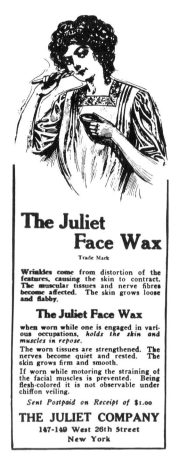

**The Juliet
Face Wax**

Trade Mark

Wrinkles come from distortion of the
features, causing the skin to contract.
The muscular tissues and nerve fibres
become affected. The skin grows loose
and flabby.

The Juliet Face Wax

when worn while one is engaged in various occupations, *holds the skin and
muscles in repose.*

The worn tissues are strengthened. The
nerves become quiet and rested. The
skin grows firm and smooth.

If worn while motoring the straining of
the facial muscles is prevented. Being
flesh-colored it is not observable under
chiffon veiling.

Sent Postpaid on Receipt of $1.00

THE JULIET COMPANY
147-149 West 26th Street
New York

FIG. 200 : Advertisement from *Vogue, c.* 1912.

The newest thing for the nails was a box of 'five gilt-stoppered bottles full of
all sorts of polishing, bleaching and softening preparations' — a nail pomade,
a cuticle softener, a nail bleach, a nail polisher, and a rose tint 'for those whose
nails are apt to be a trifle pale'. A liquid polish, Vogue reported, was gaining in
favour. It was simple to apply, gave a brilliant gloss and 'the slightly rose tint
which betokens health'.

In February Vogue reported with ladylike enthusiasm on a new rouge which
was 'a prepared bit of soft cloth which, when rubbed on the face, produces an
exquisite tint that varies in depth according to the gentleness or vigor with
which it is used; it washes off easily and will outlast several ordinary sized
cakes of rouge'. The cloth came in a box with mirror and cost thirty-five cents.
In March they confided that they had found a liquid rouge in 'a really wonderful shade' which blended with the skin marvellously 'when applied with any
degree of skill. It spreads evenly,' the reader was assured, 'so that the tell-tale

edge may easily be avoided'. It cost one dollar a bottle. In April *Vogue* gave instructions for mending a hot-water bottle.

'The critical women of Boston', according to a 1912 advertisement, had turned almost unanimously to Mrs A. J. MacHale, whose Cherry Blossom Rouge imparted to their cheeks 'a soft, rose-like tint' which could not 'be detected from the natural'. It was available in two tints, one for blondes, one for brunettes. Mrs MacHale also sold a Primrose Balm — 'the most expensive of all toilet preparations to manufacture, and the most satisfactory to use'.

In New York the Hanson-Jenks Company, appealing to women 'fastidious in refinement', offered a box of their 'toilet requisites' (Halcyon Rose Perfume, Ilys Sachet, Wood Violet Toilet Water, Violet Toilet Soap Brut, and Violet Talcum Brut), valued at fifty cents, for only twenty-five cents in cash or fifteen two-cent stamps. 'Hanson-Jenks products have never been cheated of quality to meet price,' proclaimed the full-page advertisement. 'They are not cheap. They are expensive goods at reasonable prices. In quality only the best of the imported approach them. . . . The actual cost of the production is greater than their whole price.' A half-page advertisement for Dralle's Illusion ('the most costly perfume sold in America') boasted that 'Dralle's is too costly to send you a sample'.

Le Secret Gaby Deslys was an internationally known cosmetic (8 francs in France, 3 rubles in Russia, 6 marks in Germany, 6 shillings in England, 1 dollar and fifty cents in the United States) combining — in two tubes, a box, and a sponge — a whitener for the neck and arms, a tint for the face, and a rouge for the lips, cheeks, and nails. All could be blended together, claimed the advertisements, and applied with the sponge to give any desired tint. 'Le Secret Gaby Deslys', the prospective user was assured, 'will absolutely conceal any facial blemish . . . absolutely defies detection . . . will remain perfect for hours without being touched . . . prevents excessive perspiration and kills its odor.' The advertisement was accompanied by a large photograph of Gaby Deslys, laden with pearls and feathers, chin resting on the back of her hand, smiling coyly at the reader, and advising all women to use Le Secret.

BEAUTY AND HEALTH

In spite of frequent warnings from medical men and exposés in newspapers and magazines, women continued to gamble with their health and what beauty they had in order to look younger and more attractive. There were the paraffin injections which went wrong, resulting in unsightly lumps in the wrong places; there were skinning treatments which resulted in near-fatal infections; and there were operations which caused permanent disfigurement. A reporter for

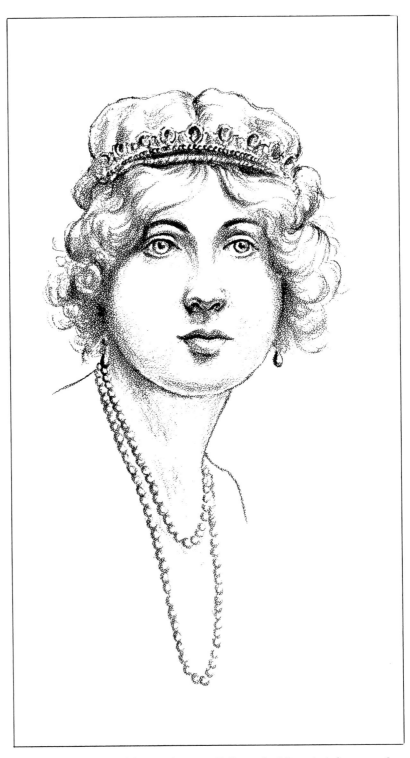

FIG. 201 : Girl with false pearls, 1913. Full, rosebud lips, dark brows, and light skin were fashionable.

the *Ladies Home Journal*, writing in 1912, tells of a young girl who, dissatisfied with the paleness of her complexion, entrusted herself to the skill of a 'beauty doctor who . . . possessed a secret of injecting into the cheeks a carmine fluid that would lend them forever the pale tint of the pink rose. . . . The fluid was injected. But it did not confine itself to the cheeks. The red colouring spread over the girl's entire face and neck. Moreover, innumerable disfiguring pimples began to appear.' In the end the girl's complexion was permanently ruined and her fiancé broke their engagement because it was clear that the young lady lacked 'those qualities which should be possessed by the wife of a man who has to earn his living'.

Despite the increase in the use of cosmetics in the United States, there were no effective government regulations to prevent misleading advertising or the inclusion of harmful substances. The government had little interest in the ingredients of a product so long as they were accurately acknowledged on the label. In 1911, as a result of a case of poisoning, some Klintho Cream was confiscated; but as soon as the manufacturer removed the words 'Absolutely harmless' from the label, the dangerous product was back on the market with the government's implied blessing. The following year another case of a woman having trouble with the same product was reported. When her face had become inflamed, she consulted her physician, who prescribed an ointment of iodide of potash. This reacted with the mercury in the cream, turning the woman's face a flaming vermilion, whereupon she consulted a second physician. The sulphur ointment he prescribed, coming into contact with the mercury, turned her skin black.

Sartoin Skin Food, manufactured in Dayton, Ohio, a product guaranteed to produce 'a soft velvety tint on the roughest of skins . . . the most effective remedy known to science for sunburn, rashes, and all skin blemishes', proved to be a mixture of Epsom salts and pink dye.

The manufacturer of Madame Yale's various beauty lotions and tonics was evidently strong on imagination and finance and weak on chemistry. The Madame Yale Excelsior Complexion Bleach, which was claimed to 'create natural beauty' and 'purify the entire skin, penetrating its remotest recesses', at a cost of two dollars per bottle, was merely a solution of borax in orange water — estimated cost, six cents. Excelsior Skin Food was a mixture of vaseline and zinc oxide coloured with pink dye and perfumed. It sold for a dollar and a half and cost about three cents. Madame Yale's Blush of Youth, according to the copy-writer, was 'as refreshing as concentrated dew, pure as purity. It overcomes all inactivity and imperfections of the skin and underlying structure; spiritualizes the expression and gives countenances the glow, luster, and beauty of child-hood, and preserves the morning of life indefinitely'. It was a mixture of water, alcohol, and glycerine, perfumed and dyed. It cost about nine cents to make and sold for three dollars.

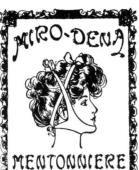

MENTONNIERE
(CHIN SUPPORTER)

A marvelous patented French invention — the one device which will positively prevent or overcome the double chin, the drooping mouth, the lines about the nose and mouth and the wilted throat. It also insures proper normal breathing and prevents throat affections caused by mouth breathing.

It is made of a special knitted fabric, both comfortable and durable, and *has no rubber to overheat, wilt, shrivel or wrinkle the skin.* It is the one Chin Supporter which always holds securely to the head.

MIRO-DENA
POUDRE LIQUIFIÈE

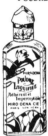

An incomparable preparation that gives a delicately clear and velvety whiteness to the face, neck and arms. More lasting than powder, and an invaluable adjunct for the day or the evening toilet.

MIRO-DENA
ROUGE VÉGÉTAL

A wonderful vegetable rouge which produces a blood coloring so perfectly true to nature as to absolutely defy detection. Shades for Brunette and Blonde.

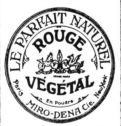

Procurable at high-class Toilet Goods Departments and Drug Stores. Pamphlets mailed upon application.

MIRO-DENA CIE.

373 Fourth Avenue, New York

FIG. 202: Advertisement from *Vogue*, 1913.

With the enactment of more effective regulatory laws, the government did finally take action against the products. It is reported that a department store salesgirl, upon being asked for one of the Madame Yale lotions, told the customer, with some apparent indignation, that the products had become very difficult to obtain because the government had done something to Madame Yale.

The author of an article on patching, published in 1912, recalled having noticed, when visiting the mother of the Aga Khan in Bombay, 'that she and her ladies not merely had painted, but also wore a patch on the lower part of their forehead and held in their hands a patch-box made of tortoiseshell to renew those which in that damp climate fell so easily'.

Dresser sets were considered almost essential in 1912, and a twelve-piece one of imitation ivory, monogrammed and selling for twenty-five dollars, contained a mirror, clothes brush, hat brush, hair brush, comb, nail polisher, shoe horn, shoe buttoner, nail file, cuticle knife, soap box, and powder box. It was recommended for summer use or for travelling since it was lighter in weight than silver and did not require polishing.

THE GENTLEMAN OF 1912

It was customary in many periods for men to perfume the hair and beard, and frequently this was more in the nature of a necessity than a luxury. But with Puritanism gradually blanketing the Western world, it was considered not quite proper for men to smell noticeably pleasant. Conformists settled for a decently masculine smell of tobacco, which many women seemed to find attractive. The prejudice against scent for men was not easy to root out, but the early years of the twentieth century saw a beginning. In 1908 the *Barbers' Journal* reported that 'the custom by men of using extracts upon the handkerchief and of faintly scenting the hair and *mustaches* began anew in England about five years ago, after nearly a generation of abstemiousness in the matter of fragrance. This fashion has attained suddenly large proportions in this country. Whereas three years ago the big perfumers were engaged in merely supplying a staple amount of certain extracts and cologne water for men who have a way of clinging to their own fancies no matter what fashions rule, now they are vying with one another in the endeavor to produce some distinct novelty in fragrance which will captivate the masculine fancy. Enormous quantities of cologne water are being sold to men as well as an ever increasing quantity of extracts. So far sachets have been tabooed by them, save in rare cases; but there are men unable to resist the alluring, evanescent aroma of a dainty sachet.'

But it was not really until after mid-century that a wide variety of men's

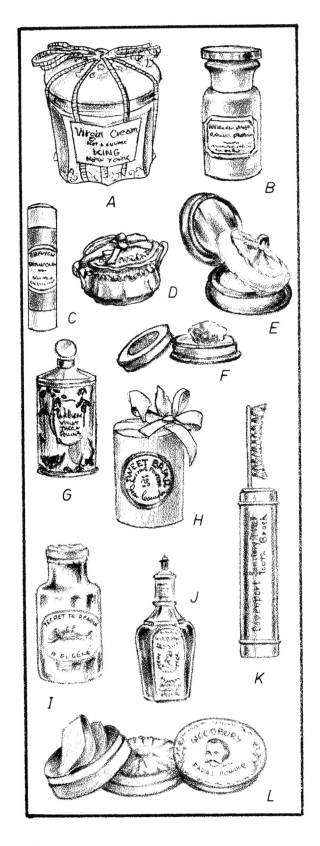

PLATE 22 : TWENTIETH CENTURY
1907–1911

A   1907. King's Virgin Cream — 'A Marvellous Skin Food and Tissue Builder'.

B   1907. Harriet Hubbard Ayer's Wrinkle Eradicator. Price, $3.

C   1907. Crayon Brillerose pour les Ongles. Stick nail polish.

D   1907. La Belle Coquette. Rouge pomade in rose-garlanded Limoges pot, by Harriet Hubbard Ayer. Price, $2.

E   1911. Silver-plated vanity case sent for 16 cents in stamps to the purchaser of a can of Williams' Talc Powder.

F   1915. Rouge paste 'from an Old Southern formula', to be applied with a sponge.

G   1911. Williams' Violet Talcum Powder in 4 scents — Violet, Carnation, Rose, and Karsi.

H   1907. Sweet Briar Dusting Powder by Jean Carrington. Price, 50 cents.

I   1911. Monte Christo Secret of Beauty. Liquid complexion powder.

J   1911. Dr Benach's Spearmint Tooth Elixer — 'As Refreshing as a Plunge in the Surf'. Price, 25 cents.

K   1911. Davenport Sanitary Pocket Tooth Brush. Nickel plate, 75 cents; silver plate, $1.

L   1911. Woodbury's Facial Powder with 'Double Box and Free Chamois'. Price, 25 cents.

PLATE 23 : TWENTIETH CENTURY
1913–1920

A   1913. Rigaud Talcum in glass bottle, scented with Mary Garden perfume.

B   1918. Jonteel Talc in black can with red, yellow, green, and violet parrot. Face powder and cold cream also available.

C   1918. Cutex Cuticle Remover.

D   1913. Dorin cake rouge in blue and gold box. Brunette, Framboise, and other shades.

E   1918. Rigaud Rouge, scented with Mary Garden perfume, 'in dainty vanity case with puff and mirror'. Price, 50 cents.

F   1919. Dorin liquid rouge, Paris.

G   1917. Gold powder compact. Price, $5.

H   1919. Paris and Boston. Talcum, face powder, and liquid rouge by Jardin. Available in Jardin de Lilas or Jardin de Rose.

I   1917. Lipstick in gold case. Price, $3.

J   1917, French. Marquise de Sévigné face powder. Price, $1.50.

K   1919. Pompeian Day Cream (vanishing) and Pompeian Bloom (rouge). The rouge was available in light, medium, and dark.

L   1917. Ivory powder box from an eleven-piece dressing-table set. Bonwit Teller, New York.

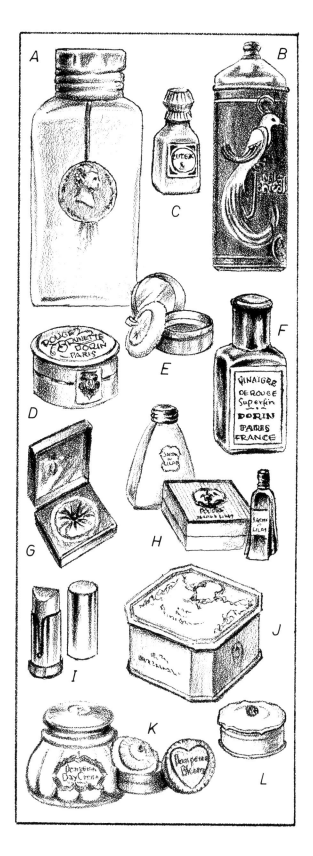

colognes with masculine names and masculine bottles began to flood the open market. And so long as they appeared to be designed exclusively for men, they met with very little resistance.

A newspaper article printed in the summer of 1912 and reprinted in the *Barbers' Journal* gives some interesting sidelights on the gentleman of the period:

'To begin with men like to smell sweet. Being ashamed to purchase perfume, they buy hair tonic. The shelf in front of every barber's chair looks like the buffet of a fancy drink fiend. . . . Having had his hair cut as he wants it, the man then has a shampoo. . . . There is the egg shampoo, the prepared egg shampoo, the tar shampoo, the patent preparation shampoo, and a combination of any of these shampoos, such as the tar and egg shampoo, and others. . . . After a man has been shaved and massaged, has had his hair cut and has been shampooed, he is ready for the finishing touches. All that has gone before is just a groundwork on which what is to follow is built.

'Suppose a man lacks color, his cheeks are white and have not the healthy peachy bloom of the simple life. The barber rubs his cheeks with rouge or a liquid preparation and colors them in this fashion.

'Suppose that the lips are not red enough or the skin on the lips is not soft, the barber rubs them with a lipstick or treats them with various softening and healing preparations.

'Suppose there are not eyebrows enough or those that are there are not dark enough. The barber either paints in new eyebrows or colors up the old colorless ones.

'Suppose the mustache is not quite brilliant enough or stiff enough. It is long enough, perhaps, but it drops and has not that jaunty, bristling, cock's-comb appearance that is admired in men's mustaches. The barber rubs it with a liquid preparation which makes it brilliant, stiff, bristly, and beautiful.

'Suppose any part of the facial geography is too red. The nose may be flowering like the scarlet geranium or the ears may be too encarmined. The barber treats the offending parts with a preparation which takes the color out of the skin.

'There are many other little processes, such as removing pimples and so on, that the man orders before the barber is through with his face. When all the small details have been attended to he usually has a rub with some sort of scented toilet water. . . .

'Having had his head and face beautified one would think that the man would be satisfied — satisfied, at least, that he had been made as pretty as the barber shop could make him. But not so. The modern barber shop has a manicure girl — many of them — and the modern man must have his fingers prettified before he trusts himself on the street alone. . . .

'The wig shop is a minor place in which the vanity of men is to be seen.

Many men wear wigs, though women do not suspect it. Many men dye their hair too. More dye their mustaches.'

NEW PRODUCTS, 1913

'The little boxes of hard powder, each with its tiny puff,' wrote the beauty editor of *Vogue* in 1913, 'have become almost indispensable to womankind.' These were first packaged in cardboard boxes (Plate 22-L), then in metal, complete with a puff and a mirror in the cover (Plate 22-E). Dry rouge cakes (Plate 23-D-E-K) had gone through the same packaging development. For years white, pink, and rachel powder had seemed adequate for any feminine complexion, but now new shades were being added — mauve, ochre, orange. And for the first time, cakes of powder and rouge were being packaged in a single box with puffs and mirror.

Other new items to help fill up a lady's purse were a three-inch celluloid tube containing a stick of rose nail polish and a celluloid nail file (price, 18 cents), a miniature celluloid hand mirror with a compartment in the back for a powder puff (price, 65 cents), and a moiré silk vanity case containing a powder puff and an oval mirror hung from a ribbon.

BEAUTY SECRETS OF THE FAMOUS

The beauty secrets of famous actresses were always in demand, and any cosmetic used by Sarah Bernhardt was naturally of interest to women on both sides of the Atlantic. The ingredients of her famous Beauty Bath were reported to be two pounds of barley, a pound of rice, six pounds of bran, two pounds of oatmeal, and a half pound of lavender. These were boiled in two quarts of water for an hour, then strained. The liquid, along with an ounce each of borax and bicarbonate of soda, was added to the water. Another recipe for Bernhardt's Beauty Bath called for a half pound of marshmallow flowers, a quarter pound of hyssop, and four pounds of bran put directly into the bath water.

There was also a Bernhardt Wrinkle Eradicator, requiring alum, almond milk, and rose water. This was to be bottled and used when needed.

In 1914 Madame Lina Cavalieri revealed her beauty secrets in a 317-page book full of advice and recipes. The dressing room, she advised, should be equipped with a large mirror, well-lighted, in order to expose every blemish. The table and the mirror frame, even if home-made and very plain, should always be white in order to give an effect of daintiness and cleanliness. 'Some women,' she wrote, 'have a fancy for draping their dressing tables in muslin or silk tied back with ribbons, or in silk finished by tassels of the same shade, each to match the

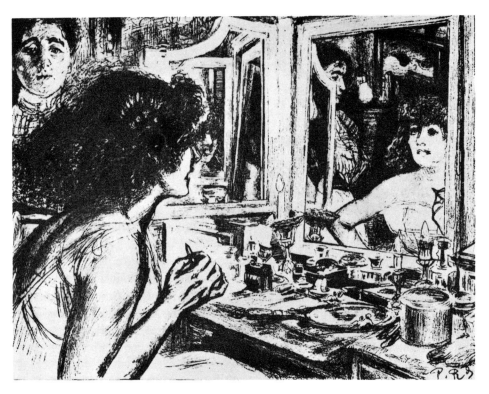

FIG. 203 : Finishing touches. Sarah Bernhardt at her dressing-table before a performance of *La Femme de Claude*.

curtains at the windows and the draperies of the bed. . . . Draperies are elegant, but besides their elegance I always see their other significance — that of dust traps. In furnishing rooms I try to put the money into rich woods **and rugs and** shun draperies. . . .

'On most dressing tables we see a brush and comb, This is the worst possible place for them. Perhaps they are there merely for ornament, to complete a handsome ivory or silver or gold set and give the spectator a sense of the completeness of the table furnishings. But the comb and brush that are in use should be carefully kept in a drawer of the dressing table or in a toilet closet, or in one of the medicine chests with which bathrooms are now supplied. . . .

'The toilet table should be furnished also with a tray or box containing the manicure utensils. The orangewood stick should be ready for cleansing the nails and pushing back the skin that is anxious to encroach upon the nails. In a drawer there should be a package of medicated cotton. In a flask on the toilet table there should be a little peroxide of hydrogen. This not to "touch up the hair", but to serve two worthier purposes. The orangewood stick wrapped round with a bit of the cotton and dipped into the peroxide — or better, the peroxide poured upon it—will quickly cleanse the end of the nail that has been darkened by dust. The peroxide is also valuable for a gargle, or to give the mouth one of the frequently necessary baths.

'In one of the little silver or ivory or enameled boxes, of which a toilet table cannot have too many, there should be a little powdered pumice stone. When the daily scrutiny reveals dark stains upon or between the teeth, apply this pumice stone by dipping an orangewood stick or a hard round toothpick into it and gently rubbing with them the stained surface. . . .

'One of the toilet bottles on my dressing table I always keep filled with rosewater. This is soothing when the face is fevered, and is always grateful and healing to the skin. In another bottle I keep a strong toilet vinegar to inhale or to sprinkle about my neck to revive me when I am fatigued.'

The toilet vinegar she used was compounded from an eighteenth-century recipe calling for honey, vinegar, isinglass, nutmeg, and shredded red sandalwood. In one of her little boxes she kept home-made pastilles of pulverized licorice, vanilla sugar, and gum arabic. Also on her dressing table was a powder box with powder made from rice flour, rice starch, carbonate of magnesia, powdered boric acid, orris root, essence of bergamot, and essence of citron, as well as a nasal atomizer, which, she said, no toilet table was complete without. The toilet table was, in fact, incomplete without all of the 'creams and other remedies which personal experience has taught you are best suited for your skin'. It is probably just as well that she kept her brush and comb in a drawer.

Madame Cavalieri used Elizabeth of Hungary's face cream, Sarah Bernhardt's skin tonic, and a recipe from a Turkish harem, requiring sweet almond oil, white wax, spermaceti, powdered benzoin, tincture of ambergris, and pulverized rice. She was very suspicious of beauty preparations sold commercially. 'Never use preparations in or upon the eyes,' she warned, 'unless you have them analyzed. Do not count the cost of analysis. What are a few American dollars or French francs or Italian lire compared with beauty! Never use any toilet article without such analysis. And even after you have used the preparation for a time, it is wise to again submit it to another analysis, for when an article has secured its vogue through excellence I am sorry to say that manufacturers oftentimes increase their profits by cheapening the ingredients and adulterating the article.'

She did not recommend any sort of makeup for the eyes. The lips, she said, should be a deep pink or a light red, at least three shades lighter than the blood.

In October the editor of *The Queen*'s beauty column advised a correspondent identified only as 'Snowdrop', that Mrs Adair in New Bond Street could supply a perfectly safe 'cream for improving the size and contour of the bust'. But Snowdrop was advised not to attempt any form of massage without expert advice. The cream was also recommended for 'scraggy, thin necks'. Mrs Adair's Ganesh Diable skin tonic was suggested for puffiness under the eyes. For extreme cases ladies were advised to resort to Mrs Adair's anti-puff lotion.

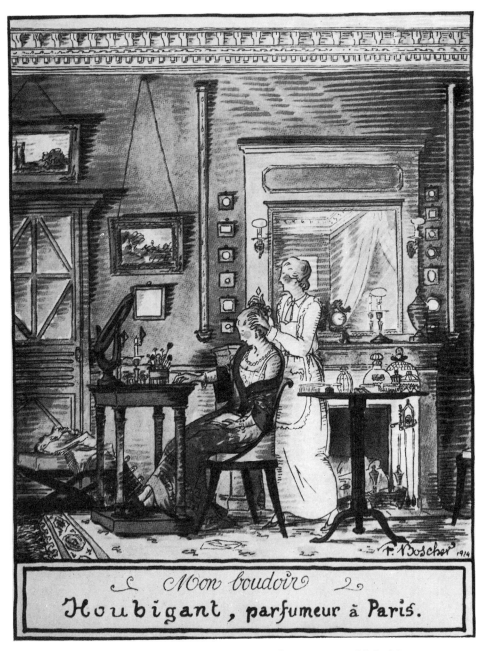

FIG. 204: Mon boudoir, 1914. From an Houbigant advertisement published in 1925.

For those wanting an inexpensive protective cream, Crême Simon was available from the local chemist for a shilling a jar. Other available creams and lotions were Crême Veloutée ('Creates a pure and beautiful skin and keeps it soft as velvet'), Lotion D'Or ('Prevents and cures open pores, blackheads, pimples, and greasiness of the skin'), and Crowsfeet Pasta ('Obliterates crowsfeet and strengthens the muscles round the eyes').

Perfumes and Cosmetics, 1915

Even as late as 1915 recipes for leaves of rouge (rouge *en feuilles*) or rouge papers were published. These were circular discs of paper covered with carmine containing sufficient gum acacia to make the colour adhere to the paper. In using the papers, one had to breathe on the rouge, then rub cotton on it in order to transfer the colour to the face.

George Askinson, in *Perfumes and Cosmetics*, recommended a liquid rouge containing ammonia, carmine, essence of rose, and rose water. After about ten days of maceration and shaking and a few more days for settling, the liquid rouge was ready to be decanted. It was used largely for the lips.

For a paste rouge, usually sold in shallow porcelain dishes, Askinson suggested a mixture of carmine, talcum, and gum acacia. An alternative recipe, giving a greenish metallic lustre to the rouge, called for carthamin (1 ounce), talcum powder (1 pound), gum acacia (1½ ounces), and oil of rose (15 grains).

Still another recipe, which Askinson claimed was exactly like the Austrian *schnouda*, required only mixing 75 grains of moistened alloxan with 1 pound of cold cream. The result was a white cream which gradually turned red after application.

Evidently there was still some demand for blue pencils for painting the veins, for Askinson retained the following recipe in the 1915 edition of his book:

> Venetian chalk....................1 pound
> Berlin blue......................1¾ ounces
> Gum acacia.........................1 ounce

To the powdered solids add sufficient water to form a mass to be rolled into sticks. For use, a pencil is breathed on, rubbed against the rough side of a piece of white glove leather, and the veins are marked with the adhering color on the skin coated with pearl white. Of course, some dexterity is required to make the veins appear natural by use of this blue color.

The Askinson book also contained recipes for toilet oatmeal, whitening cream, skin food for hands, nail enamel, nail powder, nail polish (wax), nail varnish, rice powder, pearl powder, violet powder, rose powder, pistachio powder, musk paste, skin gloss, beard wax, whisker dye, pearl water, freckle milk, skin lotion, anti-kink hair pomade, and other cosmetic preparations.

There was intense competition among face powders, and each manufacturer managed to find some reason why his was better than the others. The Henry Tetlow Company took the approach that a general toilet or talcum powder was 'not suitable for use as a face powder. Such powders, although usually pure and harmless, do not have the qualities of Henry Tetlow's Gossamer or other high-grade face powders. HENRY TETLOW's GOSSAMER is soft and "feathery." It contains ingredients that actually soften and nourish the skin, while talcum powder is simply neutral and inert. Henry Tetlow's Gossamer is translucent, allowing the natural color of the skin to show through. It never rubs shiny.' Henry Tetlow's Gossamer was made in White, Flesh, Pink, Cream, and Brunette. Colonial Dame face powder, on the other hand, promised to give 'impalpable bloom' and 'youthful lustre'. Lady Mary face powder (Figure 205) was 'so skillfully blended that each single soft flake of it exhales the fragrance of wonderful flowers', Marinello powder protected one against wind and sun, and Azurea imparted 'that youthful charm'. Djer-Kiss contented themselves with saying that 'There is much good powder — but *smart* powder is *French*'.

Most of the books of powder-papers had lost their popularity by 1915, and *Vogue* had found something new and better — 'a sterile pad of soft fiber that will not shake loose powder upon hands or clothing but will yield just the right amount when wiped or tapped against the skin. . . . The little packet measures two inches square and is very thin and is supposed to last one day. The pad is made up of several layers so that each layer can be removed as it becomes soiled'. There were five shades of powder available — white, flesh, cream, pink, and lavender, sold in packets of 14, 30, 42, 60, and 75, ranging in price from 25 cents to $1.25. Twenty-five pads of rouge could be bought for 50 cents (4 shillings). For a little extra, one could obtain either rouge or powder packets with no printing other than a monogram, from either one's personal die or an original design supplied by the company. For use as gifts, fabric-covered containers for the packets could be obtained in white, rose, blue, lavender, gold, or a flowered design.

A cosmetics package available for the Christmas season contained a jar of skin-renewing cream, another of rose-coloured paste, and a third of a white paste to take the place of powder — all supposedly from old Southern recipes handed down for generations. The rouge was sponged on and allowed to dry, then the whole face covered with a sponging of the white paste. The result was supposed to be a complexion 'delicately tinted . . . without a hint of makeup'. Each box also contained a package of sterilized papers for removing the makeup.

A weekend toilet box, recommended as a suitable gift for oneself or a very

FIG. 205: Advertisement from *Vogue*, 1915.

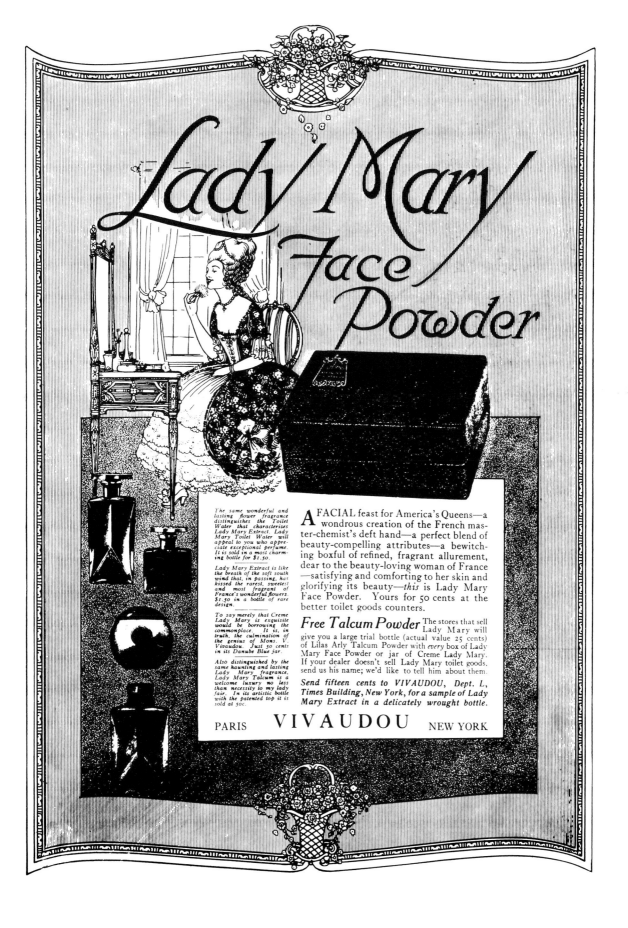

dear friend, contained several packages of sterilized gauze, a chamois cloth, 'little powdered tabs to take on a walk or a drive', a toothbrush, toothpaste, a nail file, nail polish, a lipstick, liquid rouge, an eyebrow pencil, a celluloid box of compressed powder with puff, talcum powder, soap, 'a wee sterilized puff', a tube of cream, a box of variegated beauty spots, and a mirror. The box was made of leatherette, lined with white oilcloth, and with its contents a lady would be prepared for almost anything.

The first American-made lipsticks and eyebrow pencils, both in simple slide tubes, are believed to have been made in 1915. These were probably the first metal containers for makeup.

Scarcely a decade had passed since *Vogue* had approached the delicate question of makeup with caution and even, at times, a note of apology. But caution had long since vanished when in 1915 the beauty editor wrote that 'To sit before her dressing-table at the end of a long full day in preparation for a long gay evening and be able to disregard those artificial means to youth, the rouge pot and the lip stick, is the privilege of only a few women, especially during the strenuous winter season. Naturally bright eyes, rosy cheeks, and red lips are relinquished to youth with sighs regretful but resigned, and the matron turns to the dressing-table, her high altar, where she performs those mysterious ceremonies which double her natural beauty'.

Inquiries to 'The Toilet' column in *The Queen* continued, with answers addressed to Pinkie, Iolanthe, Blue Bird, Kitty from Cork, The Last Hope, and many others. Iolanthe, it seems, had 'little red veins' which distressed her, Constance's hair was getting very thin in places, Grannie wanted a transformation which wouldn't make her look too young and fashionable, Red Cross suffered from 'flabbiness of face', and Norseland wanted to be rid of some puffiness under the eyes. All were told where to go for assistance and how much they would have to pay. Help was available, in many cases, for as little as four or five shillings.

Three months later, in an issue which showed a photograph of the Duchess of Bedford posing proudly with a large number of dead fish, Gladioli wanted to get rid of hair from the face, Tee's white hair was going yellow, Rosie blushed too much, and Shylock wanted to 'redden the lips in such a way that the colour will not come off easily'. Shylock was advised to try a 'simply splendid cosmetic called Labyl', which not only reddened the lips but plumped them up as well. It was made by Mrs Hemmings and was procurable from Cyclax for four shillings and sixpence.

A Trip to New York

In the autumn of 1915 there appeared in the *Delineator* a series of articles on current cosmetic habits of fashionable American women, written from the point of view of an unsophisticated young lady making her first trip to New York to visit a well-to-do cousin on Fifth Avenue:

'Parker—Cousin Margaret's maid—has just left me with my face covered with cold-cream and with strict orders to keep quiet while she prepares the "steamer and vibrator." Doesn't it sound mysterious?—a steamer and a vibrator! And it really is all so wonderful that I am afraid I shall not tell half unless I start very near the beginning.

'Cousin Margaret met me at the station, looking prettier and, my dear! younger than ever, after all these years. I had no time to wonder, for porters seemed to spring from everywhere; and in a few minutes Cousin Margaret, I and my various belongings were stowed away in her car and we were whisked off.'

After getting settled in her own suite full of sunshine, plants, and flowered chintz, she stretches out in a Morris chair in front of the fire, and Parker, the maid, takes over:

'When Parker had put a towel behind my head and let my hair down, I was firmly ordered to close my eyes and try to relax; but through one narrow crack I peeped at what was going on. A small linen-covered table had on it mysterious bottles, jars, bowls and pieces of linen and cotton batting. The tyrant shook my hair out and gently massaged my scalp, muttering about "young girls that never know when they have a decent head of hair and abuse it—as if a gentlewoman should ever travel with her head uncovered—without at least a veil to protect it from the cinders, which ruin the hair."

'When I was allowed to go into the bathroom a most delicious perfume, like lemon verbena, greeted me, which proved to be a soothing but stimulating bath salt. I was ordered to scrub my body as much as I liked, but to leave my face and neck alone unless I "wished to look like an old woman in a year or two". . . . Then she rubbed my cheeks, neck and eyes with a piece of ice wrapped in a linen cloth, very gently dried the skin and dusted me over with powder, shook out my hair and let me look in the glass, and I agreed with her muttered: "It may be possible to make something of Madam's young cousin after all".'

As the second installment begins, our wide-eyed young lady has just been having a shampoo. 'First I must tell you about the shampoo, for it's quite new to me. Parker, the maid, used, instead of an every-day toilet soap such as I usually seize upon in my haste, or a prepared shampoo, melted Castile soap. Then she rinsed this off with a strong infusion of camomile tea. The effect was very softening and seemed to bring out the color and gloss wonderfully. . . . Camomile tea is a refreshing drink, also. To make it one has only to buy ten

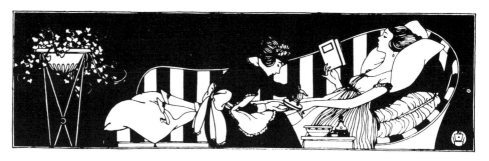

FIG. 206: Lady being manicured by her maid. From the *Delineator*, 1919.

cents' worth of camomile flowers, pour a big coffee-cup of boiling water over half of them, and steep them well. You can flavor the tea with a little sugar and perhaps lemon-juice if it seems insipid. . . .

'One of the delights of being under Parker's ministrations are the constant surprises. The other day she brought me some lip-salve that is quite the best I ever used. . . . This is the formula: Let three ounces of oil of almonds and a half ounce of alkanet soak together in a warm place until the oil is colored, then strain. Melt one and a half ounces of white wax, and half an ounce of sperma-ceti with the oil, until it begins to thicken, and add twelve drops of attar of roses. . . .

'By the way, I had to stop before I had half finished my last month's article. I meant to tell about the most wonderful treatment of the face with mud! . . . The specialist was installed in Cousin Margaret's dressing-room, surrounded with much that was mysterious. I was consumed with curiosity, so I was delighted to learn that Cousin Margaret was to be done first. The wind, sun and dust, combined with a rather strenuous three days in the country, had resulted in showing up undiscovered lines in her face that for the first time made her look her age. . . . A towel was pinned over her hair and then the skin-cleansing cream was rubbed into every crevice of her face and neck and carefully wiped off with a soft piece of cheese-cloth. Next, a delicious, smooth cold cream was rubbed in. . . .

'After the skin had been thoroughly massaged she produced a jar in which was a sort of wet clay—later, when my turn came, I found that it was not at all disagreeable, as it was quite warm when applied and was not put on so thick that I could not move. The effect was a gentle but decided astringent. Every-thing but my nostrils, eyes and mouth was covered, and the feeling was as if they were making a death-mask of my face.

'Cousin Margaret kept her mask on for an hour, but mine, owing to my youthful skin, only remained on for twenty minutes. The process of removing the "pack" was delightful. Basins of warm water were brought and cloths dipped in it were gently passed over my face and neck until every particle of mud was removed; then a pad dipped in ice-water was applied and my face was gently dried. After that a liquid astringent smelling like fresh violets was allowed to dry on the skin, followed by a lotion which is to soothe the skin. A final dusting of powder made our skin look so fresh and rested that I laughed aloud when I looked at myself in the mirror. . . .

'I must not forget to tell you about the "bath bags," for this was a new experience. When the water was drawn Parker produced a cheese-cloth bag filled with all sorts of herbs—a preparation that is used by Sarah Bernhardt and is too delicious for words. It soothes one delightfully, and at the same time tones up the system. . . . In my next talk I must tell about my manicuring experience, and some other things I've found out. It is most smart, by the bye, to affect one special perfume—an individual one if you can get it—using it for your sachets and clothes-hangers and all your possessions. As the French say, It gives one so much more *cachet*.'

BATHROOMS AND BOUDOIRS

The latest idea for the boudoir was French vitrines or glass cabinets in which to display fans, jewelery, shoes, cosmetics, or anything else that was considered displayable. V*ogue* described a vitrine which it thought would be particularly handsome atop a Louis XV commode, as having a metal framework enamelled in rose, with space beneath the curved top for a flower. V*ogue* found it 'easy to imagine the charming frivolity of the rose cabinet when it is filled with perfume jars, rouge pots, and powder boxes such as are designed by the group of Paris artists who do not scorn to place their artistic gifts at the service of feminine elegance.'

'The modern bathroom,' said V*ogue* in 1915, 'is most luxurious and usually harmonizes with the general tone of the suite to which it belongs.' The Editor then described one with Louis XIV influence as being entirely panelled with mirrors, with a 'canopy of cream lace over blue silk, gathered with garlands of pink satin roses and green leaves, over a crystal drop-light. The sunken bath of Italian marble has gold-plated faucets in the form of dragons. A long slab of marble with gold-plated supports has, besides the basin, room on each side for all the articles of the toilet; these are in gold-topped bottles, powder boxes, soap cases, and such things. There is a tendency now to use crystal appointments in the place of gold or silver appointments, and fascinating bottles, bowls, and jars are being designed for this purpose. White fur mats, to be replaced by the softest of bath mats, relieve the cold of the tiled floor.' V*ogue* also described the actual taking of the bath :

'While Madame is taking her early cup of coffee, the maid sees that the fires are lighted in the dressing-rooms and that the bath is drawn. Into the bath are often put some of those delicious bath crystals that have the effect of invigorating, or others that perhaps reduce. Some of these salts have wonderful properties; in any case they soften the water and perfume the bathroom, and this is delightful.

'Towels of every degree of softness or roughness are placed before the fire in the dressing-room. Towels that are as large as sheets are used to swath the body, while narrower towels are used to get up the necessary friction. Many Englishwomen use a small towel made of knitted tape; this makes a towel that retains to the end of its existence the roughness that is so important in promoting the circulation. When the big bowl of fragrant bath soap, the special cake of soap made with a curve on one side so as to fit conveniently into the hollow of the hand, and the bath sponges, and all, are in readiness, Madame is assisted into a bath-robe with mules to match, and proceeds to the bath.'

Then the maid puts a rubber cape on her mistress, regulates the faucets, wraps her in a warm bath sheet when she is finished, dries her off and rubs her down, applies a lotion, and finally dusts her with bath powder. After that, Madame relaxes in a reclining chair with her feet in a white fur bag while the maid massages her face and does her hair and a manicurist and a chiropodist do the rest. 'Such a regime may seem very arduous,' concludes *Vogue* sympathetically, 'but thus must one pay the price of being beautiful.'

PRETTY POISONS

According to *Everybody's Magazine* in December 1915, fifty million dollars' worth of cosmetics were being sold annually in the United States. 'Yet,' the magazine points out, 'there is little effective legislation to prevent the manufacturers — who are men — from poisoning and defrauding their women customers.

'Large numbers of "skin-foods" examined by scientific friends of womankind have been found to contain large quantities of wood alcohol. It is a poison of great dangerousness. Large numbers of "beauty-washes" and "face-enamels" have been found to be heavily loaded with "flake white". This is really carbonate of lead, a poison so violent that it produces a disease with a name of its own—"plumbism". . . . Many "wrinkle lotions" are selling at two to four dollars a pound. They consist of Epsom salts. You can buy a pound of Epsom salts for five cents.

'Population in the United States, from 1900–1910, increased twenty per cent. The sale of cosmetics — including skin-bleaches and toilet-vinegars and the rest

—increased one hundred per cent. We have maintained in these pages that social reform and political activity are not de-feminizing our female citizens. The United States Public Health Service proves that we were right.'

IN DEFENCE OF MAKEUP

In *McClure's Magazine* in 1916, Richard Le Gallienne defended the use of makeup. Referring to a friend who refused to go out with a girl because she was wearing powder, he wrote:

'I suppose that there are other human anachronisms like my friend still existing here and there, survivals from the days of the thumb-screw and the ducking-stool, but they must be very lonely, and I hardly know where they would look for wives. For, of all the ages in the world, this would seem to be the age of the powder puff and the vanity-box. . . . It is, I think, for the most part an innocent vanity. The innocence of the powder-puff has been discovered. One remembers from old novels, and indeed from novels not so very old, what a stir used to be made by the advent in a prim village community of some pretty lady, who must be very naughty and "French", because it was evident that she powdered; or — horrors! — even painted.

'And, indeed, one does occasionally encounter a pretty woman who retains a curious moral objection to the powder-puff, and who, even in summer heat, prefers her face to shine with its natural emollient. It is the old Puritan fear of ribbons and laces still in the blood. Happily, for the eyes of the beholder, these feminine throw-backs are rare, and the fair majority are more considerate in avoiding the "jar" to those "in front" which comes of a skin whose imperfections a touch of powder would decently cover. For it is not necessarily vanity that brings out the powder-puff, but a courteous regard for the esthetic sensibilities of others. . . . Natural beauty, indeed, may be regarded as so much raw material which the artist has the right to adapt and enhance. Of course, there will always be silly women who think of nothing else but their looks, and there will always be bad artists who over-do the thing. One has too much reason to plead with women for more, rather than less, art in their decorative effects. Perhaps if they were to sign their complexions — as other artists sign their pictures — they would take more care of and pride in them. Certainly some complexions are such masterpieces that one often longs to know the name of the artist.'

In 1916 English women were making their faces pink, white, or cream with Saunders' Face Powder, advertised to preserve 'the Beauty and Freshness of Youth in extreme age', and cleansing their skin with Ven-Yusa, the Oxygen Face Cream, promoted as the 'equivalent of an oxygen bath'. They were filling in their 'scraggy necks' with Mme Verdi's tissuefood and caring for their discoloured teeth with Jewsbury and Brown's toothpaste in pots and tubes. Ladies wanting to turn their hair as white as their teeth were sent to Messrs Dubosch and Gillingham, who also provided transformations with 'clever partings'. While Mrs Adair was selling the Ganesch chin strap for the 'prevention of a double chin at home', Mme Rubinstein was providing single-treatments-with-advice. A thirty-five-year-old woman with ugly, black hairs on her chest by-passed Mme Rubinstein and went straight to *The Queen* for advice. She was told to buy a jar of Haroffe.

ADVICE FROM VOGUE

'Happy is the woman,' wrote *Vogue*'s beauty consultant in 1917, 'who possesses for her dressing-table some old inlaid shell which has become fashionable again. The real shell is almost priceless but, fortunately for the woman of good taste, there is a modern ware of amber celluloid with a very pleasing resemblance to old amber and with an exquisite inlaid border in blue, black, and skilfully inlaid gold and which at once suggests the old-world atmosphere and harmonizes delightfully with any setting. It would be particularly good in a yellow room furnished in mahogany.

'From France come lovely bits of embroidery and lace, yellow with age and rich in their suggestion of the aristocratic old houses to which they once belonged. On a cover made of such a cloth, a toilet-set of this inlaid wood is rich and effective; the set may be bought in a number of pieces. There is a large tray, a small one, a shoe-horn, a large clothes-brush, a hat-brush, a powder-box, and a quaint clock. These, with all the other details of the toilet-set, may be ordered to suit one's taste, and make a charming collection for the dressing-table at a comparatively small cost.'

For the latest in cosmetics *Vogue* recommended two French powders — one which came in a gold vanity case with matching lipstick (see Plate 23-I) and the other in 'a quaint box covered with blue or pink brocade with a little tray to match, and one of those geisha brushes with which Japanese women apply just enough powder'. *Vogue* called the latter 'a particularly pretty conceit'.

For the swimmer who wanted to come out of the water looking her best, there was a liquid waterproof rouge 'so perfect in its results that its bloom cannot be distinguished from that of a healthy skin'. It came in a tube with a tiny silk sponge, both in a rubber-lined silk bag.

Vogue's Shoppers' and Buyers' Guide for October held out hope in abundance for many women — *Pate Grise* ('for aging & ugly hands'), *Ferrol's Magic Skin Food* ('for filling out hollow & wasted necks'), *Undetectable Rouge* ('an interesting & instructive treatise' from the Rosebud Company), and *Olive Robart* ('a

1917 Trial Beauty outfit of Alternating Pat Pat Creams, Spat Spat muscle raiser, San San water softeners, & Poudre Matinee').

For the serviceman overseas, *Vogue* suggested a khaki case containing talcum powder, shaving stick, ribbon dental cream, and a cake of soap in a rubber case, all for sixty cents.

In November Bonwit Teller advertised an eleven-piece ivory dressing-table set with relief carved three-initial monogram for $23.50 (£10). Included were a hair brush, cloth brush, hat brush, mirror, comb, puff box, hair receiver, nail polisher, button-hook, nail file, and combination jewel box and pin cushion. The cushion was available in pink, blue, or old rose velvet. For filling the powder box (see Plate 23-L) they recommended Marquise de Sevigné powder, in Blanche, Rose No. 1, Rose No. 2, Rachel No. 1, Rachel No. 2, Naturelle, Mauve, or Mouresque.

'Even the dressing-table,' wrote the *Vogue* beauty editor in 1918, 'is influenced nowadays by a war income, and simple materials, such as chintzes and quaint cottons, are much used as summer covers for the few toilet accessories that are permissible on the smart dressing-table. In the country house, if white dimity is used for curtains at the window and on the mahogany four poster of the restful and simple bedroom, the necessary touch of colour may be given by the gay cretonne on the dressing-table, used under glass if one prefers. The generously proportioned glass powder-box has a covered top to match, while the glass tray is framed in the cretonne and the various boxes and trinkets are covered to correspond.'

But the following month she described a somewhat more elaborate dressing room 'made from a long rather narrow passageway with a window at one side. At the doorway and the window were used the palest of green glazed chintz with an entertaining design of cerise and brown Chinamen swinging from impossible branches. This was edged with a two-inch binding of cerise taffeta. The walls, painted a soft beige tone, were a pleasant background for an old walnut French dressing-table with its accompanying tall crystal bottles, and a full-length lacquer mirror was painted to exactly harmonize with the cerise of the chintz. A pair of Chinese figurines on black lacquer wall brackets and the smallest of black lacquer screens placed at the doorway leading to the hall, completed a room of great distinction.'

For women who had ivory dresser sets, and they seemed to be the most popular kind to have, Ivory Cream (in a thirty-five cent tube) was designed to remove all discolourations and keep them in perfect condition.

Vogue suggested that after cleansing the face with cream in the morning, one should use a liquid powder with 'a smooth clinging whiteness that in no way resembles an enamel'. It was supposed to have 'the invigorating effect of a tonic'. As a final touch to the makeup, *Vogue* recommended a touch of cream rouge.

Health-Glow Water Proof Rouge, advertised as the 'color of rich glowing blood' and guaranteed to last throughout the day, was available in 'tube form in fancy (silk) case (with application pad) for shopping bag' or in liquid form in bottles. The price in either case was seventy-five cents. Madame Hunting-ford's rouge, paste or dry, was available for fifty cents and her English Beauty Powder for eighty-five cents. Laird's Bloom of Youth ('In Miladi's Boudoir for over 50 years') sold for seventy-five cents.

Advertisements for Dorin's Rouge (Plate 23-D), available in two shades, stressed the appearance of health the rouge would give, as well as its use by conservative women. 'To remove all trace of fatigue,' the reader was advised, 'most women will need also when traveling, a box of Dorin's Rouge Brunette or Rouge Framboise. These compact rouges are so subtle in the shade, so impalpable in fineness that their use is evident only in the effect of health and well being which they produce. Dorin's Compactes are not "make-up" in any ordinary sense. They are first aids to daintiness and beauty used by the most conserva-tive women of France and America. They are valued by women prominent in society and philanthropy, leaders in the learned professions, mothers of families, wholesome college girls and others who appreciate that half the secret of beauty is a fresh and radiant complexion.' In other words, Dorin's Rouge (Brunette or Framboise) seemed ideally suited to all women everywhere. Samples of rouge and powder were available for six cents in stamps.

In spite of the changing times, Papier Poudré was still being advertised. It was available in three shades — white, rose, and rachel. One was advised to look for the word 'Lehcaresor' on the front cover of the book.

For the woman whose nostrils were too wide, *Vogue* suggested a nasal clamp 'formed so as gently to shape the sides of the nose without impeding the breath-ing'. The device was fastened over the ears with an elastic band and 'adjusted over the nose with small screws'. The price was five dollars.

Cyclax of London was offering (in addition to a muscle restorer which did not require exercise) an Instant Beautifier, which was supposed to revive the skin 'immediately, rendering it charmingly white and smooth'. All of this was to be the result of 'a momentary application'. The price was five shillings. One of the specialities of Mrs Adair (of New Bond Street) was Ganesh Lily lotion, a liquid powder, said to be 'extremely good for the skin'. It was made in a variety of shades. And in the same issue of *The Queen* in which these adver-tisements appeared, 'Aunt Alice' complained of 'hair coming out very much on the forehead'. She was advised to get a toupee.

FASHIONS OF 1919

In 1919 women weren't sure whether they wanted to be tan in the summer or not. Celia Caroline Cole, the *Delineator* beauty columnist, thought they should be. 'Just a nice, comfortable, careless tan,' she advised, 'is what every woman ought to have in Summer if she wants to help her skin all she can. It is becoming to nearly every one in light Summer clothes, and it is good for the skin. And you can always take it off in September with very little expense or trouble. . . . But,' she added, 'if you really must be pink-and-white and para-soled, there are one or two good vanishing creams, harmless light rice-powder, and always an astringent and a good, pure bleach you can use.'

In September Mrs Cole set out to reveal 'the innermost secrets of the smartest and most approved New York specialists'. Their secrets for beauty involved a clean skin, plenty of rest, an eye cup (for salt water eye baths), a pair of tweezers (for plucking stray hairs), an eyelash ointment, skin-food, muscle oil, cold cream, and faith. Mrs Cole and the smart specialists appeared to be not quite ready for makeup. And yet only a month later we find her advising 'a touch of the eyelash paste here, a bit of rouge there, possibly a splash of henna or bleach shampoo on top. And there you are, all in harmony and yet all tuned up to a higher key.' On the same page as Mrs Cole's column there is an adver-tisement for Tetlow's Pussywillow Talc de luxe — designed to harmonize with Pussywillow face powder, Pussywillow rouge, and Pussywillow toilette cream. And that represented Pussywillow's complete line of products. A free sample of Pussywillow Face Powder would be sent on request.

Pompeian (Plate 23-K) was one of the big names in cosmetics in 1919. They advertised a Day Cream ('Keeps the skin smooth and velvety'); a Beauty Powder ('Adds a lovely clearness to the skin') in white, brunette, and flesh; Pompeian Bloom ('A rouge that is imperceptible when properly applied') in light, medium, and dark; and a talcum powder. The Pompeian lipstick was yet to come. Each item sold for fifty cents.

In a later column Mrs Cole advised business women always to keep within easy reach 'some absorbent cotton and a small bottle of astringent, and a jar of cold-cream. Wet the cotton in cold water, squeeze it out tight, then wet it with the astringent and the cold cream on top of that and wipe your face with it. Dry it finally with a Japanese tissue; it will pay you to get a package, they're just the thing for an office. If you'll do that, you can sit in an office until you're seventy, and you won't spoil the texture of your skin, and if you can *pat* it morning and night, you'll keep your color too. . . .

'There are lotions that will make that upper lip virgin white, and if you won't want to buy a lotion, put on a certain little mixture of camphor and peroxide and ammonia and keep putting it on. There are cures for liver-spots, and a good petroleum jelly at night and salt-water baths in the day will make eyelashes grow where none ever grew before.'

Mrs Cole's parting words to the working girls of America are probably as appropriate as any in bringing the decade to a close before plunging into the Roaring Twenties:

'As I said at the beginning, I think you're perfectly wonderful. I sing a hymn of praise whenever I think of you and think a little prayer that in the midst of the click of the office now and then you will dream a wee, short dream of ruffled curtains at the window and a blue-and-white kitchen and a cedar-chest and a pale-blue-silk bassinet!'

19 · *The Twentieth Century 1920-1930*

In the gloaming, oh my darling,
When the lights are dim and low,
That your face is powder-painted,
How am I, sweetheart, to know?
Twice this month I've had to bundle
Every coat that I possess,
To the cleaners—won't you, darling,
Love me more and powder less.

ANONYMOUS

'Even the most conservative and prejudiced people,' wrote the beauty editor of *Vogue* in 1920, 'now concede that a woman exquisitely made up may yet be, in spite of seeming frivolity, a faithful wife and a devoted mother. Like eating and speaking and dressing, making up has well-bred and vulgar possibilities. The woman who is innately tasteful will not powder to extreme nor daub her lips with a too vivid crimson. The crudities of a whitewashed face upon which the colour flares out like the spots on a clown's cheeks, appear to her in their true character, discordant, jangling. Conspicuous make-up goes hand in hand with other vulgarities. The woman who uses overwhelming perfumes and too much jewellery, whose voice is a shade too loud, will, inevitably, have her eyebrows shaved to abnormal thinness and contorted shape and her lips painted flamboyantly scarlet. . . .

'The whole art of make-up is first to know oneself. . . . If one's lashes are short and scattered and one's eyes lack particular distinction, a careful darkening of these lashes will give an impression of greater thickness and will add size and depth to the eyes. The rest of the face should be untouched, save for the tasteful dusting of powder. Too much make-up takes away expressiveness from the face. It is far better to make it all lead up to or set off one special feature. If the mouth is well-shaped, an accent of red will enhance its charm and concentrate attention on it. . . . Pretty fingers may be touched with rose to call attention to their slenderness. A dark skin may be made distinctive by a blending powder and a rich red rouge. Too often, dark women powder their faces white and rouge them baby pink, and this produces a most incongruous effect in comparison with the olive colour of their necks and hands.

'There is not a woman living who could not increase her piquancy and charm by a little dash of artificiality, for there is a lure, a fascinating flavour about it, so long as it is elusive. . . . So out upon the dressing-table come the little jars and boxes, and concealment is no longer a necessary act in connection with one's lip-stick. There are so many creams and lotions, rouges and powders

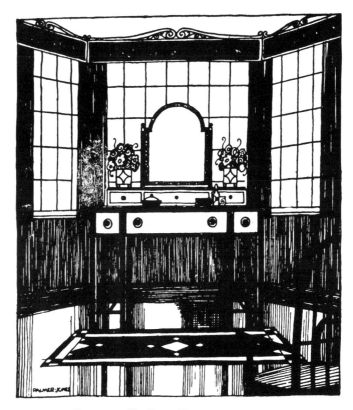

FIG. 207: Dressing-table. From *Vogue*, 1920.

that delight with their little jars and boxes and bottles, that actual knowledge
is necessary to guide one in a choice of cosmetics. . . . If one chooses the best
and uses it well, one may possess — or very nearly possess — the world-sought,
infinitely precious secret of eternal beauty.'

Even men were caught up in the wave of beautification. In 1920 the *Barbers'
Journal* carried a surprising news item for Cleveland: 'It's here at last — the
eyebrow plucking parlor for men. James Macaluse, proprietor of a barber shop
at East 115th Street and Superior Avenue, announced his intention of conduct-
ing a plucking establishment in connection with his regular tonsorial work.
"I've had a number of men come in recently and ask where they could get their
lashes drooped or their brows weeded out and run into nice curves," he said.
"I'll practice on the first one, and then after a time I'll get the knack of pulling
'em out gently," he said.'

In December, readers of *The Queen* were deluged with suggestions for possible
Christmas gifts — toilet sets mounted in enamel from Dickins and Jones, manicure and vanity boxes 'covered with fancy silk and trimmed with gold lace and

miniature silken rosebuds' from Penberthy, hand painted glass and silver powder jars from Harrods, Shem-el-Nessim face powder from Grossmith, and Old English Lavender soap from practically anybody. An Oriental perfume called Phul-nana promised to bring 'the languorous sweetness of the East . . . from the sun-kissed slopes of India . . . to our dull, fog-ridden shores'.

MAKEUP IN 1921

'Not so very long ago,' reminisced *Vogue* in 1921, 'the woman who frankly admitted that face powder was indispensable to her was apt to cause an elevation of conservative eyebrows; while she who went so far as to be even under the suspicion of using rouge was regarded as a person of considerably more than questionable taste. Nowadays, however, the situation is so changed that it has become very nearly imperative for every well-groomed woman to understand the right use, not only of powder, but of rouge, as well.'

Powders were available in such shades as peach, henna, sunburn, Spanish-

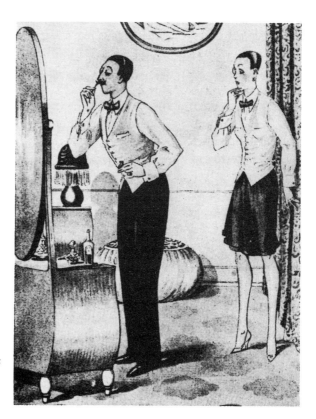

FIG. 208: The moustache comes back! Newspaper caricature, Berlin, 1926.

rachel, flesh, orchid, cream, and pale green, a Paris favourite. V*ogue* suggested that shades be mixed. For a complete makeup they recommended that a foundation cream be smoothed on and wiped off twice and a dark powder applied to the upper part of the face 'to give brilliance to the eyes' and a lighter powder to the lower part. Powder on the neck should match the skin. 'Then a little powdered rouge should be dusted on the cheeks and the whole blended together by a gentle brushing with a tiny brush of softest camel's-hair. The finishing touches are given by deftly brushing the eyelashes and eyebrows and finally by applying an accent of carmine to the lips.'

In October V*ogue* described a method 'for removing tan and other blemishes'. The treatment, in a Fifth Avenue salon (probably Dorothy Gray's), began in a comfortable armchair with one's feet on a soft cushion. Then a thick brownish bleach was spread on the face, neck, and arms and left for about fifteen minutes or until it began to smart, When it was wiped off and a less powerful white paste bleach was spread on and eventually removed. This was followed by an application of 'delicious skin foods', which were patted on 'with a rhythmic, dancing movement of the fingers that race swiftly and lightly over the face and neck'. After about an hour and a half, the lady, now a shade or two lighter, was sent out to face the world with 'the inevitable hint of rouge' on her cheeks and lips and a dusting of peach-coloured powder, carefully brushed out of the lashes and brows. After five or six more treatments, all traces of the suntan should be gone. And so would twenty-five dollars.

In this same year a sample of Hinds Honey and Almond Cream could be had for two cents. And for ten cents one could obtain a Home Try-out Package, containing, in addition, Hinds Cold Cream, Disappearing Cream, Face Powder, and Talcum. Twelve cents in stamps would bring a Glazo Minute Manicure set delivered to one's door.

The motoring enthusiast could obtain, for $76.40 (about £32), a black leather travelling case containing twenty-two preparations 'for the protection of the skin against the ravages of the sun, wind, and dust'. These included a protective lotion, a bleach cream, face powder, lipstick, and liquid, cream, and dry rouge.

The classified advertisements in V*ogue's* Shoppers' and Buyers' Guide for November listed a number of interesting items, including *Dr. Pavlova's Skincharm* ('keeps face perpetually youthful'), *Sagging Cheeks Lifted* ('Device concealed by hair'), *Eyebrow and Eyelash Coloura* ('imparts expression'), *Primavera Company* ('Old World Secret of Invigorating Salts'), *Sara Rejuvenator* ('women will never have lines while using this tonic'), and *Ill Shaped Noses* ('quickly made perfect at home nights'). Then there was the *Roll-Off Reducing Cream* at six dollars per pound — presumably per pound of cream.

In 1921 in London one could buy a Lady's Attaché Dressing Case covered with pigskin, lined with silk, and fitted with solid silver toilet and powder jars, ivory brushes, a leather-backed mirror, and a pair of manicure scissors for

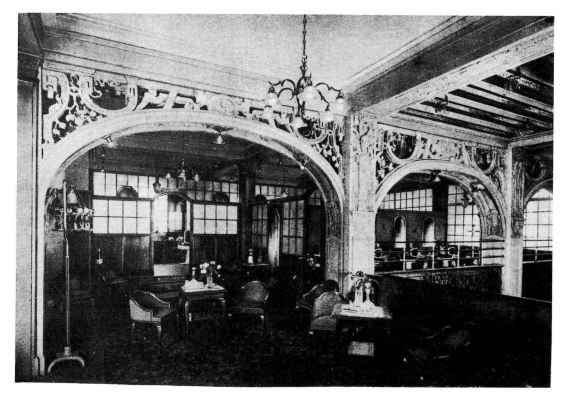

FIG. 209: Beauty salon in Berlin in the 1920s.

£11 5s. More elaborate cases sold for £27 15s. 6d.

In October Helena Rubinstein was back in London, busily promoting her products and her services. 'Complexions :- cultivated or camouflaged? What shall it be?' asked her copywriter in a half-page advertisement in *The Queen*. 'If you wish merely to play make-believe with your complexion, there are to accomodate you hundreds of more or less pretentious "make-up parlours" all the way from the lofty West End districts to the humbler sections of London.

'It is just as well to be outspoken.

'But if intelligently you are looking for something that will make your complexion loyal and your own, then your choice is very small, indeed.

'And it *is* so small because in that entire feminine activity known as beauty cultivation there is in reality only one person who warns you against the fallacy of confusing the complexion with the skin.

'That person is Madame Helena Rubinstein, and she states pointedly that if you take care of your skin, your complexion will take care of itself. . . .

'It is, indeed, just as well to be outspoken.

'But the treatment means *proper* treatment. It means proper treatment for *you*. In London and in Paris, from New York to San Francisco, and in the Antipodes, the name of Madame Helena Rubinstein stands for beauty — beauty awakened, developed, constant, triumphant, not camouflaged.

'Where Royalty rules and Society dictates, where Professions demand perfection of profile and face-oval . . . there the art that is Madame Rubinstein's asserts itself. There Madame Rubinstein is recognized as the beauty Specialiste *par excellence*, because she in fact specializes. She cultivates the skin, induces it to work as by Nature's law it should, to unfold the wondrous panoply of its beauty.

'Her reputation is not a thing of yesterday or to-day, is not merely a thing of printer's ink and print paper, but it is cherishingly traced back in the memory of the mothers and grandmothers of the debutantes of to-day.

'Having just removed her Paris establishment to new, larger, and more commodious quarters, at No. 126, Rue Faubourg Saint Honoré, and 38 Rue de Penthièvre, MADAME RUBINSTEIN IS NOW IN LONDON with a wide range of new and fascinating preparations and Treatments. *She is assisted again by that same noted Continental Doctor whose rare cleverness in aesthetic surgery has been the sensation of many a London Season.*'

Madame could be consulted personally in Grafton Street.

The firm of Yardley, which could trace its origins to 1770, opened its first New York branch in 1921. Published in this same year, *The Woman's Book* ('contains everything a woman ought to know'), though it included detailed information on postal rates, proof reading manuscripts, buying coal, teaching a parrot to talk, and cleaning fish, managed in its more than seven hundred pages never once to mention cosmetics.

But by now most books on beauty were generally permissive, though cautious, in their approach to makeup. Naturalness was still essential. In *Physical Beauty* Florence Courtenay writes that 'to make the eyes look wider and fuller a tiny touch of black in the corners is effective. Do not, however, be too free with the eyelash pencil. And do not use a black pencil if your hair is brown, use a brown one. Blonde eyelashes and eyebrows are not beautiful, as a rule, and it is permissible to darken them. . . . The lips *should* have a natural rose hue — but at times the lipstick has to help out forgetful Nature. Now the lipstick cannot be considered unless in its relation to rouge. Most people use rouge paste badly — and while using rouge is not a crime, using it badly is — because they do so without consideration for their own natural *color*. What is more ridiculous than to see a woman flush through her rouge and present on one and the same cheek two distinct shades of color, real and artificial. The rouge used for the face — it should be applied rather high on the cheeks and shaded off gradually — should be matched by the shade used on the lips. Hence, let your lipstick match your rouge exactly. Most women need no lipstick — not that this prevents their using one. . . . Dyeing is a hair crime. In most cases it destroys the light, shade, and luster of the hair, and usually — unless so subtly done as to be past detection — it is a hallmark of vulgarity'.

COSMETIC AIDS, 1923

The year 1923 saw the invention of Kurlash, a tool for curling eyelashes. It seemed fairly complicated to work, took ten minutes to do the job, and cost five dollars, but it was an enormous success all the same. Thirty years later a greatly improved Kurlash did its work in thirty seconds and cost only a dollar.

Vogue's Shoppers' and Buyers' Guide for April 1923 carried advertisements for Fernol's Magic Skin Food ('unexcelled for filling out hollow and wasted necks'). Madame Berthe's Zip ('positively destroys Hair with roots — no electricity or caustics'), Sagging Cheeks Lifted ('wrinkles smoothed out and the contour restored'), and Kitty Gordon's Egyptian Treatment ('remarkable for removing wrinkles and tightening the muscles').

In a regular feature on beauty and cosmetics, the editor wrote:

'It is a far cry from those Puritan days when one's complexion was considered a gift from Heaven, not to be trifled with and still less to be altered or exchanged. . . . It will soon be an equally far cry to the days not so long ago when skins were so artificially coated and creamed and powdered that naturalness was all but stifled. . . . Beauty specialists of today, while they promise no glittering impossibilities, guarantee to make the skin healthy and, in this way, to realize the highest possibilities of the individual.'

All of this was by way of introducing several new products — a lemon soap (seventy-five cents a cake), nourishing cream (two dollars a jar), a lotion to remove it (two dollars a bottle), a face bleach (two dollars a bottle), cereal compresses (two dollars a package), and an astringent for sagging chins (three dollars and fifty cents). *Vogue* gave no trade names but offered to purchase the items for any reader who sent in her cheque.

In this same issue there appeared a quarter-page advertisement for the Lionel Compact ('Opens and Closes with a Snap'), described as 'a cleverly contrived square, leather-like case (Plate 25-C) that eliminates clasps and broken finger nails. It opens easily, and at the slightest pressure, closes firmly. It contains a large mirror and a lamb's wool puff perfumed with the exquisite fragrance of Golliwogg de Vigny.' Powder was available in rachel, white, and natural.

Elizabeth Arden offered a 'Muscle-Strapping Skin Tight Treatment' which 'rejuvenates weary tissues and muscles, freshens faded cheeks and makes you the lovely and glowing picture that you would like to be'. In addition, selected products were listed as 'Particularly Helpful in this Season' — Venetian Ardena Skin Tonic, Venetian Cleansing Cream, Venetian Orange Skin Food, Venetian Muscle Oil, Venetian Special Astringent, Venetian Satin Liquid, Savon Kenott ('The Smoker's Dentifrice') and the Double O-Boy Compact.

Eau de Cologne 4711, which could trace its origin to the eighteenth century, was still popular and in 1923 was being recommended for clearing up pimples and blotches.

In 1923, with the flat-chested look in fashion, English women were writing to *The Queen* for advice on how to reduce the bust. One young lady, who signed herself 'Hydrant', was advised 'to be very careful'. Avis, who was fat and equally out of fashion, was reminded that 'lying late in bed in the mornings after an early cup of tea with bread and butter, sitting about in easy chairs, and so on, conduce to undue flesh formation'. For double chins, unfashionable for more than a century, women were sent for a special treatment to Elvira, who was evidently so well known in London that no address was given.

For rough, dry skin — never fashionable in any age — Pond's Cold Cream ('only 2/6 for a big jar') was recommended. And for the fashionable powdered look, a Mrs Lawrence provided Japanese Lily Powder in a variety of shades, including one which was 'just the flesh tone of the normal English face'.

For years, particularly on the Continent, women had quietly been having repairs made on sagging faces. The whole thing, it was said, had been started in Paris by a surgeon who was attempting, at the request of an aging actress, to restore her youthful appearance through surgery. He took a few tucks in strategic places, sent her home to bed, and in a few days she reappeared looking years younger. Word got around, and women kept getting younger. In all such cases the flesh eventually sagged again, but since the operation could be repeated, this was not considered too great a drawback. One unidentified actress of the time was reported to have had her face lifted seven times.

In the wake of World War I, with soldiers needing surgical repairs for aesthetic reasons, plastic surgery was being openly recommended to English women for improving on nature and for removing the signs of age. Those women unfamiliar with the face-lifting process, which tended to be discussed in whispers, were being cautioned that the operation required the services of a competent surgeon and must not be entrusted to charlatans. The Hystogen Institute in Baker Street was considered a reputable place to go for facial surgery.

In the December 6 issue of *The Queen* the Violet Nurseries in Sussex advertised special Christmas presents for the toilet table — bath crystals, boxes of soap, perfumes, sachets, and 'the dearest little circular pincushion'; the Crown Perfumery Company offered Crab Apple Blossom perfumes; and Dubarry packed up a whole box full of their toilet preparations. Men's toiletries were limited, and for a Christmas box 'for husband or brother' the Messrs. Pears could provide only a bar of shaving soap, a sterilized brush, solid brilliantine, and a cake of transparent soap. This was advertised as 'the gentleman's casket'. The ladies' companion piece, covered in cretonne, contained talcum powder, cuticle cream, 'and other good things' — all for eight shillings and sixpence. The gentleman's was only six shillings and sixpence.

It was reported about this time that the annual sales of talcum powder, cold cream, rouge, lipstick, and face powder in America amounted to $750,000,000 (£312,500,000) or approximately $15 for every woman in the country. This did not include perfumes, toilet waters, and soaps. The statistics disturbed the editors of *Nation*, who grimly set about alerting readers.

THE LITTLE RED BOX OF COURAGE

'We are interested in the philosophy of that $750,000,000,' they wrote. 'Last summer in a large and respectable women's magazine we read an affecting article entitled The Little Red Box of Courage, and in it we found packed the secret philosophy of the rouge-pot—a philosophy so terrible, so cynical, so blood-curdling that we have had to comfort ourselves with the thought that while the dippers into the pot are many, its prophets are few. The argument ran something like this: The world is a dark place, full of wars and injustices, of dying babies and devastated lands. Old standards have crumbled, old enthusiasms are dead. The mind faints and the heart fails before the demands life makes upon them. What is there left to encourage us, to give us cheer in the midst of harassing reality? And the answer is: The Little Red Box of Courage. . . . They find in that little box sheer immorality and sex allurement. . . . But allurements that are bought by the women of the country for $750,000,000 leave us cold. If they are vicious it is because they caricature nature and joke about beauty; if they are immoral it is because they indicate a terrible, humble distrust of a woman's self. But chiefly they are neither immoral nor vicious. They are pitiable. Is it anything less than a confession of fear to plaster on these masks of red and white? . . . The women who paint and alter their reflections in the mirror distrust themselves—they are, though often enough quite unaware of it, a little afraid of life as they meet it.'

Having got this off their chests the editors may have felt better; but if they expected it to change the habits of a single woman, they were merely being naive. Now that makeup had finally emerged into the open after being underground for nearly a century, it was destined to remain in the open for a long time to come.

Celia Caroline Cole, writing in the *Delineator*, described the complete makeup procedure for the well-groomed woman of 1923:

'First the cleansing cream, soft, soft as whipped cream, to keep the skin smooth and fine-grained and clean. Next a bottle of skin tonic to tone up the skin and bring out the natural freshness. You either buy this skin tonic or make it out of one-third witch-hazel and two-thirds Florida water. . . . Then skin-food cream to pat under the eyes . . . and all over thin faces and necks. Then a small jar of astringent cream for the pores. And if you want to have a really lovely, silken poreless texture, you buy a little bottle of the right kind of oil and, taking a bit of the cream for the pores into your palm, mix just a drop or two of this oil with the pore cream in your palm, smooth it over your face, and leave it on all night. . . . If you are at all inclined to be plump, you should have tucked away neatly in a drawer in a little box all its own a patter or a molder or some such device to keep your chin where it ought to be, clear-lined and never doubled, and your cheeks patted or molded up and out of their sagginess. . . .

'Then the foundation cream, if you use one. If you don't use it, just smooth a bit of the skin food on again, leave it on a moment or two and then wipe it off. . . . Next the little box or bottle of rouge. Oh, yes you do! Most of you, anyway. You need it when you're tired, if you don't any other time. If you use a paste, just touch your middle finger to it and rub over the place your natural color used to be. (Don't make your cheeks just alike—they never are in nature.) Put a touch upon the point of the chin. Personally, I love a blur of it on the center of the chest where you burn in summer.

'Now an eyebrow-brush to clean the brows and lashes of powder. . . . If your brows and lashes are light, better have a small jar of eyelash paste or hard cake and sweep your brush lightly across the paste or cake and go over them again after you've got all the powder off.

'There are eyebrow-pencils nowadays of brown as well as black. A little darkening of eyebrows with a brown pencil will often give a charming accent to a blond face. One no longer grooms the brows as mercilessly as a season or two ago, but of course don't have them too careless. And, finally, the dot with the pencil in the outer corner of the eye to give the tilted-up look, if that is your type, or a tiny line to elongate the eyes, if you are that type.

'Don't use chamois skin for your powdering—you're apt to rub the powder in too hard. Get a good, fine, well-made powder and put it on with a puff or pad and it will *stick*. And keep that puff or pat as clean as your immortal soul. Match your powder to your skin—Nature knew what she was doing. Get ocher or cream face-powder if you're naturally dark; flesh, if you're blond; dead white if you want to be bizarre.'

For twenty-five cents in coin or stamps one could obtain the Armand Week-end Package containing face powder, rouge, cold cream, talcum, soap, and a booklet entitled *Creed of Beauty*. And for only a dime one could order a sample of Pert, the Waterproof Rouge. 'Women who are wise in the secrets of loveliness,' advised the copywriter, 'apply Pert also to the lips and to the tips of the ears.' The effect, they were assured, was charming. For another dime the same company would supply a sample of Winx (also waterproof), for 'darkening the lashes and making them appear heavier'.

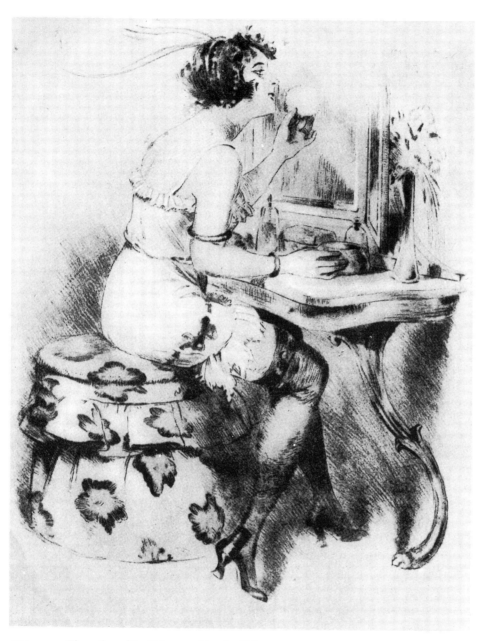

FIG. 210: The toilet table. Colour etching by Kalmar.

Painted Lilies

Men continued to write, as they had for centuries, about women's fashions. Alexander Black complained, in 1923, that the complexion had been standardized. 'It no longer needs to be earned. And in buying it there is no really embarrassing range of choice. Its elements are as portable as the elements of any other first-aid kit. Adjusting a complexion has a dressing-room origin, but it can be completed or edited anywhere. While the man pays the waiter . . . the women revises, accentuates, and cajoles, then scrupulously reviews with the aid of her vanity-case mirror, every phase of the effect; and having corrected the ravages inflicted by the meal and the napkin, completes the ritual with a lip-stick.

'Probably the lip-stick has aroused sharper critical rage than any other whimsicality of women. It can appear to have seized the feminine imagination more violently than any other specific device of fashion, and its effects, apprehended collectively, stagger an unsympathetic spectator. A whole company of scarlet lips, accompanied by a ghostly collection of white noses and shreds of negligible clothes, can indeed, be fearfully depressing to one who doesn't quite catch the joke. In the presence of so many masks a man may find that a chance woman with clean skin has an absolutely voluptuous charm. The preparation and the carrying of these masks suggest immense labor and discomfort. But discomfort is a relativity. A man doesn't feel dressed until he is throttled by a collar. A woman doesn't feel fashionable unless something hurts. It is at the excess point that fashion consciousness begins.

'In the basic grammar of the modern toilet, face powder began as a means of subduing the luster of the skin. The shining face celebrated by poetry is too raw, too elemental, for a conscious art. Especially is a shiny nose resented. "If I can see my nose," said one charming woman, "I can't see anything else." Hence the powder. The esthetic consideration is accented by association. Powdering the nose having become the final preparatory action at the brink of any imaginable experience, is to be regarded as indulgently as any other of our intrinsically meaningless, but useful, automatisms. . . . Probably such irrelevancies did not exist at the beginning of the powdering practice. If a little powder suggested difference from the common face of labor, for example, a great deal of powder became an emphasis of the difference. If a little pink on the lips could restore an effect of ripe youth, a splash of vermilion could violently rebuke the hint of a youth vanished beyond recall. Presently, as in all the arts, the primitive meanings are lost sight of in effects for their own sake. The ghastliness of accentuated lips is nowhere more apparent than in the movies. Lips too red are, after all, an understandable whimsicality. But lips in the movies are black. One can see the dark gash coming and presently is permitted to assemble the rest of the heroine.

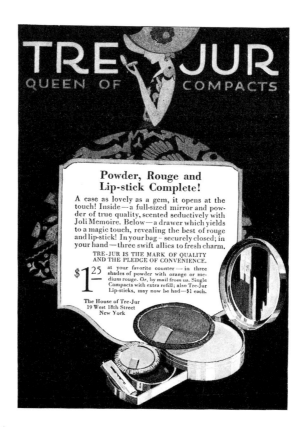

FIG. 211: Advertisement for Tre-Jur compact, 1924.

'It would be a mistake to assume that all men are revolted by these appearances. Men are notoriously fashion-bound. A man's cowardice when his woman threatens to be different from other women is too well understood to call for comment. "You've forgotten your nose," says the exacting husband, chained hopelessly to the habits of his set. And quite aside from the fashion thrall is the male enthusiasm for sex emphasis. I can recall a discussion about painted lips. One man was cynically indifferent. Two described their actual nausea when forced into the company of a bedaubed mouth. "Now, do you know," said the fourth, — I need not add that he was the youngest, — "I rather like the taste of it".'

But in the end Mr Black decides that perhaps he has overstated the case and that men should simply be reminded that there are other flowers in the garden. 'The typical remark that "all women smoke nowadays" belongs in the category with the July or August idiocy that "everybody is out of town". It is altogether likely that fewer than one woman in a thousand in the United States use tobacco. There is an equally good probability that not more than one in a thousand use a lip-stick. . . . When lilies are painted, they are meant to be

465

looked at. A certain shock is part of the expectation . . . and if the day ever comes when women lose the spot-light of an exaggerated attention, we shall have real reason to be nervous about the fate of the race.'

In 1923 the factory value of cosmetics and perfumes in the United States was more than $75,000,000 (£31,250,000), an increase of 400 percent in ten years. Nearly 10,000 employees earned close to a million dollars a month in the more than 400 cosmetic and perfume factories. Imports were in excess of $8,000,000 and exports about $1,000,000.

The increased interest in cosmetics had necessitated improved packaging — spill-proof powder containers that were small enough to carry around, rouge and powder and eventually lipstick in the same compact, elegant perfume bottles to compete with imported French ones — and the improved packaging attracted more customers. Increased sales meant lower costs and the availability of lower-priced products. A gold-plated brass compact with mirror, powder, and puff could be bought for twenty cents and a smaller compact with rouge and puff for ten cents. Lipsticks, eyebrow pencils, and even tiny vials of perfume could be had for a dime. But for the carriage trade, packaging was fancier and prices were higher. One manufacturer of a twenty-five-cent face powder, faced with competition from fifteen-cent powders, put out a new brand for fifty cents and outsold the competition. Curiously, his biggest sales were in the poorer neighbourhoods.

The makers of Pompeian cosmetics (Plate 23-K) reassured the public in 1924 that 'a discriminating use of rouge is as much a part of the well-dressed woman's toilette as the correct dressing of her hair — adding a sparkle to her eyes and life to her entire face'. Pompeian Bloom, added Mme. Jeanette (the *Specialiste en Beauté*), was available in three shades of rose — light, medium, and dark, 'as well as the new Orange Tint. The Medium shade of Pompeian Bloom is the shade that is best for the average American woman.' But, she added, with an eye on the cash box, 'many women have found the new Orange Tint especially adapted to their skin-tone — and even those women who use Medium Bloom as a general practice find Orange Tint better for their coloring during the summer months'. Pompeian lipstick was recommended for 'a delightfully natural color'.

WHITHER ARE WE DRIFTING?

This same year James H. Collins noted that it was estimated that fifty million American women were using lipstick and wondered about the outcome of their being kissed daily by as few as fifty million men. 'Is there danger,' he asked the readers of the *Saturday Evening Post*, 'that the men will be poisoned? The

New York Board of Health . . . thinks the situation worth investigating and is collecting and analyzing lipstick samples. . . . Go into the very cheapest stores in any large city and see the beauty goods piled on the counter. They take almost as much space as the kitchen ware. Go into the department stores and see the phalanxes of saleswomen demonstrating and selling face powders, lipsticks, preparations, perfumes. Whither are we drifting?

'As for the girls and women today — well, look at them! I doubt that newspaper estimate of 50,000,000 using the lipstick — doubt whether there are half that many who use the powder rag, because it has been ascertained that less than half the people in the United States use toothbrushes, and it would probably be found on investigation, that a few million have still to discover soap. But there are enough painted lips and whitewashed complexions in your community to make you wonder where we are drifting.'

In the summer of 1924 Celia Caroline Cole informed her readers that she had just discovered 'a heavenly new whitener. Not only does it whiten, but it brings that illuminated look into the skin — pearly, the good old novels call it. And it's nice'n cheap too'. Also, 'the perfect orange rouge' had just arrived — ideal for 'those who have gold lights in their skin rather than creamy, or pink and white . . . this orange rouge gives the most devastating charm. . . . And,' adds Mrs Cole, almost breathlessly, 'there's a man in our town who takes away every sign of enlarged pores and coarsened skin — and who cures acne, by the way, without a single miss ever. And does it all painlessly without acids; and he lifts and tightens the muscles in that same glorious, antiseptic, painless way without a knife — all by electricity.'

It was estimated in 1925 that American women spent nearly a billion dollars (about 417 million pounds) a year for cosmetics and beauty care. Cold cream headed the list of best sellers in the beauty shops, followed by soap, perfume, and compact powder in the brunette shade. But the well-stocked dressing table and bathroom also contained loose powder, moist and dry rouge, lipstick, toilet water, vanishing cream, tissue-building cream, massage cream, skin lotions, eyebrow pencils, astringents, depilatories, dusting powder, sachet powder, shampoo, bath salts, and clay treatments.

Kathleen Eddy, writing in the *Pictorial Review*, explained that the popularity of compact powder was a direct outgrowth of the frequent powdering of noses in public and the consequent spilling of powder down the front of dresses and coats. For loose powder, a mixture of Rachel and rose, called 'Peaches and Cream', was the most popular shade and was used for all complexions, as was 'brunette', though shades of powder designed for all complexions were available.

Miss Eddy describes a beauty laboratory she visited as being 'spotless and sanitary from the floor to the ceiling, including the dresses, aprons, and caps worn by the employees. And practically every product is carried from the first step in its preparation to the final labeling without ever being touched by human hands. The huge vats of cream, cold and vanishing; the large containers of powder, delicately tinted, suggest confections more than cosmetics.'

It was reported in the twenties that in Japan face powder was not so harmless as it had become in the West and that for the past two hundred years one of the foremost causes of infant mortality had been a disease resulting from the use by mothers of a white face powder containing lead. The disease usually appeared at about eight months and was more frequent in the summer when face powder was used in greater quantities. In cases of fatality, the body always showed traces of lead and could always be traced to face powder used by the mother.

THE MID-TWENTIES

In the mid-twenties, when makeup, applied openly and frankly, was a new and exciting plaything, most women, guided only by manufacturers' labels, were less than successful in choosing makeup which was becoming. Mary Brush Williams, writing in the *Ladies Home Journal* in 1925, quoted a friend who took the trouble to find a rouge which was just right for her own colouring:

'Everybody wears rouge too light for them. . . . That firm alone makes eight shades, and I tried every one at home by daylight and electricity too. I got sixteen shades from other houses and experimented with them as well. There wasn't any of them that seemed exactly to hit it, and I mixed them. I even tried them by candlelight. When I go to a dinner, I poke around to find from my hostess in advance whether there will be candles or dim lamps or electricity. And then I get all set for the lighting. That's how much trouble I've taken to get myself a reputation for a good complexion.'

Then Mrs Williams added a few hints of her own. 'Lip rouge,' she said, 'throws all the rest of your coloring out of proportion. If you leave the rest of your face natural, lip rouge makes you look deadly pale. And if you put on make-up to balance it, you are too artificial to suit even the college boys, who usually don't like things too simple.' She approved of a little eyeshadow but found darkening the lashes too artificial. Her big news she saved for last. 'The fashion — right from Paris,' she wrote, 'is not to look made-up any more, but natural!'

THE AMERICAN WOMAN, 1925

Early in 1925, the New Hampshire legislature, having forgotten or being unaware of the consistent failures, throughout history, in trying to legislate standards of female beauty and cosmetic practices, set about attempting to ban the use of cosmetics in the state. The project was naturally doomed to failure, and the legislators should have known better. Had they been women, the matter would never have come up — not that all women, especially conservative New England ones, approved of some women doing openly what most women had been doing in secret, but they would have been instinctively aware of the futility of such a project.

'Men,' wrote Henry Tetlow later in the year, 'are naturally the keenest anti-cosmetic crusaders. Seven American men out of ten, even today, will declare that they prefer their women barefaced, and three of the seven probably actually believe there is One Woman who never uses any makeup. At least one of the three imagines that there are women who can appear on a blindingly lighted stage without the aid of artificial coloring. . . . When the truth comes out at last, the men who Really Believed will get awfully sore. There will be gnashing of teeth and, following it, prohibitory persecution. Heretofore, the social regulators have avoided the moral issue in their attacks on cosmetics. They have grounded their case on the pernicious effect of paint and powder on the human skin. . . .

'Thus, under the Pure Food and Drug Act of 1906 (You had forgotten that there ever was such a thing! Do you remember all it was going to do for you?) the much enduring cosmetician was required to register and guarantee his goods. What they were guaranteed for or against is not clear yet. No formulae were revealed nor required to be altered.'

Nevertheless, women welcomed some assurance, no matter how nebulous, that their cosmetics were safe to use. Any assurance they had received up to this time had been worth very little.

'Nearly all American women use make-up,' continued Mr Tetlow, 'don't let them tell you different! Most of them do not use nearly enough. Many, of course, use too much at the wrong time, but that is another matter. . . . The trouble is with our climate. The sunlight on this side of the world burns the natural color out of the human skin. The ruddy-cheeked immigrant quickly fades, and succeeding generations never recover. The native North American is characteristically a revolting shade of gray. Hence, although they still do not use enough, American women use more rouge and face powder per capita than their European cousins. . . . But the characteristic North American complexion will absorb more color than a brown wall paper, and millions of American women remain afraid of color. . . . They prefer to make themselves and all who see them wretched by appearing flat and under-done.'

Mr Tetlow pointed out that white powder was still the most popular shade and that Latins would use nothing else. But the women of Britain and northern Europe preferred a yellow tint usually called rachel or cream. Americans, on the whole, preferred pink, which they called flesh, though a good deal of brunette ('a yellow powder, a sort of dirty pinkish brown, somewhat lighter

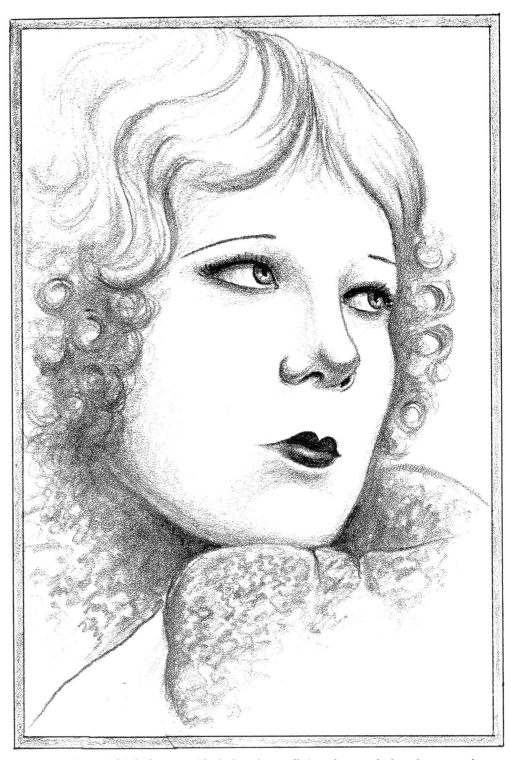

FIG. 212: The wistful look, 1925. Plucked and pencilled eyebrows, shadowed eyes, and painted rosebud mouth.

than the freshly clipped coat of a Chincoteague pony') was coming into fashion and was often used for touching up the nose, even when the rest of the face had been powdered with pink or white. Mr Tetlow also chided the blondes who made themselves up with red, white, and pink, a naturally pink and white blonde being 'something rarer than an albino'.

As for the current styles in rouge and lipstick, he found some of them quite hideous — 'especially the nameless drowned-blue and the Orangeman's Delight'. He recommended that lipstick be chosen according to what it did for the colour of the teeth.

As for quality in cosmetics, he concluded that it had nothing to do with popularity and that all cosmetics were 'just about alike, and it is as difficult and expensive to make bad face powders and rouges as it is to make the best — if not more so. As long as they will stick on and are not rough, they satisfy all the requirements of quality. It is the perfume that makes or breaks a cosmetic.'

NEW PRODUCTS, 1925

In October *Vogue* reported on a visit to a New York perfume and cosmetics shop which featured a rose jelly astringent and three liquid ones — strawberry (medium strength), opal (very light), and benzoin ('suited to double chins'). Also available were various creams, skin foods, muscle oils, and face powders. Then there was an indelible liquid lip rouge in rose or medium red, an indelible lip pomade, and liquid cheek rouge in rose, mandarin, or medium. Lescondieu cosmetics, imported from Paris, included a vanishing cream called *La Reine des Crèmes*, 'the newest and most discreet creme rouge', called *Farjole*, a nail polish named *Eclador*, and *Lipstick Tussy* (see Plate 25-H), indelible and scented. Primrose House advertised their lipstick as *practically* indelible.

Lucille Buhl's cosmetic gimmick was doubles — a face powder box containing two drawers of powder, one for day and one for evening ('By choosing the day shade, the correct evening shade is assured'), and the Vanisuthe Double Lipstick, one side cream, the other side rouge, in light, medium, or dark. *Vogue* mentioned but did not identify a double rouge compact — a gun metal vanity case with mirror and dry rouge (medium, rose, or bright) on one side and cream rouge (dark or cherry) on the other.

Lablache ('The Choice of Gentlewomen for Three Generations') had an unusually wide variety of cosmetic items on their list — loose powder, single compact (powder only), double compact (powder and rouge), triple compact (powder, rouge, and lipstick), Glove Rouge Vanity, Glove Powder Vanity, changeable lipstick (orange turning to red), red lipstick (rose, poppy, geranium), deluxe lipstick, hexagon eyebrow pencil (see Plate 24-C), toilet powder in a

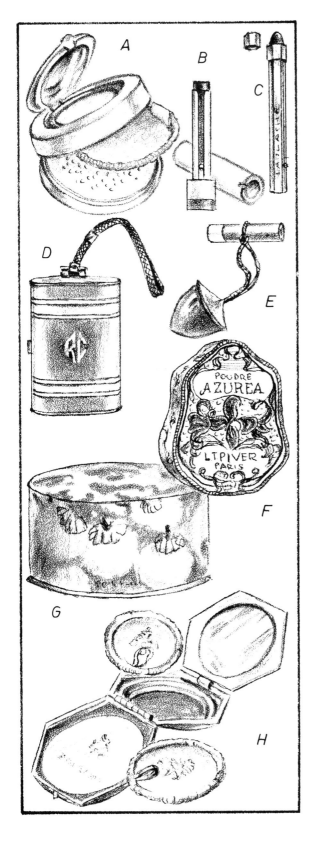

PLATE 24 : TWENTIETH CENTURY
1920–1930

A   1925. Solid silver compact for rouge and loose powder. By International Sterling.

B   1925. Terri lipstick in Bakelite case.

C   1925. Eyebrow pencil by Lablache.

D   1925. Terri vanity case with fitted compartments for powder, rouge, lipstick, cigarettes or bills, key, and coins. Also contains a mirror and comb. Leather case with white or green gold.

E   1925. Terri loose-powder vanity and lipstick in bakelite case.

F   1920. Azurea face powder, Paris. Available at least as early as 1915.

G   1927. Coty Face Powder.

H   1927. Houbigant Double Compact for rouge (4 shades) and powder (3 shades). Price, $2.50.

PLATE 25 : TWENTIETH CENTURY
1920–1930

A   1923. Solid silver vanity case by International Silver. Contains mirror, powder puff, note pad, 2 coin holders, and a compartment for visiting cards.

B   1923. Pert cream rouge. 'Orange in the jar, it turns to a natural pink as it touches the skin.'

C   1923. Lionel compact. 'Opens and closes with a snap.' Imitation leather case, lamb's wool puff perfumed with Golliwogg de Vigny. Price $1.

D   1928. Mascara and brush in sea-green metal case. By Dorothy Gray.

E   1928. Dorothy Gray liquid Cherri Rouge.

F   Dorothy Gray lipstick.

G   1928. Dunhill vanity case containing rouge, powder, puffs, lipstick, and mirror. Available in natural metal or coloured enamels. Price, $5 to $500.

H   1925. Tussy indelible lipstick, by Lesquendieu, Paris.

I   1925. Scented indelible liquid lip rouge.

J   1925. Tangee lipstick.

K   1925. Tangee Crème Rouge in glass jar.

L   Dorothy Gray vanity case, containing rouge, powder, puffs, mirror, lipstick, eyebrow brush, tweezers, eyeshadow, and mascara. Available in various colours and leathers. Price, $9 to $18.

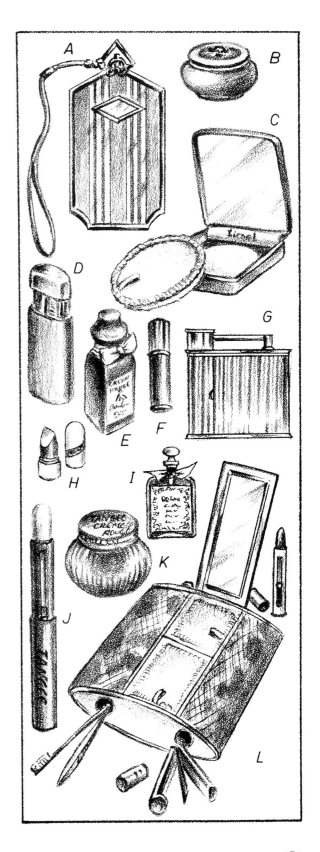

bottle, bath powder, bath salts, Beauty Rouge, face tonic, astringent lotion, vanishing cream, cleansing cream, tissue cream, and beauty cream. Houbigant was more conservative, with five shades of face powder, nail crayons, two shades of lipstick, and four shades of rouge 'for four types'.

The newest vivid shade of rouge in Paris was Red Geranium, available in lipstick as well as cream and dry rouge. Red Raspberry was also a popular shade. In powder the newest shade was called Blush, designed to replace Naturelle or Flesh.

In November, International Sterling took a half-page advertisement in *Vogue* to promote their newest solid-silver vanity case (see Plate 24-A), described by their wide-eyed copywriter:

' "Stunningest of vanities!" exclaims mademoiselle when she beholds this newest creation. So slim! So trim! And of solid silver! . . . She opens the case! It holds the very newest combination. A compartment for rouge! And then . . . another compartment with another mirror for her own choice of loose powder! A clever sifter device dusts the powder out, just as mademoiselle wants it.'

Bourjois Java face powder came in 'a tint for every type', but there were only two shades of rouge — Ashes of Roses and Mandarine. Armand's specialties were Cold Cream Powder ('dense and very fine') and Armand Peridore ('to be put on quickly'), both in six shades — white, pink, creme, brunette, natural, and flame ('double brunette'). Ingram's Milkweed Cream ('Perfect for Every Use') was still available at fifty cents a jar or one dollar for the large economy size.

Late in the year Jane Cowl revealed her beauty secrets to her public through the pages of the *Ladies Home Journal*. 'I wash with a good face cream,' wrote Miss Cowl. 'Rarely do I use water on my face, although I don't think that matters; every woman has to suit her own skin. . . . A good cleansing cream, applications of ice or cold water to stimulate the face muscles, a good powder, perhaps the slightest amount of make-up — these are all a part of good grooming.' She also spent some time each day in vigorous exercise.

Even in the twenties some women were still concocting some of their own cosmetics. Justine Johnstone mentioned to her *Ladies Home Journal* readers that she made her own eye lotion with ten cents' worth of camomile flowers steeped in boiling water.

But women who could afford it, reported Marie Wright in *The Queen*, often patronized specialists who blended individual shades of rouge and powder. Other women then demanded the same shades, whether they were becoming or not. 'The tangerine rouge, with its apricot sister, the suntan powder, that queer purplish powder only to be used at night under electric lights — these were all made in the first place for some particular woman whose skin and style they suited.'

Unlike most women, the Frenchwoman, Miss Wright noted, deliberately emphasized her worst features. 'If she has a very long nose, a mouth which is too wide, or eyes too small or too almond-shaped, or too sunken, she never grieves over the fault. She goes to a beauty specialist for advice, and she makes up and dresses to enhance that feature, to call attention to it until it comes to have a charm of its own, and gives her an individuality. She studies the best make-up to use, the proper hats to wear, the best sort of frock to enhance her style. The tragedy is that she so often sets a fashion which, while carefully adapted to her needs, is followed by other women, whom it disfigures.'

MAKING UP, 1926

Marise de Fleur, writing in *Sunset Magazine*, gives a good picture of the ideal makeup practices of 1926. It can probably be assumed that though women may have tried to follow such advice, they were not always successful. Miss de Fleur points out, to begin with, that makeup 'should be used as an accent, the delicate underlining of an individual note; long lashes darkened to increase the shadows that add depth to the eyes, lips reddened in a fair face that needs no other additional color, just the right shade of rouge and powder to combat the glare of the ballroom. . . . There is now a shade for every skin, and a shade for every time of day. To limit one shade to blondes or to brunettes is impossible. Some powders can be used by both equally, some are becoming in daylight and not at night, or the reverse, so that experiments are necessary, just as an artist tries out colors before using them on his canvas. Fair blondes can use a rose powder if the shade is pale and natural. A mauve powder is good on the average skin, giving it a clear, delicate look, and may be used either at night or by day. A dark rose powder is sometimes used by dark or medium blondes in place of rouge. A lovely effect is often obtained by using one powder as a base and another on the cheeks to give the necessary additional color, if no great amount is needed.

'Rouge should always be applied with sufficient restraint to deceive the public if possible. When the deception is apparent, the charm is gone, to a great extent at least. And usually this fault is not in the rouge but in the application. Here again there is a becoming color for each complexion, a shade that will look natural and inconspicuous while adding a depth and bloom that throws off the years by the half-dozens.

'Rouge comes in three forms, powder, liquid and paste. Powder and paste are easier for the beginner to use than the liquid, although this gives an excellent effect if well applied. A good quality of paste rouge which is now sold will last all day without renewing. All artificial color should be placed high on the cheeks to improve the contour of the face. Try to make the effect somewhat different on each cheek, as a more natural effect is gained in this way. Brush the rouge lightly over the upper part of the cheeks, rub up and out, then along the back line of the face, toward the chin but not too far down. Then erase the hard edges with the fingers. Last of all, put a light film of powder over the rouge. . . .

'The mouth now comes in for its share of attention. The shape as well as the shade can be improved by the use of a good lipstick, but discretion should govern its application. A white face in which a bright red mouth is the most noticeable accent may look grotesque rather than beautiful. If you use the lip rouge . . . apply it with the finger, following the contour of the lips, but stopping short of the corners. Accent the curve of the upper lip, but put little if any on the lower lip, as it gets sufficient from the one above, and this gives a more natural appearance.

'The color of the eyes should dictate the color of the make-up used round them. With blue eyes a blue or purple eyebrow pencil may be used to shade the lids, while brown or hazel eyes demand a purple pencil to develop their full beauty. Black eyes are lovely with a faint touch of red. Rub the pencil very gently over the eyelids and blend into a delicate shadow over the entire surface. Another faint line may be drawn under the eyes and treated in the same way, but should be even more shadowy and indistinct, or a hollow-eyed effect will result.

'In reducing the eyebrows to an orderly and shapely growth, the tweezers are the most effective weapon against the weedy growth of volunteer hairs that will appear just off the main trail. Do not reduce the eyebrows to a hard line. Leave them full and natural looking, and darken the hairs to a desirable shade with the pencil. Be careful to confine the darkening to the hairs, not allowing any to cling to the skin, as this gives an untidy look to the face and ruins the line of brow as well.'

The author recommends darkening the eyelashes, preferably with a brown liquid mascara. She adds in conclusion :

'Just as it is well to avoid the use of too much make-up, so it is wise to apply it as infrequently as possible and with some privacy, where that can be done. Every woman now-a-days carries a vanity case, or a group of little accessories to give her beauty, wherever she may be, on a minute's notice. An attractive thin compact can be obtained, carrying both rouge and a loose powder, that is a charming novelty as well as a useful necessity.'

Fashions of 1927

Early in 1927 Rose Feld, reporting in *Colliers* on current fashions in makeup, indicated that women were emerging from the period of obvious, garish makeup and going into one of more subtlety and naturalness. 'The vivid pinks and flat yellows are going,' she wrote, 'and in their place the milder flesh tints are being sold. Two or three years ago it was even considered smart and exotic to use powder with a distinct green tint. Women believed it made them look wan and interesting. A rumor had spread that Nazimova used green powder and shortly after hundreds of green goddesses appeared in restaurants and ballrooms and spread as much horror and wonder as Dunsany's gods.'

Even conservative women, reported Miss Feld, were still using bright lipstick. Mascara and eyebrow pencil were usually reserved for evening use. There were some women, she added, who actually used eyeshadow, which she described for the benefit of the unsophisticated reader as 'a dark mixture applied on lids and in the hollow of the eye to bring out its sombre radiance'. But such women, noted Miss Feld firmly, 'are being gradually laughed off the scene'. She insisted, nevertheless, that the percentage of women over twenty who used no makeup at all could 'be compared to the squeak of a mouse in a thunderstorm'.

Hazel Rawson Cades, in her regular beauty column in *Colliers*, had a few words of advice for the outdoor girl of 1927. 'Don't try to cover sunburn with pink or white powder,' she cautioned. 'Buy a shade that will tone in or try blending your own if you can't find the right shade in the shops. . . . If your face flushes with the heat, see what you can do with green powder. If you want to sport a pearly pallor at the country-club dance, experiment with one of the subtle evening orchid shades.

'Don't depend on winter rouge or indoor rouge in the glare of summer sun. . . . Vivid artificial shades look queer when you begin to flush with color of your own. If you're apt to turn a little bluish in the water . . . start your swim with a moderate application of rouge and lipstick that tone this way. You should keep in mind, however, that the present trend is toward natural effects in make-up and away from the bizarre.'

English women were still having their usual cosmetic problems and asking for help from invisible and unidentified columnists. Madge, who wanted her ears pierced, was sent to Goldsmiths and Silversmiths Co. Ltd., in Regent Street; Anemone, who was too fat, was referred to Mrs Adair in New Bond Street; and D.K.B., who was plagued with heavy nasolabial folds, was advised to cultivate a cheerful expression. For ladies who resisted this means of self help, there was a *Wrinkle Book* available for three shillings and sixpence.

Dorothy Cocks, writing in 1927 in her *Etiquette of Beauty*, typifies the relaxed attitude of the twenties, as she wonders why cosmetics always seem to be a moral issue : 'A bit of red stain on the cheeks, a fluff of white on the nose,

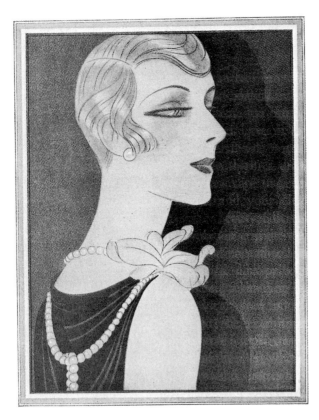

a shadow of black around the eyes, what are they to arouse the wrath of centuries of reformers? They seem such vagaries to attract such earnest attention.'

But then she goes on to make it clear that there are still a few dark clouds of disapproval left on the horizon:

'But oddly enough, even in modern times, cosmetics still cause a lift of the eyebrows in some circles. Our older generation shudders at our younger generation's frank use of the lipstick. But that very frankness makes a lipstick virtuous! It is only an immoral motive which can make cosmetics iniquitous. And in the last analysis, immorality is doing something one is ashamed to be caught doing. If we rouge our cheeks and powder our noses before every mirror we meet in public, there can be no turpitude in that! Our Victorian grandmothers, who bled themselves in private to be pale, were more vicious. . . .

'Today, good taste dictates that every cosmetic aid shall contribute to the effect of natural and healthy good looks. Rouge and powder and lip paste may be as obvious as you please, if they improve your appearance. But you show your exquisite good taste, your education and experience in the nice details of personal care, by knowing just how obvious make-up may *be* and still improve your appearance. Eyes shadowed with deep purple are cadaverous looking in the daytime. Scarlet cheeks detract from the interest of your eyes. Such rules as these govern the present use of cosmetics.'

478

Miss Cocks found liquid rouge the most natural but also the most difficult to apply. She recommended using paste rouge at home and dry rouge away from home for touch-ups. In addition to the colour high on the cheeks, she suggested a touch of rouge for pale ears, long noses, and prominent chins. She preferred the yellowish rouges, in a light tint, with lipstick to match. 'Cerise lipstick,' she warned firmly, 'is ridiculous.' But she recommended the curious practice, common in the late twenties, of dividing the upper lip into two painted halves separated by a vertical line of natural skin. Powder was expected to match, not whiten, the skin. Women were urged to search zealously for a perfect match and, failing to find it, to blend their own from available shades. As the skin tones became deeper during the summer months, so should the powder.

Miss Cocks did not approve of the fashionable plucked eyebrows nor of any eye makeup for street wear. But for artificial lighting she suggested a trace of eyebrow pencil, not too dark, a faint line next to the upper lashes, and cream on the lashes. Beading the lashes, she cautioned her readers, was only for the stage. She did not mention eyeshadow but did suggest a trace of dark powder on the upper lids.

In the autumn of 1927, in the pages of the *Ladies Home Journal*, Lynn Fontanne (Figure 214) spoke to the women of America about makeup:

'I thoroughly believe in making up the face. I don't believe in going about without make-up on. I don't believe a person looks as if she had finished dressing for the day. She will give every attention towards concealing the defects of her figure with corsets, with brassières, with what not. She will wear sheer stockings to make her ankles look delicate; she will select slippers that will hide any defect of her feet. But when it comes to her face, she leaves it plain and unadorned, its defects probably accented, its excellences lost through the lack of make-up. Too many people leave their face in the raw state it was given them. Too many women think they have done all they can for themselves when they dab on a bit of powder — a powder that probably is entirely out of tone with their coloring. Yet it is what is done to the face that decides whether a woman will give an impression of beauty or of plainness.'

Miss Fontanne then gave her own procedure in making up:

'As a base for my powder I use a very familiar face lotion. I find the powder goes on much smoother and better and stays on longer than when I use a cold-cream base. . . . I use a cream-colored powder, and on my lips I rub a light-red lip rouge — the brighter the shade, the better. I use a dry rouge on my cheeks, the same for daytime and for night, and I make it myself by combining two rouges — an ordinary brunet rouge and a light orange powder. The orange powder gives the rouge an animation it hasn't got by itself.'

But Miss Fontanne points out that what may be right for her would be quite wrong for another woman, and each should choose for herself. One of her

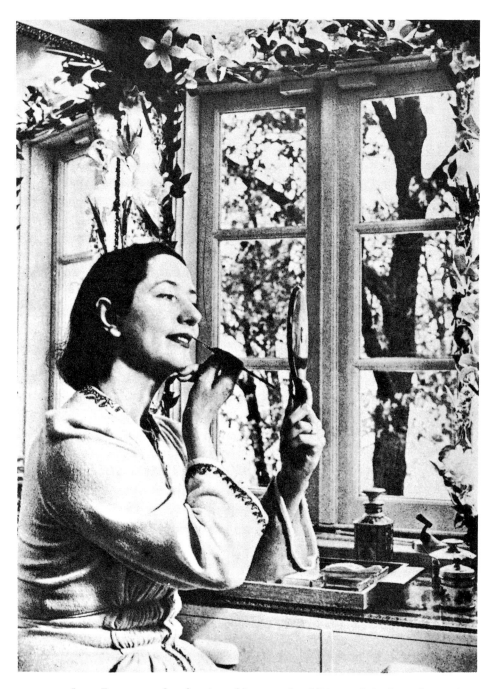

FIG. 214: Lynn Fontanne at her dressing-table, 1940. In addition to light from the window, there are fluorescent tubes and luminous glass flowers. Published in *Vogue*.

comments undoubtedly reflect the sentiments of luxury loving women through-out history:

'In my bath I shake a few drops of a bath essence which cost a great deal of money. Some accessories are expensive, yet in the end they are worth their price because they stimulate a feeling of well-being, of a sort of inner luxury which raises the spirits, which make one feel beautiful, which is half the battle of presenting a charming appearance.'

According to the U.S. Department of Commerce, nearly 30 million dollars' worth of face creams were sold in 1927, about the same in various kinds of toilet powders, and more than 11 million dollars' worth of rouge. But the cosmetic boom was not confined to the Western World. Three years after the Kremlin had organized *Glavperfume*, on the revolutionary theory that female Comrades ought to be feminine, Madame Molotov was chosen to promote the sale and use of cosmetics, which had already grown to a thirteen-million-dollar business.

BEAUTY PROMOTION, 1928

In 1928 a light skin was still considered desirable, and a full-page advertise-ment in *Vogue* guaranteed that Golden Peacock Bleach Creme would make the skin four shades lighter in three days: 'A single application will prove its powers to you. Prove them beyond all doubt or skepticism. Apply it tonight. Tomorrow your skin will be appreciably lighter. In three days it will be four to five shades lighter — no matter how dark it may be today.'

Powder was still the most important cosmetic for many women, especially those who shied away from rouge and lipstick. To cater for these conservative women and to others who were tired of garish reds and wanted something more subtle, Helena Rubinstein introduced a very pink powder which gave the effect of a pale rouge when used with an ivory powder.

Tangee was one of the most popular brands of the period. Their lipstick and rouge came in only one shade — a light orange, which changed to an intense coral pink on the skin. In addition to lipstick, cream rouge, and dry rouge cake, Tangee made day cream, night cream, and face powder. For twenty cents one could obtain miniature sizes of all six items, as well as a booklet on 'The Art of Make-up'.

In 1928 one could also mail in a coupon for a free sample of a new cleansing tissue called Kleenex ('If you still use a soiled bit of linen that rubs germs back into the skin or a harsh towel that is so quickly ruined by cream and grease, you'll find Kleenex a delightful surprise. . . . You use Kleenex once, then dis-card it just like paper.') One could also buy Stillman's Freckle Cream ('bleaches them out while you sleep'); Gouraud's Oriental Cream ('renders an entrancing, bewitching appearance that will not rub off') in white, flesh, and rachel; Pond's Skin Freshener ('rejuvenates the skin'); Maybelline ('used by millions of lovely women'); and Eversweet ('the dainty deodorant'), advertised as invigorating, healing, and antiseptic.

Princess Pat did not offer free samples, but for twenty-five cents in coin the manufacturers would send the Princess Pat Week End Set, containing 'easily a month's supply of Almond Base Powder and six other delightful Princess Pat preparations'. The latter, unidentified, were evidently to come as a happy surprise.

For only ten cents the coupon addict could obtain a miniature Glazo manicure set and a booklet by Miss Rosaline Dunn, whose association with Glazo climaxed a life 'devoted to the art of manicuring'. Miss Dunn put it this way:

'Then from Paris came the whisper that liquid polishes had been created. I tried all of them. But some of them peeled or dulled in spots. Others gave the nails an unnatural tint that was too obvious. Then just when I despaired of ever realizing my ambitions I discovered the Glazo Manicure. What a happy meeting!'

Vanity cases were an essential part of the chic woman's equipment, and *Vogue* described a new one by Terri as being 'made of black metal, with a single bright line of color at the top and a smart marcasite motif'. The vanity contained rouge, powder, lipstick, and mirror, as well as allowing space for cigarettes. Kathleen Mary Quinlan, who originated Persian Muscle Oil, also produced a silver and blue vanity case containing rouge, powder, lip salve, eyeshadow, and a mirror. Dunhill's vanity case, looking, not surprisingly, like a cigarette lighter (Plate 25-G), contained the usual rouge, powder, lipstick, and mirror and cost from five dollars to five hundred dollars (two hundred pounds). Corday's Silver Queen compact was designed to look like a flattened golf ball. Dorothy Gray had a vanity reminiscent of centuries past, containing rouge, powder, puffs, lipstick, eyebrow brush, tweezers, eyeshadow, mascara, and mirror (see Plate 25-L).

In this same year Lydia O'Leary, a young woman who had been forced to earn her living in back rooms painting gift cards, perfected and marketed a cosmetic which she had invented and developed to conceal her own disfiguring birthmark. *Covermark*, originally a heavy liquid, later a greaseless cream, was made in several shades and could successfully cover a variety of facial blemishes. It was estimated that about fifteen percent of the sales were to men.

Nail polish was also in the beauty news from time to time. 'One of the first things that the knowing American woman does upon her arrival in Paris,' wrote *Vogue*'s beauty editor, is to make an appointment for a manicure at Madame Mille's — that little place in the rue Saint Honoré which was formerly known as Carmichaël's. The excellence of Madame Mille's liquid polish and the

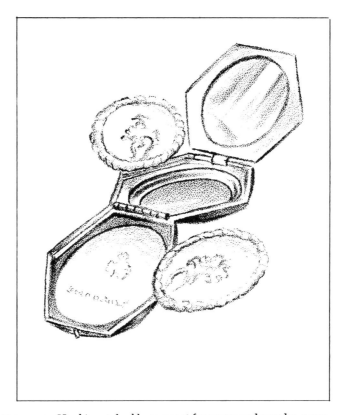

FIG. 215 : Houbigant double compact for rouge and powder, 1927.

exotic delicacy of the tint imparted to the nails have made her justly famous.'
Madame's polish was also available in New York.

THE COST OF MAKEUP, 1928

An enlightening survey in the *Milwaukee Sentinel* indicated that a little over
half of American women used rouge but that only fifteen percent used lipstick.
About ninety percent used face powder, more than used perfume or toilet
water. It was estimated that the average American woman spent about fifty
dollars (twenty pounds) a year for cosmetics and beauty treatments, less than
the average man spent for tobacco. Of course, a woman could, and some did,
spend more than half this much for an ounce of perfume; but she could also
buy an ounce of an unadvertised brand for fifty cents. The average price at

the time was only $1.86 (fifteen shillings).

But the averages were misleading since they included farm women, who spent very little, and women in the large cities, who sometimes spent a great deal. The toilet goods section of a single New York department store, according to Ivor Griffith, occupied an area of 15,000 square feet, employed forty-nine clerks, and sold three million dollars' worth of beauty accessories every year. The decisions facing a woman shopper were staggering—about 600 cold creams, 347 rouges, 1200 varieties of perfume, and 1300 choices in face powder.

In 1928 American women spent $1,835,000,000 (£760,000,000) for cosmetics, and in 1929 the figures were climbing upwards because of the sudden rage for the suntanned look, leaving women with dressing tables crammed with makeup colours that were no longer fashionable. 'Today,' wrote Betty Thornley in the autumn of 1929, 'we're all tanned—out in the sun or out of a bottle . . . and most of us will stay as we are at least through the autumn.' An American manufacturer sold 200,000 bottles of instant tan in the first ten days his product was on the market. The tan look was first taken up by Hollywood and New York's international set, but the rest of the country followed quickly.

With the tanned face came a slight decrease in the use of rouge and a shift towards the orange shades. Pink and white powders virtually disappeared. An increased emphasis on keying the makeup colours to the costume resulted in an enormous increase in the sale of cosmetics. Then, too, there were colours for daytime and colours for evening, the latter being, in general, lighter and brighter. Blue eyeshadow and blue mascara had been used to make eyes look bluer, but now eye makeup was also being keyed to the costume. Brown eyeshadow was no longer worn with brown eyes when the lady was wearing a blue dress. And the blue eyeshadow which had done wonders for the lady's blue eyes up to now had to be abandoned with a brown dress. Only with red, orange, yellow, or black dresses could the eyeshadow match the eye.

A country-wide survey in 1929 showed that New England was the most conservative part of the country in makeup, preferring cream and liquid rouges because they were more natural, and resisting any but pale lipsticks, like Tangee (Plate 25-J), which changed colour after application. Southern women used the most rouge; and, except for southern California, parts of the country with the most sun and the darkest skins preferred the lightest powder. It was estimated that the fashionable woman needed at least two lipsticks (day and evening) and four powders (two for day, two for evening), in addition to other cosmetics. Middle-aged women were advised always to use two powders—an ochre rose followed by a rachel. The new darker powders, it was said, were very popular with the men because they liked to use them, and having a good supply close at hand solved the problem of how to get them without the inconvenience or embarrassment of going into a store and buying them.

Authorities on makeup (meaning any woman who sold cosmetics or could

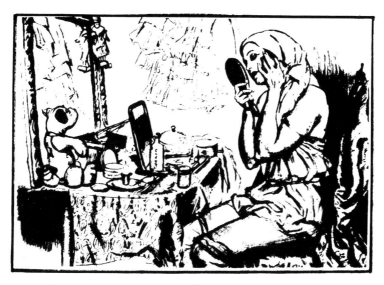

FIG. 216: Actress at her dressing-table, 1929.

get her opinions into print) were plentiful, and one of them outlined her idea of the correct way to apply makeup in 1929:

'First an orange rouge — then your powder — then a dusting of the dry rouge you usually use. . . . Outline your Cupid's bow in liquid rouge, making the mouth you'd have chosen if you could; let it dry on, then apply your lipstick. Put your eyeshadow very close to the lashes, never on the ball of the eye. Elongate the eye itself by blending the shadow out. With a suntan makeup, try brown eyeshadow first, with blue on top. More brown should be used in the daytime, more blue at night.'

The cosmetics which flooded the market in the twenties were in most cases considerably different from those of the eighteenth century, the previous peak period in cosmetic usage. Rouge was now made from carmine, carmoisine, and coal tar colours, mixed with talcum, starch, or fuller's earth, and perfumed. For dry cake rouge, gum arabic was added; liquid rouges were usually dissolved in glycerine and alcohol. Lipsticks had a paraffin base reinforced with wax or cocoa butter and tinted with carmine or coal tar dyes. But cold cream was not vastly different from that invented by Galen in the second century A.D., and according to Ivor Griffith, 'Eyebrow pencils and eyelash cosmetics are still made as they were in Egypt five thousand years ago — namely, from soot, lampblack, burnt sienna, and soap or wax and paraffin'.

POCKETS OF RESISTANCE

But the use of cosmetics was far from universal, and there were pockets of determined resistance. Griffith quotes a Dress Reform Pledge, which circulated (whether signed by anybody or not, he does not say) in Guthrie, Oklahoma, in 1928. Anyone rash enough to sign thereby promised to abstain from short sleeves (less than three-quarter length), short skirts (above the shoe tops), unnecessarily bright apparel, attractive head attire, dressing the hair, and the use of cosmetics. Those who objected to signing the pledge were directed to see 2 Corinthians XIII,5 ('Examine yourselves, whether ye be in the faith; prove your own selves. Know ye not your own selves, how that Jesus Christ is in you, except ye be reprobates').

Actress Blanche Bates, having failed to stir up any indignation in her protest to the San Francisco Board of Education about the use of makeup by schoolgirls, took her case to the country at large by way of *Colliers*. 'This might well be called The Painted Age,' began Miss Bates. 'A walk down any street in any city is much the same as watching Easter eggs rolling on the White House lawn.

'No, that is not quite true. Some degree of care and thought is given to the coloring of an egg, while the general run of faces look as if the paint had been slapped on with a trowel. And *such* paint! Every imaginable shade of red — and some shades that cannot be imagined — and, in ninety-nine cases out a hundred, the wrong shade. . . .

'The average woman of today . . . proceeds upon the happy assumption that there is no more to make-up than a paint barrel, a spade, and physical strength. And as for lights it never enters her head to make a distinction between artificial and natural. As a consequence, she makes up under an electric lamp without thought of the outside sun, and when she reaches the street, she looks for all the world like a circus clown.

'I am not leveling any wholesale indictment against paint and powder and lipsticks. I uphold the right of every woman to make herself as attractive as possible. . . . Where I dislike and resent the employment of make-up is in the case of old women and young girls. To me, at least, there is nothing more painful and pathetic than the sight of a grandmother — ancient enough to be one anyway — mincing along a public street with her cheekbones buried under a mass of crude vermilion, mascara dripping from her eyelashes, and her mouth a study in scarlet. . . .

'Even more ghastly is the spectacle of a young girl, still in her teens, going about with a compact clutched tightly in her hand, opening it every few minutes to freshen the violent crimson of her lips, to add to the blobs of rouge on her cheeks, or to plaster more powder on her nose, already gleaming like a tombstone against the background of reds and ochers. I never see the performance without wanting to grab the little halfwit and throw her under a pump. . . .

'My objection to painting and powdering and lipsticking by adolescents is that it cheats them out of childhood. A child may start on the use of a compact because "all the other girls do it", but be very sure it will not be long before its significances are understood by her. In its essence the thing is a call to vanity, and there can be no question that it leads to a premature development of the sex instinct. . . .

'If I have picked on this painting and powdering business, it is because I know of no better symbol for the joy-riding spirit of the times. Don't tell me that any decent mother approves the use of cosmetics by her thirteen-year-old daughter! Take away every other consideration involved, and the mere sight of a baby face smeared all over with rouge is enough to make any normal human being heartsick. . . .

'Let them call me old-fashioned all they please. My thirteen-year-old daughter is going to keep right on going to bed at half past eight; she is not going to be permitted to paint and powder, sit with boys in darkened movie galleries, smoke cigarettes, and attend hip-flask parties; at least, not until she is eighteen.'

MEN VERSUS PAINT

In the October issue of the *Delineator*, Frederick Collins discussed the youth movement and where it started. 'Personally,' he wrote, 'I think it started in a chemical laboratory when some scientist . . . invented a rouge that didn't show. We all remember the "painted women" of only a few years ago, with their thick scarlet rouge — the same color for every cheek! — and their gritty white powder which looked as if it had leaked out of a sack of "Minneapolis seconds." They didn't look like "nice" women, and most of them weren't. The average wife and mother wouldn't appear on the street in such a make-up any more than she would in tights. . . . But today, as my bobbed haired friend expressed it: "Lipsticks and rouge are just as respectable as collar buttons or derbies — and far more becoming". . . .

'Today in thousands of American communities, the unpainted woman is the exception, not the rule. In another decade she may be extinct. . . . The final breaking up of the prejudice against rouge seems to have followed the breaking up of the hard shell, enameled face. A scene in a recent Viennese operetta depicted the antics of a woman whose face was so firmly caked that she had to hire a lackey to register her emotions for her. She did not dare show fear, anger, amusement, or joy, lest she crack. To those who remembered the hard-boiled complexion of thirty years ago, the scene was a reminiscent scream. To the neatly tinted youngster of the present day, it was largely unintelligible. The modern woman can wear paint and express herself at the same time. . . .

'To be sure, some of the more conservative matrons teetered a while between color and pallor. They didn't like to look painted. But when chemists produced a rouge that defied detection — and osculation — the staidest housewife turned toward the sunrise and faced the new day with "the rose of youth upon her". The first results, as in the case of other youthfulizing experiments, weren't altogether promising . . . the unskilful dauber of flesh was no better than the unskilful dauber of canvas. The average output was poor. But this was only a passing phase. Beauty shops multiplied. . . . Periodicals which had hitherto ignored the existence of rouge devoted columns to showing their readers how to use it. Knowledge became power. Beauty was frequently achieved — youth approached.

'As a man, I don't like it. When I can detect paint on a woman's face, I resent it. Even when I can't see it but know it is there, I deplore it. But I find that I am noticing it less often as the skill becomes greater, and thinking of it less harshly as the practice becomes more general. And I must admit that where the job is done well, the modern woman's use of paint and powder is a tremendous factor in her fight for youth.'

Evidently other men thought so too. Although the painted women of the twenties seemed not to call forth the biting satire from men that their predecessors in earlier centuries had, the free use of paint by women of all ages in a desperate effort to recapture their youth did result in at least one mild collegiate verse :

> Tell me, pray thee, pretty maid,
> Are you sixty-five years old,
> Or am I overbold?
> Tell me, pray thee, pretty maid,
> Shall I judge you by your looks
> Or take heed to what I'm told?
> Tell me, pray thee, pretty maid,
> Are you sixty-five years old?

William Goeckerman, who seems to have been rather a glum sort, chose to rap a few female knuckles without mincing words. 'The discriminating observer,' he wrote, 'may well marvel at what an individual hopes to achieve by superficially applying some lotion, powder, or paint to certain parts of the body. . . . It is likely that the prime objective of the user of the so-called cosmetics is to convey a temporary deceptive impression of beauty and thus increase admiration. As a matter of fact, even this object is only occasionally attained, and just the opposite effect is often created. Whatever the result, if this is the motive, its

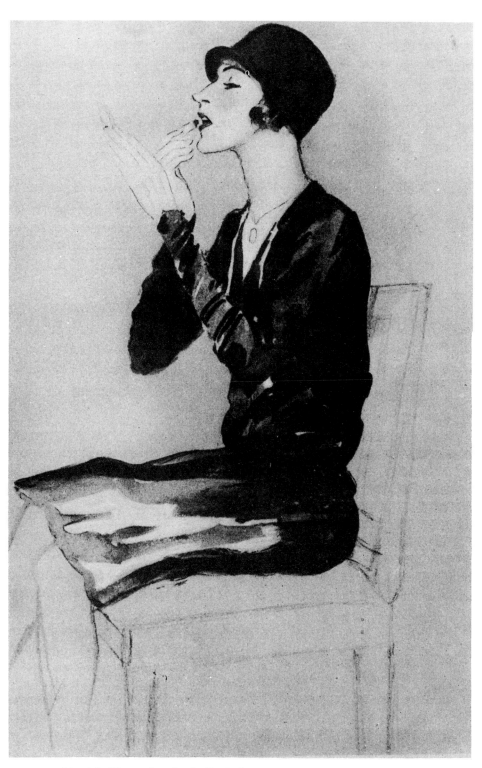

FIG. 217: Lipstick. Watercolour by Steffie Nathan, 1928.

very essence is fraud.' Mr Goeckerman also added a warning about 'the dangerous chemicals from hair washes, tonics, and dyes, shampoos, complexion powders and toilet powders, moth and freckle lotions, face enamels, toilet waters, grease paints, face creams, skin bleaches, and what have you . . . often preparations are advertised as being absolutely harmless when they contain wood alcohol, corrosive sublimate, arsenous acid, paraphenylendiamine (a toxic aniline dye), sugar of lead, lead plaster, calomel, white precipitate, resorcin, and so forth.'

In a lecture given in 1929 Ivor Griffith said that 'if there is any one phase of external decoration which is today overdone, it is in the field . . . of cosmetics. Nor is overdoing or overmaking up the only sin committed in the name of cosmetics, for this field of personal adornment is one that lends itself very easily to the wiles of the quack and the crook. . . . Kittens take two weeks to open their little eyes — but there are humans whose mental eyes seem closed long after their kindergarten days. And it is these human kittens who largely furnish the force and fashion the face of the great cosmetic splurge. For they are the believing kind who hearken to the claims of every noisy quack — and who fall easy prey to the wiles of every crook. They form the undiminishing multitude that still believes in the creative functions of hair tonics — in the face lifting, wrinkle erasing ability of creams — in one-night bunion banishers, and in two-day chest or hip removers.' He ridiculed young women who 'kalsomine, laquer, enamel, veneer, bake, parboil, porcelain finish, shellac, and electro-plate their faces with chemicals and corrosives fit only for barns, radiators, and board fences. The other day I saw a futuristic picture of Franklin Field after the ball game was over, and I said to the artist — "What are those fuzzy caterpillars streaming out of those red wren houses?" And he looked sympathetically at me and pronounced them as young men of means wrapped up in raccoon coats. But I had no need to ask him what the accompanying fusiform vermilion streams were, for I recognized them at once as the mercurochromed obtruding lips of current Cleopatras.'

3000 Miles of Lipstick

About this time an advertising agency estimated (conservatively, they said) that American women were using three thousand miles of lipstick a year, 375,000,000 boxes of face powder, and 240,000,000 cakes of dry rouge. American cosmetics manufacturers, in 1928, spent more than 16 million dollars (nearly 7 million pounds) in advertising their products, making them the third largest industry in the country in volume of magazine advertising. According to the U.S. Census Bureau, their number had risen from 39 in 1849 to 803 in 1929. The cosmetics produced had risen in value from \$355 (£148) to \$191,039,469 (about £80,000,000) a year. This does not include imported cosmetics, which in 1920 were valued at more than six million dollars, exclusive of toilet soap.

But the increase in volume of sales did not necessarily bring with it an improvement in the quality of the product. 'Some women,' said Dr Charles W. Pabst, a New York dermatologist, 'apply mixtures to their faces that would take the paint off an automobile.' He reported an increase of fifty percent in three years in cases of skin diseases resulting from cosmetics. Products in the three-billion-dollar-a-year cosmetics industry were found to contain such familiar poisons as lead, mercury, and arsenic, which had plagued women for centuries. One dangerous product mentioned was a face powder advertised not to rub off. Continued use, warned Dr Pabst, would result in lead poisoning, and the special remover provided by the manufacturer was even more dangerous than the powder.

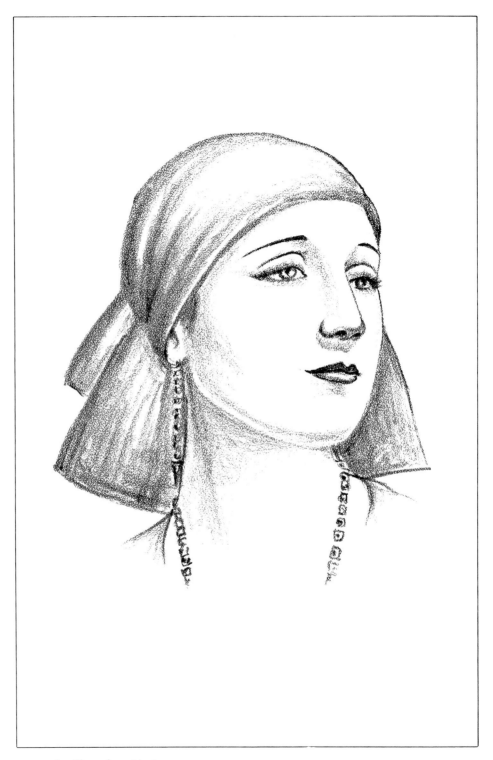

FIG. 218: The sad-eyed look, 1930.

20 · The Twentieth Century 1930-1940

Some women aren't as young as they are painted.
HELEN FOLLETT JAMESON

'The average American woman,' wrote Paul W. White in 1930, 'has sixteen square feet of skin. Her dissatisfaction with it . . . accounts for the expenditure in one year of at least $2,000,000,000.' This amount, Mr White pointed out, surpassed the total budgets of half a dozen states.

Evidently this was not enough, judging from the figures of Elizabeth E. Myers, a cosmetologist, who thought that every woman should spend at least $307 (£128) a year on keeping herself cosmetically presentable. Miss Myers provided the following breakdown:

```
 2  permanent waves, $20
26  shampoos, $26
26  special rinses, $13
26  haircuts, $13
12  hot oil treatments, $18
52  facials, $130
26  eyebrow plucks, $13
 8  eyebrow dyes, $12
26  manicures, $19.50
 4  lipsticks, $4
    rouge, $10
 4  jars cleansing cream, $5
 4  jars tissue cream, $5
 3  jars skin food, $3.75
 3  jars muscle oil, $3
 4  bottles astringent, $6
 3  boxes powder, $6
```

Even though American women had not begun to spend what Miss Myers thought they should, they were using 4000 tons of powder, 52,500 tons of cleansing cream, 26,250 tons of skin lotion, 19,109 tons of complexion soap, 17,500 tons of nourishing cream, 8750 tons of rouge, and 'enough lipsticks to reach from Chicago to Los Angeles by way of San Francisco'.

A single woman's magazine might carry advertisements for as many as sixty brands of cosmetics, selling at from $1 to $25 or occasionally as much as $200

(£83) for a jar of some very exclusive, exotic cream in an elegant jar of opaque green and silver, crystal and silver, or orchid and black.

The names were carefully designed to increase the allure. A single catalogue of the period listed such items as Camellia Cream, Special Texture Cream, Persian Muscle Oil, Astringent Cerate, Violet Astringent, Mist of Dawn Face Powder, Poudres des Perles, and Vah-Dah Eye Cream. There were sixty-eight 'beauty necessities' listed at prices ranging from forty cents for cleansing tissue to twenty-five dollars for a small urn of imported face cream — 'a triumph in the mysterious realm of the endocrines'.

The profit to be made from all of this was unusually attractive. A pharmacist could make up one ounce of cold cream (white wax, oil of almond, spermaceti, rose water, powdered sodium borate) for not more than eight cents, and he would probably sell it for twenty-five cents (two shillings). But one ounce of an advertised brand of essentially the same cold cream, differently scented and sold by the same pharmacist, might cost as much as $1.25 (10s. 5d.).

The copywriters and beauty editors were kept busy thinking up new ways of titillating women's easily stimulated desire to acquire every new beauty preparation appearing on the market. One release read:

'The whole world has gone to work to beautify the American woman. France is growing roses, Asia sending musk, England lavender, and Italy iris and bergamot. All are brought on ships to New York where manufacturers compound the fragrant, beautiful raw materials into rouge, lipstick, powders, and perfumes. The finished products are then redistributed by train and shipped to all parts of America and other countries.'

THE BEAUTY SALONS

All of the publicity and the enticing displays of elegantly packaged cosmetics drew women like a magnet to the beauty counters and into the beauty salons, one of which was described in the *Beauty Shop News*:

'The Boutique Empire motif characteristic of the exquisite "Little Shops" of Paris in the days of the First Empire . . . is retained throughout. From the street the visitor steps into a foyer in which a large wall-hanging of blue and silver, patterned in a small flower design gives color to cool gray walls and leads the eye harmoniously to the bronze framework of the door leading to the salon itself.

'The atmosphere of the salon is artistically Gallic in its effect. Touches of rose, blue, green, and gold are used throughout, set off against neutral tones of ivory and gray. The furniture is in Empire style with frames of gray-green deftly accentuated with old-gold and in varied upholsterings of toile de joie in a dominant blue pattern, mulberry silk in an Empire design of silver and blue silk figured with vari-colored flowers.

'The wall treatment is particularly noteworthy. To the left of the entrance is a large alcoved mirror in unique checker-board of mirror squares alternating with patterned frosted glass, against which is set an unusual treatment of two preening peacocks. To the right are two wall paintings by Larsson-Bernath showing two garden scenes of the French school, treated in predominant shades of soft blue which makes them an integral part of the color harmony of the whole interior.'

In such surroundings women of the thirties spent endless hours and money having their faces massaged, cleansed, nourished, stimulated, painted, and powdered. At one Fifth Avenue salon a facial cost $3.50; a youth-restoring eye treatment, $3; blackhead treatment, $5; special stimulating treatment, $10; muscle treatment, $10; arm treatment, $3; hair and scalp treatment, $3; shampoo, $1.50; and hot oil shampoo, $3. There were nearly 40,000 such shops (most of them less elegant and less expensive) across the country, organized into various groups (such as the National Hairdressers and Cosmetologists Association) to get the women away from the beauty counters and do-it-yourself makeup and into the salons. But Associations must have rules and principles and aims and charters and constitutions and conventions, and these were no exception. The National Association of Cosmeticians and Hair Artists issued the following statement of their aims and principles:

'To promote uniform legislation. To bring about a higher standard of skill and education. To educate the public and the members of the profession as to the scope and possibilities of high class service. To cultivate a friendly and co-operative spirit among all engaged in this work. To provide methods for carrying on and systematizing the business of the membership of the Association. To promote interest in and exchange ideas for the advancement of the profession.

'We believe that education is necessary if our profession is to win the position it is entitled to. The cosmetician and hair artist of the future must be efficient and thoroughly trained in all branches of the work. . . . The future will demand greater effort, more self-sacrifice, boundless enthusiasm and tireless energy if the high standard of our work is to be maintained.'

At a typical convention of one of these associations, there were contests in finger waving, marcelling, and permanent waving, free lessons in various techniques of the trade, exhibitions of new machines and methods, as well as the usual dinners and entertainments. Even as early as 1930 there were a number of well-established trade journals — *Beauty Culture, The American Hairdresser, The Beautician, Beauty Shop News, The National Beauty Shop, The Beauty Journal, The Modern Beauty Shop, The Southern Beauty Shop,* and *The Western Beauty Shop.* A single issue of *The Beautician* provided articles on 'Coiffure, Complexion, Costume Blend', 'Now the Baby Permanent', 'The Coiffure Joins the Ensemble', 'The Sun-Tan Miracle', 'Beauty Survey Shows Business Trend', 'Handsome Does as Handsome Is', 'The Hair Tells a Story', 'This Month's Ten Dollar Idea', 'Things New and Noteworthy', and 'Match the Mood with Perfume'. At this same time there were such newspaper headlines as 'Health Chief Warns in Beauty War' and 'Poison May Lurk in Lipstick Kiss'. But when one expert warned women against dangerous cosmetics, there were always other experts to pour oil on troubled waters with assurances that it wasn't really all that bad. The women, if they cared at all, preferred to believe the optimists and to go right on pouring their husbands' money into the beauty business.

Blood red nails were fashionable in 1930, and in Paris emerald green and other colours were beginning to be seen as well. In May *Harper's Bazaar* reported on 'a delightfully original ensemble Peggy Sage has created — a lipstick to match your nail polish. Strange, with the ensemble idea being the fetish it is, that no one thought of it before. Now you may match your type or your colouring by nails and lips that harmonize. An altogether intriguing idea, don't you think?' The three available shades were Lido Crimson, Riviera Red, and Palm Beach Coral.

Reporting on a visit to a friend's country house, Doris Lee Ashley listed the cosmetic items her hostess had provided. In the private bath there were tubes of cleansing cream, nourishing cream, and toothpaste, a package of coloured cleansing tissues, a new toothbrush, effervescent bath tablets, scented soap, deodorant bath powder, deodorant, and an after-bath rub. On the dressing table she found a small manicure set, including nail polish, 'a large jar of cotton powder-puffs, two small boxes of complexion powder, suntan and rachel, a cream rouge of medium tone, and a large bottle of a liquid which declared on its label that it would cleanse the skin, tone it, and provide an excellent base for powder.'

HELENA RUBINSTEIN

To Helena Rubinstein, who began by beautifying Australian women in 1902 with a batch of home-made face cream from Poland, makeup soon became a business and an art. The self-styled 'World's Greatest Beauty Culturist' appeared in 1915 in the United States, where she proceeded to amass a fortune of more than 500 million dollars. By 1960 her twenty-room Park Avenue apartment contained a valuable collection of paintings, including fourteen portraits of herself by famous contemporary artists.

'My mother,' she wrote in 1930, 'had brought us up to use a little powder on our faces but would have been horrified at the thought of rouge or lipstick or mascara for the eyes. And it was not until my establishment in London had been open for about a year that I began to give serious thought to the subject of cosmetics. . . . After many requests, I started to create my own rouges and lipsticks (powders I had always been making), the purity of which was absolutely sure. . . . I haunted the art galleries of London to study the various shades of coloring in the portraits of all ages. I also went to France, Spain, and Italy and, finally, to India, Egypt, and other tropical countries to learn more about the preparation and use of decorative cosmetics.

'I was forced to try out my creations on my own face and so gradually came to use them myself, though previously I had not used make-up at all. Very few Englishwomen at that time were brave enough to confess to the use of rouge, though many of them *secretly* touched up their faces.

'Rouge for the cheeks, and powder, were the main standbys of the toilette table, and lipsticks and mascara were practically unheard of. France, of course, has escaped these inhibitions with regard to make-up, never having come under the influence of good Queen Victoria. . . . Another reason is that French-women are willing to take more time at their toilette than the average Anglo-Saxon. . . .

'It is very fortunate that a frank attitude toward make-up has been reached in the United States within the past ten years. In this country the extremes of climate and the high speed of living tend to take the color out of the face very quickly. Even young women barely out of their teens often have a washed-out look in their faces when they are without make-up. Make-up is now put on to heighten and enhance the appearance much as one adds jewelry to a costume. It is used as a part of the decorative scheme, and hence its scope is somewhat wider than is actually necessary to secure the impression of blooming youth.'

Madame Rubinstein considered powder of primary importance in any makeup and the most indispensable item on the dressing table. But it had to be extremely fine ('sifted many times through the finest silk bolting cloth') and suited to one's type of skin. She did not advise white powder but admitted there were a few who could get by with it. For the past few years, she said, 'Paris, Vienna, and Rome seem to have preferred the darker tones in powder, a preference that has at last reached the smart women of America. I believe the chic Europeans originally chose these tones because they suggest health and out-of-doors, and also because they bring out the whiteness of their teeth. Now the whole young world inclines to the "sunplexion" tones—and they are singularly becoming.'

As for rouge, more and more women, said Madame Rubinstein, were giving up the hard-to-apply liquid rouge for compact or cream rouge. For subtle blending, she recommended cream rouge applied in dots with the third finger and blended with the second. 'For evening,' she added, 'a hint of rouge on the lobes of the ears is nice. Frenchwomen employ it almost invariably and some-times in the nostrils.' She found brilliant rouge acceptable with large eyes but not with those which were 'small, soft, and serene'. Raspberry, she found, was a safe shade for everybody, though geranium was suitable for a fair skin, brunette for the olive-skinned, and crushed rose tint for the mature woman. Tangerine, she added, was still used by a few blondes and redheads but was otherwise 'very little in favor'.

At this time Madame recommended Persian eyeblack for the eyes, applied to both upper and lower lids with the index finger, covered with fine linen. With the optional addition of a little eyebrow pencil, the makeup was done. It was to be removed with cold cream, followed by astringent.

Each day as European and American women were performing their ritual with creams, paints, and powders, women in parts of Africa, Australia, Malaya, Borneo, and other parts of the world were still staining their teeth red, blue, or black, filing them to points, or boring holes in them and inserting stubs, tattoo-ing their lips or inserting bamboo rings, or (among the Eskimos) smearing them-selves with walrus fat. The products, procedures, and results varied, but the intention was the same.

TRENDS IN MAKEUP, 1931

Vogue and *Harper's Bazaar* agreed, in 1931, that more natural makeup was the Paris fashion and consequently the fashion everywhere. 'A vivid slash of red lips,' noted *Vogue*, 'has no place in today's very feminine, individual mode. Avoid lipsticks that do not match your natural coloring.' In endorsing Tangee products, *Harper's Bazaar* said approximately the same thing. Ruth Murrin, writing in *Good Housekeeping*, echoed the plea for greater naturalness and pointed out that a much greater variety in shades of powder and rouge was available. 'One perfumer,' she wrote, 'makes eight shades of powder rouge, varying all the way from a delicate nasturtium to the brightest blush. A Fifth Avenue specialist has seven shades in compact rouge and almost as many in cream rouge. The softer, more delicate shades are the best choice for the present fashions, but one must remember that what is natural and lovely for one woman looks gaudy on another. As a general rule, orange-red rouges are more becoming to brunette and violet-red to blonde complexions.' Eye makeup was also less artificial, with the heavy black cosmetic wax being replaced by mascara in a variety of colours.

Tangee's popular Theatrical Lipstick was now joined by Theatrical Rouge. Helena Rubinstein's Lipstick Enchanté was, according to her copywriter, 'the most beautiful ever created', and her waterproof rouge was 'irresistible as a young blush', evidently available in only one shade but in either a surf green or a cerise container. Yet in this same year Dorothy Gray had seven new shades of rouge, and Marie Earle had five shades of eyeshadow.

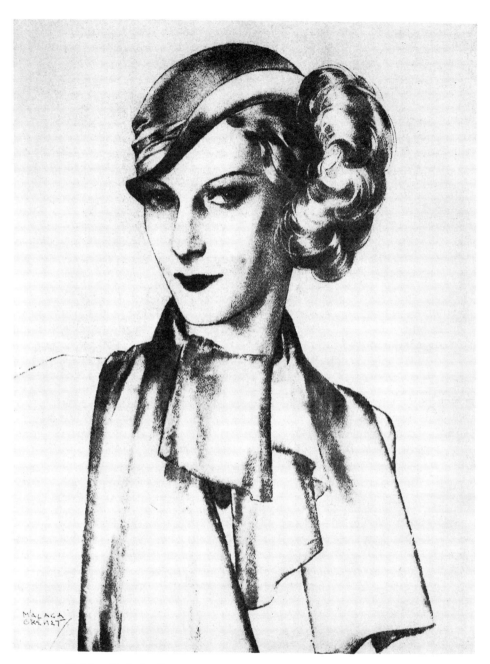

FIG. 219: **Fashionable lady of 1931.**

The summer of 1931 found Betty Thornley Stuart writing enthusiastically to the readers of *Colliers* about the latest trend in makeup — subtlety and individuality:

'The girls have done it again. . . . They've always used make-up, but heretofore the process has gone by fashion rather than by type and has resulted in something that looked more like a billboard than a work of art. All girls were adjured to do the same thing, so that we can remember whole eras like the nose-in-the-flour barrel, the twin-sunsets-on-cheeks, the corpse-face with the scarlet gash for a mouth, the recent mahogany finish all over, the still more recent feminine wave that forced even the lusty Amazon to look fragile and appealing.

'This thing is different. The keynote is individuality, the watchword subtlety. The colors, subcolors, and shadings are as delicately varied at those a painter puts on canvas. . . . Evening make-up is, of course, the chef d'oeuvre of the whole performance, though daytime effects for town run it a close second. Even the most ardent devotees of the new movement go easy for sport. . . .

'Suppose you're one of those pale non-descripts with a wedge-shaped face, lightish brown hair and eyes that are neither here nor there, unless you begin to analyze their shade. You must realize that you're slated to be extra-pale and play it up—no rouge whatever, unless the merest touch when you aren't feeling well. Your mouth should be a brilliant red. But the crux of the situation lies in your eyes . . . they can change like the sea and be just as dangerous.

'If you want to wear blue . . . your eyes should be made up with a neutral light-brown cream eye shadow, applied over the entire lid from lash to brow, shaded a bit with dark blue, outward on the lid and toward the corners. If, on the contrary, you plan to wear green, the neutral shadow should be reënforced with a touch of the same color. Mascara is to be used at all times—just the least delicate bit on the upper lashes, applied from underneath and afterward gone over with a dry brush to remove the movie effect. The brows aren't to be plucked—that is gone forever—but brushed so as to be a little thinner and flatter.'

For ice-blondes Mrs Stuart suggested 'cream rouge the color of blood' and a light indelible lipstick. For a freckled red-head she recommended, following a good skin bleach, a pastel rouge 'rather than the orange so mistakenly used by many' and a light brown eyeshadow. For all types wearing white in the summer she proposed a dark cream rouge, dark powder, 'a very, very vivid lipstick', and more mascara than usual. As for tanning, Mrs Stuart said the cult was over, and now women could tan or not as they chose.

A cable from Paris in the late summer indicated that makeup was 'quite naturalistic with reference to powder and rouge, but lips are still very brilliant and eyes are slightly more accentuated on account of the allure of new hats. Feeling against sun-tanning is growing.' *Harper's Bazaar* said that makeup would be less obvious and that 'Lovely pink and white faces with striking accents on mouth and eyes' would 'peer charmingly from the new upturned brims. . . . Rouge will be blood colour and lipstick a bit more definite, while eyes will play an important role through the subtle application of shadows and the merest suggestion of mascara.' Nails were expected to continue to be pink, though Paris approved of bright shades, especially for evening. Beauty editors were advising women that it was just as easy to have nails and lips in harmony as in conflict.

Opalescent fingernails were occasionally seen in Paris. An adaptation of this was called Platinum Tips—the application of an opaque silver polish to the tips of red enamelled nails.

In October it was reported that Madame Rubinstein had been busy in Paris creating the 'Eugénie Complexion', with which she hoped to 'bring about a happy coordination between fall faces and fall modes'. Her newest coral rouge was described as the 'essence of a nineteenth-century blush' and was supposed to be becoming to everybody. But in case of doubt, there was still her Red Raspberry (medium) and her Red Geranium (light). Her new lipsticks, one for blondes and one for brunettes, *Harper's Bazaar* described as 'brilliant without being lurid'. In addition, she had Persian Eyeblack ('the super-mascara'), Coral Nail Groom ('the smartest shade in Paris'), and a variety of creams including Water Lily Cleansing Cream, containing 'skin youthifying essence of water lily buds'.

Elizabeth Arden's autumn promotion was for her set of six lipsticks to match one's costume—Chariot (lacquer red case), Printemps (fern-green case), Victoire (black case), Coquette (black and oyster white case), Viola (blue case), and Carmenita (black and silver case). Printemps was designed as 'a charming accent for pastel frocks', Coquette gave 'a dashing touch', and Viola was supposed to 'make the skin whiter and the eyes more shadowy'.

In *The Beauty Box*, published in 1931, Helen Follett Jameson devoted most of her time to care of the face and figure but did include one chapter of miscellaneous comments on makeup. Cosmetics, she said, were not to be scorned; but without health there was 'no sixty-watt flicker in the eye, no pink velvet bloom upon the alabaster cheek, no spirit in the step'. Nevertheless, makeup was fun and the days when a beauty spree meant dipping a bit of muslin into the cornstarch box were gone forever.

Mrs Jameson advised applying plenty of powder, skimming off the surplus with a camel's hair brush, adding rouge, then more powder. For the average complexion she favoured a rich ivory tint with a trace of flesh; but for a white skin, cotton-coloured hair, and blue eyes, she rather liked mauve. Green face powder was evidently worn by some women but not with Mrs Jameson's blessing.

In order to discover where to apply rouge, the author suggested applying

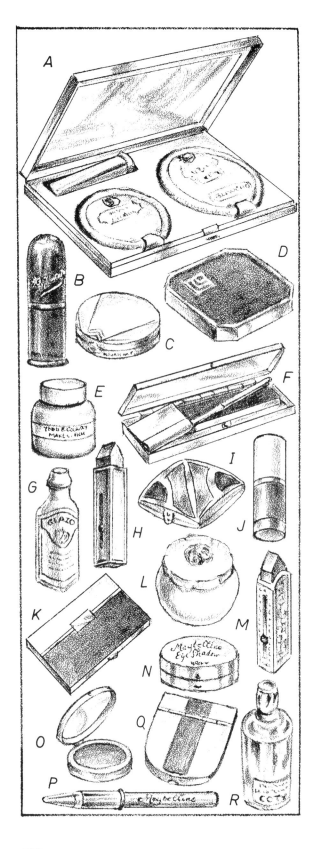

PLATE 26 : TWENTIETH CENTURY
1930–40

A 1931. Houbigant Triple Vanity with rouge, powder, and lipstick. Cover enamelled in geometric design in black, gold, and shades of either red, green, blue, or yellow. Price, $3.50.

B 1931. Jaquet Petit-Point Rouge, in 4 shades. Price, $1.

C 1931. Houbigant platinum-toned rouge compact.

D 1931. Petite Baguette rouge or powder compact, by Lucien Lelong.

E 1939. Town and Country Make-Up Film (powder base). Price, $1.50.

F 1931. Houbigant mascara in platinum-toned case with blue enamelled design. Price, $1.25.

G 1930. Glazo Nail Polish, plain or perfumed.

H 1933. Elizabeth Arden lipstick.

I 1930. Helena Rubinstein rouge and powder compact in black, vermilion, and silver case.

J 1931. Elizabeth Arden lipstick. Available in a set of 6 colours, each in a different coloured case. Price, $1.50 each, 6 for $7.50.

K 1933. Black and cream compact by Lenthéric.

L 1930. Yardley Combination Cream in ivory coloured jar.

M 1933. Louis Philippe lipstick.

N 1930. Maybelline eyeshadow.

O 1930. Helena Rubinstein Valaze Eyeshadow in blue, brown, blue-green, green, or black. Price, $1.

P 1930. Maybelline eyebrow pencil. Price, 35 cents.

Q 1933. Caron gold and black loose-powder case with lipstick.

R 1930. Coty clear liquid nail polish.

PLATE 27 : TWENTIETH CENTURY
1935–1940

A   1939. Ski lipstick, by Antoine. Price, $1.50.

B   Kurlash. For curling eyelashes.

C   1939. Daredevil lipstick, by Dorothy Gray. Price, $1.

D   1939. Daredevil cream rouge, by Dorothy Gray. Price, $1.25.

E   1939. Daredevil compact rouge, by Dorothy Gray. Price, $1.

F   1939. Revlon lipstick. Available in Sky, Windsor, Sun Rose, Bravo, Jueltone, Red Dice, Chilibean, Trinigar, and Mahogany. Price, $1.

G   1939. Gold vanity with diamond clasp by Black, Starr & Frost-Gorham. Price, $135.

H   1939. Cinema Sable Fountain Lip-Brush in ebonite case. Also available in gold or silver-plated case and in several shades of lip colouring. Price, $1.

I   1939. DuBarry cake rouge vanity. Price, $1.

J   1938. Max Factor's Pan-Cake in black and white plastic box.

K   1939. Coty pressed powder vanity in red and gold case. Price, $1.

L   1935. Vanity case by Kathleen Mary Quinlan.

M   1935. Louis Philippe Angelus Rouge Incarnat. 'A brilliant beautifier for lip and cheek that will not rub off.' In Framboise, Poppy, Sun Orange, Pandora, Light, and Medium. Lipstick available in the same colours.

N   1935. Duplé vanity by Volupté. For powder and cigarettes.

O   1935. Devon Milk Cleaner in ivory complexion bowl, by Kent of London. Price, $1.25.

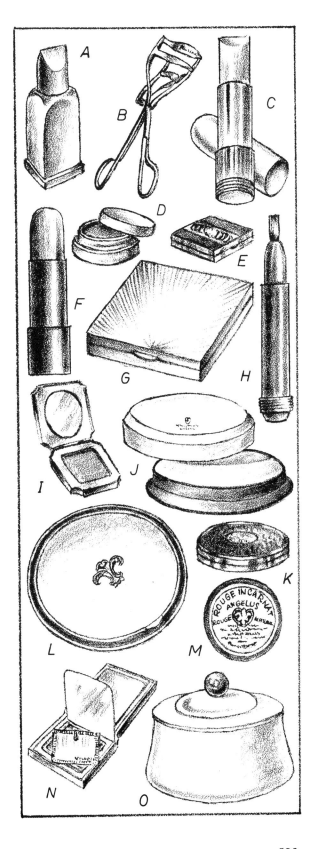

cold compresses to the face for five minutes, then noting which areas became pink. 'Some women', she observed, 'aren't as young as they are painted.' And she warned that painting a withered skin only called attention to its condition. But she liked a bit of rouge on the eyelids. The newest rouge colour in 1931 was yellow red, the purple reds having passed out of fashion, along with poppy-red cheeks and lips. The girl of the period used ivory or rachelle powder, little or no rouge on her cheeks, and no more than a faint 'suggestion of raspberry cream on her lips'. Eyeshadow in blue, mauve, green, or brown was acceptable. Mrs Jameson liked mauve with golden hair; and though brown greasepaint was becoming popular with brunettes, she preferred the latest fashion — faint purple, maintaining that it added 'a mysterious and exotic air'. Natural or peroxide blondes were wearing green, and white-haired women with good complexions often used grey. The result, Mrs Jameson assured her readers, wasn't as terrible as it sounded.

Brown mascara was recommended for darkening the eyebrows and brown pencil for extending them if they were too short. They were supposed to be narrow and very long. Often they were dyed.

Chinese red and orange lipsticks were out; raspberry was in. And since naturalness was fashionable, lipstick, in a shade to match the rouge, was to be applied sparingly. Too much makeup, warned Mrs Jameson, 'makes a woman look wild'. Temperance was the watchword, especially for faded beauties, who could not afford to wear 'flamingo-colored lips, eye shadows, and cheek smears'.

In *Your Face and Figure*, Lilyan Malmstead devoted only one page to makeup, her cardinal rule being, the less the better. Miss Malmstead suggested a light rouge for blondes, dark for brunettes; but for 'the appearance of smartness and refinement', she recommended lipstick and no rouge at all. She also suggested regularly squeezing the upper lip with the thumb and forefinger and pushing it upward towards the nose, presumably to give the mouth the bee-stung look popular at the time. She disapproved of plucking the eyebrows into a thin line.

LETTER FROM LALLA

In 1931 *Household Magazine* sponsored what they called a beauty contest, offering twenty-five dollars as the first prize for the best letter 'telling about the toilet articles you use, including brand names and reasons for your choices'. What the basis of selection' was to be was not specified; but judging from the winning letter, it may have been based on the greatest number of items mentioned. In any case, the letter, most of which is quoted here, does give us a good picture of what the American woman was doing to her face in 1931:

'Speaking of the servants of my dressing table, I shall tell you first about a

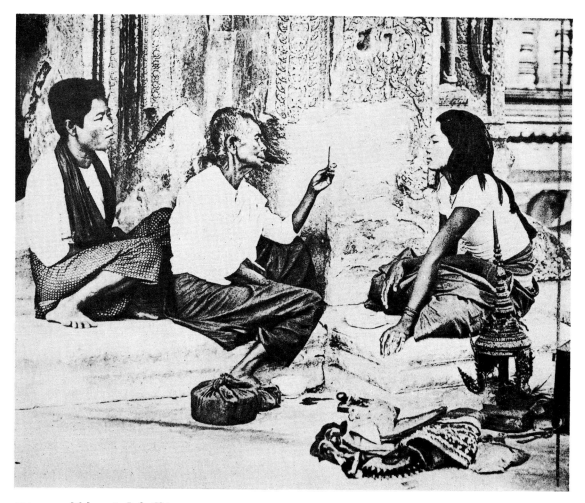

FIG. 220: Makeup in Indo-China, *c.* 1932.

pink and black hat-shaped box containing a flesh-colored face powder with a cold cream base. It is Armand's. Because of the heaviness of this powder and its unusual mellowness and delightful fragrance, I have been unable to find its equal anywhere. Hot weather affects it but little. The shiny nose is covered to stay. Armand's goes on smoothly and it stays on. To my mind, those are the two biggest factors to consider in choosing powder. I find that I need no powder foundation when using Armand's.

'I also have a preference for Armand's cold cream rouge. I use a soft orange shade, finding it most becoming to my natural coloring. As in the case of the powder, it goes on smoothly and stays until removed. Constant retouching is not necessary. It does not clog the pores and thus cause blackheads and pimples.

'In lipstick, I find Tangee all that it is advertised to be. Its orange hue changes to a red that blends with the natural coloring of my lips. Its rich creaminess is soothing.

'Eye lashes and brows come next in consideration. First I apply Three Flowers non-liquid brilliantine to lashes and brows, after which I apply Tangee mascara (black). The brilliantine keeps the eye lashes from becoming brittle when the mascara is used and also gives them a gloss. This particular brilliantine has a delightful fragrance that lingers. Tangee mascara does not make the eyelids smart.

'Now for the care of my skin. To begin with, I use Ivory soap because I have an easily irritated skin and the extreme mildness of this soap causes no irritation or dryness.

'For an astringent I use only Listerine. I tried this after reading the advertisements and found it effective, cooling, and freshening.

'Occasionally I use Boncilla face clay, which is beneficial in removing blackheads and minor skin blemishes, and is a general skin freshener. Boncilla lemon cream is efficient as a skin food and bleach combined. For general cleansing, I prefer Boncilla pink cleansing cream. It is superior to many cleaners in that it both loosens and absorbs dirt from the pores.

'I like Pond's cleaning tissues for removing creams, excess rouge, lipstick, and the like. They are extra soft and absorbent.

'I prefer Coty's bath powder, salts, talcum powder, sachet, toilet water, and perfume because of their lasting fragrance. I use the Styx odor in every one possible.

'I am partial to Hinds Honey Rose and Almond cream for my hands.

'For my nails, I have never used anything except Cutex — liquid polish and remover, nail white, and cuticle cream. These have been satisfactory and I have had no reason to try another brand.

'Because I am troubled with dandruff, I use Fitch's dandruff remover shampoo, and find it helpful. For a hair rinse, I prefer Golden Glint. It brings out the reddish glint in my hair, making it soft and shiny. Wildroot is my tonic, chiefly because it is effective in checking dandruff and leaves the scalp refreshed and clean. I keep the waves set in my hair with Jo-Curl.

'I prefer Delatone cream for removing hair under and on my arms. It is less irritating to my skin than other depilatories, and pleasant to use because of its snowy whiteness and pleasant odor. For a deodorant I use liquid Odo-ro-no.

'I use a Prophylactic tooth brush, because it massages the gums as well as cleans the teeth. Iodent tooth paste is favored because my teeth are hard to whiten, and because it leaves a sweet, pleasant, tingling sensation of perfect cleanliness in my mouth. Listering is my mouth wash. When it is impossible to use a mouth wash, I use May Breath, as it is reliable, satisfactory, and convenient to use.'

What Lalla Cleone Hocton, the creamed and painted May-breath siren who wrote the winning letter, received as her reward, was not specified.

The treatment rooms in the new Richard Hudnut Salon, according to *Harper's*

Bazaar, were 'masterpieces of charm and convenience, each in its own colour scheme, with such engaging combinations as brown and gold, blue and coral, or green and rose'. One room had 'henna walls, turquoise-blue drapes, and black and silver woodwork', and another had 'chalk-white taffeta hangings against walls of lobster-red'.

A New Colour Consciousness

Women in 1932 were still struggling with the bewildering variety of new reds available in rouge and lipstick—cherry, ruby, geranium, American beauty, crimson, magenta, cerise, raspberry, plum, blush-pink, rose, salmon, coral, vermilion, gold, orange-tan, blood orange, and many others. Beauty editors were continually cautioning women about choosing the right shade for both complexion and costume. 'I have discovered' wrote Ruth Murrin in *Good Housekeeping*, 'that when the average woman buys a lipstick or a new pat of rouge, she asks for the medium shade; a very dark brunette asks usually for dark, and a fair blonde for light rouge—a fact which accounts for much misguided make-up. . . . The effect to strive for in using all make-up is naturalness and harmony—not so easy, but much prettier than it sounds!'

Referring to the American girl of 1933, *Vogue* called their approach to the makeup box 'frank and frankly artistic. They use it, not so much to cover up anything as to enhance what they already have. If they have anything particularly stupendous confronting them, they reach instinctively for a lipstick. They try everything once and most things twice and have many pet theories up their sleeves, but none that can not be broken down. They tried ruby nail varnish and stuck to it. The blue-eyed ones are now painting their eyelashes blue. Not a few of the most genuinely fascinating blinkers here about are artificial ones, glued on. They never do their hair in exactly the same way for more than six months at a time without experimenting, unless they are having babies, and then they usually let it run for nine. The hair-dresser is their friend and confidant. They go to him with the regularity of a clock. . . .

'In these days showmanship is everything. If the nose is a bit long or the mouth a bit vast, you can make offending features palatable and do so. In fact, these little idiosyncracies are sometimes dished up as the rarest charm. Of the five most conspicuous and successful beauties in New York right now, one has freckles generously sprinkled across her nose and is much too tall to dance with the average man. Another has to wear pincushions for lack of poitrine. Another has a definite cast in one eye, so that she can never be photographed front faced. Two of them have long, sallow faces with hatchet chins. Another has, we regret to say, rather large legs, and a fifth would have been called, a decade ago, nothing but a bag of bones. . . .

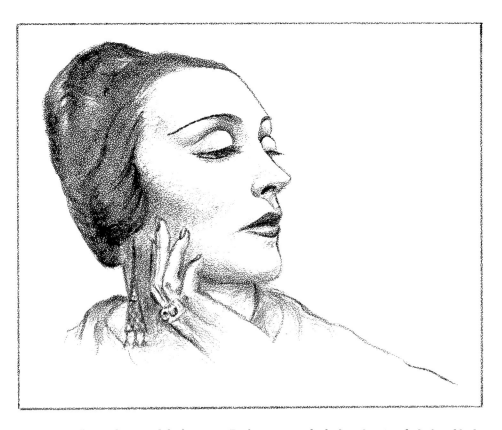

FIG. 221: The sophisticated look, 1933. Eyebrows are plucked and painted, lashes blackened, and lips and cheeks reddened.

'Beauty to-day . . . is no longer left to fate. It is born more often than not in the mind of a homely little girl looking in the mirror at herself for the first time seriously, gritting her teeth, and making up her mind that she is going to launch a thousand ships as well as Helen.'

Nothing, decided *Vogue*, was more significant for women than their lipsticks: 'If we were perpetuating the gestures of the twentieth century for posterity, putting on lipstick would head the list. An ode could be written to it, and to the way in which it serves as a staff for our morale, as well as a beautifier of our faces. It has come to a point where gentlemen have even developed preferences in the very taste of lipsticks.' Older women and conservative ones usually preferred lip-salve to lipstick. Lipstick tissues were available in packets.

Casually brushing aside thousands of years of painting the eyes among the ancients, *Vogue* referred to eye makeup as 'the newest of all the cosmetic sciences . . . and the most fun'. But they warned against the thin, plucked eyebrows popular in the late twenties and allowed only 'the faintest tint of mascara' or the mere touch of an eyebrow pencil.

Eyeshadow was available in 1933 in blue, green, violet, brown, black, silver, and silvered colours. For grey-haired ladies, *Vogue* recommended silvered blue shadow with blue mascara on the lashes. The effect, they promised, would be beautiful without being artificial. Mascara, liquid or cake, could be had in blue and blue-green as well as black and brown. There were also false eyelashes 'of bewildering length' and eyelash irons for curling one's own. Eyebrows could be professionally dyed if one wished.

For evening wear Elizabeth Arden suggested blue-green eyeshadow and dark blue lashes tipped with black. To go with this, one might wear her Victoire cream rouge and Viola lipstick (a bluish red) with Poudre de Lilas. The Arden manicurists were experimenting with using one colour of nail polish over another, for what *Vogue* called 'a very new effect'. The editor was particularly pleased with violet over cyclamen with 'pale, slender hands and a white evening gown'.

For Christmas *Vogue* suggested a Richard Hudnut brown-and-cream enamel vanity case containing dry rouge and loose powder, both with puffs, and a miniature lipstick.

DANGEROUS COSMETICS

In July 1933, according to *The Survey*, American drug and cosmetics companies bought $800,000 worth of radio time to advertise their products. In the absence of laws or regulations concerning the advertising of cosmetics, they were free to make fanciful claims for products which might be harmless at best, but possibly dangerous. Later in the year, in the wake of reports of a number of cases of eye afflictions resulting from the use of harmful eye cosmetics, New York City prohibited the 'sale and use of any eye cosmetics known to contain harmful ingredients'.

Despite all of this, the editors of *Hygeia* wrote that harmful ingredients were not likely to be found in the better grades of cosmetics, that the presence of lead in face powder was no longer greatly to be feared, and that, barring allergies of a few individuals, the colours used in rouge, lipsticks, and eyebrow pencils were relatively harmless.

Stimulated by considerable prodding from the American Medical Association, Consumers Research, the book *100,000,000 Guinea Pigs*, and other publications, the American government showed renewed interest in including cosmetics in new pure food and drug legislation.

Charles Lerner, writing on cosmetics in 1934, wondered whether they really made an ugly woman better looking. 'If she has a large nose,' he decided, 'or a prominent chin, powder will not improve either. Should her lips be thickened or otherwise unsightly, lipstick only adds to the unsightliness. Tampering with the lids and lashes causes, too often, a weird or freakish appearance when seen from a short distance. I have always maintained that natural ugliness is far more beautiful than artificial beauty. A face loaded with cosmetics produces a masked or false appearance . . . the exaggerated quantity of cosmetics that some women smear on their faces sometimes almost becomes repulsive to the average observer.'

In April 1934 the 'Beauty Editress' of *The Queen* reported on a new method for colouring and decolouring the cheeks 'by scientific means', which she termed 'almost a miracle'. For rosy cheeks a colouring compound was 'gently impregnated beneath the skin' of a pallid anesthetized lady. If she wished, she could also have her 'thin and forbidding lips' reshaped into a winsome cupid's bow.

For those who already had too many roses in their cheeks, the colour could be removed in five days. A red nose, it was claimed, could be made 'absolutely white and natural-looking'. There were no before-and-after photographs accompanying the article.

Although women had long since abandoned chicken-skin gloves, the Ideal Home Exhibit in London featured Dekur Sebum gloves of rubber lined with rubber sponge. Impregnated with Dekur lotion and worn twenty minutes a day for a fortnight, they were supposed to make the hands 'as smooth as the face'.

For ladies with rough faces there was Dekur Turtle Oil face cream, guaranteed not to grow hair. It was recommended for wrinkles and acidity under the eyes.

Christmas in London, 1934, brought a variety of gifts — Hand Bag Mascara in a silver and black case ('Does not sting or run or cake the lashes'), a Herbal Mask ('For a New Holiday Face'), a Special Lotion for Shiny Nose ('Soignée faces simply can't live without it!'), and Everywoman's Beauty Box ('a marvellous bargain and a joy to own'). The box contained Cleansing Cream, Beautifying Skinfood, Beauty Foundation Cream, Skin Toning Lotion, and powder.

BEAUTY SECRETS

Metropolitan opera star Gladys Swarthout, in an interview for *Colliers*, revealed her makeup secrets, which were passed on to the public by Marie Beynon Ray:

'Miss Swarthout, a brunette, uses a mere fingertip of a paste rouge, cherry red, rubbed in till it's almost invisible, then a film of powder the color of her skin — basque, a dark powder with a rose tinge — and most of that brushed off with a camel's-hair brush. If she finds herself looking the least bit powdery, she

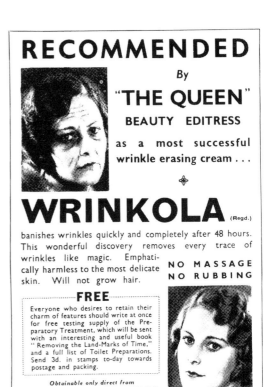

FIG. 222: Advertisement from *The Queen*, 1935.

begins all over again. Then she rubs a mere nothing of eye-shadow in the upper lids—a deep maroon. Invisible though it is, it has its effect. The lips are the one spot where the chic lady really lets herself go. No lipstick has ever been made too red.

'Here there are many schools: the one which holds that the lipstick should match the rouge, which should be the natural color which shows in the cheeks when they are pinched; the school which maintains that the lipstick should be changed according to the time of day, the season of the year, and whether one is in town or country.'

Miss Swarthout herself subscribed to another theory:

'When it comes to lipstick, I'm positively frivolous. I vary the shades to harmonize with the colors of my clothes. I saw Mrs. Alan Ryan recently when she had actually *matched* her purse, her nails, and her lips—all three a deep, dark cherry red, very effective.'

Miss Swarthout used an 'almost natural' liquid nail varnish rather than 'those deep-dyed, bloody nail varnishes that have flooded the country'. And she left her eyebrows much as nature made them, plucking only a few stray hairs.

511

THE MID-THIRTIES

By the mid-thirties, the manufacture of cosmetics was no longer a hit-or-miss process, and new products were seldom marketed, at least by reputable companies, without exhaustive tests. Suntan creams and lotions were patch-tested on women's backs with ultra-violet light, face creams were put into ovens and refrigerators to make sure the ingredients would not separate or crystallize should they be left too long in the heat or cold, and they were aged for months or years to find out if they would turn rancid. The *Ladies Home Journal* reported on equally rigorous tests for nail polish:

'In a certain nail polish factory there is a complete manicure salon where an expert manicurist sits all day giving manicures to the women who work in the plant and offices. . . . She uses a stop watch to time the seconds it takes the polish to dry. Instruments on the walls measure the temperature and humidity of the room. . . . She reports on the consistency, spread, and shine of the polish. She reports how the polish has worn after intervals of one, three, and five days, whether it still sparkles, whether it has rubbed off evenly, or peeled off in bits, whether the color has streaked. If it has worn poorly, she must find out what her client has been doing with her hands in the interim. If there seems to be no excuse for the polish's wearing badly, that batch goes back to the laboratory and none of it reaches you.'

After passing all the laboratory tests, samples of the product were given to women employed by the manufacturer. If they liked it, it was then tried on women outside the company. If they approved the product, it was tested in other parts of the country. Then it might be sold in a single store to see if women would buy it. If they did, it then went on sale throughout a city or state. And passing that test, it was made available at beauty counters throughout the country and sometimes abroad.

The contemporary Japanese makeup, as described by *Vogue*, evidently varied little from the traditional makeup seen in the Utamaro woodcuts (see Chapters 12 and 13). It began with 'a cream or lotion, then a liquid white over which is sprayed a fixative. . . . Rouge, very peach blossom in colour, is placed at the temples, under the eyes, and on the eyelids to encourage a bulging convex shape and a slightly excited expression. Powder is put on again, so much on the upper lip that it sometimes half disappears as though it had bitten into a rice-cake. On the lower lip . . . she applies a dark and violet rouge. It is a dry rouge, held in a small saucer or shell, and she wets her finger to apply it—only on the lower lip, strangely enough. It leaves on the lip a golden reflection with a touch of violet. This rouge is called *beni*.'

Vogue enthusiastically recommended the Youth-Molde combination head band and chin strap (see Figure 223) which served to keep the hair in place and

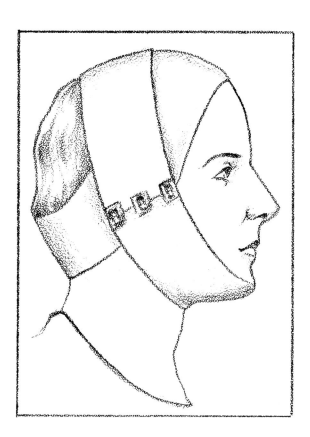

FIG. 223: Youth-Molde head band and chin
strap, 1935.

supported sagging muscles at the same time. *Vogue* suggested that it be used while reading or writing or even all night if one wished.

For an elegant Christmas gift Helena Rubinstein offered a makeup box containing compact rouge, cream rouge, lipstick, eyeshadow, mascara, eyelash grower, eyebrow crayon, face powder, Herbal Eye Tissue Oil, and Town and Country Foundation.

The well-groomed look in makeup for 1936 is exemplified by a series of questions in *Good Housekeeping*:

'Does your skin look fine-textured and has it a vibrant, healthy tone?

'Does your powder give it a dull, velvety finish?

'Is your cheek rouge — if any — so delicately applied that it is hard to tell whether the pink is due to art or nature?

'Do your lips look softly red?

'Do your eyes keep their proper place as the most important feature of your face?

'Do your complexion and your costume complement each other in a friendly fashion?'

The woman who could answer all questions affirmatively might then feel free to relax until the styles changed.

In 1936 Russia's *Glavperfume*, still under the supervision of Madame Molotov, produced 85 million bottles of perfume and cologne, 70 million 'packets of cosmetics', and 300 million cakes of soap (an average of two bars per Russian per year). But despite the inadequacies in production, the industry had shown enormous growth since its beginnings in 1924 and in 1935 showed a profit of 84 million dollars (35 million pounds). Moscow's New Dawn perfume factory, employing 12,000 workers, produced 220,000 bottles of perfume a day. There were 15,000 items available from *Glavperfume*, luring customers with such catchy brand names as Red Moscow, Progress, Express, and Kremlin.

In the United States there were still no adequate controls over the sale of cosmetics, and women were still being disfigured and poisoned while the dangerous cosmetic they had used remained on the market to tempt other victims. According to *Hygeia*, one woman died and several others were totally or partially blinded as a result of using *Lash Lure*, which continued to be sold openly at cosmetic counters. *Koremlu*, a cream depilatory containing thallium acetate, more often used as a rat poison, was forced into bankruptcy by an accumulation of damage suits, not by any government action. But public sentiment for workable controls was increasing and would eventually bring results.

THE ENGLISH DEBUTANTE

Early in 1937 English debutantes preparing for the Coronation were also taking lessons in makeup. A beauty specialist who boasted of having Royal clients described one of the debutantes, coming in with her mother for lessons, as having 'eyes so made-up that she was exactly like a ring-tailed monkey at the Zoo. Her fine skin was literally plastered with powder, her rouge was one shade, her lipstick another — and the trouble was that she thought she knew *all* about make-up, thank you'. Clients were given lessons in marriage, cleansing the skin, makeup, matching nail varnish with lipstick, and changing the shape of the face to suit one's hat.

Since Queen Elizabeth, like Queen Mary, disliked obvious makeup, the debutantes were expected to strive for a reasonably natural look. In the court-yard of Lansdowne House there was set up a special beauty bar with a makeup expert in attendance. There the girls could touch up their makeup at a long sycamore-topped table fully equipped with items considered necessary for correct makeup. There was even a choice of colours — pale rust nail varnish for brunettes or delicate pink for blondes and brown eyeshadow for brunettes, mauve for blondes, and green for the mousy-haired. The eyeshadow was permitted only for evening wear.

For the 'muddle-headed young person, capable of using her skin food as a foundation for powder and her lipstick as a face rouge', salons packed makeup in cases with explicit instructions on how to use it. Debutantes wearing Renaissance dresses in the evening were advised to keep their makeup pale with emphasis on eyes and lips, whereas Regency dresses called for something 'more audacious'.

The final results of all of this flurry over debutantes' makeup were not reported.

COSMETICS FOR MEN, 1937

In 1937, the year that Yardley opened its first beauty salon in London, it was estimated that the upkeep of men's faces in the United States came to more than $200,000,000 (£83,000,000) spent in barbers' shops, some $30,000,000 more than was spent by women in beauty shops. In addition, there would have been a sizeable amount spent for home use of shaving creams, blades, lotions, and other cosmetic items that men would never admit to using.

Beards at the time were out of fashion, and most of the millions of dollars were spent on their prevention. The average American male, reported *Fortune*, 'drops nearly five ounces of hair on the barbershop floor every year and about an ounce down the bathroom drain. And nothing is done with this waste tonnage, which is as heavy as ninety streamlined trains of the Burlington *Zephyr* type. Back in the last century barber artists used to create portraits and landscapes with barber sweepings. Today art moves forward in other forms and the sweepings are incinerated.'

Shaving cosmetics included lather creams, brushless creams, cakes, tablets, bowls, sticks, powders, and liquids. After-shaving lotions in a variety of scents were available in barbers' shops and at toilet counters. For special facial treatments men sometimes secretly patronized women's beauty shops, some of which were anything but secretive about encouraging their patronage.

For more permanent changes, plastic surgeons pared down noses and chins, pulled back ears, corrected harelips, tucked up sagging jowls, and generally made life more pleasant for a number of men and women with major or minor disfigurements.

THE LATE THIRTIES

In 1938 Elizabeth Arden had twenty-nine salons in operation throughout the world — nineteen in the United States. In the six-floor New York salon (renting for about $70,000 a year), one could get a half-hour facial for $2.50 or a paraffin bath for $10. An average morning's beautification cost from $15 (£6) to $20 (£8). In addition, there were 108 cosmetic items to choose from, packaged in 595 assorted jars, bottles, and tubes. The gross income from all of the Arden enterprises, according to *Fortune*, was nearly $4,000,000 (£1,625,000) a year.

Perhaps the most significant development of 1938 was the appearance of Max Factor's Pan-Cake, the first water-soluble cake foundation. The name derived from the fact that it was a cake makeup in panchromatic shades for film. But as it grew in popularity for street, stage, and television, the range of colours expanded to meet the demand. Other companies produced their own cake makeup, and before long women everywhere were appearing with uniformly flat, chalky, beige-to-tan complexions, often with a clear line of demarcation somewhere between the front of the neck and the back. Women, like actors, sometimes forget that they are ever seen from the rear.

Harper's Bazaar found that Schiaparelli's new autumn lipstick shades, keyed to the fall fashions in clothes, gave one's mouth 'the almost indecent allure of Gaugin fruit' — Schiap (a bright, yellowish red), Incarnat (a true red), Fragile (bluish pink), Shocking (intense pink), and Pruneau (the colour of crushed plums).

Eyeshadow sticks were new in 1938.

To a great extent Hollywood set the makeup fashions in the thirties. In a full-page advertisement in *Vogue*, the makers of a lip brush called Cinema Sable (see Plate 27-H), appealed directly to the desire of the average woman to look like a movie star: 'The difference between YOUR lips and those of the glamorous cinema star is that YOU use a blunt lipstick, while SHE uses a lip-brush. HER lips are glorified by a definite, sharp, clear outline, made with a fine sable brush and a certain kind of very concentrated cream color. CINEMA SABLE is a fountain lip-brush with the color right inside its pretty body. Very simple to use . . . it will draw *real* cinema lips on you with all the deftness of a Hollywood make-up man, so that YOUR lips will appear as perfect and as beautiful as those you see on the screen.'

In this same year Mary Pickford, following the lead of Constance Bennett and Josephine Culbertson, entered the cosmetics field as president of Mary Pickford Cosmetics, Inc. Mrs Culbertson, with the estimated 15,000,000 bridge players in the United States clearly in mind, specialized in care of the hands. But she did not work actively at selling her cosmetics. Constance Bennett, on the other hand, made personal appearances at department stores all over the country, and her business flourished.

American women in 1938, according to *American Mercury*, bought 52,000 tons of cleansing cream, 18,000 tons of nourishing cream, 27,000 tons of skin lotion, 20,000 tons of complexion soap, and 2500 tons of rouge. These and other cosmetics cost them $400,000,000 (£162,500,000).

The universal use of makeup brought with it problems in etiquette un-

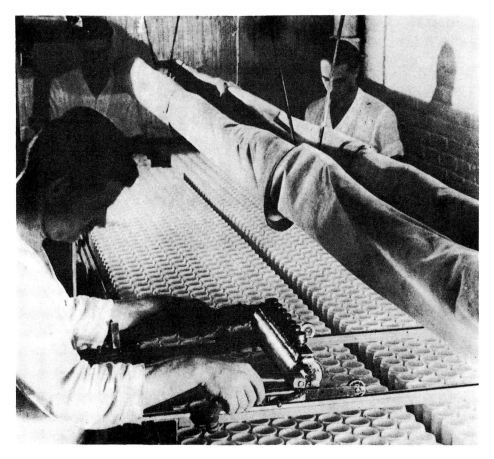

FIG. 224: Filling jars with Ardena cleansing cream, 1938.

dreamed of a few decades earlier. The application of lipstick and powder in public had come to be tolerated, even by men, so long at is was done discreetly and only when necessary. But men did not like lipstick to be applied in public with a brush, and they did not like rouge to be applied in public at all. Women who seemed otherwise reasonably well bred combed their hair at restaurant tables, left lipstick smears on napkins, towels, and glasses, and powdered their noses with dirty, greasy powder puffs from messy vanity cases. The experts advised — pull yourself together before you go out, then leave yourself alone in public.

Christmas gifts advertised in *The Queen* in 1939 included Glovlies ('The medicated night gloves') for 2s 11d, Lanalol Hair Food ('actually made from hair-growing glands') for 2s 6d, Eye Masks ('The ideal inexpensive gift') for

4s 6d, and a five-piece brush set in royal Worcester china, two matching scent bottles and one powder bowl for a total of £17 15s. The eye masks were recommended to counteract the effects of 'black-out nights and stuffy rooms, high winds and dimmed lights'. The hair food was enthusiastically endorsed by a Kentish lady whose 'hair was frightfully thin and came out by handfulls'.

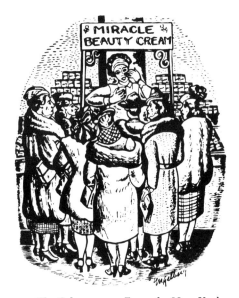

FIG. 225 : The Saleswoman. From the *New Yorker*, 1940.

21 · The Twentieth Century 1940 - 1960

Most of it doesn't do any good anyway.

C. A. WILLARD

'Paint your lips as an artist would,' advised *Vogue* in 1941. 'Use a brush. Use two shades of lipstick. . . . Dramatize a good mouth. Put blue-red on the upper lip, orange-red on the lower. . . . With your summer tan, in bright sun, try bright orange on the upper lip, brownish orange on the lower.' The lady in Figure 226 is following *Vogue's* advice.

There were now 629 items in the Rubinstein line — 78 powders, 62 creams, 69 lotions, 115 lipsticks, 46 perfumes and toilet waters, and a variety of rouges, eyeshadows, and mascaras. Madame used very few of them on herself, preferring to devote her energies to beautifying other women, but she did find time to put on Aquadade foundation, Town and Country face powder, blue-green eyeshadow, black mascara, and lipstick on both lips and cheeks.

Her newest perfume, chosen after she had rejected some eight hundred samples, was, she declared, 'a heavenly scent'. So it was called Heaven Scent, given an angel-and-cloud motif, and launched by means of five hundred pink and blue angel-decorated balloons attached to five hundred wicker baskets, each containing a small vial of cologne, dropped from the roof of Bonwit Teller's Fifth Avenue store. A millionairess with an eye on the pennies, Madame Rubinstein was a genius at promoting herself and her products and liked to be photographed in a white smock in a laboratory, where she was presumably stirring up new concoctions to beautify the women of the world.

The first Food and Drug Act in the United States since 1906 went into effect in 1940. Since it now covered the field of cosmetics, it was called the Food, Drug, and Cosmetic Act and covered all cosmetics involved in interstate commerce. A number of states passed similar laws to plug the loopholes. A display of corrosive eyelash dyes, poisonous freckle creams, and hair dyes containing lead or silver would make it clear to even a casual observer that the law was long overdue.

The law was designed to prevent adulteration, misbranding, and deceptive packaging. In other words, no cosmetic introduced into interstate commerce was permitted to contain poison or any other harmful substance; it could not promise to eradicate wrinkles, restore natural hair colour, or anything else it could not actually do; and it could not be packaged in false-bottomed jars. In addition, coal tar dyes were strictly regulated and thoroughly tested on mice before being approved. Hair dyes dangerous to the eyes or likely to cause allergic reactions had to be so labelled. Misleading advertising had already been prohibited under the Wheeler-Lea Act of 1938.

The Food and Drug Administration suggested as a guideline that certain names of products were regarded as unwarranted and misleading. These included contour cream, crow's foot cream, deep pore cleanser, eyelash grower, eye wrinkle cream, hair grower, rejuvenating cream, scalp food, circulating cream, muscle oil, nourishing cream, pore paste, skin conditioner, skin food, skin tonic, tissue cream, and wrinkle eradicator. Many companies predicted that such restrictions would destroy the industry. But the industry adjusted and survived and began to provide the public with better quality and more accurately labelled products.

Makeup in Wartime

In 1941, according to the *New York Times*, Americans spent more than half a billion dollars (more than 200 million pounds) on cosmetics. This included twenty million dollars' worth of lipstick and sixty million dollars' worth of cold cream. Reactions to this wartime expenditure varied. New York's Mayor LaGuardia hedged but said that in any case he didn't like 'that red stuff on fingernails', and Joseph Maloney, a soda jerk, thought it was 'an awful lot of lettuce to spend on a woman's face'. C. A. Willard of the Cosmetics Branch of the War Production Board found it hardly justifiable, then added: 'Most of it doesn't do any good anyway'.

But a chemical engineer who was interviewed thought it was probably less than men spent on smoking and had better results. A flight instructor decided it was well worth it. He said that every girl in his shop wore makeup, and it gave him a lift every time he went in. A seaman thought it was a bit too much and that the girls ought to taper off, especially on smeary lipstick. A Coast Guard lieutenant didn't mind so long as it didn't interfere with the war, and he had no desire to find out how women would look without makeup.

Dr Iago Galston considered makeup as essential to a woman's morale as a pipe to a male smoker's and figured that prohibiting it might cost the country millions in decreased efficiency. He also pointed out that the current trend was towards buying higher priced cosmetics, even though cheap ones were readily available.

It appeared for a while in 1942 that the war was going to deal a severe blow to the cosmetics industry. In the United States the War Production Board issued, in July, an arbitrary classification of cosmetics according to essentiality, thus severely limiting production. In October the order was revoked, the Board

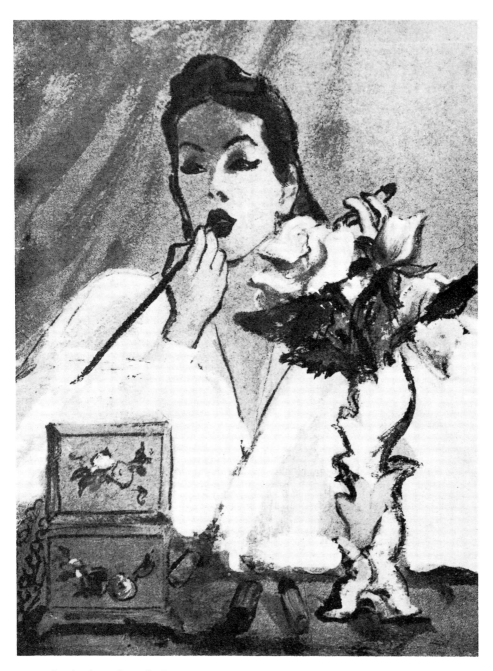

FIG. 226: Applying lipstick. From *Vogue*, 1941.

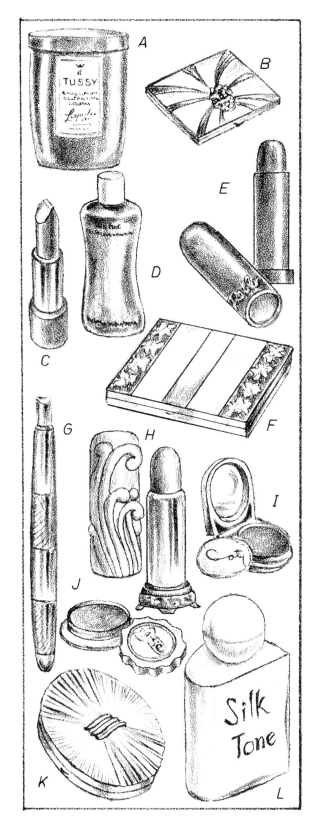

PLATE 28 : TWENTIETH CENTURY
1940–1950

A   1943. Tussy Emulsified Cleansing Cream. Price, $1.

B   1948. Jewelook compact in bronze and silver, by Elgin-American. Price, $9.95.

C   1943. Tabu lipstick in plastic case.

D   1948. Helena Rubinstein Sun Tint — 'Turns fair ladies into bronzed beauties'. (Name was later changed to Tan-in-a-Minute.)

E   1943. Revlon Cherry Coke lipstick in red plastic case.

F   1946. Elgin-American compact. Price, $1.50.

G   1948. Harriet Hubbard Ayer lipstick.

H   1946. Chen-Yu Jade Stick (lipstick) in jade green and gold case. Price, $2.

I   1943. Coty rouge in plastic compact.

J   1946. Hattie Carnegie rouge in plastic case. Price, $1.25.

K   1948. Gold-finish compact with loose powder sifter, by Evans Case Company. Price, $3.

L   1948. Helena Rubinstein Silk-Tone liquid foundation in 6 shades. Price, $1.50.

PLATE 29 : TWENTIETH CENTURY
1940–1950

A 1947. Prince Matchabelli lipstick, available in regular and queen size. Metal case with black or aqua panels. 5 shades, including Fuchsia Tulip.

B 1947. Lenthéric lipstick.

C 1947. Ballpoint lipstick by Chanel, in 6 shades.

D 1947. Goubaud sable lip brush.

E 1947. Tiffany lipstick brush in gold case. Price, $16.

F 1947. Sutton lipstick in brass case, available in 9 shades. Price, $1.

G 1941. DuBarry lipstick in Emblem Red. Price, $1.

H 1941. DuBarry rouge compact in Emblem Red. Price, $1.

I 1947. Powder puff in a tube, by Henri Bendel. Tube holds both puff and powder. Remove cap, push up the base, and the puff, powdered and ready to use, opens out like an umbrella. (Tube — in a different design — is also shown closed.)

J 1941. Chanel lipstick.

K 1947. Revlon's Fashion Plate cream cake foundation, applied with the fingertips. In 12 colours — the newest one, Cinderella's Pumpkin.

L 1941. Tangee lipstick in natural, red-red, and theatrical red.

M 1944. Coty Sub-Tint foundation in light, medium, and dark.

N 1943. Chen-Yu lipstick in Golden Mauve, Powder Blue, Fuchsia, Flame-Swept Red, Exotic Pink, Dragon's Blood, Ruby, and Black Rose. Price, $1.

O 1941. Hampden Powd'r-Base. Tinted foundation. Price, 50 cents and $1.

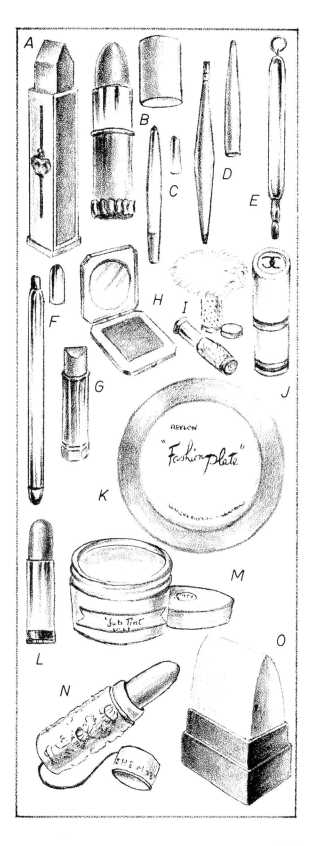

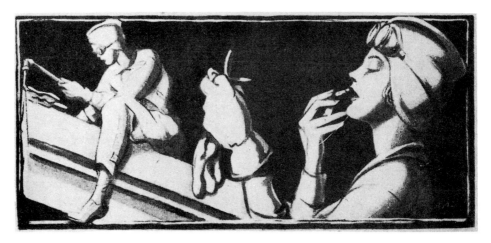

FIG. 227: **War work, 1942. From the *New York Times*.**

evidently having had its fill of deciding the relative importance to women of skin cream and mascara.

But there were still shortages to deal with. The severely curtailed supply of alcohol meant more perfume and less cologne. Reduced supplies of fats and oils and the complete unavailability of glycerine meant that if production was to be continued, substitutes must be found. Manufacturers supplemented their dwindling supplies of nitrocellulose for nail enamel with film scrap.

But packaging, which was often more important in sales than the product, proved to be the most difficult. Metal containers and closures had to be replaced by something. Since plastic was in short supply, paper was tried but proved a poor substitute. Glass was too expensive for low-priced items. But despite the problems, manufacturers continued to spend about twenty percent of their income on advertising, still playing up glamour and romance but also emphasizing the importance of keeping war workers looking their best.

In England the beauty editor of *The Queen* wrote that 'Women in the Forces and on other National work will be particularly interested in Max Factor's Pancake Make-up, which is very quick and easy to use and will stay on the skin for many hours'. Pan-Cake (Plate 27-J) was not exactly new, having been used for films, but Max Factor was just beginning to make it available in colours suitable for street wear — or, as *The Queen* put it, 'in six lovely shades, ranging in tone from a pale flesh tint to a deep warm tan, and all . . . in keeping with the colouring of the Women's Service Uniforms'. There was a final note that it might be difficult to obtain Pan-cake 'owing to the restriction of supplies, but the reward for the trouble you have taken in getting it will be well worth while'.

For a while, at least, leg makeup seemed to be a practical and relatively inexpensive answer to the wartime stocking problem. But instructions for 'How to Put it On and Take It Off Nicely', published in *Good Housekeeping* in 1943, make it fairly clear why women went back to nylons when they could get them:

'1. Before you begin, rub your fingernails over a cake of soap so that the tips of the nails won't be filled with brown.

'2. To avoid splashing makeup around the bathroom, stand on a newspaper and put one foot on the tub.

'3. Cup your hand, pour out enough to cover the entire leg, and press hands together. Starting at the foot, spread the color with a round-and-round motion of both hands. . . .

'4. Work fast, concentrating on covering the surface before the makeup dries. Use a light touch; heavy pressure makes streaks.

'5. When the leg is covered, lightly pat it with the fingertips of both hands, paying special attention to spots where color is uneven. When the makeup seems to stick to the fingers, stop patting.

'6. Never try to patch spots after the makeup is dry. The results will be streaky.

'7. If you dress before the leg is dry, pin up your skirt with pinch clothes-pins to keep it from rubbing off the color.

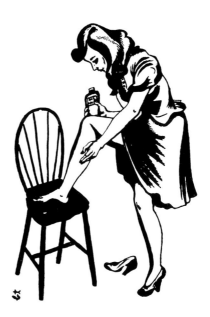

FIG. 228: Applying leg makeup, 1944.
From the *New Yorker*.

'8. If you get caught in the rain and the makeup spots, wait till the skin is dry, then rub the skin briskly with your hands or with tissues to blend the color.

'9. Stand in the tub. Rub soap to a generous lather on your hands, and with them wash your legs. Rinse thoroughly. Then take a shower as usual. In this way there will be no brown stains on soap, washcloth, or towels, no splatters on the shower curtains or floor.'

The following year the *New York Times* reported good news in leg makeup. The problems which came with early versions of the product had been solved, and women need no longer worry about streaking and rain splotching, but they did need two quick hands to get the makeup on before it dried. It was available in lotions, creams, tints, sticks, and even a paint-filled mit to be rubbed on.

In regard to the requirements of the ideal dressing table, a lady quoted by the *New York Times* asked for a working surface shallow enough so that she could get close to the mirror, plenty of drawers, conveniently placed, a perfume and nail polish resistant finish, a good light, and, if possible, a swivel seat. Mary Roche, the practical-minded *New York Times* reporter, suggested 'a pair of unpainted night stands or plastic-coated, paper-covered chests' topped with a heavy board, a sheet of plate glass, or a slab of marble, a good mirror with a bed-lamp attached, and an old piano stool.

COSMETICS FOR MEN, 1945

By 1945 there were more than a hundred manufacturers of men's toiletries, grossing about $50,000,000 a year, with an advertising budget of $10,000,000, and by 1946 the number of manufacturers had doubled. Returning G.I.s, having been conditioned by overseas gift packages, marched right up to toiletries counters and bought strongly scented colognes without a second thought, and the boom was on.

In the autumn of 1946 Dr Herbert Rattner, writing in *Hygeia*, took note of this increase in men's use of cosmetics in an article forthrightly entitled 'Cosmetics for Men'. 'The war,' wrote Dr Rattner, 'has given a real impetus to the sale of cosmetic sets for men — it was an excellent solution of the problem of what to send to the man in service. Cosmetic sets have now become the popular gift for the man in the family. While the packages are designed to appeal to women, the scents used in these articles are designed to appeal to men. They are of heather and fern, grasses, and resins, so-called virile rather than delicate scents and they are named so as to appeal to men, too, the names suggesting somehow the outdoors, tanbark, leather, athletics, fishing, or hunting. Even soap is now made in large "man-sized" bars.'

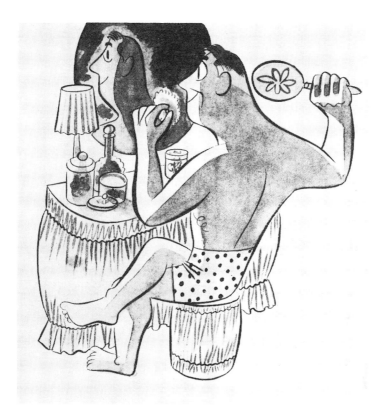

FIG. 229: The cosmetics revolution, 1946. From *Hygeia*.

Any cosmetic or toilet article with the word *shave* in it had a good chance for quick acceptance by men, even when as strongly scented as Old Spice. Hardly a man could be found who would admit to using face powder, but he openly and happily used 'after-shave talc', which he applied clumsily with his hands, scattering powder all over the bathroom. To use the far more practical powder puff would have been considered effeminate. Dr Rattner predicted that as soon as this prejudice against the powder puff was overcome, men would switch to women's face powder, which adheres better than talc but cannot be conveniently applied with the hands.

Most face powders contained some talc to give the desirable 'slip', zinc or magnesium stearate for adhesiveness, zinc oxide, titanium oxide, or kaolin for covering power, and some sort of perfuming ingredient, which occasionally provoked allergic reactions. Dr Rattner considered a good mineral face powder 'the least harmful to the skin of all cosmetics' and of some protective value. He did not, however, endorse cake makeup, a mixture of powder and grease or gums, which he considered likely to clog the pores.

As for the 'scientific blends' of face powder frequently dispensed 'in a department store by a woman with a nice complexion, dressed in a nurse's uniform who stands behind a counter on which are placed several bowls of powder of different shades', Dr Rattner pointed out that the mixing might prove artful but was in no sense scientific and could be expected to produce no cosmetic miracles. Nevertheless, the unscientific blending continued to be popular (see Figure 230).

After-shave lotions, since they contained the magic word, were acceptable to men, and it was only a short step from there to colognes, still in what were considered to be masculine scents. With a sharp eye on profits, manufacturers provided attractive gift sets containing both after-shave lotion and cologne, along with after-shave talc in matching container.

Face creams were used by men in connection with facial massages and were more acceptable when called 'massage creams'. In addition, men used shaving cream, shaving soaps, scalp lotions, hair dressings, hair dyes, and deodorants. Any cosmetic used to colour the face was simply not discussed.

THE MID-FORTIES

In 1946 American women spent nearly thirty million dollars (more than twelve million pounds) for five thousand tons of lipstick, of which nearly six million dollars went to the government for luxury taxes — or, as *Life* pointed out, enough to pay the President's salary for seventy-seven years.

The lipstick manufacturing process, as reported from a study of the Tangee factory, began with pouring and mixing the coloured pigments, oils, waxes, and perfumes in enormous stainless steel vats, steam heated to about 190°F. After the mixture was tested and approved, lipstick moulds were filled from faucets in the vats and cooled. After the moulds were opened, the sticks were sorted and inspected, then set into the metal containers in which they were to be used. These were then individually inspected and boxed for shipment.

Despite the war, overall sales of cosmetics in the United States had increased sixty-five percent since 1940 (from $400 million to $600 million) and promised to increase even more rapidly in the future, this in spite of the unavailability of many essential ingredients. Before the war, American manufacturers had imported jasmine, rose, tuberose, and orange absolutes, oil of neroly petals, and oil of lavender from France; civet from Ethiopia; orris and bergamot from Italy; vetivert Java, citronella Java, conanga Java, and patchouli from the Dutch East Indies; geranium African from Algeria; vetivert Bourbon, ylang Bourbon, geranium Bourbon, and Bourbon vanilla beans from Madagascar and Reunion Island; otto of rose from Bulgaria; and oak moss from Yugoslavia. In order to

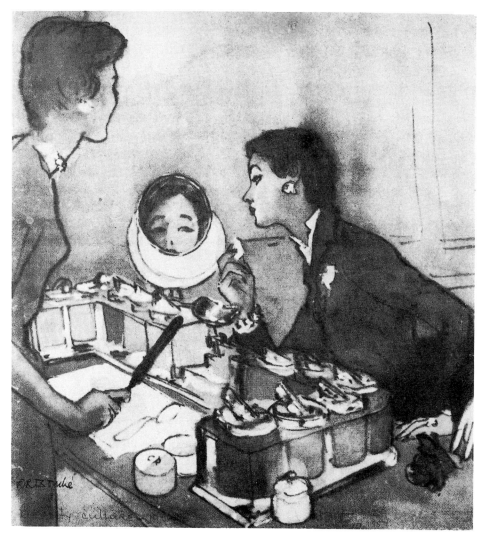

FIG. 230: Blending face powder. Typical scene at a cosmetics counter. From a Charles of the Ritz advertisement in the *New Yorker*, 1954.

conserve and extend available stocks of these ingredients and develop substitutes, a scientific advisory committee was set up through the Toilet Goods Association, and the results of research were shared through the industry.

In 1942 restrictions were placed on the manufacture of cosmetics by the War Production Board, but as a result of pressure from the industry, the restrictions were lifted except for critical raw materials. The discovery of the morale-building values of cosmetics in war plants may well have contributed to the decision and certainly helped the cosmetics industry in the war and post-war years.

Predictably, prices of raw materials increased markedly. Attar of roses, which had been available for as low as $4 an ounce, rose to as much as $40; and jasmine absolute went from $400 a pound to more than $2000. But ingredients such as lemon oil, sassafras, wormwood, terpineol, and peppermint were obtained from domestic sources, and such synthetics as ylang ylang, hydroxy citronella, bergamot, and phenyl ethyl alcohol (a rose scent) replaced many imports.

Evelyn Green Haynes, evidently feeling that not much had happened to women's beauty image since the twenties, wrote in *Vogue* that a 'new kind of beauty' had at last arrived. 'The gentleness of the new beauty,' she said, 'is reflected in make-up. Foundations will now be used with a feather touch — lightly, lightly. They will be used for their original purpose: to hold powder and not to drown the complexion. And they will be chosen in delicate, normal colours. Powders, pale pink or peach or gold, will be smoothed on sheerly. . . . And the lipstick to use with this will have only a part of former intensity. The lips, outlined surely and cleanly and naturally, will reflect a pastel of red: pink or coral. And now, if one has never used eye-shadow and mascara before, one might. And if one has always used them, one might use them a little more sparingly.'

Later she amplified on this in a speech before the Fashion Group of New York, emphasizing the importance of a flawless complexion. 'I think,' she said, 'there are many young women today who, ever since they used make-up at all, have been so busy building a heavy false face over their own that they've never thought much about the complexion underneath.' Foundations were meant to hold powder, 'not to give the face the texture of a piece of felt. . . . Over the foundation goes a light-coloured powder — in a pale pink or peach or gold tone.'

The lipstick colours were to be much lighter than they had been, with emphasis on rosy pinks, pale corals, and 'diluted tawny shades'. Because of the lightness of the face, eye makeup and rouge were to assume more importance. Nail polishes, said Mrs Haynes, would follow the lighter lipstick colours.

THE LATE FORTIES

For the well-groomed woman of 1948, Hazel Rawson Cades recommended 'a smooth base and a film of powder to give an illusion of lovelier texture to your skin, well-placed rouge . . . a clean-cut lipstick job . . . a touch of mascara on the upper lashes, and a bit of shadow or pomade on the lids'.

In 1948 Gala of London was advertising Lip Line — a long, thin lipstick for outlining the lips, then filling them in. Additional tubes of various colours were available to slip into the original case. The House of Rimmel had a similar lip pencil 'in a slim gilt case' and looking rather like a streamlined fountain pen. It sold for seven shillings and sixpence with refills for four shillings and a penny. Three new colours — Pink Purple, Pink Ice, and Dangerous Red — supposedly could be 'worn by everyone'.

Gala's lipsticks were available in a variety of colours — Cock's Comb, Lantern Red, Heart Red, Heavenly Pink, Blaze, Chestnut, Red Bunting, Ballet Pink, Cyclamen, Red Sequin, Sea Coral, and their newest one, Precious Ruby ('A fabulous colour, deepest, darkest ruby, aflame with blue fire; smoother than velvet . . . to curtain your lips with magic; royal, rich, romantic'). Gala powder was available in Lotus, Nectarine, Honey, Rio, and Sarong. Goya at the same time was advertising its new Grandee lipstick in Goya Pink, one of seven shades, and 'twice the size of ordinary lipsticks'.

In the autumn *The Queen* warned its readers about wearing their summer-tan makeup with 'the new donkey browns and greys', which would surely give them 'an unhealthy, sallow tone'. Strong lipstick colours were recommended — dark grape red, Arden's Red Cactus, Yardley's Copper Red, Pomeroy's Almond Blossom, Factor's Clear Red No. 1, and Gala's Ballet Pink. Lipsticks tinged with blue were supposed to give 'that coveted delicate look'.

October found H. T. W. Housefield defending women's use of cosmetics in an article in *The Queen*. 'I am surprised to learn', he wrote, 'that we are still so immature that we have not yet got used to women using cosmetics. Heavens above! Cosmetics were as essential as clothing even in the Pelasgian civilisation. But some education authority, I hear, has recently been grilled because it suggested that senior girls on leaving school should be taught how — discreetly — to make up their faces.

'We hear much about the decline in marriage and the increase in divorce. Would it not, therefore, be sensible to educate young women to fulfil their proper place in society by becoming more attractive — and more useful — to men? *Of course*, teach girls to make up properly — and to wash and brush their hair and to clean their nails and to cook.

'The prettiest girls are the most difficult to instruct, I am told. When a damsel has a lovely natural complexion, conceit leads her to believe that she need not ever try to do anything to improve or to preserve it; so it is the really pretty girl, feeling temporarily anaemic, who arrives with one cheek so red one fears she has been slapped, and the other almost ghastly pale.

'Forty or fifty years ago, they tell me, a gentlewoman might, without offence, dab a trifle of fuller's earth upon her nose when it shone over-much after lawn-tennis. But she dared go no further. Regarding some of the feminine noses that appear in public vehicles to-day, one wishes even for a dab of that primitive powder to make them tolerable.

'If we were properly grown up as a nation we should instinctively know that clothing, soap, cosmetics — even scent in strict moderation — are proper

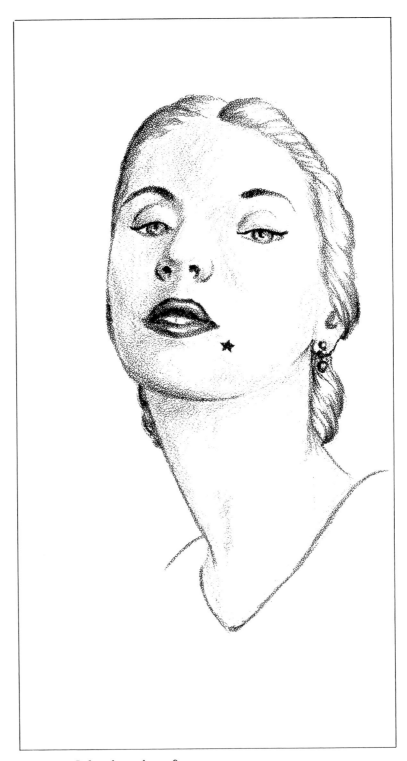

FIG. 231 : Girl with patch, 1948.

methods whereby a person may enhance her potential attractiveness to other persons.'

In the United States there were new makeup foundations. 'Who but Helena Rubinstein,' rhapsodized Helena Rubinstein's copywriter, 'with her dynamic imagination and years of cosmetic research would pulverize millions of silk filaments . . . homogenize them with velvety creams and rich oils . . . to capture all the spectacular beauty of silk in two fabulous new make-up foundations — like no other foundations on earth!' The two new foundations were Silk-Film, a cream foundation in a flat plastic case, and Silk-Tone, a liquid foundation in a clear glass bottle (see Plate 28-L). Both were available in six shades.

For the second time in the century beauty patches were being revived (Figure 231). They were available in boxes of one hundred black silk cut-outs of circles, triangles, squares, diamonds, hearts, stars, half-moons, arrows, cloverleafs, and human figures, which were supposed to be worn one at a time in order to call attention to one's best feature. But if those responsible anticipated another century of patching, they were to be disappointed.

For the summer of 1949 *Vogue* predicted orange-red lipstick, coral rouge, beige powder, pale green eyeshadow, dark green or brown mascara, and brown eyebrow pencil.

THE PAINTED LOOK

The winter of 1949–50 saw the beginning, in Paris, of a revolution in eye makeup — the doe-eyed look. As in the twenties, when lipstick suddenly became respectable, the new painted eyes — shadow, eyebrow pencil, mascara, and, most important of all, eye lining — were aggressively unreal. The painted look was in, and those who cried out in alarm at the little black or coloured lines around women's eyes and prophesied the imminent disintegration of modern society, never dreamed of what the next twenty years would bring. Hollywood, surprisingly, was on the side of the alarmists and dubbed the new eye makeup the Bride-of-Frankenstein look.

The trend in 1950, according to *Vogue*, was towards lighter skin, darker lips, and no rouge. Cake powder compacts were back. With the new emphasis on the eyes, the market was flooded with mascara, eyeshadow, and lining pencil, all in related shades. With their Blue Frost eyeliner, Revlon suggested Fresh Violet mascara, Mauve Frost and Fresh Violet eyeshadow; or Ice Blue mascara with Ice Blue and Silver shadows. Titian mascara and Green Frost and Evergreen eyeshadow were recommended with Walnut eyeliner. For the exotic touch one might try Evergreen eyeliner, Pistachio mascara, and Pistachio and Gold shadows.

Sales in eye makeup rose dramatically. Nieman-Marcus in Dallas sold as

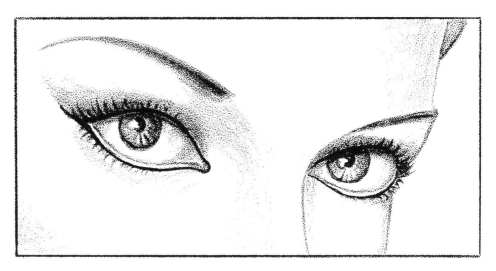

FIG. 232: The doe-eyed look, 1950. Eyes are lined with pencil, upper lids shadowed, eyebrows pencilled, and lashes darkened with mascara.

much in the first two months of 1950 as they had in the entire preceding year. And the sales of Aziza, a small company specializing in eye makeup, rose 215 percent. The Aziza (meaning 'darling' in Arabic) firm traced its beginnings to 1920, when chemist Nina Sussman mixed up a batch of mascara in her Paris kitchen. It was not until the depression that the Sussmans decided to sell Nina's eye makeup to augment their dwindling income. Aziza products became well established in Europe, but the German occupation of Paris in 1940 brought about a move to New York, where the Sussmans made a new start with a cooking pan in a small room on West 22nd Street. By 1950 they had moved uptown with a staff of seventeen, including son André, a former paratrooper, who proved to be extraordinarily successful in demonstrating eye makeup.

In June 1950 the *New Yorker* reported on a visit to Helena Rubinstein's Wonder School to observe a class in eye makeup. Dr Gould, a red-haired woman from Vienna, presided over the pink-walled room and the dozen ladies who were learning what to do with their eyes. 'I am coming here when there is the World's Fair,' she told the reporter. 'Do not inquire about me further.' Then she proceeded to explain the eye work:

'With the short hairdo now fashionable, there is more of the face than there was before. So naturally, there is more of the eyes. Now must the eye be exotic.' This she proposed to accomplish with shadow, mascara, and pencils, using two shadows, not one, the colours depending on the complexion and the costume. 'We pencil the corner of the eye upward to make it almond-shaped, add a spot of rouge we are wearing over the eyelid, put on the mascara, which comes in all kinds of colors, and what we have is terrific.'

In the autumn Hazel Rawson Cades, ignoring the new exotic eye makeup, cautioned her presumably conservative *Woman's Home Companion* readers to apply mascara only to upper lashes for the most natural effect and warned that eyeshadow was meant to *be* shadow, not a colour accent, and should be used sparingly.

In 1951 English women were wearing Coty's London Lilac lipstick, having their face powder individually blended by Charles of the Ritz, confidently plastering their faces with the Cyclax 10-Minute Beauty Mask, and softening their hands with Dubarry's Crème Shalimar. To whiten their hands they were advised to shake them loosely from the wrist.

They were also still using the century-old Powdered Violet Oatmeal by Rimmel. Dissolved in the wash basin, it was supposed to cleanse, soften, soothe, and remove blemishes. Rimmel also made a Violet Oatmeal Face Pack and Violet Oatmeal Soap. Women who found cosmetics inadequate to meet their needs could try the Pifco Vibratory Massager which was advertised to be 'both pleasant and beneficial'.

The London fashion for spring was the Golden Look, featuring such makeup colours as Double Peony, Cock's Comb, Calypso, Red Banana, Moon Lustre, and Touch of Genius.

Women on both sides of the Atlantic were using Elizabeth Arden's Surprise Lipstick, which was supposed to have 'the come-hither of pink, the persuasiveness of rose, the courage of red', and to turn every woman it touched 'into a softly glowing beauty'.

The use of cosmetics was no longer restricted to adults. 'Before World War I,' wrote Veronica Conley in 1951, 'if a girl was discovered actually using face powder, the scandal spread through social circles like a grass fire. Of course, lip and face rouge were worn only by show girls and entertainers. In the twenties, however, along with short skirts, raccoon coats and the Charleston, came a new attitude toward cosmetics. The industry has been slowly but persistently snowballing ever since. Today the reins of social custom have been greatly loosened and, to a commercial eye, the potentialities of the teen-age market are tremendous.' But Miss Conley herself was less than enthusiastic about teenage makeup and urged careful guidance.

About this time a survey of teenagers indicated that two-thirds of them had worn lipstick and ninety percent had worn nail enamel since they were fourteen. Eighteen percent had started using nail enamel before they were ten. The colour preference was, first, for clear red, then medium blue-red, dark red, light rose, and clear.

In spite of a variety of shaving preparations and talcums designed specifically for men, sales were not exactly flourishing, and it was discovered that a good many of the preparations purchased by women as gifts were never used. Social custom still decreed that any toilet article used by a man must in no way suggest femininity in packaging, smell, or physical characteristics. Cosmetics manufacturers had their eyes on the future, but they had to move very slowly. For one thing, they were careful to refer to 'men's toiletries', not 'men's cosmetics'. But within the acceptable limits, the number of available items was increasing.

'Today,' wrote Miss Conley, 'good grooming has become as important a social prerequisite for men as for women. As a result, the demand for such items as shaving preparations, soaps, shampoos, hair dressings, hair lotions, deodorants, and antiperspirants has increased. The use of cosmetic items other than these is insignificant. . . . Bear in mind that the cosmetic habit is not as well established in men as it is in women. Therefore, before investing in men's toiletries, know the preferences of the man they are intended for. He will not be converted to the use of a different type of product simply because he received it as a gift. He will either discard it or ignore it entirely.'

A few months later, in 1952, Miss Conley pointed out what most women already knew — that they had a greater psychological dependence on lipstick than on any other cosmetic. 'The importance of this cosmetic to women all over the world,' she wrote, 'was forcibly brought out during World War II. Lipstick was frequently mentioned as ranking high on the "most-missed" list by those whose existence afforded only the barest necessities. Navy nurses evacuated by submarines from Corregidor included a lipstick among the few personal items they took with them.'

FIRE AND ICE

This same year Charles Revson, president of Revlon, stated that makeup 'has finally gotten around to individuals. Nowadays, each woman develops her good points in her own way. Look-alikes are passé.' Before Christmas Revlon launched a full-scale and enormously successful advertising campaign for its new shade of lipstick and nail enamel called 'Fire and Ice'. *Business Week* called it one of the most effective advertisements in cosmetics history, combining 'dignity, class, and glamor'. This memorable advertisement, which was designed to reach every user of cosmetics throughout the country, showed a dark haired model in a dress of silver sequins with a scarlet wrap in front of a glittering background. 'Are you made for "Fire and Ice"?' asks the copywriter. If you can answer *yes* to eight of fifteen questions ('Have you ever danced with your shoes off?' 'Do you close your eyes when you're kissed?'), he assures you that you are. If you can't, then presumably you may as well drag along with whatever you've been using. But since the Fire-and-Ice girl was 'the 1952 American beauty with a foolproof formula for melting a male', most women with any hope in their hearts would no doubt try very hard to score at least eight. And hope, accord-

PLATE 30 : TWENTIETH CENTURY
1950–1960

A Max Factor Pan-Stik.
B 1957. Revlon Nail Enamel.
C 1953. Cyclax lipstick.
D 1959. Elizabeth Arden eyebrow pencil.
E 1950. Pond's Angel Face. Makeup foundation.
F 1959. Max Factor Mascara Wand in Jet Gray.
G 1950. Revlon Lip-Mirror. Price, $1.50.
H 1959. Max Factor Eyeshadow Stick. Price, $1.25.
I 1959. Innoxa Liquid Satin foundation in 5 shades.
J 1958. Helena Rubinstein Mascara-Matic. Automatic, waterproof mascara in black, brown, navy, royal blue, emerald green. Price, $2.
K 1957. Show-Case lipstick by Du-Barry. Black, white, or gold case. 10 shades. Price, $1.25.
L 1958. Dew-Kissed lipstick by Helena Rubinstein. Newest colour, Bed of Roses. Price, $1.35 to $5.
M 1959. Ultima skin cream by Revlon. Price, $20 and $12.50.

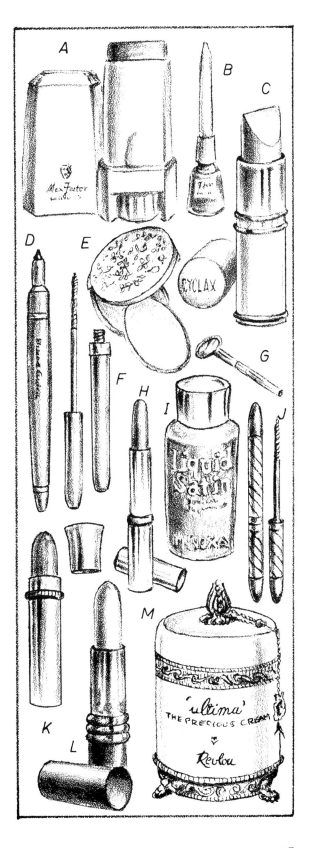

ing to vice-president Martin Revson, was what Revlon was selling and what every woman wanted to buy.

He was probably right, for the formula worked then and it continued to work, for high-school girls, grandmothers, and all women in between were in the market. 'Women are living longer,' said Revson, 'and they are no longer satisfied with being Whistler's Mother. . . . You have to sell by touching all the facets of the emotional side of a woman. Most women lead lives of dullness, of quiet desperation. Cosmetics are a wonderful escape from it — if you play it right. And we play it by giving the idea that Revlon girls only go out at night.'

For making cosmetics truly a part of fashion, Revlon was eager to take the credit. Having decided that lipstick and nail enamel lasted too long, they started bringing out a new shade every six months instead of once a year. This, *Business Week* pointed out, 'involved a couple of really high hurdles. First, to sell the new item, Revlon had to convince women that it was in line with the new fashions. Second, it really had to be in line with the new fashions. . . . The difficulty with that was that the whole selling campaign had to be planned so far in advance that no new fashions were even on paper. Revlon had to anticipate styles — and do it accurately. . . . But to those who decide . . . it's no mysterious secret. All you have to do, they say, is sense the changing moods of American women, and you can tell what the styles will be.'

In the case of the Fire-and-Ice campaign, which followed Paint-the-Town-Pink, Revlon's four owners sensed as early as January 'a growing rebellion among American women. They had grown tired of the prevailing mode — the tiny waist, a girdle that made them sit and walk formally.' But Revlon decided that the new mood resulted not from the discomfort, but from jealousy of European glamour girls who were being imported for movies, plays, and nightclub engagements. By autumn, reasoned the four, it would be time for 'the natural, free-flowing look that is the touch of the mermaid'. For the perfect colour, they examined, so they claimed, nearly five thousand shades of red, from which they chose 'a lush and passionate red, the richest red the company had ever made'.

Then, in order to name the colour, the Creative Planning Board took over, and from their hundreds of suggestions, the owners chose the one which 'suggested the rich red of rubies and the expensive glamor of diamonds' — Fire and Ice. As for the universality of the appeal, the group reasoned, 'Every woman is made of Fire and Ice, though too many of them don't realize it. It is up to us to make every woman know it.'

Once the basic decision was made, there were endless details to be worked out — the psychological quiz and the questions to be used, the selection of the right model, the designing of the costume, the colour photograph. Then the promotion had to be planned. On April 5 Revlon's fashion director had a conference with *Vogue* executives, who agreed to co-operate with the glitter-and-glamour theme in their editorial approach for the November 1 issue and in arranging for window displays in prestige departments stores throughout the country.

On November 2 the first newspaper advertisements appeared, followed immediately by window displays in 9000 department stores, drugstores, and beauty salons. According to *Business Week*, 'push money was being paid to sales girls everywhere to suggest Fire and Ice to customers at cosmetics counters'. The result was the largest volume of sales Revlon had ever achieved for a single colour.

The four owners of Revlon (three Revsons and a Lachman) organized the company in 1932 in a small back room on New York's West 45th Street in an era when lipsticks came in light, medium, and dark. Beginning with an initial outlay of $300 for a batch of nail enamel, Revlon was grossing $68,000 three years later and, it was estimated by *Business Week*, probably $25,000,000 by 1952, with their products being sold in 73 countries.

In the spring of 1953, the Coronation year, *The Queen* charted suitable makeup colours for fair or dark Englishwomen for day or night. According to the magazine, in the daytime an untanned blonde should wear Arden's Rose Rachel base, Pink Perfection cream rouge and lipstick, Pearly Green eyeshadow, and Neutral powder over Special Mat Foncé, Arcancil's San Colour mascara, and Peggy Sage's Coronet nail lacquer. At night she should switch to Yardley's Blonde Feather Foundation, Cherry cream rouge and lipstick, and Pink Pearl powder, Factor's Theatrical Green eyeshadow and Brown-Black mascara, and Chen Yu's Imperial Flame nail lacquer. Then, if she developed a summer tan, she would have to buy a complete new set of makeup—Cyclax Bronze Velvet Glamour Tint, Gay Morning rouge and lipstick, and Summer Gold powder, Max Factor's Grey eyeshadow and Brown mascara, and Gala's Sea Coral nail lacquer. If, in a rash moment, she were suddenly to become a brunette, she'd have to begin all over again.

Perhaps remembering great grandmothers who surreptitiously heightened their colouring with a moistened red ribbon, Elizabeth Arden suggested scraping a black velvet ribbon with a razor blade to make a little pile of black fluff, then dipping a brush, wet with mascara, into the fluff before applying it to the eyelashes. The result was supposed to be velvety lashes.

For a smoother makeup Harriet Hubbard Ayer recommended applying nearly everything with foam rubber sponges, including foundation, powder, rouge, eyeshadow, and mascara. Even lipstick was to be blotted with one. Aziza proposed two shades of mascara, the darker one for the outer corner of the eye.

In London in the spring of 1955 Dorothy Gray was promoting Elation Makeup Film and Pink Mink lipstick, both of which, according to the copywriter, would go splendidly with everything. Lancôme, on the other hand, offered a wide range of foundations and thirty-eight shades of lipstick 'from the palest coral rose to the deep exotic reds'. There were nineteen shades of cream eyeshadow for day and evening wear, six of them irridiscent. Advertising their products in London, Lancôme stressed the fact that they were 'made only in Paris'.

At the same time Elizabeth Arden was offering English women the opportunity to 'combat sagging contours, dry skin, puffiness, wrinkles, and jawline heaviness' with 'only the uplifting touch' of their own hands and two guineas' worth of Firm-Lift Treatment Lotion, Firmo-Lift Salon Treatment Oil, and Ardena Vitamin Oil. 'Years,' they were assured 'seem to lift away.' Cyclax of London promised to do much the same thing through regular use of their soap (daily), Skin Food (nightly), and Special Lotion (weekly). No prices were given.

THE MID-FIFTIES

After years of glamourizing movie stars into painted wax dolls, perfect in every detail, Hollywood, perhaps largely through the influence of Ingrid Bergman and imported foreign films, switched to the Natural Look. Eyes and eyebrows were accented but not painted, lips were lighter, hair was more casual, and even a few imperfections, such as freckles, were sometimes allowed to show. The Harlow hair, the Crawford mouth, the Dietrich eyebrows—all were a thing of the past, and one's favourite movie star was supposed to look like a girl who, if one were lucky, might live next door.

Max Factor's contribution to the cosmetics market in 1954 was a flesh-coloured makeup stick called Erace, to be used for hiding dark circles under the eyes or other skin discolourations. It was used occasionally by men as well as women. Max Factor Sr., a Polish immigrant wigmaker, started in Hollywood beautifying the film stars and compounding new powders and greasepaints in more becoming colours. When the stars began wearing his makeup off screen as well as on, he was in the beauty business for good. Before long he was back in the hair business as well, making toupees and wigs for men and women all over the country. One of Factor's greatest successes was Pan-Cake makeup, which in 1953 sold more than ten million cakes.

After a period of paleness due to the banning of cosmetics, Hungarian women were once again blooming with colour. The Communist bosses, evidently unable to cope with the black market in smuggled rouge and lipstick, opened state-owned beauty shops in Budapest. But the government-produced cosmetics proved to be of such inferior quality that women returned to the black market, leaving the government little choice but to import cosmetics, which they sold for as much as twelve times the price of the local product.

Paris originated the Mandarin makeup, but the influence soon spread. For those who wanted to go all the way, the outer ends of the eyebrows were

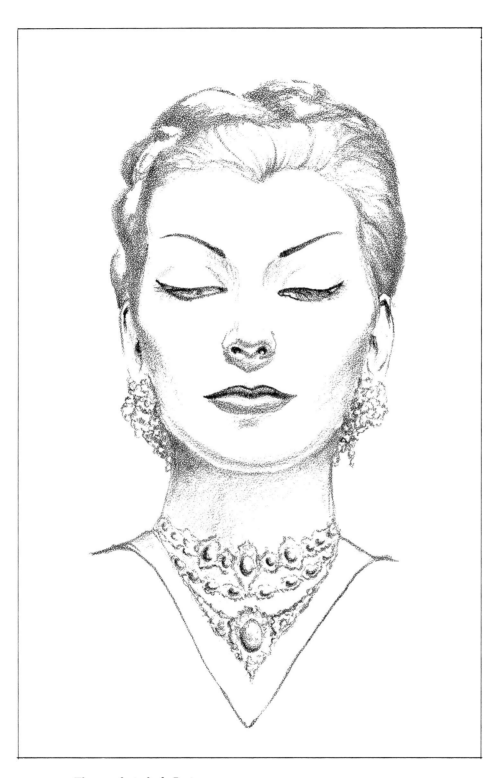

FIG. 233 : The mandarin look, Paris, 1955.

entirely plucked out and new brows pencilled on in a great upward and outward sweep. The foundation was pale, with no trace of pink, and the eyelids, up to the brows, were plastered with white. The eyes were lined with an upward sweep at the outer corners, following the line of the brows. Powder was pure white. The upper lip was small and sharply defined; the lower one was full and sensual. But few women went all the way. Most of them modified their usual makeup or adapted elements of the new look which happened to appeal to them.

One of the newest cosmetic ingredients in 1955 was the highly advertised import, royal jelly, the food of the queen bee. From the extravagant claims in the advertisements and the prices charged ($15 an ounce for a cream containing the jelly), one would never have suspected that there wasn't a shred of evidence to show that royal jelly could benefit the skin. But women, ever hopeful, bought it anyway, convinced by the high price, if nothing else. Presumably, anything that expensive *had* to be good.

Aerosol containers for cosmetics were news in 1956 and promised to revolutionize the application of a number of toiletries. This was only one of many scientific advances in cosmetics, resulting from the hundreds of thousands of dollars being spent for research. The huckstering was as blatant as ever, but more often than not, it was based on solid scientific improvement of the product.

By the 1950s few women were making their own cosmetics, and few writers were recommending the practice. Veronica Conley pointed out in 1956 that formulas for cold cream were readily available and could in some cases be used for home production. 'However,' she added, 'it is highly improbable that money can be saved or that a product can be produced approaching the elegance of commercial cold cream. Formulation of this cosmetic in the kitchen is time-consuming and the purchase of raw materials in small amounts very costly. Considerable skill and experience are required to select a compatible perfume and ingredients of appropriate quality. If the purpose of making a cold cream at home is to save time and money or to produce a superior product, the success of the venture is improbable.'

In March 1956 English women were advised to get a thorough spring cleaning in order to rid themselves of 'all the winter's dust and smog'. Turkish baths at the Dorchester Hotel and the Porchester Hall (Ladies' days were Tuesdays, Thursdays, and Fridays) or wax baths from Elizabeth Arden or Maria Hornes were recommended. Women who found the baths too strenuous could go to Lancôme for a dry massage, Charles of the Ritz for a Vaperzone Cleanse, Cyclax for mask and toning, and Yardley's for their Standard Treatment.

At the behest of a Hungarian plastic surgeon, Jesuit Father Virginio Rotundi expressed the view of the Church that beautification of women through plastic surgery might be either good or evil, depending on its purpose. To counteract out-and-out ugliness or to make it possible to earn a living was certainly permissible. In fact, suggested Father Rotundi, there was nothing really sinful about wanting to improve one's appearance. 'It does not seem to me exaggerated to say,' he added, 'that sometimes plastic surgery has brought back peace to estranged marriage couples. . . . When confessors tell their penitents that face lifting is a frivolity and is condemned without reserve by the Church, they are . . . wrong.'

In April 1957 *Queen's* beauty expert, Claire West, got quite carried away by the advent of spring. 'We whisk out our spring palette,' she wrote, 'and boldly mix our azalea and camellia pinks, tender greens and yellow, the blues and lilacs of scylla, anemone, and immortelle. We build up our spring make-up on two basic English complexions, regardless of the colour of the hair. They are the apple blossom petal skin, and the apricot, or tea rose petal skin. In each case, and for every age and type of skin, we advocate a colour foundation, although the debutante will wear it for special occasions only. If chosen with discrimination, it brings out the sheen of a flower petal plus the warmth of your natural pigment. It lubricates and makes you look truly radiant. Wear little or no powder over this, the caked look can only date you. If you must have it, dust it on lightly so as to give you the look of an untouched peach. We like a mere trace of light rouge, if any, to match the lips. Eyebrows are natural, or drawn thick and short with matching pencil, grey or fawn. Blue eye make-up with dark eyes is a novelty. Apply lipstick carefully with a brush.'

For the fair skin Miss West recommended a warm foundation colour — Lancôme's Douceline Foundation, Soleil Couchant or Revlon's Touch-and-Glo in Creamy Ivory; for the golden complexion, Revlon's Dusty Rose Foundation or Lancôme's Supple Foundation, Pampero, with powder to match. For eye-shadow, she liked a touch of gold with sun dappled brown eyes, Algue Chatoyant with green mascara, or Violet Argent by Arden, which, she promised, would turn 'dark eyes to pools of shadow'. She also suggested Arden's deep tulip lipstick called Rosa Aurora, her Desert Pink, Dior's N.9., and Lancôme's Capucine. And then, concluded Miss West, you can lean back and rejoice and 'forget about it till repairs are needed'.

September found Joan Price writing in *The Queen* that the new fashion colours called for 'warmer, more vital-looking make-up'. The pale Spring lipsticks had been replaced by glowing orange pinks and reds. The emphasis was still on the eyes. For the latest technique she quoted Elizabeth Arden:

'Great play is made with eye shadow, the use of blending browns Brun Clair and pale Cher Or up and out, towards the brows, with the colour Emerald or Opal Blue on the front of the lids. Eyebrow pencil, grey or brown, should be feathered between the top lashes to give an intense shadowed effect rather than a hard line. Complexions, peach, achieved with rachel toned foundations and powder and for the mouth an exciting new shade called New Fashion applied to look full but not square in a smiling curve.'

In November *The Queen's* classified announcements offered readers assistance in removing superfluous hair (Electro Cosmetics Ltd.), developing the bust (Butibust, Dept. BC45), and clearing up spotty complexions (Rebelle, Haute Coiffeur). Katherine Corbett was prepared to pierce ears and treat red veins and moles; Delia Collins offered to take care of acne and warts; and Jules (who had 'studied as a sculptor') felt it was 'his right to style Madam's coiffeur to suit the contours of her face'. In Scotland Xavier Giralt of Glasgow, who wanted 'to equip women for the battle of charm', declared confidently that his methods of hair styling were 'nearer the aesthetic conceptions of a fine art than ever before'.

English women were conditioning their faces with Raymond's new Vitamin A Skin Food, Dorothy Gray's Cellogen Cream, Gala's Lemon Cleanser, Anne French's Milk Cleanser, Rose Laird's Liquid Lather and Cream Masque, and Dorothy Gray's Throat Cream. To protect their skin after it was conditioned they might choose Elizabeth Arden's Velva Moisture Film, Revlon's Moon Drops, Hudnut's Basic Dew, or Charles of the Ritz's Revenescence.

In the Christmas issue Miss Price warned that lipstick should be played down and applied with a lighter touch, sometimes under a dusting of powder, and that all of the coral and flame tones had replaced the blue pinks in popularity. Foundations were cooler and a shade lighter than the natural skin tone.

A study of a group of American college girls in 1957 showed that 99.7 percent used lipstick and 79.4 percent used face powder. About half of them used eyebrow pencil and mascara, though not regularly, and still fewer used rouge and eyeshadow. The general attitude towards makeup seemed to be expressed by the opinion of one girl: 'I prefer natural beauty to artificial beauty, but I also prefer artificial beauty to natural homeliness.'

So-called experts recommended that of the twenty or so shades of lipstick available, a college girl buys only two — a pink, coral, or light clear red for classes and a deeper shade for evening. The use of cheek rouge was not encouraged; but if lack of colour seemed to require it, a delicate pink or coral was suggested.

The autumn news in *McCalls* focused on eye makeup easier to apply — irridescent eyeshadow in stick form, cream mascara in a tube, and charcoal pencils instead of black. The pattern of application was still much the same, however — shadow close to the lids and blending upwards and outwards, a pencil line close to the lashes on the upper lid, ending in an upward and outward sweep, mascara, and lightly stroked-on eyebrow pencil.

Although American men were keeping quiet about their burgeoning interest in grooming, there were revealing statistics available. Census information indicated that whereas in 1949 women's beauty parlours had been grossing nearly $13 million a year more than barbers' shops, by 1953 men were spending $2 million more than women on grooming. They were, in fact, spending close to $500 million (£200 million) a year in barbershops. This included not only haircuts, shaves, and shampoos, but manicures, facials, and scalp massages. By 1957 disguised beauty parlours for men were beginning to appear. The Groom Shop in New York featured mud packs (called 'facial packs'), massages, hair tinting, and similar services. Skin creams could be purchased there for home use. As for scented shaving lotions and colognes, American men were spending about $27,000,000 (£11,000,000) a year, slightly less than a third of the amount spent by women. But figuring by the gallon, they used more. Each year showed a marked increase in the percentage of men using deodorants, hair grooming products, and shaving lotions. Not only that, but moustache wax was making a comeback.

THE LATE FIFTIES

According to *Vogue*, the new face for 1958 meant softer eyes ('grey eyeshadow, grey eyebrow pencil, a smoky mascara') and brighter mouths ('with true-red, orange, pink-orange lipsticks'). This was in February. In May, *Vogue*, always reaching for something new, came up with the idea of an undercoating of coloured face powder—blue (for blondes), green (for redheads), yellow (for brunettes), and pink (for grey hair)—topped with a more normal flesh-toned powder. For blondes, for example, the plan went like this: 'Ivory-coloured foundation. Pale-blue primer-coat powder. Lighter ivoried topcoat powder. Lipstick and nail enamel, true pink. Eyeshadow a stepped-up version of the primer-coat blue. Bright blue mascara. Brows stroked with blue and grey.'

About this same time Max Factor was advertising Pink 'n Orange hi-fi lipstick—'not pink! not orange! Max Factor's outrageous new color creation that captivated all Paris! . . . The soft flattery of pink plus the brilliant excitement of orange—all in one shade. It's bold. It's feminine. It's the shade Paris says will make him yours.'

In May *Vogue* also pointed out that a natural look did not mean an absence of makeup but, on the contrary, more *making up*, if not more makeup—that is, greater skill in blending colours and modelling the features. One should not, *Vogue* cautioned, 'undervalue the use of eye make-up in natural good looks; properly used, it gives the eyes a look of being brighter, bigger, more wide-open. . . . Plan on using a soft, rather full brush; at least two colours of eye shadow, one of them white. Work the colours on a palette . . . then stroke your brush through the white shadow and begin at the inside corner of the eye. Follow deftly across the lid and close to the lash, adding your mixture—newest additive is amber—as you progress. At the outside corner of the eye bring the colour up and tap the edges out softly on the flat between the eye-corner and the lip of the eyebrow.' Mascara was becoming lighter and muted, with gold and silver spangling for evening.

Many of the new makeups contained guanine, a crystalline substance occurring in fish scales, guano, and other animal excrements, giving a shimmering lustre to the surface of the paints and powders.

In the summer *Time* devoted one of its cover stories to the ritual of feminine beautification, American style. 'With a clink of vials and a wafting of odors,' said *Time*, 'the mysterious rite begins. It is 6.45 a.m., and her husband is still abed, but pretty Mrs. James Locke sits before a mirrored table in her three-room San Francisco apartment, her blonde hair covered by a filmy nylon cap. Over an array of multi-scented bottles, sticks, jars, and tubes, Jean Locke hovers like an alchemist. She cleans her skin of night cream, anoints it with icy water — and for one brief moment shows her true face. Then, slowly, comes the metamorphosis.

'Over her face she spreads a foundation cream, creating a pale and expressionless mask. She caresses her cheeks with a liquid rouge, slowly adding color to her face, tops it off by gently patting on a flesh-colored powder. She shadows her eyes with turquoise, dabs a few drops of perfume behind her ears, at her elbows, temples, and wrists. With a dark pencil she shapes her eyebrows to give an artful lift to her expression, brushes her eyelashes with a penlike wand to emphasize her blue eyes. Finally, twenty minutes later, she spreads on the finishing touch — an orange lipstick to match her fingernail polish.' Ready now to face the world, she goes off to her secretarial job in an advertising agency.

Mrs Locke and every other woman in the country had no lack of romantic or adventuresome-sounding cosmetics to choose from — Pond's Angel Face, Revlon's Love-Pat, Factor's Creme Puff and Cup of Youth, Rubinstein's Red Hellion and Tree of Life, Neushaefer's Torrid and Pink Passion. The products and the services purchased in the United States in 1957 cost about four billion dollars, and it was estimated that ninety-five percent of women over the age of twelve used at least one beauty product. Milwaukee's Kolmar Laboratories produced 2800 shades of lipstick and used 20,000 formulas for cosmetics. There were 220,000 beauty salons in the United States, and more than five million Americans patronized reducing salons and health clubs.

Revlon employed more than seventy chemists in a continuing search for new products and ways to improve on old ones. Rubinstein advertised such exotic ingredients for her cosmetics as the juice of water lilies (supplied by nuns in Paris and London) and extract of human placenta (source unrevealed). Lily Daché sold a face powder containing pulverized pearls, and Estée Lauder used turtle oil in 'the most expensive facial preparation in the world'. She asked and got $115 (£48) a pound. When royal jelly was introduced in a face cream, cosmetics houses swarmed to their laboratories, busily putting it into everything they could think of, including lipsticks. But saner minds warned that the women who paid high prices for the stuff were getting royally stung. By 1958 it was still possible to pay fifteen dollars an ounce for cream containing seventeen cents' worth of royal jelly, but it was also possible to pay one dollar for the same amount.

Hair was no longer dyed—it was rinsed, tinted, or bleached, and three out of ten women did it. Although most of them may not have advertised the fact, neither did they try very hard to hide it. Hair colouring, whatever it was called, was now respectable. Roux marketed a five-minute hair rinse; and hair spray, only seven years old, was bringing in $84,000,000 (£35,000,000) a year.

Most of the cosmetics were sold by a relatively small number of well-known names—Elizabeth Arden, Helena Rubinstein, Max Factor, Revlon, Pond. Elizabeth Arden studied to be a nurse and opened her own beauty shop in 1910, eight years after Helena Rubinstein appeared in Australia with her batch of cold cream; and by 1958 she was grossing an estimated $15,000,000 a year from her beauty preparations, her chain of salons, and her Maine Chance ranches, 'magic isles' where cares and worries were supposed to vanish—at least until one stopped to think about what it was all costing.

Time described a woman's day at Madame Rubinstein's New York salon, said to be patronized by 74,000 women a year:

'First, she is told to change into a black leotard, given paper slippers and a white robe to wear. Her medical history is solemnly taken. . . . After doing exercises in front of a Ph.D. from Vienna ($12), she hops into a thirty-minute bubble bath with froth three feet high ($5). Her skin is then defuzzed of superfluous hair by a wax treatment ($26). She can have an infra-red treatment . . . at $10 or a paraffin application at $15 to lose a pound or two. Then comes a facial, in which her face is coated with cream . . . massaged . . . and sprayed with a salty liquid for "disturbed skin" ($9). To top it off she goes to a treatment by Michel, who sketches the hairdo he thinks best for her, gives her a permanent, then fluffs, smooths, and fusses her hair into place ($35). The final touch: she can have artificial fingernails applied for $17.50.'

Miss Arden and Madame Rubinstein ('First Lady of Beauty Science') were not the friendliest of rivals and, it is said, never met. Employees of one establishment had a way of turning up at the other one at a higher salary. In 1938 Arden got Rubinstein's sales manager, and the following year Madame hired Miss Arden's ex-husband and general manager. 'I think,' Miss Arden is quoted as saying, 'this is the nastiest business in the world. There are so many people in it, and they all just copy me.' Charles Revson of Revlon said he didn't meet competition—he crushed it. Miss Arden's opinion, reported by *Time*: 'I just don't like that man'.

The fierce competition did little to reduce prices. The average lipstick selling for one or two dollars cost about six cents to make. A similar product could be bought at Woolworth's for twenty-five cents or less, but most women preferred to pay the higher price. One manufacturer admitted to a 900 percent markup on some products. A cheaper line, he said, simply wouldn't sell as well.

In the autumn English women were dividing their attention between thoroughly shadowed eyes and vivid lips. Helena Rubinstein decided that her Bed of Roses Lipstick was perfect for all occasions and recommended blue and green eyeshadow for dramatic effect.

For Christmas in England in 1958 men and women were getting and giving black plastic nail brushes decorated with penguins, feathered evening masks by French of London, Yardley's Shower Talc and Shaving Stick, mahogany shaving mirrors, 4711 cologne and soap in a wicker basket, drums of Morny Dusting Powder, gift vouchers from Rose Laird, Max Factor's Busy Man's Bar, Imperial Leather Shaving Bowls, Omy Soap and Dusting Powder, perfumed body foam, a new flower-scented Araby soap (triple milled), and a pigskin document case filled with Arden for Men preparations which sold for £38 10s.

In 1959 the Christmas issue of *The Queen* contained advertisements for Innoxa Cream Powder ('keeps your skin dewey-fresh every minute you wear it'), Rose Laird's skin treatment ('not sold indiscriminately'), Helena Rubinstein's Real Silk Face Powder (each box contained 'one whole mile' of silk), Guerlain's Ambrosia Emulsion ('the complete rejuvenating beauty treatment'), Placentubex ('gives your skin a thrilling *younger* look'), Kigu's Musical Compact ('in silk-lined presentation box'), Jacques Fath's lipstick ('in 12 wonderful shades'), and — for the woman who had everything and wanted more — Asprey and Company's 18ct. gold vanity case ('set with diamonds and rubies') for £440.

The newest cosmetic for men was Man-Tan, a colourless solution of dihydroxyacetone, which turned the skin a yellowish tan or brown after a few hours' contact. Additional applications resulted in a deeper tan. The DHA, a form of sugar, combined with proteins in the skin, causing the colour change. The colour could not be washed off but faded gradually. It did, however, rub off slightly on shirt collars, and it was extremely difficult to get an even tan by using it. Man-Tan was quickly followed by other less expensive brands, some in cream form, all of which worked the same way.

22 · The Twentieth Century 1960-

Makeup for men is here. Just don't call it makeup.
—PAUL D. BLACKMAN

For the English 'man of action' who wanted, as well, to be both 'well-groomed and immaculate', Zygmunt suggested as Christmas gifts their Ambassador cologne and talc with a 'distinctly masculine aroma'. The gift was supposed, according to the advertisements, to give him extra confidence and 'that added something that will make their evening together, a dream and an enchantment.' No prices given.

Perhaps as an antidote to the highly touted hormone creams, Skinfare promised to transform the whole texture of the English skin with a natural food guaranteed to contain no hormones. After an initial investment of only nine shillings and sixpence, this natural miracle was to take place in just twenty-one days.

Like all makeup companies, Yardley of London was concerned with improving the skin as well as concealing its flaws. 'Leave things to chance,' they warned, 'and you lose the radiant petal-smooth look of a perfect skin'. Their solution was a trio of preparations consisting of cleansing cream, skin food, and freshener. 'Use them all,' the women were promised, 'and your mirror will show a skin to rival the rose in smooth and flawless beauty'. The cost: sixteen shillings.

For autumn, Gala of London was promoting 'the golden gift of radiance' through using Mutation Mink on the skin, soft Mutation, tawny Sable or Burnished Gold on the lips and nails, with Gala gold and pearly brown on the eyelids. For some reason the eyes of the Gala model were bloodshot.

Custom beauty bars were more in evidence in 1960. They tended to specialize in new, original, or exotic makeup ideas along with special blends for each customer. Jon Pierre, according to *Mademoiselle*, provided a green Neutra-tone foundation to screen out the natural complexion colour and to 'prepare the way for a second foundation colour of your own fancy. Lavender Neutra-tone is effective over a fading sun tan or a sallow complexion, and it adds a lovely translucence to normal skin tones. Shad-A-Way is a pale green camouflage cream that covers shadows and skin discolourations.'

Coty's newest contributions to eye makeup were an automatic eyebrow pencil with a sharpener in the cap, a liquid eyeliner in fifteen colours, and the Duo-matic—a spiral-type mascara wand in one end, an eye crayon in the other, both refillable.

The newest lipstick colour from Paris was brown — light or dark, yellowish or reddish, sand or cinnamon. For the woman who didn't care for brown, there were varying shades of coral, amber, or apricot. The cupid's bow was de-emphasized, and the lips were gently curved with a tiny upsweep at the corners.

The Natural Look, which keeps reappearing from time to time when women react against excessive painting, was said to be in fashion in 1961, but the naturalness was relative. The hundreds of new paints and gadgets for applying them were not discarded — they were merely used with a little more subtlety. Eyes were still lined and shadowed, with the coloured shadows (True Blue, Pale Mauve, Star Sapphire) often covering the entire eye area — a challenge to any girl who was really trying to look natural. *Mademoiselle* suggested pencilling in a coloured beauty spot near the eye, preferably blue, using two colours of eye-liner (say, dark blue and turquoise, one above the other), coloured mascara or liquid eye-liner on the underside of false eyelashes.

The 1960 brown lipstick shades were being replaced by pink and golden tones — Bold Peach, Sunbronze Coral, Honey Bee, Pink Jonquil, Lilac Pastel. Foundation tones might be Cream of Pink, Pêche Rosée, or simply Beige. The newest liquid foundation colour from Cyclax of London was called Amber Velvet — 'a daring, dramatic shade that adds a dash of new excitement to your look. Goes perfectly with matching Amber Velvet Beauty Pressed powder or with Cyclax Enchanted Mist face powder, in Regency Pink. . . . Match with smooth creamy Cyclax lipstick in Coral Reef or Pink Allure.'

Vogue's midsummer eye makeup for evening included 'short, fringy eye-lashes . . . black lines drawn close behind the upper lashes from eye-corner to eye-corner and not a jot beyond; dark, eyelash pomade slicked on sparingly over a coat of pitch mascara'; or, in another version — 'silvered shadow, triangled down from the in-corner of the brow and swept along to the outer edge of the eye . . . a thin smudge of whitened silver under the eyebrow'.

In 1961 Revlon introduced Eye Velvet, a new fluid matte eyeshadow in a tube (Plate 31-L). 'Better than dry powders that cake,' proclaimed the copy-writer. 'Better than smeary sticks that settle in creases and fade.' It was available in twelve imaginatively named if unlikely shades — Blue Snowdrop, Teal Blossom, Brown Ash, Turquoise Petal, Fresh Emeralds, Lilac Heather, Bluebud, Aqua Fern, Fresh Emeralds Lamée, Lilac Heather Lamée, Bluewillow Lamée, and Aqua Fern Lamée.

In May *Time* took a hard, jaundiced look at New York's 'latest, most pre-posterous beauty shop . . . a designer's powder-puffed version of what Pompeii would have looked like if Revlon had been running things before Vesuvius decided to end it all'.

What Revlon actually provided, for the woman who could afford it, was a day of luxury, with fountains, music, flowers, manicures, pedicures, hair sets,

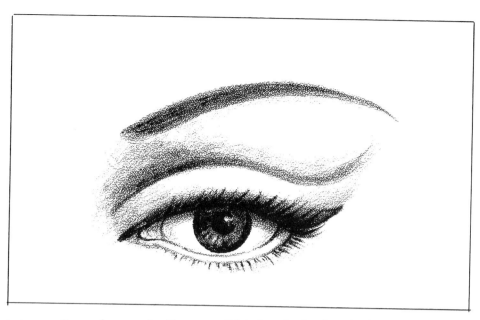

FIG. 234: Eye makeup, 1961. The upper lid is heavily lined with charcoal black, high-lighted with pale aqua, and shadowed with umber brown. The brow is pencilled with charcoal black.

permanents, makeups, Swedish showers, lunch, and a bath of one's choice in a sunken marble tub. One could arrive in the morning with dog and evening clothes, slip into a simple pink creation with gold slippers for the day, and leave sans dog and day wear, both of which would be delivered to one's home.

The *New York Times* reported that under the ceiling, painted like a night sky, there was a splashing fountain 'flanked by murals of Pan and gamboling satyrs'. There was also a long Pompeiian pool with underwater lighting and at pool's edge occasional hassocks where ladies could sit and dangle their toes in the perfumed antiseptic water. For the gregarious, the salon could be a place to meet one's friends and gossip—the equivalent of a Roman bath, but the cost was considerably higher.

In spite of all the elegance, the comfort, and the coddling, *Time* discovered one unsuspected trap for the unwary. One customer, strolling from the 'taupe-gold champagne Rotunda Reception Hall toward the Pompeiian Plaza', was so busy taking in the decor that she fell into the Pompeiian pool, where she was presumably perfumed and antisepticized at the same time.

The new makeup look for autumn included softer eyeshadow, starting on the sides of the nose and heaviest in the crease between the eyeball and the super-ciliary bone forming the eye socket—basically the same shadows used in theatrical makeup for aging the eye. Lipstick colours were striking ('poppy

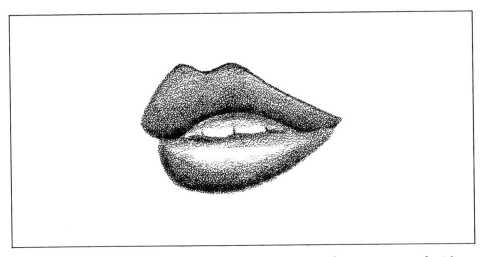

FIG. 235: Uplifted lips, 1961. The outer corners of the upper lip are overpainted with an upward lift.

pinks, vermillions, clovery mauves'), and a permanent smile was painted on by giving the upper lip a lift at the corners (Figure 235). Foundations were warm beige or cream, lightly applied. Eyebrows were often covered by the hair.

Vogue's evening makeup suggestions for 1961 included a cream or lotion skin conditioner, a tinted foundation sparingly applied, and a liquid white foundation around the eyes. 'Then, with coloured grease shadow, draw a line just at the eyelid crease, smooth and blend it slightly upward—leaving the actual lid and bone-area near the brow uncoloured by anything but the white foundation.' This was followed by a delicate application of the popular subtle rouge tints and a first coating of lipstick, shaping the lips in natural curves. Then the brows were darkened with liquid liner, mascara, or pencil. After a thorough application of transparent powder, the grease shadow could be set with a matching shade of powdered shadow, the eyebrows cleared of all powder, liquid eyeliner applied 'in a fairly narrow line at lash edges', the eyelashes darkened with mascara, and the lipstick reapplied over the powder. The whole thing could then be patted with a slightly damp sponge to remove any powdery look.

Dr Glen J. Sperandio, an associate professor of pharmacy at Purdue University, in searching for new ways to make cosmetics safe, hit upon the idea of making them from food. Dr Sperandio and his assistants had, he reported, formulated an effective skin lotion largely from peaches and cream (a natural for some alert copywriter, one would think), and an anti-chapping cream from tapioca. He also, according to *Science News Letter*, made a liquid makeup from chocolate syrup and mashed potatoes. If any company beat the competition and succeeded in buying Dr Sperandio's chocolate and potatoes recipe, their advertising department kept very quiet about it.

In 1962 Helena Rubinstein offered, for thirty-five dollars, a Day of Beauty, beginning with a weighing-in and quick check-up with the resident doctor, who made up a chart, then a half-hour bout in the exercise room, with more notations on the chart. This was followed by a body massage, lunch, and a facial massage, with discussions of skin problems and still more information added to the chart, then a shampoo, new hairdo, manicure, and pedicure. Finally, makeup artist Peter Bradford took over and did half of the face, letting the client do the other half for practice, and making some final remarks on the chart. It was now some six hours later, and the lady was presumably irresistible and ready for anything.

The latest in eye makeup was stick eyeshadow in matte and regular finish and a case of multiple cake shadows (Plate 31-F) from Cutex. Lanolin Plus offered a Shadow-Plus Compact, containing five shades of pressed powder shadow — three pastels plus gold and silver. Revlon's Eye Velvet (Plate 31-L), a matte shadow in a tube, was made in eight colours. Mascara was available in cakes, tubes, and spiral brush applicators (Plate 33-A). Some was waterproof, some not.

Fabergé packaged three colours in a kit with mirror and brush (Plate 32-C) for five dollars. Available colours were Aqua Marina, Burnt Sienna, Cerulean Blue, Ebony Green, Lavender, Slate Black, Ultramarine, Verdigreen, Alabaster, Antique Gold, and Silver Leaf.

The new trend in lipsticks, according to *Vogue*, was 'toward clear, bright, outspoken colours. The reds are true reds, the pinks practically essence-of-pink.' In line with this, Coty's new shades included Pure Apricot, Pure Honey, Pure Mango, Pure Cherry, Pure Cranberry, Pure Strawberry, Pure Pumpkin, Pure Watermelon, Pure Orchid, and Pure Peppermint.

In February *Mademoiselle* tried to explain to the novice the new technique of modelling the face with highlights and shadows — after the cream or liquid foundation, a natural rouge in one of the newest shades (brick pink, terra-cotta, coral), then a tiny bit of rouge (cream, stick, liquid, dry) pressed along the underside of the cheekbones with the fingertips. 'For correcting as you color, blend up to the corner of the eye and out to the ear lobe.' This was to round a long face. For the reverse effect, 'blend up and down, concentrating color in the center of the cheeks but fading off to the outer corner of the eye'. There were additional instructions for other deficiencies, including circles under the eyes.

For discoloured teeth, Kopal, a white tooth enamel was guaranteed to give a 'flawless smile'. And for the girl with an unsteady hand or uncertain eye, there were plastic shapers for lips and eyebrows.

The movie version of *Antony and Cleopatra* almost inevitably brought about the Egyptian Look, which *Look* reported (based on two Michel Kazan versions) as meaning lips boldly painted, the lower one fuller than the upper, eyes heavily lined with black and shadowed with Nile green or highlighted with

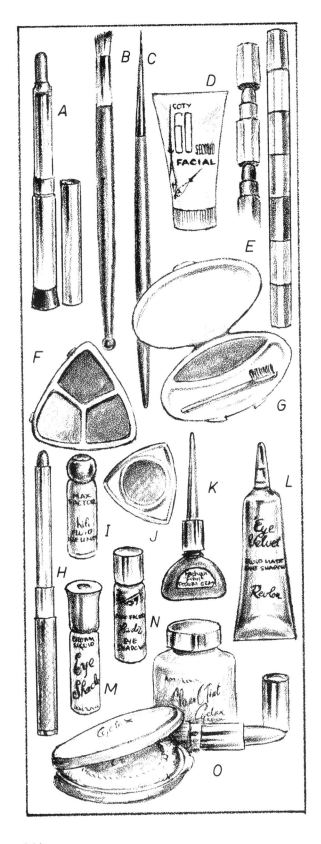

PLATE 31 : TWENTIETH CENTURY
1960–1962

A   1962. Helena Rubinstein Fashion Stick lipstick. Newest colour, Red Hellion.

B   1961. Eyeshadow brush by Martha Lorraine. Price, \$1.25.

C   1961. Eyeliner brush by Martha Lorraine. Price, \$1.

D   1961. Coty 60-Second Facial. \$1.50.

E   1960. Tussy Shado-rama — 6 eye-shadows in 1 'lidstick'. Colours — silver, turquoise, mauve, sapphire, emerald, and blue-violet. Price, \$1.75.

F   1962. Cutex triple eyeshadows in clear plastic case.

G   1962. Cutex cake mascara.

H   1961. Dorothy Gray Fashion Lipstick in 12 shades. Price, \$1.50.

I   1961. Max Factor Hi-Fi Fluid Eyeliner, available in 13 shades.

J   1962. Cutex cream shadow in clear plastic case.

K   1961. Dorothy Gray Fashion Finish nail enamel.

L   1961. Revlon Eye Velvet in coloured plastic tube. 12 shades.

M   1961. Elizabeth Arden liquid eyeshadow.

N   1961. Max Factor Powder Eyeshadow in glass bottle.

O   1961. Cyclax of London pressed powder, Glam-O-Tint liquid foundation, and lipstick.

PLATE 32 : TWENTIETH CENTURY
1962–1964

A   1963. Revlon Sculptura lipstick.
B   1963. Triangular lipstick by Fabergé.
C   1962. Fabergé Eye Colour Kit. 3 eyeshadow colours with mirror and brush.
D   1962. DuBarry Crème Paradox, a night cream in an elegant container.
E   1964. Makeup brushes for rouge, eyeshadow, lipstick, eyeliner, mascara, and eyebrow darkener.
F   1964. Caramel Lip Glacé by Fabergé.
G   1964. Eyebrow brush.
H   1964. Coty Airspun cream powder compact with lipstick. The powder was available in 12 shades and the lipstick in 42. The Duette compact was made in black, pearlized white, and gold-tone metal.

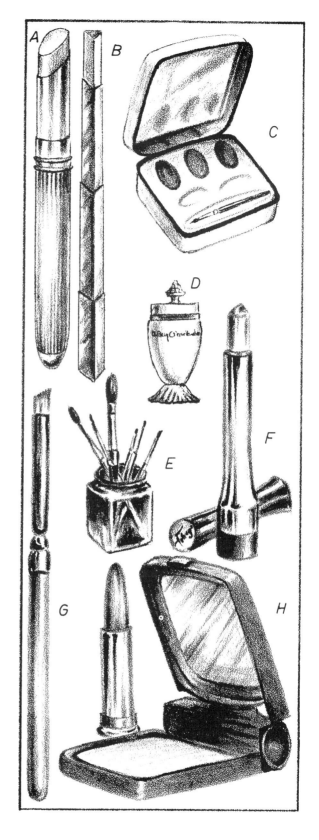

white, and eyebrows heavily pencilled with black. (See Figure 236.) The Egyptian Look was not overwhelmingly popular in its extreme form, but it did have some effect on the general trend in makeup.

The Golden Look was in for summer — golden tan or beige foundation, coral, amber, or orange lipstick, charcoal or brown eyebrow pencil, brown, black, or blue mascara, and blue, blue-green, or blue-violet eyeshadow.

FASHIONS OF 1963

Rouge was news in 1963 — all over the face. The new rouges — usually called blushers — were in the form of pale liquid washes, pots of frothy cream to be applied with a dampened sponge, moist rouges in tubes, and brush-on rouges in cakes. These subtle shades of rouge were blended over the brow, into the hair-line, under the chin, on the neck, and even on the cheeks. The result was supposed to be a natural and exhuberantly healthy glow, as if one were per-petually running to catch a bus. Hazel Bishop's rouge-in-a-tube was called Fresh'n Bright; Fabergé's was Rosy Glow Extraordinaire; Elizabeth Arden's potted cream was a delicate Faint Blush. Germaine Monteil offered a liquid blusher in 'cool mauve to spicy-pink to warming dusky pink'. Revlon's Blush-On cake, applied with a thick, stubby brush, proved to be the most popular of all, and in a few years makeup counters would be filled with hundreds of tints and shades of brush-on cakes of rouge and eyeshadow.

The doe-eyed look was going out, and the eye-liner (brown or greyed rather than black) was thickened a bit in the centre of the eye and not angled upwards at the outer corners, in order to give a rounder effect. Eyebrows were also rounded. Eyeshadow was softer and greyer and concentrated in the fold, the lid itself being light. Lips, though still light, were becoming pleasantly pink. Rouge was delicately and subtly 'blushed' on. *Vogue* called it the raffiné look.

In 1963 *Consumers Reports* published the results of tests of twelve brands of automatic mascaras (first introduced in 1958) in both black and brown. These were wand applicators of both the screw and the brush types. The investigators had no clear-cut preference between the two types, finding both convenient and practical. But they did have preferences in brands.

It was reported by the *Drug Trade News* that in 1963 American women spent $398,900,000 in keeping clean, $194,210,000 in smelling attractive, $91,680,000 in colouring their hair, $613,400,000 in keeping their hair in con-dition, $133,590,000 in caring for their skin, $116,130,000 on their hands, and $457,110,000 (£190,000,000) on makeup.

In November *Time* reported on two new male beauty parlours in New York: 'The big news in the skin game is that it's getting masculine to be feminine.

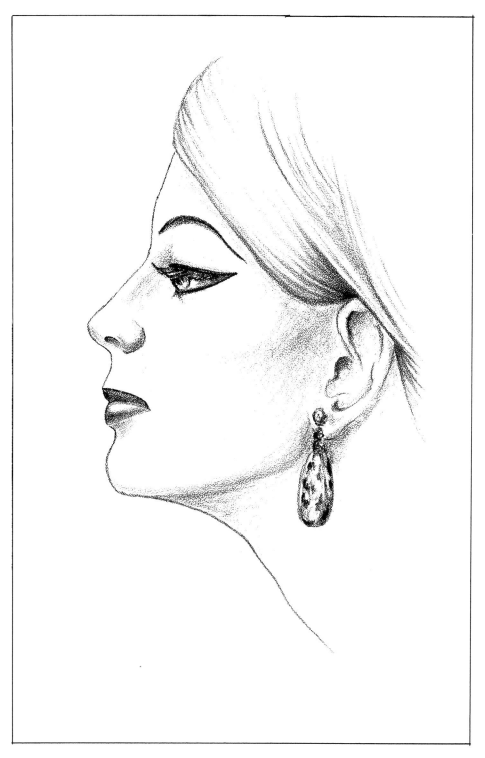

FIG. 236: The Egyptian look, 1962. Adapted from a Michel Kazan conception. Eyebrows are blackened and extended, eyes heavily lined with black, upper lids shadowed with Nile green and highlighted with white, eyelashes blackened with mascara, and lower lip painted fuller than the upper.

The leathery look in men is Out. Creams and cleansers, powders and pomades, hair-tinting combs, face-tightening masks, nail lacquers, hair sprays and sweet-smelling stuff in all sizes, shapes and prices are booming in the male market, and the cosmetics industry is rushing to repackage its female products into something for the boys. . . . Beautician Aida Gray has branched out from her female trade in Beverly Hills to open two masculine beauty parlors . . . where she has facilities for facials, massages, instant skin-tanning and eyebrow tinting. "In the past year or year and a half," chirps chic, French-born Aida, "there's been a tremendous rise in men's cosmetics. I got into the male line when I discovered that about 50% of my customers had husbands who were using their beauty creams. We sell green powder for ruddy skin and blue powder for sallow skin. We don't sell them powder puffs, of course." Manufacturers and retailers were reluctant to try to explain the shift in male habits, though they were quick to take advantage of it. As one busy and happy buyer put it, "Men have just decided not to smell like men any more. They want to smell good."

SEAL FUZZ AND COW'S BLOOD

In January 1964 *Life* reported on a developing interest in cosmetics among 381 Eskimos in the village of Gambell on St Laurence Island. An enterprising hunter and ivory-carver, John Aningayou, intrigued by an advertisement for cosmetics saleswomen in the Anchorage *Times*, sent ten dollars for a sample kit for his wife. She posted the literature on the door of the GI Quonset hut to stimulate interest, then proceeded to teach herself how to use the strange and exotic preparations. When she was eventually ready to demonstrate the new products, the villagers, including a few men, crowded into the Quonset hut, smelled and handled the jars and bottles, watched a young village beauty being creamed and painted, and decided that Studio Girl face cream was better than rancid seal oil.

Although Adeline Aningayou did not always follow conventional application procedure (she used baby seal fuzz for applying makeup and dampened caribou moss for removing it), whatever she did proved to be so successful with the women that she ordered a supply of men's toiletries. Since the men grew the scantiest of beards and customarily plucked them out with pliers about twice a year, the before-and-after shaving lotions were not in great demand. But no doubt Adeline eventually figured out a way to get round that. After all, the Mister After-Shower Spray was a sell-out among the non-bathing villagers.

The newest attempt to combat wrinkles resulted in a preparation made from cow's blood — cheap to make, expensive to buy. Helene Curtis reached the

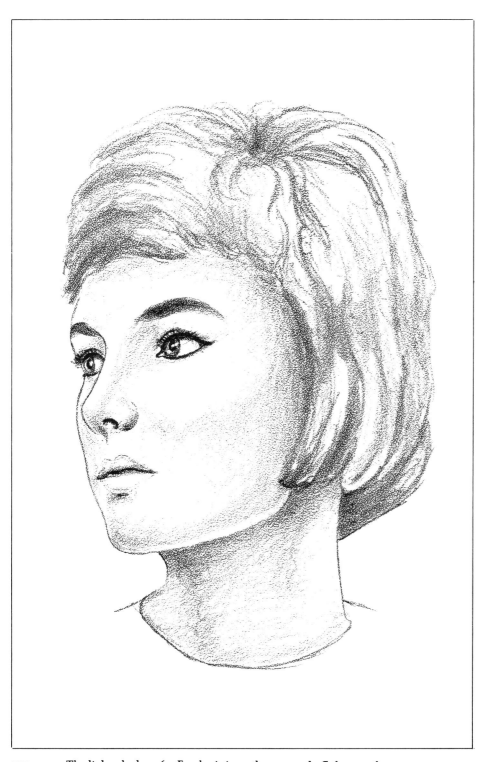

FIG. 237: The lipless look, 1963. Emphasis is on the eyes and off the mouth.

market first, in February 1964, with Magic Secret, which sold for twenty-five dollars an ounce. The tiny gold fifth-ounce bottles provided twenty wrinkle-smoothing facials. Magic Secret was followed by Coty's Line Away, Revlon's Liqui-Lift, and others, some of them, taking advantage of the advertising done by the large companies (five million dollars by Helene Curtis, it was reported), selling at a considerably lower price.

The lotion worked its magic in about fifteen minutes and lasted for eight hours — unless the lady had the misfortune to get caught in the rain, in which case she found herself in much the same predicament as the eighteenth-century ladies whose enamel ran under adverse conditions. Should this happen, fifteen minutes in private could restore the damage.

Mademoiselle's big news for 1964 was extravagant eyelashes — 'big, beautiful, battable, believable' to go with 'a paled and pouty mouth, a blush of modest proportions — a face that could have been lifted from a Victorian valentine'.

First, there were the black mascaras — brown-black, blue-black, green-black, grey-black, golden-black, then the lash-lengtheners, and finally the false eyelashes, applied lash by lash and good for about three weeks and costing up to twenty dollars, or more commonly applied in the conventional strip. The most expensive ones (up to eighty dollars a pair) were made of mink, sable, seal, or human hair. Real enthusiasts were known to wear as many as three pairs at once. Some eyelashes were made in a two-toned or tweed effect — double eyelashes of two different colours — green and brown, blue and black, brown and black, green and blue, henna and brown — any combination. They were available in New York for eleven dollars a pair, nineteen dollars if custom fitted. Mascara wands had developed into lash lengtheners, applied in the same way. Revlon's was called Fabulash. False eyebrows were also available as well as a brush-on eyebrow makeup.

Fingernails were pale in 1964 — tallow, ivory, tan, pearl, quicksilver — sometimes clear, sometimes frosted.

In England, according to *Queen's* Joan Price, emphasis was on the natural look, with skin visible through the makeup. Helena Rubinstein, in order to make a trio of *Queen* cover girls as beautifully natural as possible, used Opaline Coverfluid, Opalescent powder, Silk Tone Liquid Rouge, brown eyeliner, brown Long-Lash mascara, Black Pearl eyeshadow, Rose Baccarat lipstick, and Rose Tone nail lacquer.

For the natural look, the skin, Miss Price insisted, 'must be fed a high protein diet'. But the proteins, instead of being eaten, as one might reasonably expect, were put into makeup and skin creams — milk in Lentheric's Special Formula Skin Food, the 'biologically active ingredients' of peaches in Innoxa's Living Peach, watermelon in Dr Payot's Crème Hydriana, and wheatgerm in Arlane's Crème Naturelle, which also contained hops, juniper, gooseberries, apricots, cucumbers, and pith of the Elder tree.

There was a minor flurry of caramel-flavoured lipstick (Plate 32-F). 'Just slick delicious Caramel Lip Glace over your regular lipstick,' urged the Fabergé copy-writer. 'Watch this marvelous new burnt-sugar glaze sweeten your lips with honey'd tones . . . turn them tawny, toasty, terrific!' Cutex echoed: 'Sssshh! Don't say a word! Just kiss . . . and *it* tells. Yes, Caramel Kiss actually *tastes* of caramel.' Fabergé also offered Graype and Pistachio. Evidently these taste-treats did not start a revolutionary trend.

THE SCULPTURED LOOK

The sculptured look was getting underway in 1964. Young Lady Esther offered three basic colour schemes — Gold Vapour, Misty Mauve, and Balmy Bronze, which were supposed to create the illusion of shadows and highlights. In the Balmy Bronze group, recommended for autumn, there was a 'foundation to enhance (or simulate) an August tan, bronzy eyeshadow to warm the eyelids, mocha lipstick for highlighting, and tawny powder for final polish'. But actually modelling the face to bring out the bones required varying shades of foundation colour, rouge, and eyeshadow and was at that time left largely to the experts.

Women everywhere were brushing on nearly everything but their founda-tion colour. The traditional brushes for mascara and lipstick had now been joined by slender brushes for liquid eyeliner, chubby ones for brush-on rouge, similar but smaller ones for brush-on eyeshadow, and slanted ones for colouring eyebrows. (See Plate 32-E.)

According to *Mademoiselle*, 'anyone who sticks to pure naturalism is simply not going to meet the competition. . . . Rouges and blushers are used whole-heartedly and nearly whole-facedly. They go all around the periphery — hairline, cheekbones, jawline, chin — making a fine frame for the features. . . . Lodes of gold and silver struck for the first time in daytime makeup. The gold intensifies tawny makeups; the silver does the same for pink-and-whites. Prospect for both in powder, foundation, eyeshadow — even lipstick. . . . Counterpoint coloring: A pure pink-based makeup worn with an offbeat orange sweater, for instance, or tawny coloration with a fragile-pink dress. The idea being that me-tooism in makeup is out, and that colors come across more strongly in contrast.' In line with the new colouring, Fabergé had just brought out a new gold lipstick.

Mademoiselle's model used to illustrate the new trend wore a sweater the colour of burnished brass and a DuBarry foundation 'on the cool side of pink. . . . Her lipstick, one of DuBarry's six new shades, Glissando Pink No.7 — swirled with orange in the tube, swirled with light when it's on . . . the brows brushed and browned with Brush-On brow liner; the lids finely lined in black, then silvered by an all-over pearling with Pearl Glacé.'

The new makeup for autumn was what *Mademoiselle* called 'subtle extremism'. Instead of enamelled eyes and no lips, the golden look was the fashion. 'The gold is hazed with smoke,' said *Mademoiselle*, 'gilds you to tawniness, not glitter. There's a light and luminous eyeshadow called Holiday Highlight. A pale, lights-up powder, Holiday Gold. And a lipstick, also known as Holiday Gold, in . . . a deep goldy-bronze.'

Coloured lipstick was back — 'pearly lipsticks, marbelized lipsticks, lipsticks flecked with gold or silver'. Some were flavoured. Tussy's Two-Tone Golden Wonder provided two shades in one, the darker used for outlining.

Mademoiselle described an Elizabeth Arden makeup illustrated in their October issue: 'The eyes are subtly sculptured, in alternating stripes of White and Smoke Sapphire eyeshadow. The Black liner extends over the corners of the eye, and a dash of White Shadow in the corners creates the look of a larger eye. In the balance, the mouth is tinted a warm, rich Sepia Pink.'

Although cosmetics packaging was becoming increasingly elegant, women who could afford to sometimes preferred to dip into the past for one-of-a-kind containers or holders for their twentieth-century paints, powders, and brushes. *Vogue* reported on a few of them — a yellow enamel Fabergé cigarette holder made into an eyebrow pencil, a makeup sponge set in gold with turquoises and coral, a collection of eighteenth-century marble balls used as stands for hairpieces, an antique Indian hand warmer of perforated brass now used to carry makeup.

The revolution-to-come in men's cosmetics got a strong boost in the mid-fifties when American college men in Paris began buying a chic cologne called Canoë, unobtainable in the United States. Finally, in 1959, Dana took the plunge and imported 4000 bottles, which were sold out in 61 days. For the 1963 Christmas market, Dana imported 43 tons of Canoë.

Swank, a jewelry company with more cosmetics foresight than the perfume manufacturers, brought out an exotic cologne for men in 1963 and called it Jade East. The commercials showed a Chinese girl bathing in a fountain in a tropical setting. 'She senses your presence before you speak a word,' intones a male voice. 'It's something about you that excites her. Perhaps the Jade East you use.' In other words, the advertisers were trying the same technique that had proved so successful with women. And it worked. In the first six months they sold $700,000 worth of Jade East and two years later were expecting to sell more than twenty million dollars' worth.

The success of Jade East roused well over a hundred other companies to look for the hidden gold in the bottle of scent, and soon department stores all over the United States had special toiletries counters for men. Salesmen were advised by a trade publication to develop a special vocabulary, stressing such words as 'tantalizing, crisp, suave, vigorous, robust, virile, manly'.

'The liquids,' reported *Life*, 'are all deep greens, reds, and browns. The bottles

PLATE 33 : TWENTIETH CENTURY
1964, 1965

A 1964. Maybelline Ultra Lash Mascara — 'Builds, colours, curls, separates'. Price, $1.

B 1964. Gilt bamboo-handled lipstick brush and gilt shell pressed-powder compact by Givenchy.

C 1964. DuBarry cake shadow, applied with moistened brush.

D 1964. Blush Brush by Scandia.

E 1965. Dior lipstick.

F 1965. Dior nail enamel.

G 1964. Grand Illusion makeup by John Robert Powers.

H 1964. Max Factor Fine Line lipstick in gold and white tube.

I 1964. DuBarry automatic eyebrow pencil.

J 1965. Hazel Bishop Spotlight lipstick, with white centre for highlighting. Beige, peach, blush, and pink.

K 1965. Makeup brush by Angel Face. Fits into Brush-Alive Compact.

L 1965. Brush-on rouge in two shades.

M 1965. DuBarry Glissando marbellized Eye Color Stick in blue, grey, turquoise, lilac, and taupe.

N 1965. Sponge-tipped applicator for pressed powder eyeshadow. By Helena Rubinstein.

O 1965. Dorothy Gray Brush Stroke eyeshadow compact and brush. Tray of shadow slides out and brush pops up.

P 1965. DuBarry Glissando makeup with foundation, highlight, shadow, and silk sponge.

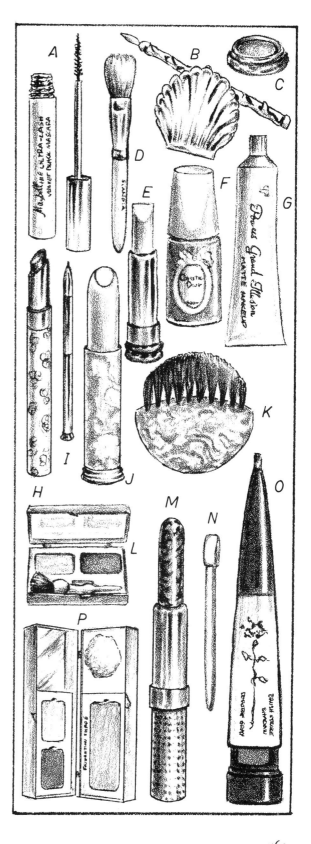

—short and sturdy with big wood or gold tops—are covered with symbols like horses, boats, Indians, swords, and stock tickers. They have brand names such as Extra Dry, Big Shot, White Knight, Executive, Tidal Wave, Secret Service, Branded, Gravel, Stampede, Waterloo, Tycoon, and, of course, 007. . . . Most of the colognes are 85% alcohol mixed with a wide variety of sweet perfume ingredients such as citrus, lavender, floral extracts, and many "woodsy, mossy" derivatives.' The scents were strong and long-lasting and, boasted one manufacturer, 'If there's a fellow in the room with our scent on, you know it!' Prices were usually about five dollars for four ounces, but a few were much higher.

The success of cologne sent manufacturers scurrying to their conference rooms and their laboratories to work on hair sprays, hair colouring, face creams, coloured foundations, and mascara for men. But some executives remained cautious, among them Dana's Richard Livingstone. 'There is a great tendency in this business to rush something like this,' he said. 'My fundamental fear is that if the industry goes too fast and tries to force on the public ideas it isn't ready to accept, the whole campaign may backfire. Men will reject the whole idea and go right back behind that closed bathroom door.'

Men's beauty parlours, though they were never called that, were now becoming popular with executives, who wanted to relax to quiet music and regain a little youth with a hair wave; an eyebrow tint, or, at Madison Avenue's Jerry Spallina's, a Sudden Youth facial—a latex mask brushed on over an oil base and good for a few wrinkle-free hours. At Eddie Pulaski's, down the street, the same thing was done with a Sudden Veil Lift.

THE EXOTIC LOOK

With makeup becoming increasingly complex, makeup men were beginning to be in demand. Elizabeth Arden's Pablo, a young Italian nobleman with a flair for imaginative design, garnered a good share of the publicity and most of the prominent customers. He was straightforward with the press. It was his opinion, as quoted by *Time*, that 'Pink foundation is awful, green eyeshadow is vulgar, eyebrows are hateful, dark lipstick is obsolete'. He was interested mostly in eyes—'the only part really worth making up'. In a makeup described by *Look*, he began with a thorough cleansing and moisturizing, then applied foundation 'tapering to a mere film at the sides' and lightly powdered. For a deep-set look in the eyes, he shadowed the crease between the lid and the eye-socket bone with dark brown and highlighted the lid and the bone under the brow with white. He applied more white at both inner and outer corners of the eye, pinpointing it at the inner corner, sweeping it up at the outer. He lined the eyes

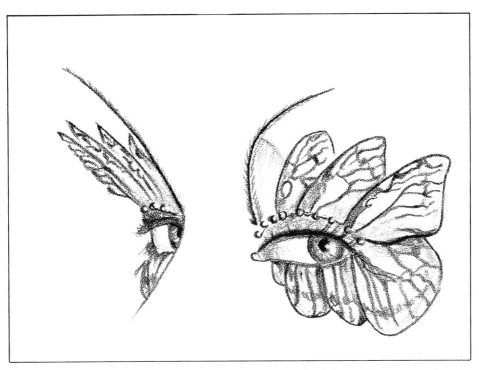

FIG. 238: Butterfly eyes, 1964. After a design in *Vogue* by Pablo of Elizabeth Arden.

with black, beginning with a thin line at the inner corners and building it up toward the centre and outer corners. Mascara, false lashes, and a touch of dark on the brows completed the eyes. Lips were 'naturally defined but underplayed'.

As for the exotic, theatrically stylized eye makeups which brought him quick attention in New York (see Figure 238), he was appalled that women actually wanted to wear his jewelled, checkered, feathered, flowered eye designs, some of which took as long as five hours to apply. At twenty dollars a half hour, that could run into money.

For the anything-but-natural look in eye makeup (Figure 239), *McCall's* suggested (1) upper lid heavily lined with midnight blue and creases around eyeball with brown, upper lid highlighted with silver and brow bone with beige, sides of nose shadowed with taupe, and lashes heavily blackened with lash-building mascara; (2) taupe liner on upper lid and in crease, beige highlights on lid, silver under brows. For the rest, suggestions centred around beige foundation, pink or coral lipstick, and perhaps a blusher on the cheekbones.

The pale look (or, as *Time* put it, 'The Big Fade') seemed to have reached its peak in 1965. Lips had begun to disappear in 1961, then colour from the cheeks;

now it was the eyebrows' turn. They were bleached, covered with foundation, painted beige, or concealed with bangs. The idea, which had been growing steadily for a number of years, was to focus attention on the eye itself. To this end even the lids were highlighted, eyes were heavily lined, and double or triple eyelashes were worn. The fact that a dark shadow over the eye and long, pencilled eyebrows help to enlarge and therefore beautify the eye was completely lost sight of. Even tans were out of fashion. Instead of Rubinstein's Tan-in-a-Minute, the chic woman bought Elizabeth Arden's Sun Bloc to keep her skin pale at the beach. The result, at a distance, seemed rather like two exotic, furry-legged spiders slowly sinking into a bowl of custard. But like all fads, it would soon pass.

Mademoiselle's autumn report on the new trend in makeup stressed the moulded look, tawny colours, and shine. Colour was back in lipsticks (Honey, Burn, Bricktop, Glistening Pink), and eye colouring emphasized greys and browns in place of black, along with metallic shadows. Among the new items were Germaine Monteil's gold and silver Eyelash Tippers to give the effect of 'a thick fringe starred with snowflakes'. A model with Revlon makeup was wearing Bricktop lipstick frosted with White A La Carte. Her eyes were lined with Charcoal Grey cake liner and shadowed with Dove Grey Eye Velvet. A triangle of white extended beyond the corner of the eye 'to draw out the eyes' and five long lines were drawn diagonally down from the eye, presumably to give the effect of lower lashes. The actual effect was of five brown lines and a white triangle.

A Yardley advertisement included instructions for the 'London Look', which began with Fluid Film Foundation, cream rouge, and complexion powder. As for the eyes, 'Lashes should be positively dripping Yardley's Brush-On Eyematique. In brown, to soften the look. . . . Again in brown, outline eye with Yardley's Cake Eyeliner. Then with Yardley's Stick Eyeshadow, draw a topaz line clear across the ridge of the lid. Soften edges. Above and below this line blend in Yardley's dry white eyeshadow'. The brows were to be pencilled, following the natural shape. Five lipstick colours were available — Chelsea Pink, Pinkadilly, Dicey Peach, Nippy Beige, and Nectaringo. These were to be topped with Basic Slickers, Frosted Slickers, or Sunny Slickers.

Vogue's new look for November 1965 (designed by Revlon's makeup man) was a mauve-white complexion with mauve and pistachio eyelids and pistachio eyelashes turned down instead of up. But apart from this exotic makeup, inspired by a snakeskin, *Vogue* predicted, in its customary Vogue-ese, '*darker lipstick*, and let's forget the image of black-cherry lips. The new dark-red lipsticks are a today-invention. What they're loaded with is light. Light blazing away beneath the colour; light lustre-ing the surface, always. *Only* light prevents red lipstick from being the same tired old red trying for a comeback. And among red lipsticks, *only* the new reds look right. . . . But don't think the

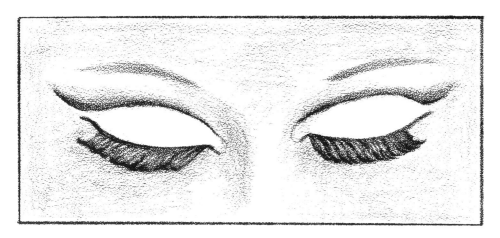

FIG. 239: Eye makeup, 1965. The upper lids are heavily lined with black, brown, or dark blue and highlighted with white; the crease above the lids is deeply shadowed with brown or taupe; the lashes are heavily coated with mascara, or false eyelashes are used; the eyebrows are underplayed.

darker lipstick, with all that goes with it (a whiter face, a determined maquillage) is out to *tromper* the great hold enjoyed by what we've come to think of as *life-coloured makeups*. These makeups, warmed by the blood, and based on glow, remain the cleverest, the sneakiest makeup approach in history because what they affect has such an unaffected mien: the look of health and happy juices.' *Vogue* also predicted the return of red nail enamel — on the little finger only. For the others they suggested a wash of gold. This was not one of *Vogue*'s more successful predictions.

Eyes, according to *Vogue*, were 'cleaning up. Shadows are made less haunting; even eye-liner works a little differently — it's lash-coloured and painted so closely to the roots of the lashes that it fits them almost like dye.'

Mary Quant, England's Queen of the Mods, had her own line of cosmetics strikingly packaged. She was tired, she said of fancy pink and gold plastic containers. The line included Starkers, a liquid foundation in two shades, 'suitable for all colourings'. Face Shapers, she said, 'is for doing all those face-modelling things and is a browny-pink rouge shadow, together with a pearly, ivory-coloured powder'. In addition, she had a Brush Lipstick in six pale tints and 'a brilliant half-and-half lipstick called Skitzo' (Plate 34-D). For highlighting she used a cream called Face Lighter. Mascara was available in both cake and liquid form with a big brush so one could 'pile the colour on to the lashes'.

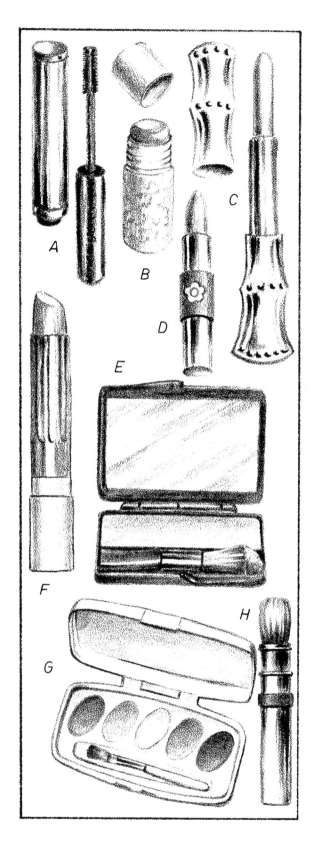

PLATE 34 : TWENTIETH CENTURY
1966–1968

A Spiral brush mascara.
B Revlon Face Gleamer. Makeup stick in plastic tube.
C Givenchy lipstick in 18-carat gold-plated bamboo case.
D 1966. Mary Quant Skitzo Lipstick.
E Clairol Soft-Blush, with cake rouge and brush.
F John Robert Powers Face-Makers, for shading and highlighting. Available in several shades of red as well as a variety of flesh tones from very light to dark.
G 1968. Coty brush-on eyeshadow in 5 shades with brush.
H 1966. Mary Quant Face Brush.

New Trends, 1966

The good news in London for 1966 was that the no-lips era was at an end (actually it wasn't). Also, bright reds for nails and lips were once more in fashion. As usual, the manufacturers came up with intriguingly exotic names for the new colours — Sea Orchid, Dawn of Spring, Mexican Fire, Silver Amber, Red Fox, Sun Gold, Wild Pink, and Jet Red. For the eyes there was Pearly Striking Blue, French Navy Blue, Gold, French Grey, Smoky Grey, Smoky Sapphire, Cactus Green, Blue Jade Cream, Turquoise, Vert Doré, and many others. But most of the imagination seemed to be exerted on naming foundation colours — Naturelle Veiled Radiance, Beige Jonquil Veiled Radiance, International Beige Veiled Radiance, Sport Light Veiled Radiance, Sport Dark Featherlight Foundation, Sun Gold Basic Sheen.

By spring eye modelling had become more colourful and even more obviously painted. Colours tended to be light and bright — fern green, sky blue, sunshine yellow — accented with deep blues, browns, and blacks. In eye makeups for *Mademoiselle*, Elizabeth Arden's Pablo, who in 1965 considered green eyeshadow vulgar, used touches of aqua green at the inner corner of the eye, lined the lids with dark brown cake liner above and dark blue pencil below, highlighted the bone under the eyebrow with Sun Gold, and sketched in lower eyelash shadows on the skin with brown. (See Figure 240-B.)

In another eye makeup (Figure 240-C) we find pale yellow highlights and forest green eyeshadow in a triangular frame of brown liner. The upper lid is lined with black; the eyelashes are dark brown.

In line with the fashion for colour in lips and nails, Estée Lauder had forty-one shades of nail lacquer ready for summer. One of them, called 24 K Gold, actually *was*, and it sold for two guineas a bottle.

With skirts up and bare knees not especially alluring, one thing led to another, and summer madness found the knees being decorated with plastic jewels, beauty spots, winking eyes, painted sunbursts, psychedelic designs, or a simple touch of rouge. Pablo of Elizabeth Arden, with a taste not all makeup artists shared, called it 'a dreadful consequence of incredible fashion' and refused to have anything to do with it.

But makeup for the whole leg was back, at least for a while. And even if you didn't want to call attention to your knees, you could paint or cream your legs with a suitable shade of beige or tan and reshape them (within strict limits) by brushing on a brown powder. Estée Lauder provided a whole kit just for legs — Satinée Shene (a pink lubricating lotion), Waterproof Leg Makeup (a cream in two shades), Slim-Leg (the brush-on powder), Knee-Glow (a powder rouge), and a collection of jewelled mouches.

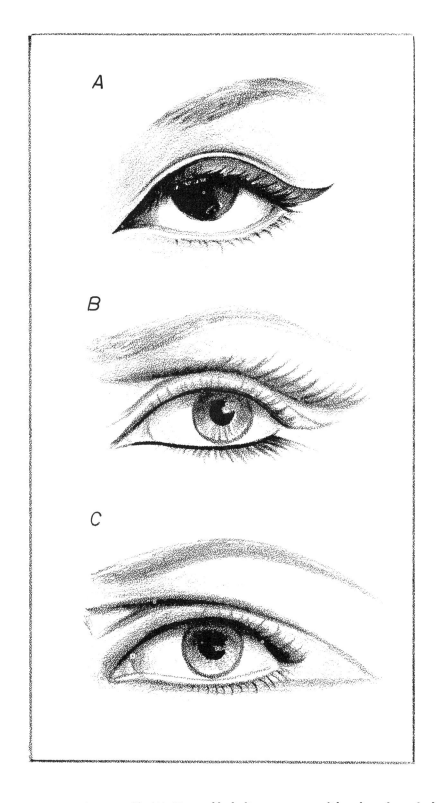

FIG. 240: Eye makeup, 1966. (A) Heavy black liner on upper lid, coloured eyeshadow, natural brows. (B) Upper lid lined with dark brown cake liner and lower one (inside the lashes) with dark blue pencil; eyelash shadows sketched in with

CONTOUR MAKEUP, 1967

In 1967 street makeup took its cue from stage makeup, with emphasis on modelling the face with highlights and shadows to give the illusion of a more interesting bone structure than one actually had — to tone down whatever one had too much of and bring out what one needed more of. The almost stupefying variety of tints, shades, tones, and hues were applied with brushes, sticks, sponges, buffers, pencils, and fingers. Brush-on eyeshadow came in paired colours, one dark and one light, or simply in a number of shades, all in one case. Clairol advertised thirteen pairs of colours. John Robert Powers introduced his Face-Makers in lipstick-like gold and white cases. 'In seconds,' said the advertisements, 'these ingenious little sculpture sticks will stroke on a beautiful interplay of highlight, shading, and colour that makes you look perfect. They make contour makeup as everyday-simple as lipstick. Want chiseled cheekbones? Classic nose? Less chin? They're yours . . . in a quick stroke and a blend.' What the copywriter did not mention was that the quick stroke and a blend, if it were to accomplish its purpose, would require a reasonable amount of skill; and the quicker the stroke, the more skill would be needed.

In a promotion gimmick ostensibly designed to meet this problem for the non-professional, DuBarry advertised a paint-by-numbers system requiring at least a dozen colours (and thus a dozen separate cosmetic items to be purchased) for every female face. Their recommended procedure was to sponge on a foundation colour, then to add Highlighters and Shadowers 'to provide beautiful contours', just as professional makeup artists had done for years in corrective makeup for the stage. Rouge was brushed on and lips painted on and the whole dusted with 'luminescent Face Light', which presumably meant powder.

The eyes required an entire system of their own, involving Colour Cake Liner in black or brown, eyeshadow stick to emphasize the deep parts of the eye socket, Colour Cake Shadow or Brush On Powdered Eye Shadow on the lid itself, Neutre Colour Cake Blender for highlighting the superciliary bone under the eyebrow, Brush On Brow Liner or Eyebrow Pencil for shaping and accenting the brows, and, 'for evening glitter', a little Glacé on the lids. The stunning green eyes of the beautiful model used in the advertisements were accented with black, green, brown, and ivory. Applied by a professional makeup artist, the result was both striking and glamorous. The do-it-yourself jobs observed on the street were not always so successful.

FIG. 240 *contd.*
> brown; aqua green shadow at inner corner of eye; sun gold highlight on bone under brow. (C) Forest green eyeshadow in a triangular frame of brown liner; upper lid lined with black; eyelashes dark brown; pale yellow highlights.

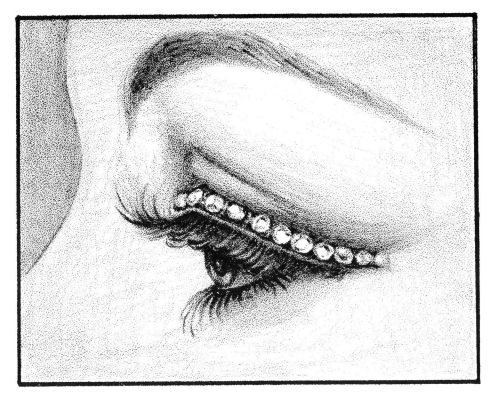

FIG. 241 : False eyelashes with rhinestones, 1967.

GLITTER AND GLINT

It was a year for glitter and glint, not only in clothes, but in makeup as well. Helena Rubinstein introduced lipstick in 'three precious-metal tones. . . . Bronze Rage! Silver Rage! Gold Rage! Plus three shades that hint of glint, rage with *color*. Pink Rage! Orange Rage! Flame Rage!' And for the eyes — 'Shadow shades that reflect the shimmer of your smile. Bronze Rage! Silver Rage! Gold Rage! Start collecting. A girl just can't have enough!' The Aziza copywriter was also describing their new eyeshadow — 'Golds never before made-to-melt with color. Blue-gold, green-gold, gleamiest gold-gold. Aziza golds to steal the nightlight.' Bonne Bell, disdaining the gold rush, simply made a lot of lip glosses in unexpected colours — mint, grape, orange, pink, toffee, and lemon. The blue-eyed, pink-lipped blonde in the advertisement looked as if she were about to eat her stick of lime.

Elizabeth Arden emphasized the glint but not the gold with her Northern Lights for her 'new glacial look'. It seems that Arden's Pablo had 'designed this

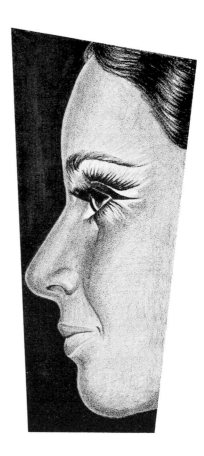

FIG. 242 : The bizarre look, 1967. High-fashion makeup
designed for *Harper's Bazaar*. Skin tone is
tan, with coral pink lipstick and no rouge.
Eyes are accentuated with false eyelashes as
well as decorative painting in black, white,
and a touch of coral.

many-splendored gamut of glacial colors for winter. He flicks light on your complexion with new Illusion Foundation. Shapes it with Arctic Pink blusher.
Frosts eyes with the northern range of Creamy Powder Eye Shadows and finishes
the look with a polar pink lipshade called Northern Lights.' The model, wrapped
in silvery-blue fur, looked very handsome indeed — and interestingly glacial.

   Vogue's trends for 1967 included more golden tones, with gold instead of
silver highlights, accent lipsticks (lilac, apricot, gold), yellow or gold eyelids,
transparent blushers, and shiny eye liners.

THE POLISHED LOOK

The cosmetic news for autumn was the polished look. 'Moist. Just born. Just
dewed with shine,' said *Mademoiselle*. 'That's the way skin should look this fall.
And that's the way it will look, judging by what the cosmetic big guns are
blasting off with this month. Hardly a chemist is now alive who hasn't
developed a pretty face polish of his own.' The man at Yardley, reported the
magazine, had come up with something called Face Slicker in 'three creamy

shades—City Beige, City Pink, and City White'. For the country girl—nothing. The three Yardley Slickers could be worn all over the face 'for a kind of supershine or as gleamers. Along the cheekbones, maybe, or at your temples and along the hairline. Earlobes, too, if you're feeling kittenish. City Pink's best by day; either of the others . . . is nice by night'.

Revlon's Face Gleamer in a round swivel stick (Plate 34-B) was available in Blush, Peach, and Tawny, as well as a 'highlighting stick of pure gleam'. Revlon proudly claimed credit for inaugurating the polished look and sprinkled full-page, full-colour advertisements liberally throughout women's magazines and New York theatre programmes. 'Dapple your cheeks with it,' urged the copywriter. 'Glisten your chin with it. Highlight *everyplace* with it. Your whole face turns on. Youngs up. Blushes. Beams. Timid types may stop at cheekbones. Avant-gardes stop at nothing.' At this same time Max Factor was advertising his new Counter-Shine to bring about 'the end of the shiny face'.

Some months later *Queen*'s Joan Price was writing enthusiastically about Revlon's Face Gleamers—'the latest development in the modern concept of rouge. Its old image was a doll-like dot of pink or crimson in a matched-to-lipstick tone that over-developed on the skin and appeared unnatural. . . . The trend today towards natural make-up has meant a swing from a matt, powdered finish; the skin looks younger without it.' The accompanying model, fairly natural-looking except for the eyes, was made up with 'Ultima II Mauvesse Under Make-Up Nutrient Creme, Aurora Beige Cremefoam Make-Up and Translucent Face Powder, and Blush Face Gleamer. *Eyes*: Ultrafall Private Eyelashes groomed with Charcoal Brown Ultima Lash Make-Up, and Ultima Patina Eyeshadow. *Lips*: Mister Melon Moondrops Lipstick'.

TANNERS AND TONERS

By 1967 most of the major department stores in large American cities had special counters for men's toiletries, featuring a wide variety of colognes, deodorants, after-shave lotions, fancy soaps and talcums, skin conditioners, tanning creams and lotions, and skin toners. More and more manufacturers of men's toiletries were adding exotic scents, face creams, and coloured skin cosmetics to their more conventional products. Among the toiletries suggested for men in the Christmas 1967 issue of *Harper's Bazaar* were a relaxing bubble bath by Givenchy, Aramis's *Spray Shower Oil*, Braggi's *Sauna Splash*, a spray-on talc from Woodard or Aramis, a colourless lipstick from John Robert Powers or Roger and Gallet, *All-Weather Hand Cream* by Aramis or *High Altitude Cream* by Bonne Bell. These were just to keep him clean and soft and pliable. Beyond that, to counteract any winter paleness, there was Fabergé's

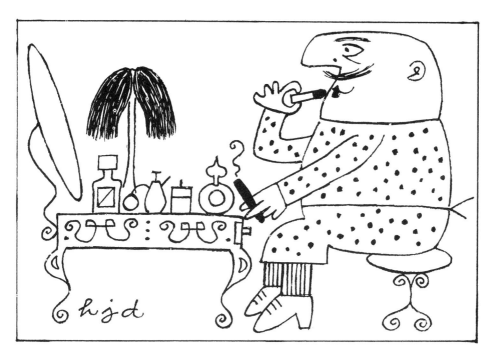

FIG. 243 : Cosmetics for dear old dad. From the *Chronicle*, San Francisco, 1968.

Brut After Shave Tan (guaranteed not to rub off on the collar), Braggi's *Face Bronzer* ('moisturizes as it goes'), Bonne Belle's *Snow Tan* (a bronzing cream capable of providing 'a full-fledged bronze burnishment with moisturizing'), and John Robert Powers's *Look Fit* (for a 'young, heathful, natural-looking color'). For cover-up jobs there was Braggi's *Cover Tone* or Aramis's *Protein Face Talc* in natural skin-tone shades. For bedtime and all-night wear, one might choose a *Shape-Up Skin Conditioner* from Baxter of California ('to smear invisibly over his growing-craggy countenance before he tucks himself in'), *Nightcap Facial Massage* from Braggi ('It's in there pitching all night long'), or *Double Action Cream* from Aramis (for 'moisturing and conditioning while it smoothes the manly brow'). Should all of this fail to revive one's man, *Harper's* suggested 'a face tuck for him by your own understanding plastic surgeon'.

FOCUS ON EYES

In January 1968 Joan Price, writing in *Queen*, assured her readers that false eyelashes—real hair, synthetic hair, or fur—were for *everyone*. For round eyes she advised real hair, trimmed short at the inner corners; and for deep-set eyes, well-trimmed, long-in-the-centre fur lashes. Almond shaped eyes, she said, required straight, shaggy-trimmed lashes, long at the outer corners, short at the inner. Demi-lashes worn on the centre of the lids were ideal for prominent eyes.

With major emphasis still on the eyes, styles of eyelashes continued to multiply. In a full-page advertisement in the *New York Times Magazine* (see Figure 244), one manufacturer illustrated twenty styles, including Natural Fine, Natural Medium, Natural Heavy, Natural Triple, Natural DeLuxe, Natural Shaggy, Standard Medium, Standard Heavy, Standard Spikey, Standard Shaggy, Mini Lash, and Glitter Lash. Most of these were available in black or brown, some in black and brown mixed. The Glitter Lash could be had in gold or silver or patent-leather black. A special lash was available for lower lids.

From time to time inventors have dabbled in the cosmetics field and come up with something original enough to warrant government protection. U.S. patent no. 3,363,242, taken out by Frederick E. Glaser of Chicago, was for a method of turning feathers into eyelashes. Mr Glaser, observing the lack of variety and originality in women's false eyelashes, turned to feathers; and by spreading a small strip of resin or adhesive to the feather barbs before separating them from the shaft, he was able to attach them to the eyelids in the usual way but with a somewhat different effect.

TRAVELLING LADY

In the early days of the automobile, women swathed themselves in veils and even wore tight-fitting goggles to protect their eyes. Nevertheless they finished the ride covered with grime. In 1968 women were still faced with the problem of pulling themselves together after a long trip. In an article entitled 'Beauty on the Road', *Hair and Makeup* recommended stocking one's glove compartment with saturated cleansing pads, tissues, hand lotion, moisturizer, hair spray, perfume or toilet water, a small cake of soap, a disposable face cloth, cleansing cream, and some hair rollers. Other arrangements would presumably have to be made for items normally kept in a glove compartment.

In order to arrive in top condition, the reader was advised to 'go limp for ten minutes', refresh the face with skin lotion, renew lipstick, slip on a curly wig, wear a wrap around print over her shift, and add a bit of jewellery. It was also suggested that a woman with a fancy car but no wig might plug in her electric curlers and give herself a quick set.

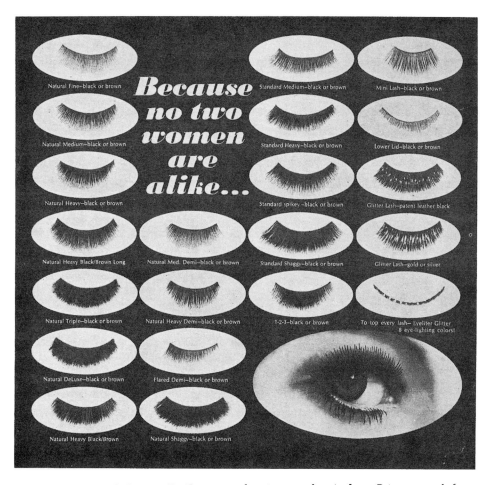

FIG. 244: False eyelashes, 1968. From an advertisement by Andrea. Prices ranged from $4 to $12.50.

Revlon's newest makeup for 1968 was called Demi Makeup. 'Determined', says *Vogue*, 'to deliver the look of less makeup without the loss of makeup's kindly ways, Revlon went to quite a lot of trouble to study the "structure of naturalness" and to formulate this in cosmetics for the entire face. . . . A fresh palette of thinner eye shadows and lid-lighteners. Silkier new translucent lengthening mascara. A batch of remarkably delicate liquid eyeliners . . . a translucent Brow Lightener.' Curiously, the result of all this determined naturalness was a heavily made-up *Vogue* model with lots of blue and white paint over the eyes, lashes stuck together in clumps from black mascara, an obviously shadowed nose, and aggressively whitened lips. The model used for Revlon's advertisements was more skilfully made up, but the green eyeshadow was hardly natural.

In February *Queen* reported on the newest Estée Lauder cosmetics for skin-care — Wrinkle Stick (to be used over makeup for touch-ups as necessary), Dry Dry Skin Creme (a peach-tinted cream for wearing under makeup), All Day Throat Creme ('made with swan oil'), All Day Eye Creme ('need not be massaged into the skin'), Whipped Cleansing Creme ('contains turtle oil'), and Dry Dry Skin Astringent ('an ice-cold toner'). This information is accompanied by a reasonably natural-looking girl with casually messy hair and goggles. 'Her complexion', we are told, 'is Golden Sun Go-Bronze, with Sun Beige Tender Make-Up Tint, and Liquid Glow Tint Highlight 1 on cheeks. Her eye make-up is Turquoise Liquid Shadow Tint, highlighted with Candlelight Pink Eye-shadow Glow and Black French Beauty Mascara. Her lipstick is Honeyspackle Peach.'

John Robert Powers's Beautique Collection featured Fluid Gold Moisture Control ('an all-day moisture bath'), Bedtime Beauty (a silky, gossamer-light cream'), Throat Creme ('to save your own neck'), Eye Lift Cream ('use the merest film under makeup'), Pick-Up Masque ('just the kind of new spirit your skin needs after a busy day'), Crème de la Crème ('shadows don't show'), Lip Gloss ('wets your lips with a high-fashion moist look'), Pressed Powder Compact ('a translucent powder for perfect touch-ups'), and Pearl Lustre Makeup (a cloud-spun cream that lights your face with flickers of flattery').

It was never clearer than in the spring issue of *Queen* that the days of light, medium, and dark lipstick was decades gone. The model facing the Beauty page was reported to be wearing an exotic-sounding lip makeup called Peach Butter-milk Super Jewelfast 22 Special. What she *appeared* to be wearing was no lip-stick at all and a rim of buttermilk on her upper lip. Elsewhere on her face were to be found Buttermilk Cream Satin Foundation, Sable Peach Spun Satin powder, White-hot Soft Cream Powder, and Fancy Rose Soft Echo rouge. Three lines jutting outward from her eyes were doubtless made with Soft Chinchilla eye-liner.

A BUSINESS OF MOONBEAMS

In its June 3rd cover story on cosmetics, *Newsweek* began by describing what might well be the climactic scene in a late-night horror movie:

'A slim woman, quiet, purposeful, bends menacingly over the lovely young girl laid out on the examining table. She reaches for a pair of electrodes; she soaks their padded tips in water to improve the contact. She flips switches, a machine hums, the girl's eyes widen. The woman moves closer. Now she touches the electrodes to the plump, youthful cheeks — and suddenly, shatteringly, the girl's face disintegrates into spastic horror. Cheeks jerk and jump, eyes twitch,

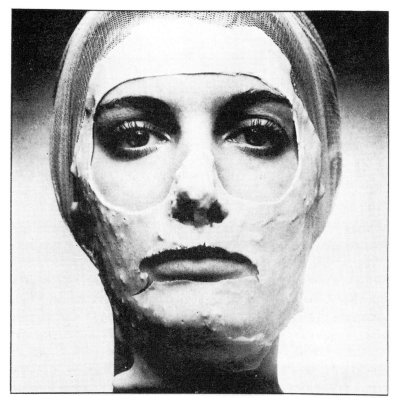

FIG. 245 : Fresh Beauty. Skin conditioning mask by Max Factor, 1969.

lips writhe. "It hurts," the girl slurs. The woman, relentless, smiles. She moistens her lips, speaks in a soft foreign accent. She says, "This stimulates the facial muscles to tone and firm, and to increase the blood circulation." '

Just another young lady having a facial and doing her bit to keep alive a seven-billion-dollar-a-year industry — 'a business of moonbeams', a buyer at Henri Bendel's called it, 'and the payoff comes, *Newsweek* added, when a lady of a certain age meets an acquaintance who has just finished four hours at the beauty parlor. In one sweeping, microscopic glance, the first lady takes it all in : dyed hair fluffed to the size of a basketball and rigid with spray; eyebrows plucked and shaved; eyesockets smeared with color; the foundation, the blusher, the toner, the powder, the pale and bloodless lips. "You look nice," she decides, and the second lady is amply repaid for her time and money.'

Four hours spent in a beauty salon was not considered excessive, and an occasional all-day series of treatments at one's favourite beauty palace was looked upon as a luxury, sometimes even a necessity. There were even those, according to *Newsweek,* who spent all day *every* day at Elizabeth Arden's Fifth Avenue salon. This was one of New York's more elegant establishments, but there were reportedly some 230,000 others in the United States. A cosmetician in one of them was quoted as saying that he put on 'whatever was supposed to be going on that week. Sometimes,' he added, 'I've made people look awful. I would say to myself, "My God, what have I done." Then, of course, I would tell her how absolutely devastating she looked.'

Women still insisted on paying as much as they could afford for their cosmetics — up to $3.50 for a lipstick with ingredients worth six cents or less and $150 for 11½ ounces of a beauty cream, ingredients and actual value unspecified. For the woman whose beauty problems seemed to be beyond the scope of ordinary cosmetics, no matter how expensive, there were various kinds of injections, face lifts, and the removal of the outer layer of wrinkled skin by either chemical or mechanical means.

In September two Mary Quant men, Derick and Digby, flew to New York from London to teach American women 'how to be bare-faced beauties' with the help of the Mary Quant line of makeup, including Cake Liner ('for the soft line'), Eye Gloss ('for the new naked-er eye'), Shadow Shaper ('makes tricky shadow-shaping easy'), Eye Shapers ('twin pressed shadows, one always pearl white'), Liquid Shadow ('marvelous smoky-smudge colors, plus white, silver, and gold'), Lip Shaper Pencil ('does what it says'), Nail Bullion ('glittering with 24 ct. gold leaf and shiny silver'), Loads of Lash ('10-inch strip of fine, feathery lash. . . . Help yourself to just what you want'), Paintbox ('Mirrored, 2 Brush Lipsticks, 3 Eye Shapers, Cake Liner, Block Mascara, all those special brushes'), and Vamps, Miss Quant's 'wildest', most 'uninhibited' eyelashes, guaranteed to 'lead any good man astray'.

THE SPOTTED LOOK

With sunglasses and eye makeup both very much in the fashion news, Courrèges suggested spotted eyes to go with pale amber glasses — a brown shadow in the hollow between the upper lid and the brow bone, mascara on the lashes, and small-to-large brown or black painted polka dots surrounding the eye. For the girl unfortunate enough not to have her own freckles, it was suggested that she paint some on. 'But don't wear coloured lipstick,' she was advised. 'It spoils the naturalness.'

The so-called natural look was, in fact, still in vogue, with variations. 'This year we're all transparent,' a New York career girl was quoted as saying, 'just like last year we were all frosted.' And, added *Newsweek,* she was going to be all wet, with the fashionable gleamers and the resultant moist look — a look which women had for a century or more gone to some trouble to overcome.

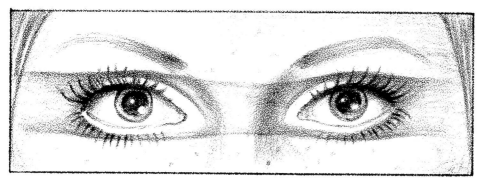

FIG. 246: Ribbon of blue eyeshadow and painted freckles on a high-fashion cover girl, 1969. After a makeup by Pablo of Elizabeth Arden.

In the spring of 1969 what might have been (but was not) called the Raccoon Look was achieved, among the ultra-fashionable, by surrounding the entire eye with coloured shadow. This trend did not fade quite so soon as one might have expected, and we find the cover girl on the October issue of *Harper's Bazaar* wearing not only painted freckles, but a one-inch-wide stripe of blue eyeshadow running straight across both eyes and the bridge of the nose, then fading away at the hairline (Figure 246). Sonja Knapp, director of the Paris fashion house of Ungaro, used Day-Glo paint to dab bright spots of colour like polka-dot tears around the eye (see Figure 247). At Grès, according to *Vogue*, one model used a thick coating of silver on the bone between the brow and the lid, whereas Cerutti's mannequins outlined their upper lids in black, 'fading into grey, softened by a pink halo, and lit up by a white triangle at the outer corner. . . . At the Italian collections, many of the mannequins had enormous, dramatic eyes spiked with spidery lashes—sometimes a double row on each lid. In contrast, hair was smoother, heads noticeably smaller'.

Although light eyebrows were fashionable, many women followed their own instincts, with brows full and dark, greyed and powdered, arched or straight, sprayed or waxed, thin and painted, or even shaved off completely. For those who kept theirs on, *Vogue* recommended a 'warily-formulated powder' applied with a 'keenly-angled brush'.

Madame Benhima, wife of the Moroccan ambassador to the United Nations, left hers naturally dark and full (Figure 248). Her eye makeup, reported *Vogue*, began with home-made kohl (a powdered navy-blue stone mixed with herbs) applied with an ivory kohl stick. Madame Benhima pointed out that in her own country the kohl was considered beneficial as well as ornamental and was even used on babies and small children. She spent about ten minutes loading her lashes with cake mascara. She used a grey shadow on the lid, darker at the outer corners. Above that she applied a mauve shadow, darkest at the inner corners. For evening she blended a stripe of white above the grey shadow and another below the eye.

High-fashion models, interviewed about their makeup ideas, veered toward the bizarre. Penelope Tree wanted to shine at night, with 'a sort of translucent pale-blue skin, pale-mauve skin, or skin the colour of the inside of a conch shell, a colour that has tints of pink, mauve, blue, silver, green' with eyeshadow in deep tones of the base colour. A brunette, she thought, 'would look marvellous with terra-cotta skin and orange shadow beneath the eyebrow'. Having just finished chopping up silver sparkles in the meat grinder and mixing them into her powder, she reported that another girl had used the silver sheen on her face as a mirror to apply her lipstick. Verushka, on the other hand, declared that away from the camera she liked to look 'absolutely natural' — just a little blue or green under the eye, some red brown at the hairline and on the chin, and a 'very very narrow' brown stain around the outside of her lips. Patti Harrison, who liked blue mascara and two colours of eyeshadow, sometimes used poster paint for striking effects.

Glamorous celebrities were still lending their names to new cosmetic lines. Zsa Zsa Gabor enthusiastically promoted her own cosmetics, including Figure Cream ('a petal pink cream . . . to use on the bust, tummy, hips and thighs'), Skin-tight Facial Masque (with the delectable fragrance of strawberries'), Liquid Makeup ('has precious porositones which allow the skin to breathe'), Formula Z Lipstick (in two dozen shades), and Brush-on Eyeshadow in Dahlia Blue, Summer Lilacs, Brown Zinnia, Gardenia Beige, Aquapetal, and Jasmine Lime. The October issue of *Town and Country* featured a model wearing Zsa Zsa Ltd. makeup — 'over Honey Finish Liquid Makeup, a light dusting of Soft Finish Face Powder, Shade 2. Her suggestion of a blush is pure attractive artifice: Muted Peach Delicate Creme Colour, highlighter-blusher-shader all in one. More color for her well-shaped lips: Peach Cordial Formula Z Lipstick. To enhance her large, soft eyes: Light Focus Eyeshadow (Brown Zinnia and Aquapetal), Wet Black Eyeliner, Light Focus Brow Colour . . . the final, poetic makeup touch: a fringe of Gypsy Lashes all around.' The final result was a strikingly handsome, tawny look.

The newest form of rouge was Transparent Blushing Gel by Ultima II — a tube of gel tinted Clear Pink, Peach, Amber, or Red. 'One trembly gel droplet on the fingers' the advertisement read, would provide 'a pulse of color so real it could only come — before today — from a pleasurable tug at the heart'.

Anticipating a hot summer, Fabergé introduced Ice Sticks — solid cologne on a stick. The principle was as old as the ancient Egyptians with their blocks of solid perfume placed on the head at banquets and allowed to melt with body heat. Only the packaging was new.

The late September issue of *Queen* devoted eight pages, including its cover, to the latest in beauty masks — or mud packs, as they were once called. Designed

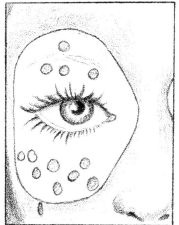

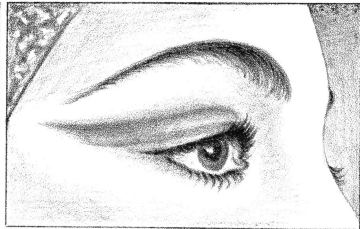

FIG. 247: Decorative eye make-up, 1969. Pearl grey area around the eye, with cerise dots outlined in black. The eyebrow is underplayed.

FIG. 248: Eye makeup of Mme Benhima, 1969. Grey and mauve shadows, white highlights, and heavily applied mascara.

to remove impurities and close the pores, most of them were quick-drying products with a wax or gelatine base, and having done their job, some of them could be removed intact. Elizabeth Arden's was a soft, white cream; Max Factor's, a powder to be mixed with water; Guerlain's, a light jelly with a vegetable base; and Harriet Hubbard Ayer's, a Strawberry Cream mask with a scent of fresh strawberries. Other masks contained honey, vitamins, minerals, royal jelly, wintergreen, hexachlorophene, and orchid pollen. The beauty editor of *Queen* spoke well of all of them.

It was hardly news that women were still having their faces lifted or peeled or sometimes entirely remodelled. But along with the increased emphasis on masculine beauty, men were doing the same thing. Face lifts, eyelid lifts, nose jobs, dermabrasion, and hair plug grafts were becoming increasingly popular in combating the effects of age.

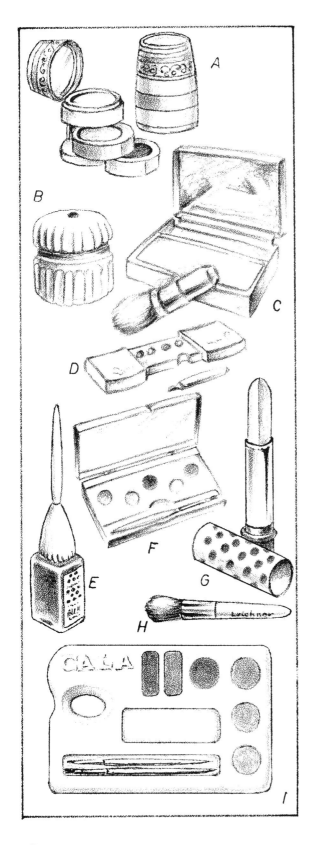

PLATE 35 : TWENTIETH CENTURY
1967, 1968

A   Yardley's Heartbreaker — eye compact containing mirror, highlight, shadow, and liner.
B   Dorothy Gray Eye Cream.
C   Lanolin brush-on makeup.
D   Lancôme palette.
E   Helena Rubinstein Vinyliner — liquid eyeliner with brush.
F   Lancôme cosmetic colouring box.
G   Helena Rubinstein's Lipshine — half gloss, half colour. Available in 6 shades.
H   Leichner's Blusher Brush.
I   Gala's Pick and Paint Eye Palette with liner and shading brushes and 4 shadows in green and aqua or mauves and blues. Price, £1 3s. 6d.

MAKEUP FOR MEN

According to *Vogue*, men were spending fifty percent more on hair preparations than they had ten years ago, twice as much on clothes, and ten times as much on colognes and cosmetics. And the ones who were doing it were no longer considered effeminate or dandyish but were, as often as not, business executives and professional men whose public image needed constant attention. One Wall Street tycoon reportedly carried his own cosmetics kit (including cake powder against unwanted shine on the nose) not to war, as did one Persian general, but to his weekend golf and tennis dates. And he insisted that his handkerchiefs be sprayed with cologne before being ironed.

To break down masculine resistance, to help persuade women to buy for men what the men would be reluctant to buy for themselves, and to sell more than one product at a time, most of the manufacturers of men's toiletries offered their wares in attractive cases, travel kits, or masculine-looking boxes. The *New York Times* carried Bloomingdale's advertisement for 'Fabergé's indispensable groomers in trim-take-along cases tailored to fit a glove compartment, desk, or suitcase'. The well-groomed, pleasantly scented man might choose either the *Brut Jet Set* with Lotion, Creme Shave, and Spray Deodorant or the *Brut Smart Set* with Lotion, Primer, and Spray Deodorant, either for $5. The *Brut After Shave Tan*, 'the instant-on, instant-off tanner and conditioner in a plastic tube' was referred to as 'another indispensable'. All were available at Harry's Bar in the toiletries department.

Aramis (an Estée Lauder brand) offered a selection to suit nearly any man or any Christmas budget: *Aramis Executive Lunch Pail* (five 'grooming agents' in a small lunch pail for $15), *Aramis Grooming Plan* (After Shave and Cologne for $10), *Aramis Envoy* (Travel Soap and After Shave for $3.75), *Aramis Corduroy Field Kit* (four plastic bottles for $17.50), *Aramis Master Plan* (a handsome stand-up compartmented box with twelve 'grooming agents' for $85), and half a dozen other combinations.

Men's colognes, the first item really to break through the barrier of Victorian (or Edwardian) masculinity, had become too numerous for anything more than a token listing—Chanel's *A Gentleman's Cologne, Russian Leather, Eau de Monsieur Balmain, Jade East*, Guerlain's *Habit Rouge*, Millot's *Partner*, Victor's *Silvestre*, Fragonard's *Zizanie*, Dana's *Canoë*, Jean D'Albret's *Écusson, Brut, Tiger, Numero Uno, Vetyver, Russian Leather, Royall Lyme, Kanøn*, Capucci's *Pour Homme*, and the Nine Flags collection of nine bottles from nine countries, boxed in plastic foam.

Altogether there were more than two hundred products available, including night creams, day creams, eye pads, and wrinkle removers. All of these cost the American man nearly 600 million dollars (250 million pounds) a year—the result of a steady and determined process of education through salesmanship and the use of circumlocutions. 'Makeup for men is here,' said Fabergé's Paul D. Blackman. 'Just don't call it makeup.'

A Touch of the Bizarre

In 1970 permissiveness in makeup hit a new peak, with no apparent restrictions on either colour or design. In London models were using a variation of poster paint around the eyes and watercolours on the face, toning it with grey and mauve. One model painted rainbows around her eyes, reddened her lashes, and streaked her hair with green. *Vogue* featured a dark haired model with eyebrows bleached to a pale yellow. She was wearing a hammered medieval neck-sculpture and apparently nothing else. Elizabeth of Toro, a dark skinned New York fashion model, began her makeup with a dusting of gold powder, and Naomi Sims, another black model, applied Fabergé's Clay rouge to her cheekbones, under her eyebrows, around her hairline, and on her chin. For a polished look she used Borghese Florentine Umber on the chin, temples, and forehead, with gold on the eyelids.

In March *Vogue* featured a gleamingly tanned model with matching lips and a pale green grease covering her eyebrows and applied a bit splotchily around her eyes. The gleam came from Max Factor's Face Glazers ('chubby sticks so translucent you can see the dawn coming up through them'), with Clear Bronze on the face, Clear Peach on the cheeks, and Geminesse Green 16 eyeshadow powder around the eyes. Another model used small dots of various shades of blue and green around the eyes and on the brows and the lashes. Combined with intense pink rouge, generously applied, the effect was, to say the least, eye catching.

In the spring, fashionable faces were designed not only to catch the eye but to rivet the attention. One — a doll-like face of the Twenties — was all in shades of pink and red — pale pink skin, with red under and on the eyebrows and on the cheekbone, raspberry lips, and a red beauty mark near the nose. Another beauty — the Marchesa Anastasia Ferrari di Collesape — managed to look thoroughly Irish with freckles, a golden skin, pink cheeks, natural looking lips, green eyebrows, and Kelly green and yellow around the eyes. Actress Sophia Loren appeared in Egyptian-cut wigs in emerald green, burnt orange, delphinium blue, and butter yellow.

For a short time women were painted at both ends. In May *Vogue* featured three feet decorated by Chilean makeup artist José Luis, using Givenchy designs. One foot was 'pink and white, festooned with coral, lapis lazuli, chunky little golden nuggets and rondels, curves of gold galloon'. The toenails were lacquered

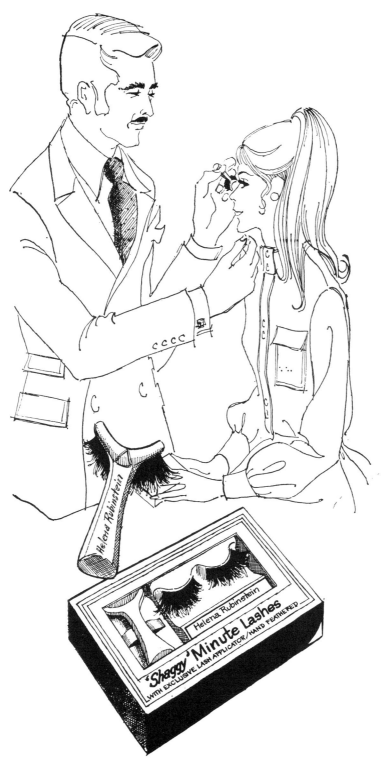

FIG. 249: Applying Helena Rubinstein's Minute Lashes. From a *New York Times* advertisement for a demonstration at Macy's cosmetic boutiques, with 'fine master makeup artists' in attendance.

coral and crusted with gold. The second foot was decorated with stripes of coral and lapis lazuli, golden beads, and a large circle of coral. The nails and the heel were sprinkled with gold dust. On the third foot, the sole was 'lacquered Chinese red, with white and navy slipper stripes, gold and silver sparklers everywhere'. But the fad did not really catch on.

Midsummer madness hit the makeup world in July with high-fashion models painting their faces to match their wildly colourful clothes. *Vogue*, for example, featured a makeup with triangles of pink and yellow on the forehead, green eyebrows, more yellow under the eyes, rose pink on the chin, cheeks, and lips, and the nose apparently shadowed with deep beige. 'Whimsical' was *Vogue's* word for it. Equally whimsical was a pearl-white face with unblended patches of blue-violet smeared over the eyebrow area, with deep shell pink on the cheeks, chin, and lips, and even around the eyes. On the stage, pink is used around the eyes to age and weaken them, but this was presumably not the intention. A third model wore an all-over golden bronze look, marred only by diagonal stripes of white and yellow war paint exploding from the eye area and covering the brows. The emphasis in all of the makeups was clearly on the bizarre rather than the beautiful.

To keep up with the colour explosion — or to encourage it — Revlon was making frosted lipsticks (Luminesque Lipfrosts) in seventeen shades, including Apple Polish, Snowsilver Rose, Copper Mine, Iceblue Pink, String of Pearls, Salmon Ice, Ginger Glaze, and Mirrored Mauve. Alexandra de Markoff, who boasted that her Countess Isserlyn was 'the world's costliest makeup', announced nineteen shades of lipstick 'ranging from barely perceptible to startling'.

'Startling' was perhaps the key word for fall, with both hair and makeup rivalling the wildest excesses of ancient Rome. Imagine, if you can, hair touched with green, forehead and nose bright lemon yellow, cheeks deep pink, lower jaw fuchsia blending into a purple neck, and — thanks to the miracles of optical science — one eye green and one eye violet. All on the same face. Other heads and faces of fashion featured rainbow hair streaked with orange, yellow, green, blue, and pink; eyelashes a jumble of blue, green, and yellow; flat, decorative patches of coloured paint placed more or less at random on the face; and a great blob of purple surrounding the eye and sending off rays in all directions.

PLATE 36 : TWENTIETH CENTURY
1969–1971

A   Lovestick by Love Cosmetics.
B   Ultima II Gelstick.
C   Bill Blass Peel-Off Pick-up Mask for Men.
D   Aramis Instant Bronzing Stick for men. A transparent gel, available in 3 shades of tan.
E   Elizabeth Arden Colour Control Blusher/Toner. For toning the entire complexion and adding colour to the cheeks and temples.
F   Clinique blusher, available in six shades.
G   Charles of the Ritz cheek pommade. Clear gel in marble compact.
H   Estée Lauder lipstick.
I   Satura Algene face cream by Dorothy Gray.
J   Etherea brush-on eyeshadow.

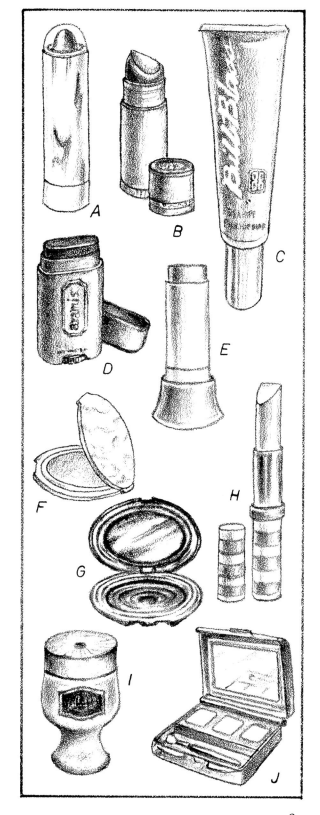

23 · *The Twentieth Century:*
The Seventies to the New Millennium

I always say beauty is only sin deep

SAKI

THE SEVENTIES: FLAPPERS, FAIRIES, DOLLS AND PUNKS

Theatricality came from fashion and influenced pop. One of the decade's most memorable images is David Bowie's *Aladdin Sane* 1973 album cover. Elizabeth Arden's Pierre La Roche painted Bowie's *alter ego* Ziggy Stardust Kabuki-white with an asymmetric red lightning flash edged with blue from forehead to jaw. However, a full three years earlier British *Vogue* had featured model Sue Baloo with lightning bolts of lapis-lazuli blue over clownish Revlon Ultima II Dresden Peach Crème Foam translucent powder. Such bizarre and startling colours were to persist throughout 1970.

The same year saw the first 1920s revival maquillage, with a doll-like face painted in all shades of pink and red. Skin was pale pink with red under and on the eyebrows and on the cheekbone, raspberry lips and a red beauty mark near the nose. It was the beginning of a nostalgic Roaring Twenties mood in high-fashion makeup that lasted for the first half of the decade. Films set in the 1920s and 1930s — *The Boyfriend, Cabaret, The Great Gatsby* and *Murder on the Orient Express* — were to inspire the Art Deco revival.

Inevitably there had to be a backlash against the madness of high-fashion makeup. Women were beginning to rediscover what most of their grand-mothers' grandmothers had once believed: that beauty comes from within as well as without. In the 1970s self-improvement took various forms: yoga, transcendental meditation, psycho-cybernetics or self-hypnosis, for instance. With an increasing emphasis on good nutrition, more and more people were eating a balanced diet of natural foods.

Along with all this — and perhaps resulting from it — came a flood of back-to-nature cosmetics that offered the possibility of making skin healthier instead of merely more presentable. Ingredients such as wheatgerm, papaya, cucumber, avocado, sesame seed, almond, date, lemon, grapefruit and egg, as well as a variety of vitamins, were not unusual. There appeared to be scientific evidence to indicate that a good many of them might prove beneficial to the skin, perhaps vindicating the usefulness of some ancestral recipes.

Particularly enterprising women even revived make-it-at-home cosmetics by rinsing their hair with strawberry juice, washing their hands in lemon juice, shadowing their eyes with blueberry juice, staining their lips with raspberry juice and tinting their legs with coffee. Milk baths, it was reported, could be made with powdered milk, and butter would protect the hands while gardening.

Mary Quant was on top of the trend, launching her Special Recipes collection in 1972 with the slogan 'Now you can be a little more natural and a lot more beautiful' and stating: 'Everyone should have a chance to buy cosmetics full of natural ingredients. So says Mary Quant who has packed a pantry-full of nature's ingredients into tubs and bottles to make you more beautiful.' If you wish to find the inspiration for Anita Roddick's Body Shop philosophy of the next decade, look no further than Mary Quant. Special Recipes lipstick was made with mineral and vegetable colouring only, and one of the basic ingredients was beeswax. Quant's foundation palette was Cool Clover, Pale Putty, Middle Earth, Natural Ochre and Nut Brown.

Fontarel Clean Make-up boasted, 'You no longer have to ruin your skin to make yourself look beautiful', while Boots No. 7 toasted their Country Colours range with 'Here's mud in your eye.' So confident were No. 7 in the back-to-nature movement that an advertising campaign as late as 1977 declared: 'Once in a while it's only natural to have egg on your face. And marigold and wheatgerm and oatmeal and purified water.' The company added: 'We put a whole egg in every one of our Marigold Extract masks because its natural goodness is said to soften dry skin.'

In November 1972 'Vogue says to be pretty, you must be natural.' Natural, however, did not mean a face touched only with soap and water. Max Factor announced 'a new programme of face care inspired by the fresh, clean beauty of Sweden'. To achieve that fresh, clean beauty with Swedish Formula required the following sackful of cosmetics: 'Fair Beige Purified Complete Make-up Foundation, Dreamy Sky Purified Eye Shadow Crème, Caramel Kiss Lipstick and Frosted Golden Amber Brush-on Blusher.' 'Beyond the Pale' read *Vogue*'s cover line. Beyond a joke was most women's response.

Acknowledging the movement away from chemicals, British *Vogue* told its readers to 'Go Back To Nature' in October 1973 and ran recipes for pot-pourri pillows, a peaches-and-cream facial, a cucumber-and-elderflower astringent, almond cream and marigold water. Do-it-yourself beauty was, however, financial suicide for the cosmetics houses and fashion magazines alike. So, ultimately, fashion paid lip-service to the trend, then perversely provided a host of cosmetics without which 'natural beauty' was unachievable.

Figures courtesy of Britain's *Financial Times* of the time reveal that very few women actually seemed to practise DIY beauty regimes. According to *Financial Times* journalist Sheila Black (writing in her April 1971 *Vogue* column), 'Women are spending all right. Lips cost us about £8 million a year, hair something like £140 million, of which about £100 million goes to the hairdressers. Eyes — £5.7 million a year. Complexions — about £15 million a year to cleanse, treat, moisturize, and what you will. Perfume — more than £20 million, deodorants more than £5 million, and there is still about £15 million for bath oils, essences, talcs and foams, for suncreams and protectives, for body creams and foot creams. Throw in nail varnish, hand cream, vaginal deodorant and a few borderline bits and pieces and you and I and our friends spend something like £235 million a year.'

One trend popular in the fashion magazines of 1971 was the highly painted doll look. Of the fashionable face of 1971, British *Vogue* declared, 'Her face will be painted like a new doll's' — and marionette makeup was born. Products that sounded as though they belonged in the playroom rather than the bathroom cabinet emerged, and it was Mary Quant who once again led the trend. 'Dip your fingers in my colours,' read her advertisement for Quant's new Greasepots, 'and give your eyes and lips a shine.' Greasepots came in the following nursery colours: Inkpots, Pinkpots, Honeypots, Plumpots and Olivepots. Quant never lost the naïve spirit of youthful flower power, and in some respects the doll face was a hangover from the Swinging Sixties, with her 'Face in the Clouds' lip colours named Sundown, Sky Blue, Cloud Pink and Moonshine and her Jelly Baby gel mascara.

Biba, too, endorsed the doll image, naming a peach face powder China Doll Foundation and recommending complementary peach lip gloss and powder blush. Barbara Hulanicki's Biba boutique cosmetics featured purple nail varnish, mahogany lipstick, black face gloss, prune watercolours, yellow foundation and a paint box containing six shades of powder, two watercolours, ten shades of face gloss, five brushes and an applicator for the fashionable face of 1971. American *Vogue*, meanwhile, featured a 'sensational' makeup on a Cardin model whose cheeks were rouged with Carita's red lipstick bang in the centre of each cheek.

Around this time deep, lustrous fruit shades of lip colour were prevalent, such as Yardley's Damson Lustre and Sugar Plum Lustre, Mary Quant's Prune and Grape Crush, Elizabeth Arden's Mulberry Glisten and Revlon's Grapevine, Estée Lauder's Cranberry and Mulberry. Attention-grabbing colours for the eyes included Estée Lauder's eyeshadows in Plum Raisin and Earth Brown, Mary Quant's Marooned Jeepers Peepers shadow and Max Factor's Seascape Grape. Mascara was equally colourful in shades such as turquoise, lavender, raspberry, navy, plum and burgundy.

The doll was to give way to the Walt Disney princess in 1972, with British fashion's number-one makeup artist Barbara Daly recreating Disney's Snow White look for *Vogue* using Mary Quant cosmetics. 'Apply Pinky Blushbaby on the cheeks. Lips are Red from Box of Crayons, sliced over with Jampot

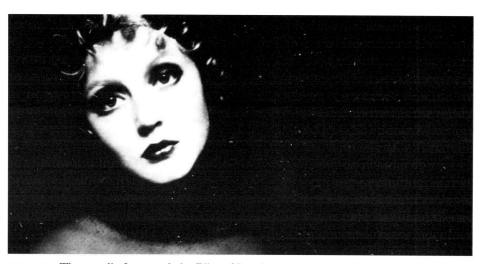

FIG. 250 : The angelic face, made by Biba of London with some of their 1971 makeup
range. Display showcard.

Greasepot. Eyes are bright under Soft Green Eyetint, Soft Blue Eyetint and
Black Tearproof Mascara.'

The glorious technicolor face did not let nature get in its way. What could
be more cartoon-like than Gala's Fashion Dazzler Eye Catchers in yellow
and lime or Dazzle Doll Cheeks in yellow, green or pink? Quant also advocated using crayons made by companies such as Caran d'Ache (applied over
foundation and blended with the fingers) as cosmetics.

The clown — or rather Pierrot — joined the doll and the cartoon look as a
major 1970s high-fashion trend. The Pierrot face was created for British
Vogue's 1975 Christmas cover using Max Factor Germinesse products by
makeup artist Richard Sharah, who would recreate the Pierrot face for David
Bowie's *Scary Monsters* album and video in 1981. The mask-like foundation
was achieved with Warm Honey Enriched Moisturizing Makeup shaded with
Cherry Blush Crème Blush. The eyes were shadowed with Charcoal Bur-
gundy and Sunlight Eye Shadow Powders and Brownish-Black Cake Liner.
A sumptuous Cupid's-bow mouth was created using Rich Mahogany Frost
Cream Lip colour.

The garishness of all these makeup fads and fashions was perhaps best
explained by *Harper's Bazaar*'s Eugenia Sheppard. Beauty was out, she said,
and excitement was in. 'To be called pretty', she told the readers of *Harper's
Bazaar* in 1971, 'has been the next thing to a downright insult for a long time.
It is early Gish and gush and much too pastel for these tough times. Beautiful
is stronger, but it smacks of Atlantic City beauty contests and double-page
advertisements in living color. It sounds all too static, regular and establish-

ment. . . . Exciting is the adjective that's replacing pretty and beautiful, as the ultimate praise for an attractive woman. Excitement is movement, noise, turbulence and today.' An exciting woman, added the journalist, 'is no classic beauty with a perfect set of features. Her eyes, nose, mouth, taken separately, may be nothing to write sonnets about. But they add up to something fresh and provocative. . . . Exciting offers much more scope for variation and originality than beautiful or pretty ever did. . . . The most exciting thing about exciting is that anyone can participate and, with a flair for self-expression, win the game.' A lot of woman participated, but not all of them won.

The Art Deco revival was due largely to three influential movies: *Cabaret*, *The Great Gatsby* and *The Boyfriend*. The leading ladies – Liza Minnelli, Mia Farrow and Twiggy respectively – were the icons of this nostalgic fashion moment. As *Cabaret*'s Sally Bowles, Liza Minnelli took false eyelashes (applied to both top and bottom lid) to their greatest lengths since the 1950s, enhanced by soaring, streamlined eyebrows and a diamanté beauty spot planted high on the cheek. Fashionable eyebrows of this era were severely plucked, then pencilled into fine Minnelli arches or faded out like Mia Farrow's.

By September 1972 Maybelline were advertising Just Lashes – long Liza falsies made from real hair. Vintage fashion illustrator and costumier Erté was painting nails for *Vogue* in divinely decadent chequerboards and green lacquer. Vogue beauty editor Felicity Clark advocated 'peaches and green' as the colour palette to emulate Liza's glittering nightclub pallor. 'Think beauty . . . say Green,' exhorted Max Factor, who painted the eyes with Aqua Factor Brilliant Green blended with Aqua Pearl Frosted Aqua Factor, Soft Green Linemaker and Brown Comb-on Mascara.

By March 1973 the flapper and Art Deco revival gained momentum as British *Vogue* urged: 'Imagine you've been chosen to play Daisy in *The Great Gatsby*: hollow your cheeks. Eyes are huge and the lips a tiny bow of a mouth.' Mia Farrow's Daisy was a delicate pastel dream shot in soft focus. The ideal model to bring the Farrow face into fashion was Twiggy, who, having starred in the 1920s pastiche film *The Boyfriend*, was already associated with the Roaring Twenties look. This demanded a rich, creamy complexion with softest, misty pastel accents. The Daisy face was delicate and patrician: echoing the fashion illustrations of the era by Erté, George Barbier, Georges Lepape and Paul Iribe. In April 1973 Twiggy appeared on the cover of British *Vogue* made up by Biba, who created her Art Deco face with China Doll No. 3 Foundation and Metallic Peach Contour Powder with China Doll loose powder and Pansy Face Gloss. Her eyes were made up with New Khaki Face Gloss on the lids, Cream Runny Gloss under the brow and Brown Mascara. On her lips were Metallic Peach lip colour and Metallic Peach Lip Colour Gloss.

Charles of the Ritz went 'back to the simplicity of flower pastels' with Primrose Pink Eyeshadow and Sweet Buttercup Frost Geranium Lips. Coty even boasted of Coty Air Spun Make-Up, 'We'll make your face look as though you did it with fresh air.' If foundation had become any paler or more ethereal the face would have vanished altogether.

In a 1972 interview Charles Revson admitted, 'Products don't change as fast as colours; and colours don't change as often as you think.' The trick, to quote American *Vogue* editor Diana Vreeland, was 'to give 'em what they never knew they wanted'. The soft-focus face was all about the way one applied cosmetics rather than the product itself. Basically, the look was a peachy-pink makeup palette applied as delicately as an airbrush to appear soft-focused. It was inspired by the dreamy, soft-focus fashion photographs of Sarah Moon (who shot Biba's makeup campaigns in the early 1970s). Naturally it took more products to achieve the soft-focus face than it did to create the mask-like doll, cartoon or clown look.

In 1973 *Vogue* advocated that its readers 'pale the rouge and brighten the lips', while the major makeup houses pearlized as many products as they could to enhance the shimmer and glow of the soft-focus face. Boots No. 7 introduced the new face with the following products: 'Honey Tone Skin Tone Foundation and Honey Tone Translucent Pressed Powder are coloured with Pink Puff-a-Blush Powder Blush. Eyelids are a deep sea green with Teal Green Nature Eyes shaded with Wild Aqua and Wild Teal Pearl Shadow Sticks. Teal Green Lashsilk Mascara and Fresh Raspberry Wild Pearl Lipstick complete the look.'

The soft-focus face reached an extreme in 1974 when all colour was faded to the point of being a variety of flesh tones. Charles of the Ritz designed a makeup of exclusively peach, pink and cream colours: 'Apricot Cream Veillessence with Chili Peach Blushing Pommade, Translucent Powder, Bare Buff Lights Blushing Powder, Premier Coral Liqui-Crème Lipstick with Frozen Pombeige Lip Pommade.'

In December 1974 Twiggy appeared on the cover of British *Vogue* in a homage to Cinderella, Holly Hobby and Titania all rolled into one. Shot by Barry Lategan, Twiggy wears Zandra Rhodes's fairy-princess dress and ethereal Estée Lauder makeup applied by Barbara Daly: 'Sparkling Beige Country Fresh Face Powder, Geranium Soft Film Compact Rouge, Persian Sea Pressed Eyelid Shadow, Twilight Glow Colour Wash, Raven Black Lustrous Roll-on Mascara tipped with Tropical Green, Red Flame Lip Pot Glossamar.'

The year 1975 was a turning point in fashion and makeup. The revival of Liberty prints and the continuing popularity of Laura Ashley's retro flower-sprig print cotton dresses saw florals rather than pastels and pinks as the inspiration for makeup artists. Richard Sharah was the English master of this new prettiness. Using Coty Originals, he made up *Vogue*'s February cover girl with Peach Pearl Transparent Face Make-Up, Tawny Russet Protein Gel

Blush, Totally Transparent Powder, Orange Peel Lipstick and Nail Enamel. Eyes were adorned with Turquoise Powder Shine with Light Green under the brow and Brown Protein Mascara and Automatic Eye Liner.

'Pick flowers from the make-up garden . . . learn to paint morning, noon and night,' exhorted *Vogue*. 'Now your face can bloom with the brilliance of spring flowers. Ingredients: hyacinth blue, willow green and pale violet eye shadows, primrose and silver-birch highlighters. The accent for the complexion is fresh, girlish and dewy. To emphasize the delicacy of their foundation, Gala name it Beige Barely Barely There Foundation, to be worn under Swiss Candy Cream Blusher and Soft Beige Sheer Finish Compressed Powder.'

Cosmetics houses borrowed colours from fruit and flowers. Helena Rubinstein produced Bikini Peach Silk Fashion Lipstick, Mary Quant made Choosy Cherry lipstick and added a range of Tiddlypinks to her iconic Jeepers Peepers eyeshadow collection. Charles of the Ritz unveiled Stormy Orange Liqui-Crème Lipstick, while Orlane's lipstick was Blackcurrant, Clinique's Black Honey and Love's Radiant Raspberry.

This mood of innocence went hand in hand for most of the 1970s with the decade's darker side. Fashion was flirting with the exotic. In January 1972 British *Vogue* declared 'Gaugin got the message' and invited Gil of Max Factor to recreate a Tahitian beauty's face. 'Gil brings South Sea surf and warmth to the January 1972 face with Moisturized on Beige Whipped Cream Make-up, Honey translucent powder and Pinki Cake Rouge . . . adding brilliance of Hibiscus flowers to lips with Sunset Rose Lipstick and Californian Transparent Lip Gloss and to the eyes Clear Red Crème Rouge.'

The Orientalism and exotica that featured largely in Art Deco was soon absorbed by the 1970s revival. Twiggy's era was almost over as more exciting, exotic models — Iman, Pat Cleveland, Grace Jones, Beverly Johnson, Tina Chow, Marie Helvin and Gia — took centre stage. In December 1973 the bronzes and golds of sinuous Art Deco figurines were the inspiration for Christmas makeup by Ultima II featuring 'Blush of Gold Blushing Crème and Patina Shadow Pure Gold blended with African Violet and Silverspun Pink and Spungold Coca Super Luscious Lips'.

British *Vogue* championed Polynesian model Marie Helvin and the allure of rich colours against tropical skin. Even Aryan blonde models Jerry Hall, Cheryl Tiegs and Christine Bolster were tanned a deep mahogany (although the Californian blonde would not become fashion's favourite girl until the 'let's get physical' 1980s). For now, fashion encouraged exotica, particularly the Arabian fantasy kaftans and scarves by Thea Porter, Bill Gibb and Zandra Rhodes. Arabian exotica reached its peak when Yves Saint Laurent produced his 1976 Ballets Russes collection inspired by the costume designs of Leon Bakst.

The icon was Scheherazade (as portrayed by Marie Helvin in British *Vogue*). 'This is prettiness carried a little further, with makeup intense and vivid, jades and rubies, shined with pomade, cheeks dusted more pink-and-white and an Arabian Midnight garden from Thea Porter.' The face, designed by Richard Sharah, used Charles of the Ritz products: 'Tangerine Liqui-Frost Lipstick, Jade Eye Shadow Pommade and Ritzy Sapphire Eye Shadow Pommade glossed with Roseshine Eye Shadow Pommade and Oyster Gleam Dusky Taupe Satin Liner and Tawny Brown Brow Colour.'

In June 1975 British *Vogue* set the new rules of makeup in stone. 'Change, experiment, think again: not just a different makeup, a radically different makeup . . . the point to remember is to keep it simple and don't get too much going on at the same time.' To demonstrate this new restraint — the decline of theatricality — the magazine introduced three new faces. First, 'the brilliant new rouge, the strongest colour on your face, travelling upwards from the cheekbones. With this play down the lipstick.' Second, 'The new area for eye shadow is under the eyes and outwards or in hazy spots at the outer corners only.' Lastly, it suggested using 'less eye makeup and more lipstick and a paler and finer mascara'. The lesson concluded, 'Decision: know a look when you see it, know how to get it, know where to stop.'

Barbara Daly, who later went on to design Lady Diana's makeup for her wedding day in 1981 to Prince Charles, demonstrated the new look. 'Make up your face like this. Rouge that is a real colour winged upwards from cheekbones to ears and brushed on in curls above the eyes; the colour rising through the outer edges of the eyebrows. Face powder is dusted on top. Palest eye shadows are dappled together. Light rather than shadow around the eyes and a light mascara. Lipstick that's bright and nail polish that's pale or vice versa.'

Bright-red lipstick made a comeback during this decade. An iconic *Vogue* cover was born when Eric Borman photographed Bianca Jagger for the March issue 1974. Wearing an Art Deco veiled cloche hat, Bianca Jagger pouts, wearing blood-red Dior Burnt Magenta lipstick painted in a Cupid's bow by celebrity makeup artist Serge Lutens. Dior also unveiled Les Carmins — 'the really reds for your lips and nails'.

'Everyone's into the red,' declared British *Vogue* in September 1974, which put a redhead on its cover wearing Estée Lauder's Blazing Red Lustrous Nail Lacquer and Blazing Red Lipstick. Not since Revlon's Fire and Ice had the colour looked so convincing. Sophisticated, mature glamour was back after over a decade of dolls, Pierrots, fairies and clowns. The disco face was coming together with primary colours as bright as an Andy Warhol screen print, erasing romance and whimsicality with the drama and sexual tension of cocaine and champagne nights at New York nightclub Studio 54.

Until Way Bandy emerged on the New York fashion scene in the mid-1970s, makeup trends were fast and loose. But it was he who really shaped the 1970s high-fashion boogie-nights face. Bandy was the pioneer of the airbrushed look and revolutionized makeup by using very few products to achieve his disco-diva face. He eliminated the fancy-dress colours from 1970s makeup and introduced a grown-up, sultry New York nightlife glamour. Bandy was the first cosmetics superstar in the 1970s and painted the faces of Liz Taylor, Lauren Hutton and Marisa Berenson as well as models Iman, Rosie Vela, Gia, Rene Russo, Beverly Johnson and Patti Hansen.

The Way Bandy face demanded a little foundation, powder, blush, eyeshadow and lipstick in a neutral palette of pinks, beiges, browns and flesh tones. Bandy mixed unconventional products together such as foundation, moisturizer and mineral water to achieve a weightless base and blended his foundations with eye drops to tighten the pores: rather like stretching a canvas before an artist starts painting in oils. Bandy favoured liquid cosmetics, mixed at home and carried to the studio in two black lacquered Japanese baskets.

Although he is largely remembered now for partying with Halston and Andy Warhol at Studio 54, for naming his dog Smudge (in honour of his airbrushing aesthetic) and always being perfectly made up himself, Bandy's legacy is the immaculate glowing pale complexion, strong red lips and smoky-eyed face that proclaimed 1970s glamour. It was a face that was to be revived twenty-five years later by his disciple Kevyn Aucoin for Gucci.

Punk was the decade's biggest anti-fashion statement — not that you would have known it in the fashion magazines. Like a surprise sock to the jaw, punk seemed to emerge from nowhere. It bubbled up in the London clubs in 1976 and 1977 before exploding into street culture as bands such as the Sex Pistols and the Clash rose to fame. Cultural commentator Ted Polhemus first acknowledged punk in the Christmas 1977 issue of *Vogue*: 'The year hair stood on end with fluorescent dyes, the year of war paint: we add to the excess of punk publicity by looking at the origins of ferocious adornment and provocative non-verbal communications.'

The godfather of punk (and manager of the Sex Pistols) Malcolm McLaren and designer Vivienne Westwood, his co-conspirator, between them created the punk look. An icon of the movement was the safety pin, famously skewered through the Queen's nose in a 1977 Sex Pistols T-shirt designed by Westwood and McLaren. Just as clothing was slashed and customized, punk faces were pierced and tattooed. Ears, lips and noses were mutilated with multiple piercings joined by ball bearings or chains. The look owed more to African tribes than to the usual teenage rebelliousness. 'Anyone who can stick a safety pin through their nose, cheek or ear must be something to contend with,' said Polhemus of the Sex Pistols' Johnny Rotten, Sid Vicious and their tribe.

Punk was angry, nihilistic and anarchic — a rebellious response to the jingoism surrounding Queen Elizabeth's Silver Jubilee. Punk makeup was designed to scare. It was a form of tribal war paint using predominantly black cosmetics on a white, pasty face. Colour – acid yellows, flamingo pink, electric blues and neon greens – was largely reserved for hair, even though punk aristocrat Jordan's hair featured two black triangles drawn from each eyebrow to hairline and filled in with red blush, while X-Ray Spex singer Poly Styrene drew neon-red lines over each brow to gruesome effect.

A very crude version of the Egyptian cat's eye makeup popularized by Liz Taylor and Barbara Streisand in 1962 was a bizarre borrowing for punks. Black eyebrow pencil was applied to the top and bottom lashes, meeting in a cat's-eye line. As punk developed, the cat's-eye line was used as a boundary inside of which the entire eye socket was coloured in and blackened with eyebrow pencil. Sue Catwoman, another key member of the punk aristocracy, coloured in her cat's eyes with acid-green shadow.

There was nothing artful about punk makeup application. Blood-red lipstick was applied as if the wearer had been smashed in the mouth, while mascara and dark eyeshadow gave the impression of a black eye. Punks even simulated bruises using black, deep purple and yellow blush. Punk was a working-class British phenomenon, and the proliferation of inexpensive makeup ranges in the 1970s (including Outdoor Girl, Rimmel, Boots 17 and Miners) made war paint available to all.

Zandra Rhodes was the first designer to absorb punk and translate it for the high-fashion customer. September 1977 British *Vogue* told its readers, 'If you haven't a rag to your name, there is new Zandra Rhodes jersey ripped, slashed and blue stitched into her own personal vision of punk.' The designer said, 'It's the first time the seventies have shown themselves.' The following year Richard Sharah created a *haute couture* punk makeup for Zandra Rhodes's advertising campaign with two tasteful purple zigzags on the forehead.

Punk set a precedent for youth cults and street trends, challenging high fashion, and from now on one informed the other. As mainstream fashion makeup moved into a new decade, Way Bandy's face remained pretty much unchallenged. It was up to the New Romantics, the Goths and a cross-dresser called Boy George to provoke change.

THE EIGHTIES: THE DYNASTY DECADE FROM NEW ROMANTICS TO THE RISE OF THE SUPERMODEL

As a new decade approached, fashion looked to distance itself from anything that echoed 1970s disco decadence. Healthy replaced sexy as the glass of fashion, with British *Vogue* painting the January 1980 cover girl with a glow of Clinique Gold Rub Colour Rub, Cinnamon Soft Pressed Eyeshadow, a touch of Charcoal Blue Eye-Shading Pencil and natural Glossy Brown Brush-On Mascara. Lips were Golden Raisin with Honey Raisin Gloss. Only the colours that nature intended for faces were encouraged. The message was to enhance but not to disguise.

The cosmetics houses promoted a healthy, zestful natural beauty. An enthusiastic Estée Lauder promised 'Transatlantic colours. Clear, clean, high-energy freshness for eyes, lips, cheeks and fingertips'. Revlon commanded: 'Listen! It's the pulsating new colour rhythm from Revlon. Pink lips and a touch of purple on the top lid.' Max Factor recommended 'innocent cheeks with Fragile Ivory Cream Makeup'.

Fashion magazines turned away from the studio and took to the great outdoors for inspiration. Early 1980s cover girls appeared almost devoid of makeup. Estée Lauder unveiled 'the Great American Desert Colours', and Revlon gave us 'new colours that boldly reach for the Western sun' called Sundance Colour. Of course the boom in foreign travel, fake tan and sunbeds now meant that all-year-round tans were not just the prerogative of the jet set. Sun-kissed skin did not need makeup to glow, and the cosmetics houses had to pander to a trend that potentially threatened their future.

In July 1980 the king of fresh-faced fashion, Bruce Weber, photographed a British *Vogue* cover with only waterproof mascara and natural lipgloss on the girl's sun-kissed face. The new generation of models were wholesome natural blondes, such as Cheryl Tiegs, Christie Brinkley and, later on, Cindy Crawford. These girls promoted the sun-kissed glow promised in 1980 by Princess Galitzine's Sun Tan Blusher, Elizabeth Arden's Les Scintillants, Coty's Sunshimmer range and the booming market in low-factor suntan oils led by Bergasol, Piz Buin and Hawaiian Tropic. 'Pretty new colours only look good on clear skin,' said December's *Vogue*. 'Camouflage is fine as a temporary measure, but proper skin care is essential.'

The new beauty philosophy did not stop at being kind to oneself, even though the fitness fad epitomized by Jane Fonda's workout ran like a melody in a minor key throughout the decade. Brands such as Beauty Without Cruelty and the Body Shop promoted products not tested on animals, while Revlon, L'Oréal and Christian Dior lined up behind them to champion ethical beauty. The decade was in danger of starting on a politically correct and puritan note. The beauty philosophy was cleanse, energize and protect, rather than paint, flirt and party.

The high-gloss hedonism of New York's Studio 54 had come to an end in 1980 when owners Steve Rubell and Ian Schrager were jailed for tax evasion. High fashion was cleaning up its act. However, the underground London club scene was about to unleash a new youth cult that celebrated unnatural beauty. From 1980 the New Romantic movement percolated in the Blitz, Hell and Billy's, where club-scene queens Leigh Bowery, Steve Strange, Boy George and Marilyn patented gender-confusing, feminine nightclub faces.

'In 1981 Steve Strange's post-Punk, New Romantic world of frills and furbelows was diametrically opposed to the old ethics of the new wave because of its hedonism and glamour,' reported *Vogue* journalist Caroline Kellett. 'Although partly a reaction against dressing down and the image of self-effacement and violence, which punk had deliberately projected, it shared the same roots in extreme stylization . . . the New Romantic movement was the most radically stylised youth cult since punk.'

The boys led the way. 'With makeup I could certainly look exotic,' says Boy George in his autobiography *Take It Like a Man.* The aspiring singer mixed Kabuki with 1930s Hollywood glamour: creamy porcelain foundation, gloss-red pouting Jean Harlow lips, soaring eyebrows drawn into Joan Crawford arches and Diana Vreeland hot-red blush from temple to the hollow of the cheek. When George burst on to the mainstream pop scene in 1981 he was mistaken for a girl. The tabloids christened him a 'gender-bender'.

The godfather of New Romanticism, David Bowie, peopled his *Ashes to Ashes* video with Blitz club habitués and had makeup artist Richard Sharah paint him as Pierrot with red, magenta and azure eyeshadow, a beauty spot and seagulls painted on his temples. Bowie claimed to have been taught Kabuki makeup techniques in Japan by one its stars, Tomaso Boru. In an interview with *Mirabelle* magazine Bowie revealed that he used white liquid base applied with a damp sponge, Elizabeth Arden's Eight Hour Cream on his lips under pearlized pink lip gloss and blue mascara.

Although teenage boys copied their New Romantic idols Duran Duran's and Spandau Ballet's pancake foundation, Japan's David Sylvian's frosted pink lip gloss, Adam Ant's white skunk stripe across his nose and Boy George's triangular pencilled eyebrows, the gender-benders' influence eventually shaped mainstream fashion in makeup for women. Boy George was the first man to grace the cover of *Cosmopolitan* magazine with immaculate diva makeup reminiscent of Lana Turner as painted by Max Factor's Hollywood Makeup Factory in the 1950s. By 1985 Boy George's makeup owed more to *Dynasty* queens Joan Collins and Linda Evans than to underground clubland.

Dynasty arguably influenced fashion in makeup more than any magazine or catwalk makeup artist. The US television serial ran from 1981 to 1989 and, for many, christened the decade. Clothed by Nolan Miller, the *Dynasty* divas brought back a level of perfection in makeup unprecedented on the small screen. Collins's villainess Alexis Colby wore primary coloured makeup as stark as a Disney witch: porcelain matt foundation, scarlet glossed lips, fiery-red blush and smoky eyes outlined on upper and lower lid with black.

Alexis's most striking feature were scarlet manicured talons shown to great effect as the character waved her signature cigarillos at her adversaries. Revlon understood Collins's fashion clout and made her the face of their perfume Scoundrel with the slogan 'Practically inspired by me'. Meanwhile, to emphasize her sugary character Krystle Carrington, Linda Evans wore a faceful of pinks, apricots and ambers plus the ubiquitous blue eyeliner popularized by Princess Diana.

Although the most famous woman in the world by 1981, Diana did not come into her own as a fashion icon until the 1990s. The women who epitomized the 1980s 'greed is good', 'excess is more' decade were Collins and her *Dynasty* co-stars, Paloma Picasso, Jerry Hall, First Lady Nancy Reagan, Margaret Thatcher, Ivana Trump and Madonna (then in her Marilyn Monroe phase). The rule they all obeyed was to wear only scarlet lipsticks such as Charles of the Ritz Garnet, Revlon's Red Diamonds, Elizabeth Arden's Scandalous Scarlet and Christian Dior's New Look Red. As *Vogue* proclaimed in September 1986, 'The fashion face, day and evening, has a cooled-down glamour that comes from the drama of a resonant red mouth with the subtlety of chiaroscuro eyes against a luminously pale skin. The big news is the dramatic mouth.' Even bigger news was a return to the unplucked, thick eyebrows made popular by Madonna and Cindy Crawford. Like Marilyn Monroe, both women also chose to make a prominent facial mole a beauty spot rather than attempt to cover it up.

Airbrushed Hollywood glamour gave makeup artists Tyen and Serge Lutens the green light to bring heavy makeup back into the fashion magazines. Lutens, creative director of Shiseido from 1980, lived in Japan and painted Dragon Empress faces for Shiseido's advertising campaigns. The images were ravishing and unachievable to all but professional makeup maestros. He and Chinese native Tyen, the creative director of Christian Dior cosmetics, were masters in the art of airbrushed complexions. Their faces were creamy, flawless blank canvases upon which Lutens would paint Cleopatra eyes and Geisha lips and which Tyen would veneer with frosted metallic shimmer. The makeup was perfect, yet mask-like. Tyen's pink, lavender and ice blue shimmer pastel faces looked as though the makeup had been blown miraculously on to the model in a cloud, while Lutens's brushwork was as precise as a Japanese woodcut.

By 1987 New York makeup artist Rick Gillette declared that he lamented 'the way it has become acceptable to see extremely overdone women. Basing the ideas of makeup on soap opera heroines creates a look more glitzy than glamorous. It comes from television mainly. There's very little restraint. I look for balance.' Gillette believed that 'we're getting back to a makeup look, not a mask. A paler face can be scary . . . it doesn't have to be that pale.' Needless to say, the power-dressed 1980s woman did not agree. Restraint, like lunch, was for wimps.

'Fashion is bringing the face into sharp focus,' said Chanel's director of cosmetics Dominique Moncourtois. 'The new look has been compared wrongly

PLATE 37 : TWENTIETH CENTURY
THE 1980S

A   Chanel's Les Tentations de Chanel
     Compact.
B   Helena Rubinstein's Lash Impact
     Volumatic Mascara.
C   Estée Lauder's Golden Shell
     Compact.

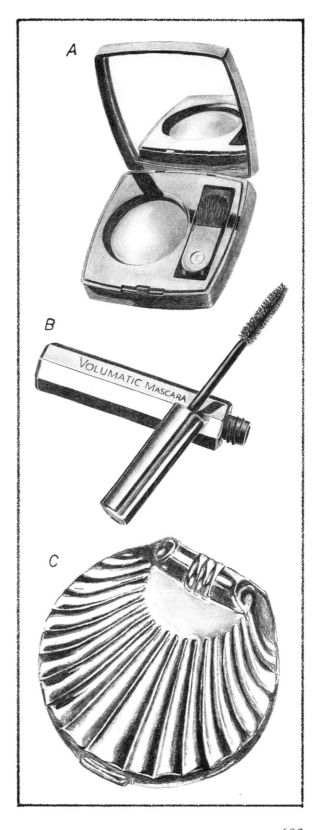

to that of the 1960s, which relied on a certain exaggeration and heaviness of application. Then it was a matter of how many lashes you could get on, how dark you could make the crease, how pale the face and lips. The impression was one of artless naïvety. Today's look, by contrast, is more polished and more professional. The main point is to be elegant.'

In the same year Dior's Tyen advised: 'Brighter makeup shades are necessary: olive green and plum shadows and yellow lipstick – yes, yellow. It's not a shocking as it sounds.' Colour came back but not the 1960s naïve, crazy application of playschool primaries. In a makeup for *Vogue*, Lancôme's Fête Sauvage collection featured eyes painted sapphire, jet, amethyst and jade, with lashes in Caribbean blue and lips shimmering in silvered bronze.

Strident jewel-brights were a major feature of makeup collections by Dior, Yves Saint Laurent and Chanel. Saint Laurent sold loose powder in gold compacts glittering with coloured semi-precious stones. The dominant makeup trend in 1988 was 'everyone's favourite' sky-blue eyeshadow, which *Vogue* deemed 'best over a lid defined with soft greys, charcoals and, the newcomer to the lids, primrose yellow. March sky blue is especially good with palest peach lips.'

The bright-red lip was no longer the rule, and 'sherbet colours the new palette: a bright wash of matt colour to bright eyes and cheeks are back in focus. Toning down winter's stark red lips to the new warm corals and candy pinks of Spring' was British *Vogue*'s recommendation. Blusher was not to be brushed along the cheekbones in flushes of colour but dabbed on to the apple of each cheek in pure pink to peach. On the eyes fuchsia gave way to clematis,

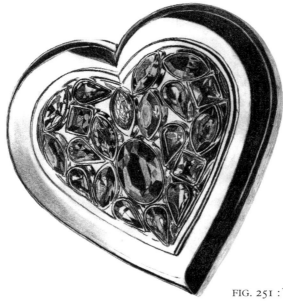

FIG. 251 : Yves Saint Laurent's Jewel.

candyfloss or blossom pink blended with violet and lilac. Light, creamy foundations were replacing tinted moisturizers, and 1940s-style pressed powder in a compact made a comeback.

In September 1988 British *Vogue* introduced 'the World Class Models of '88': Tatjana Patitz, Linda Evangelista, Cindy Crawford, Estelle Lefebure, Karen Armstrong and Rachel Williams. As it turned out, the latter three did not make supermodel status, being eclipsed by Claudia Schiffer, Karen Mulder and Naomi Campbell. But the rise of the supermodels brought with them a young generation of makeup artists who would eventually reject the mask-like makeup of Tyen and Lutens. Working with such spectacular raw material, Kevyn Aucoin, Linda Cantello, Stephane Marais and François Nars could create new faces as fashion approached the 1990s. Inspired by Way Bandy, Aucoin airbrushed smoky greys around the eyes from brow to lower lid, blanking out the lips with ghostly pinks and hollowing the cheeks with Anthracite or Mink Blush. The look was soft but strong.

THE NINETIES: SUPERWAIFS, ROCK CHICKS, ICONS AND THE ECO-FRIENDLY FACE

In January 1990 Peter Lindbergh photographed the five top models in the world for the cover of British *Vogue*. Shot in black and white, the subtle brushwork of Stephane Marais on Christy Turlington, Linda Evangelista, Tatjana Patitz, Cindy Crawford and Naomi Campbell called for calm after the *sturm und drang* of vulgar, aggressive late-1980s makeup. Revlon's advertising director Tim Delaney said: 'Society has moved through a period of conspicuous consumption, but we're now seeing the end of it. Wealth, profit and ambition have proved to be false gods.'

The supermodels were the decade's new goddesses and, thanks to Music Television (MTV) on cable and satellite and the glossy magazines, the new celebrities. The world was on first-name terms with Linda, Christy and Naomi and followed their image changes obsessively. Gerald Marie, supermodel super-agent and husband of Linda Evangelista, said: 'The thing about this group is that each has developed her character and that shows through her face. They're still in the business of selling dreams, but these days no one wants their dreams projected on a blank doll.'

Until Grunge turned fashion back from butterfly to caterpillar in 1992, the supermodels led fashion and accelerated the turnover of beauty trends to unprecedented speed. Between 1990 and 1991 chameleon model Linda Evangelista famously changed her hair colour from brown to champagne-blonde to Titian, then back to baby-blonde. Every *Vogue* cover saw Linda reinvented by a clique of makeup maestros including Kevyn Aucoin, Mary Greenwell, Stephane Marais and François Nars.

Champagne-blonde Linda of June 1991 is made-up by George Newell with nothing more than natural matt foundation, a touch of black mascara on the upper eyelids and soft-red lipstick. By October Titian-red, Marcel-waved Linda was painted like a classic 1950s *haute couture* model by Mary Greenwell. Her peaches-and-cream flawless skin was achieved with Aurora Crème Make-up, Natural Luxury Powder and Fuchsia Powder Blush. The 1950s feline eyes had false lashes on the upper lids and were painted with black liquid liner, Noir-Blanc Dual Eye Shadow and black mascara. On the lips Greenwell used a deep-garnet Chanel red.

In March 1992 *Vogue* Linda Cantello continued the 1950s *couture* mood in makeup with Christy Turlington. Turlington, possibly the most naturally beautiful of the supermodels, is made up with Chanel's 'perfect orangey-red Rouge de Minuit Lipstick', soaring arched black eyebrows, heavily coated black false lashes and pink blush. The look was completed with a black beauty spot. So when, twenty months later, *Vogue* declared that 'Glamour is back' you were left questioning where it had gone.

Nevertheless, Linda Cantello, photographer Nick Knight and the ubiquitous Evangelista finally moved glamour away from prim 1950s *couture* makeup for a famous November 1993 *Vogue* cover. Using Lancaster, Cantello lightened Evangelista's base makeup with Transparent Blush Powder. Transparent lipstick, in Amaryllis, moved the emphasis to strong, feline eyes heavily outlined with Black Pen Liquid Eyeliner and Black Rich Mascara. A smudge of kohl around the cat's eye completed this sexy, strong face. It was two years too early for fashion.

It would be unfair to lay the blame for the supermodels' demise on the fragile shoulders of Kate Moss, but it was she who largely took the rap as leader of the new superwaifs. She was the mascot of a neo-realist school of fashion photography that rejected glamour in favour of 'Grunge' — a world-weary, disillusioned and apathetic anti-fashion movement of the young.

British *Vogue* readers in 1993 were shocked by Corinne Day's images of skinny teenage Moss modelling underwear in a squalid council flat. These controversial pictures prompted President Clinton to condemn 'heroin chic' in fashion four years later. By then the London-based style bibles *The Face*, *i-D* and *Dazed & Confused* had created a new group of fashion anti-heroines, including punk aristocrat Stella Tennant, Karen Elson (dubbed Le Freak), Erin O'Connor and Amy Wesson. They were to 1990s fashion what Nirvana's Kurt Cobain and Courtney Love were to 1990s pop music.

Reassessing the *Vogue* pictures, readers today may consider that Kate Moss actually looks rather wholesome. She is made up with a touch of pink blush, pinky-brown eyeshadow and a matching matt mouth. The look was juvenile rather than junkie and one that Calvin Klein exploited when he made Moss his new face in 1992. Along with Jil Sander and Helmut Lang, it was Klein who introduced minimalist make-up to the runway. 'I especially love doing Helmut Lang's shows and Calvin's,' said Dick Page, the king of the unmade-up look. 'I'm known for minimal makeup, but there are times Calvin even wants less than I would do. That's exciting.' 'The beauty I love is in people who look real,' said Klein, 'a beauty that is pure, natural and not glamorized.'

Working with photographer David Sims and hairdresser Guido, Page was the definitive 1990s makeup artist who dared to voice the sacrilege that 'There is no such thing as natural makeup. As soon as there is makeup on the face it is not natural.' With the superwaifs as his models, Page demonstrated a new way of making up the face with sheens of clear slick, grease and gloss. Lips would be untouched but for gobs of Vaseline or Kiehl's Lip Balm No. 1. Page put nothing but transparents on the face, preferring to let natural beauty shine through his gloss and grease smeared on to eyelids, lashes and cheeks.

Instead of eye makeup the natural school advocated nothing more decorative than the new under-eye creams such as L'Oréal's Revitalift Eyes anti-wrinkle firming cream. Accentuating natural beauty was the key, and technology had advanced sufficiently to tint contact lenses and enhance green, amber and sapphire irises. More extreme contact lenses producing cat's-eye effects or even featuring Union Jack motifs were embraced by fashion stylists but largely rejected by the public which, ultimately, makes fashion happen.

The bare face made way for other means of expressing personal style. Model Stella Tennant was one of the first girls to appear on the catwalk with her nose pierced. Pierced tongues, nipples, eyebrows and lips added a punk element to the rebellious Grunge era, as did the proliferation of tattoos.

Of course the makeup houses knew that only young natural beauties such as Kate Moss or Stella Tennant could get away with greasing on to bare skin. Hence a boom in 'nude' makeup saw the launch of what remains Yves Saint Laurent's best-selling product: Touche Eclat (or Radiant Touch). This light-reflective concealer, sold in an iconic gold click-top tube with a paintbrush applicator, was formulated to hide under-eye discolourations and circles. Clinique's Dramatically Different Moisturizing Lotion launched in the early 1990s and by 2003 sold one unit every two seconds around the world. Clarins, too, launched Le Teint Mat Multi Eclat Matte Finish Foundation in the new nudes.

In 1993 Kevyn Aucoin developed the most influential nudes collection, the Nakeds, for Ultima II. 'It's the modern approach to make-up,' declared Ultima II's advertisements. 'Nineties beauty is about the face of the individual. It's about using colour that complements rather than covers, that

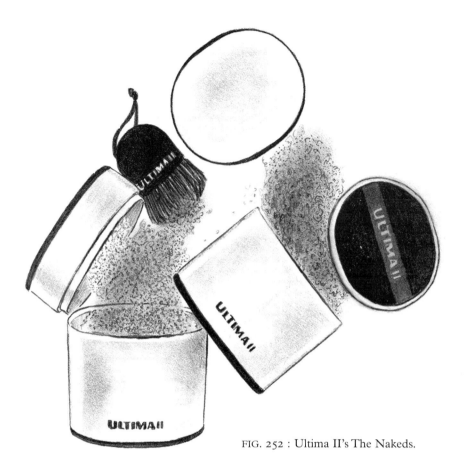

FIG. 252 : Ultima II's The Nakeds.

enhances rather than changes. Suddenly, we don't want to look made up; we want to look like ourselves, only better.'

The Nakeds tapped into the caring cosmetics trend of the 1990s — a hypo-allergenic, fragrance-free palette of nude colours based on skin tones. The collection included six tones of lip colour, matt eyeshadows, silky cheek colours 'that recreate the natural glow you get from a brisk walk' and trans-lucent loose and pressed powders to absorb oiliness, moisturize and protect from the sun. The look, according to Ultima II, was 'utterly believable'.

Comparing beauty in 1995 with the 1970s, *Harper's Bazaar* editor Liz Tilberis said, 'Although we use lots of products and spend money on them, we live in a very unmade-up-looking age. [In the 1970s] I'd get upset when a beautiful girl would come into the studio and the makeup artist would apply so much makeup to her face that the model would actually look worse on the set than when she first walked in the studio. Today, makeup pros put on much less makeup. The beauty of the model, rather than her makeup, comes through.'

In 1995 the January cover of British *Vogue* said a final farewell to Grunge with a perfectly coiffed Kate Moss naked but for Max Factor Black Stretch Mascara, Orchid Mist Cerise Lipstick and matching Diamond Hard Nail Enamel. Bubblegum pink was back. François Nars even formulated a shocking-pink lipstick which he christened 'Schiap' as an exact match of the 1930s couturier Elsa Schiaparelli's signature shade. Picking up where she left off in 1993, makeup artist Linda Cantello knew that bare-faced chic had had its day.

It was Cantello who revived Way Bandy's smoky-eyed, slick-lipped 1970s rock-chick look for Tom Ford's first Gucci collection in 1995. Gucci was all about a harder-edged modern glamour and Ford stylist Carine Roitfeld and Cantello found smudgy kohl and kajal eye pencils darker and sexier than the liquid eyeliners that dominated the first half of the decade. Max Factor and Shiseido were the first to reissue the kohl pencil. By 1996 heavy black liquid eyeliner was being painted into the Cantello cat's eye (upper and lower lid) in *W* magazine. The complexion was still left relatively untouched, while the eyes or lips were emphasized with dramatic makeup — frosted pale pink Mod lips with rock-chick cat's eyes by Dick Page in a 1996 *Harper's Bazaar* portfolio shot by Mario Testino.

Testino photographed the decade's two greatest fashion icons, Madonna and Diana, Princess of Wales, for *Vanity Fair* magazine. November 1996 saw a Testino portfolio of Madonna in her movie role of Eva Peron. Made up by Sarah Monzani using Estée Lauder's Face of Evita collection, Madonna recreates the Argentinian First Lady's dictatorial glamour with Perfect Lipstick Tango Lips, Coral and Neutral Eyeshadow and Perfect Liquid Eyeliner on the top lid plus black mascara. By far the most influential feature of Evita/Madonna was her finely tweezered eyebrows shaped into a perfect arc and darkened with a bitter-chocolate-coloured pencil. It was a look Max Factor repeated when Madonna became the face of Max Factor Gold in 1999.

Testino's fashion portfolio of Diana appeared in *Vanity Fair* the month before she was killed in a Paris car accident. Made up by Tom Pecheux using Lancôme, we see the Diana face that so many women of her generation tried to copy. The complexion is allowed to shine through and the actual makeup is minimal: Le Kohl Poudre in Fumée Noir on the eyes and on the lips Rouge Idole Indelibly Divine Lip Colour in Sacré. The face is soft, natural but unmistakably enhanced by a makeup artist with the lightest yet deftest touch.

The sainted Diana was a pioneer in her belief system of 'well-being' that encompassed mystics, masseurs, yogis and health gurus. The concept of well-being — and protection from an increasingly hostile world — dominated advances in the cosmetics industry in the 1990s. The troika of Japanese cosmetics houses Shu Uemura, Kanebo and Shiseido owed at least some of their popularity to the Japanese obsession with protecting pale skin. Kanebo was the first company to put an ultraviolet filter into its face powder, and this worked to the Japanese company's advantage now that the whole world was worried about sun damage to the skin. 'In the Nineties beauty has changed,' said Shiseido UK Managing Director Sam Sugiyama. 'Beauty in the future will have to be inside and out, and mental health is going to be much more important.'

Under the banner 'High technology with the human touch', Shiseido unveiled Bio-Performance Synchro Serum, claiming to heal stressed skin in fourteen days. Paving the way for Crème de la Mer in 2000, Kanebo's La Crème boasted that, at £260 a jar, it was the most expensive moisturizer in the world. Companies such as Aveda (meaning Knowledge of Nature) leaped on the holistic bandwagon, with founder Horst Rechelbacher saying: 'What we're doing isn't New Age, it's ancient. We're going back to natural laws and gain our knowledge from the world's shamans and herbalists.' It was an approach echoed by skin-care companies such as Melbourne-based Aesop, Philosophy, Benefit, Kiehl's and La Prairie.

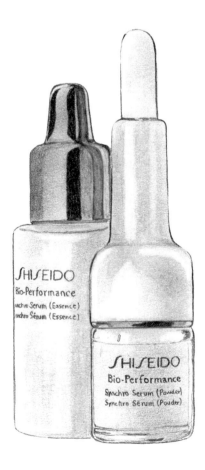

FIG. 253 : Shiseido's Bio-Performance Synchro Serum.

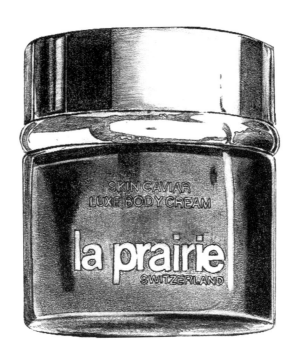

FIG. 254 : La Prairie's Skin Caviar
Luxe Body Cream.

Sudanese model (and Mrs David Bowie) Iman had a more political agenda when she launched the skincare and cosmetics collection I – Iman with the manifesto 'For too long women of colour were an invisible consumer.' 'I believe that women of colour are the women of the world,' she said. 'Native American, Hispanic, Asian, Indian, African and Middle-Eastern.' Although companies such as Prescriptives had expanded their colour range to include dark skin, it was Iman who cornered the fashion makeup market for women with black and brown skin.

From the late 1990s a new school of black rappers, led by Puff Daddy, Lil' Kim, Mary J. Blige and Missy Eliot, introduced Ghetto Fabulous fashion to the world. As role models for a generation of teenagers, the first ladies of Hip-Hop brought Nail Art out of the ghetto and into high-fashion magazines. British *Vogue* featured a spread of fake fibre talons embossed with Chanel Cs, Louis Vuitton LVs and Gucci GGs and painted with nail polish. The arrival of manicure-bar chains such as Nails Inc. to the UK made manicured, polished nails mainstream.

The cosmetics houses were quick to absorb the Ghetto Fabulous trend. MAC (Make-Up Artist Cosmetics) adopted a rebellious and bipartisan approach. Canvassing drag queen Ru Paul and singers kd lang, Elton John, Mary J. Blige and Shirley Manson, MAC launched their Viva Glam lipstick range with all profits going to AIDS research. MAC's 'glam cosmetics with a conscience' philosophy was totally right for the right-on late 1990s, as was their slogan 'All ages, all races, all sexes, all MAC.'

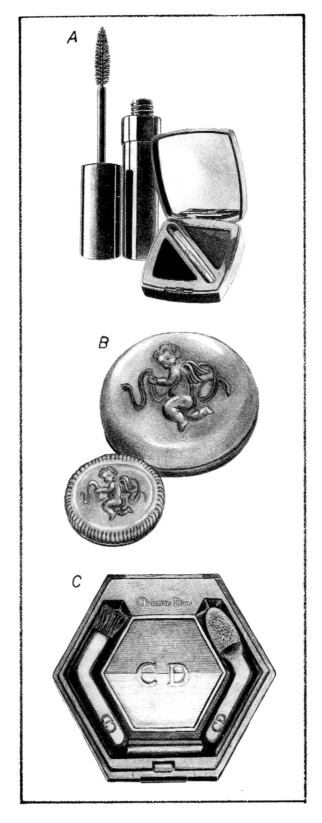

PLATE 38 : TWENTIETH CENTURY
THE 1990S

A   Chanel's La Ligne Et Cils Magiques.

B   Lancôme's Dry Blusher Cakes.

C   Christian Dior's Just Duo.

24 · Into the Twenty-first Century to the Future

Botox is the aspirin of the decade.
AMERICAN *VOGUE*, AUGUST 2002

In December 1999, British *Vogue* looked forward to 'beauty for the 21st-century girl', while Japanese cosmetic visionary Shu Uemura predicted 2013 as the year when science would defeat the ageing process and, ergo, the cosmetics industry. 'From then on, human beings can expect to live a long, young and beautiful life, thanks to technology, botany, biology, biotechnology, the development of natural and cultural sciences and the practice of meditation as in yoga and Zen.'

By August 2002 American *Vogue* was profiling Dr Frederick Brandt, the Botox king of Florida and New York, and citing an American Society of Plastic Surgeons' report that 855,846 patients had undergone Botox injections in 2001 alone. 'Are we fast approaching an ageless society?' asked *Vogue* writer Lynn Snowden. So pervasive was plastic surgery and Botox — the process of paralysing facial tissue with Botulinum toxin type A — that the very future of cosmetics was in peril, as was the billion-dollar market in anti-ageing creams that Charles Revson dubbed 'hope in a bottle'. Ironically, the resistance movement to unnatural beauty saw serum, moisturizer and makeup as a lesser evil than invasive surgery.

After nearly a decade of minimal makeup, holistic remedies and cod-scientific formulas, makeup had nowhere to go but retro. A return to innocence was vital to seduce a culture wise to the surgeon's knife, the dermatologist's syringe and the fashion-magazine editor's digital airbrush. Makeup rode the wave of millennial optimism and went back to a wild, child-like palette not seen since the 1960s.

All the boutique brands that launched in the 1990s now gathered momentum with unashamedly girlie packaging, kaleidoscopic colours and products as playful as Mary Quant and Biba. In May 2002 British *Vogue* announced 'a return of hippy chic' with Kate Moss's face painted in crayons with psychedelic flowers. Nicole Kidman appeared in September 2001 *Harper's Bazaar* as a flower-power hippy chick with Christian Dior Diorific red lips and a sunset of pink and pale yellow painted from eyes to ears using Dior's Crayon Eyeliner in Lemon Mousse.

Makeup houses were given cute names to entice the inner child and make cosmetics appear naïve again: Pretty Pretty, She She Cosmetics, Sugar Cosmetics, Pinkie Swear, Too Faced, Smashbox and Tarte. Too Faced gave us

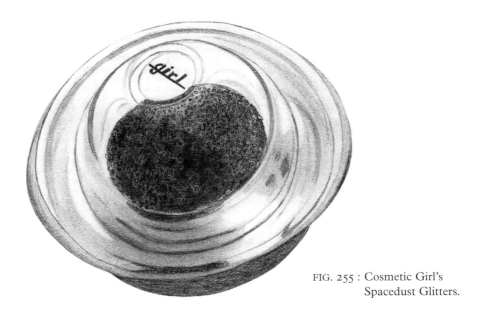

FIG. 255 : Cosmetic Girl's
Spacedust Glitters.

pots of Kitty Glitter 'to add disco ball fire', applied with a powderpuff tied with a pink satin bow. Cosmetic Girl's Spacedust Glitter came in a flying saucer-shaped clear jar and a sparkling palette of Starbaby White, Stratosphere Blue, Celestial Pink and Flamingo Pink Pluto. The Strand sisters' Pixi range included pink Lipglam Sugar Shine and Eyeglam Eye Glaze, with packaging spattered with stars.

Just as London led the way in the 1960s, so the city again took the lead with high-fashion makeup. *Pop*, a biannual fashion glossy magazine, launched in 2000 with a neon revolution. The airbrushed look, reminiscent of Athena posters from the 1980s, demanded full-face maquillage in slick, glossy colours. Lips dripped glossy colour, while electric greens, blues, fluorescent pinks and neon yellows were airbrushed around the eyes and cheekbones. MAC's advertisement in *Pop* featured three-inch false eyelashes dripping with neon rivulets of orange, purple, green and cerise liquid eye gloss.

February 2003 *Vogue* heralded a 'citrus spring' with Lancaster Luminizer Magic Lipglosses in Vibrant Anis and Vibrant Orange, nails lacquered with Christian Dior Addict One-Coat Nail Colour in Orange Tick and eyes shadowed in Shiseido The Make-Up Silky Eyeshadow Duo in Fire Sky (white and orange). A pink as vulgar and shocking as Yves Saint Laurent's Pure Transparent Lipstick in Ultraviolet had not been seen since Schiaparelli. Taste had nothing to do with it.

Nowhere was the look more extreme than in March 2002's issue of *Harper's Bazaar* where a model with a Mary Quant asymmetric bob and a Carnaby Street flat cap was made up with stripes of Estée Lauder Eyeshadow

Quad in Citrus and Shocking Pink and lips in hot-pink High Shine Lip Lacquer. In July 2002 *Harper's* featured a face with Shiseido's Electric Red The Make-Up Lipstick overlaid with Translucent Gloss Lipstick, matching the lips with Kevyn Aucoin Curling Mascara in Black Red and Madina Milano Absolute Eyeshadow in Pimento. Cheekies Crème Blush by Benefit was painted on cheeks in Crazy In Love Pink and toenails matched fingernails in Clinique's Glosswear Nail Enamel in Orchid Blast. As well as all shades of pink, yellow made a strong comeback with Giorgio Armani's line of cosmetics developed by Pat McGrath, featuring a canary-yellow eyeshadow painted from upper eyelid to eyebrow.

By 2002 fashion in the twenty-first century had finally turned from retro 1980s Athena poster to the future. But it was a future first seen through the eyes of 1960s space couturiers Paco Rabanne, Pierre Cardin and André Courrèges. The palette was all about metallics on a dazzling white complexion. From fluorescents this was just a small step. Shiseido commanded its followers to 'be radical with colours empowered by Advanced Luminous Technology'. In a 2001 advertisement the model's eyes were rimmed with black panda shading, while her chalk-white skin shimmered with silver. Upper and lower lids gleamed gold and imperial purple with MAC's Paints in Mauvism and Graphito.

Pat McGrath, the directional makeup artist who painted catwalk faces for John Galliano's Christian Dior shows, cut eyebrow shapes in gold metallic paper, appliqué'd them to models' faces and traced 24-carat gold leaf around their eyelids. In November 2001's *Harper's Bazaar* makeup artist Gucci

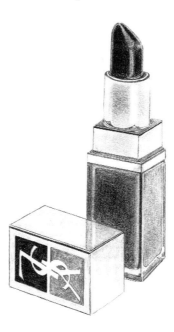

FIG. 256 : Yves Saint Laurent's Pure Transparent Lipstick
in Ultraviolet.

Westman used MAC to paint eyes with lightning flashes of metallic plum and silver, finishing the space-age look with Pro Lash mascara and violet eye pencil. The moon of a nail was painted in silver Octavia Bernadette Thompson nail polish and finished with Glittering Prune. By June 2002 *Harper's* had coated the entire upper lid with gold glitter, encouraging the readers to 'take this look from fantasy to reality with MAC Pigment Colour Powder in Gold'.

By August 2002 makeup had reached extremes even Barbarella would have found *de trop*. *Harper's* 'Shock of the New' feature showed an eye made up in black-on-silver polka dots using Chanel's Basic Eye Colour in Argents.

THE FUTURE

There is an argument that the cosmetics industry has never been as vibrant as it is today. With Tyen as creative consultant, Christian Dior cosmetics got bang up to the moment with products such as the Street Chic Lip Palette in a silver compact that attaches to wrist, bag or belt with a riveted strap. Major fashion houses such as Calvin Klein, Giorgio Armani and Prada first entered the cosmetics market in this century: Klein with strong, simple lines packaged in minimal clear Perspex and Prada selling 'scientific' beauty products such as Reviving Balm in capsules more suitable to pharmaceuticals than makeup.

High-technology serums, applied beneath moisturizer, are the 21st-century miracle products designed to stymy the Botox needle and the surgeon's scalpel. Unveiled in 2003, the £65-a-tube Timeless serum by Erno Laszlo has been dubbed 'the liquid facelift'. The Timeless formula boasts that it can repair and stimulate new growth of collagen, slow the destructive enzyme process that ages skin and energize and improve the skin's clarity. Another fast fix is Prescriptives' silicone-based Magic Invisible Line Smoother gel that claims to work like Botox without the needle, while British *InStyle* magazine calls Clarins' Beauty Flash Balm 'Cinderella in a tube' for its morning-after face-saving qualities. The secret of 21st-century preventive treatments is maximum results for minimum effort. Clinique's Repairwear Intensive Night Cream, Lotion or Serum aims to recharge tired or damaged skin while you sleep, while Shiseido's Renewing Serum claims to work best under a day moisturizer. In 2003 La Prairie formulated six serums for specific conditions: anti-wrinkle firmer, hydrator, retexturizer, illuminator, oil controller and de-sensitizer, while Clarins' Total Double Serum boasts forty-two ingredients to defy Father Time.

But while new products have been released almost daily, beauty today also

PLATE 39 : TWENTY-FIRST CENTURY
THE 2000S

A   Christian Dior's Street Chic Lip
     Palette.
B   Calvin Klein's Concord Silk Suede
     lip tint.
C   Prada's Reviving Balm.

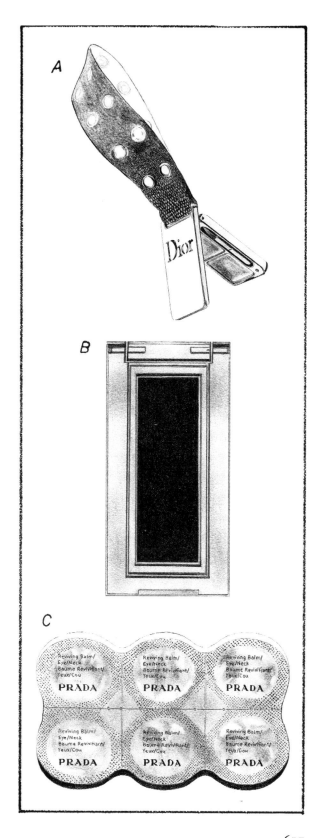

has its pantheon of classics. The industry is seeing classic products that are 'keepers', such as Maybelline's Great Lash Mascara and Estée Lauder's Pure Colour Nail Lacquer, emerge in a business known for its capriciousness. Lancôme's Juicy Tubes Ultra Shiny Lip Gloss sold 165,440 units in the UK alone in 2002. Now eleven years old, Yves Saint Laurent's Touche Eclat con-

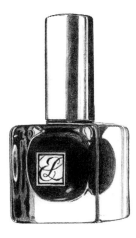

FIG. 257 : Estée Lauder's Nail Lacquer.

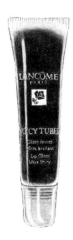

FIG. 258 : Lancôme's Juicy Tubes.

cealer sold 300,000 in the UK in 2002. One of the first light-reflective formulas, Touche Eclat has earned its nickname 'the magic wand', and using shimmer to conceal is now the rule rather than the exception. Laura Mercier's Secret Camouflage concealer is presented in a compact to allow exact match-blending, while Revlon's Skinlights Face Illuminator sheer shimmer liquids come in Natural Light, Peach Light and Pink Light.

Tanning, too, is here to stay, despite increasing anxiety about sun damage to the skin. The boom in celebrity culture coincided with 'secrets of the stars' makeup tips, and none was more accessible than St Tropez fake tan. The full-body St Tropez tan has become a byword for faking it, even though Clarins' Radiance-Plus Self-Tanning Cream-Gel is the connoisseur's choice of self-tan for the face.

As we approach 2004 the makeup industry looks built to last. The great cosmetics houses of Estée Lauder, Elizabeth Arden, Helena Rubinstein, L'Oréal, Revlon, Clarins, Clinique and Maybelline all survived. New blood invigorates august houses such as Lancôme (Fred Farrugia) and Yves Saint Laurent (Linda Cantello). Fashion houses Prada, Helmut Lang, Jil Sander, Calvin Klein, Giorgio Armani and Anna Sui successfully entered a seemingly crowded market. A new establishment is emerging from the specialist brand arena with Shu Uemura, Sisley, MAC, Trish McEvoy, Stila, Tarte, Laura

Mercier, François Nars, Bobbi Brown and I — Iman. Boutique brands Urban Decay, Hard Candy, Philosophy, Benefit, Space NK and Kiehl's continue to thrive, while cheap-and-cheerful street-style brands such as Rimmel freshened up with new face Kate Moss, urban party-queen colours and a new logo, Rimmel London.

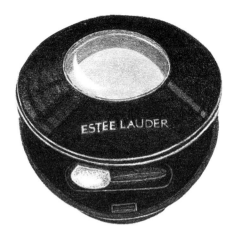

FIG. 259 : Estée Lauder's Color Intensity Microfine Powder.

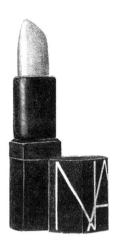

FIG. 260 : François Nars Lipstick.

EPILOGUE

Not since 1992, when the supermodels fell, have fashion magazines championed the model cover girl. Celebrities currently sell fashion magazines, and publicists do not encourage their charges to be used as blank canvases for high-fashion makeup artists to paint. The cover of March 2003 British *Vogue*, however, suggests that the classic makeup cover girl is coming back. The journal dared to present a cover featuring model Natasha Vojnovic with a faceful of glorious Versace cosmetics: glowing Fluid Moisture Foundation, peachy Glam Touch Blush and neon-pink Wet Lipgloss Lipstick. The look was modern and yet echoes the work of great makeup artists such as Barry Lategan, Way Bandy and Kevyn Aucoin. The wheel, it seems, has once again turned towards the art of beauty.

Indeed, indeed, there is charm in every period,
and only fools and flutterplates do not seek reverently
for what is charming in their own day.

MAX BEERBOHM

Bibliography

'Aids to Beauty, Real and Artificial' (in *Cornhill Magazine*, March 1863)

Alberti, Leone B. — *The Arte of Love; or, Love Discovered in an Hundred Severall Kindes*; William Leake, London, 1598

Alexander, William — *The History of Women* (3rd edition); C. Dilly and R. Christopher, London and Stockton, 1782

Ancient British Drama, The; printed for William Miller, London, 1810

Anstey, Christopher — *The New Bath Guide* (6th edition); Fletcher and Hodson, Cambridge, 1768

Art of Beauty, edited by 'Isobel'; C. A. Pearson, London, 1899

Art of Being Beautiful, The: A Series of Interviews with a Society Beauty; Henry J. Drane, London, 1902

Ashley, Doris Lee — 'Catering to Beauty' (in *Pictorial Review*, August 1930)

Ashton, John — *Modern Street Ballads*; Chatto and Windus, London, 1888

Ashton, John — *Old Times*; John C. Nimmo, London, 1885

Asquith, Lady Cynthia — *She Walks in Beauty*; Heinemann, London, 1934

Aucoin, Kevyn — *The Art of Makeup*; Harper Collins, London, 1996

Aucoin, Kevyn — *Making Faces*; Little Brown and Co., London, 1999

Ayer, Harriet Hubbard — *Harriet Hubbard Ayer's Book*; Home Topics Book Co., New York, 1899

Bailey, David — *Models Close Up*; Channel 4 Books, London, 1998

Barker, William — *A Treatise on the Principles of Hair-Dressing*; printed by J. Rozea, London, *c.* 1786

Basten, Fred E. — *Max Factor's Hollywood: Glamour, Movies, Make-up*; W. Quay Hays, Santa Monica, California, 1995

Baudot, François — *A Century of Fashion*; Thames and Hudson, London, 1999

Bayard, Martha — *The Journal of Martha Bayard, 1794–7*; Dodd, Mead, New York, 1894

Beaumont, Sir Harry — *Crito; or, A Dialogue on Beauty*; R. Dodsley, London, 1752

Beauty: Its Attainment and Preservation; Butterick, New York, 1890

Beauty and How to Keep It (by a Professional Beauty); London, 1889

Beauty's Aids; or, How to Be Beautiful; L. C. Page and Co., Boston, 1901

Beerbohm, Max — *A Defence of Cosmetics*; Dodd, Mead, New York, 1896

Begy, Joseph A. — *Practical Handbook of Toilet Preparations*; William L. Allison, New York, 1889

Bettenham, J. — *The Art of Beauty: A Poem*; R. Francklin, London, 1715

Binder, Pearl — *Muffs and Morals*; Harrap, London, 1953

Bjork, Angela and Daniela Turudich — *Vintage Face*; Streamline Press, Long Beach, California, 2001

Black, Alexander — 'Painting the Lily' (in *The Century*, August 1923)

Boehm, Max von — *Modes and Manners*; Harrap, London, 1935

Boettiger, Karl August — *Sabine; ou, Matinée d'une Dame Romaine à sa Toilette*; Chez Maradan, Paris, 1813

Boulenger, Jacques — *Sous Louis-Philippe: Les Dandys*; Nouvelle Collection Historique, Paris, 1932

Bouni, Thomas — *Problems of Beautie and All Humane Affections*; printed by G. Eld for Edward Blount and William Aspley, London, 1606

Boy George — *Take It Like a Man: The Autobiography of Boy George*; Pan Books, London, 1995

Brathwait, Richard — *The English Gentlewoman Drawne Out to the Full Body*; printed by B. Alsop and T. Fawcet for Michaell Sparke, London, 1631

Brinton, P. G. and Napheys, G. H. — *Personal Beauty: How to Cultivate and Preserve It*; W. J. Holland, Springfield, Mass., 1870

Brophy, John — *The Human Face*; Prentice Hall, New York, 1946

Brown, Bobbi — *Evolution: A Guide to a Lifetime of Beauty*; Harper Resource, New York, 2002

Brown, S. J. — *Toilet Table Talk*; London, 1856

Brown, Tom — *Amusements Serious and Comical*; Dodd, Mead, New York, 1927

Bulwer, John — *Anthropometamorphosis: Man Transform'd; or, The Artificial Changeling*; printed for J. Hardesty, London, 1650, 1653

Burbridge, Mabelle — *The Road to Beauty*; Greenberg, New York, 1924

Cades, Hazel Rawson — 'Makeup Made Easy' (in *Woman's Home Companion*, October 1950)

Carleton, Patrick — *Buried Empires*; Edward Arnold, London, 1939

Cavalieri, Lina — *My Secret of Beauty*; Circulation Syndicate, New York, 1914

Cazenave, Dr A. — *Female Beauty; or The Art of Human Decoration*; G. W. Carleton and Co., New York, 1874

Challamel, M. Augustin — *The History of Fashion in France*; Scribner and Welford, New York, 1882

Chambers's Encyclopaedia; W. and R. Chambers, London, 1860

Chambers's Journal of Popular Literature, Science and Arts

Chandra, Moti — 'Cosmetics and Coiffure in Ancient India' (in *Indian Society of Oriental Art*, Volume 8, pp. 62–145)

Clark, Sir James — *Ladies' Guide to Beauty*; Dick and Fitzgerald, New York, 1864

Cocks, Dorothy — *The Etiquette of Beauty*; George H. Doran, New York, 1927

Codrington, Robert — *The Second Part of Youth's Behaviour, or Decency in Conversation Amongst Women*; W. Lee, London, 1664

Cohen, Juliet — *Vogue Make-up*; Carlton, London, 2001

Cole, Celia Caroline — 'Romance and Red Lips' (in the *Delineator*, August 1924)

Colliers

Collins, Frederick L. — 'The Ethics of Paint and Powder' (in the *Delineator*, October 1928)

Collins, James H. — 'The Beauty Business' (in the *Saturday Evening Post*, 22 November 1924)

Conley, Veronica Lucey — 'A New Look for the American Male?' (in *Today's Health*, November 1957)

Conley, Veronica Lucey — 'Cold Cream, an Ageless Cosmetic' (in *Today's Health*, December 1956)

Conley, Veronica Lucey — 'For the Man of the Family' (in *Today's Health*, December 1951)

Connoisseur, The

Cooley, Arnold J. — *Instructions and Cautions Respecting the Selection and Use of Perfumes, Cosmetics, and Other Toilet Articles*; Robert Hardwicke, London, 1868

Cooley, Arnold J. — *The Toilet in Ancient and Modern Times*; J. B. Lippincott, Philadelphia, 1873

Cornhill Magazine

Cosmetics for My Lady and Good Fare for My Lord; Golden Cockerel Press, London, 1934

'Cosmetics with a Conscience' (in the *Ladies' Home Journal*, May 1935)

Cosmopolitan

Courtenay, Florence — *Physical Beauty*; Social Mentor Publications, New York, 1922

Cowl, Jane — 'My Beauty Secret' (in the *Ladies' Home Journal*, November 1925)

Creel, Blanche Bates — 'The Painted Age' (in *Colliers*, 2 April 1927)

Cunliffe-Owen, Margaret — *Eve's Glossary*; Herbert Stone and Co., Chicago and New York, 1897

Current Opinion

Dawson, Thomas — *The Good Huswifes Jewell*; John Wolfe, London, 1596

Dazed & Confused

De Castelbajac, Kate — *The Face of the Century: 100 Years of Makeup and Style*; Rizzoli, New York, 1995

Delany, Mary Granville — *The Autobiography and Correspondence of Mary Granville, Mrs Delany*; Richard Bentley, London, 1861

Delineator

Donne, John — *A Defence of Women for Their Inconstancy and Their Paintings*; Fanfrolico Press, London, 1925

Doran, John — *Habits and Men*; R. Bentley, London, 1855

DuBoscq, Jacques — *The Compleat Woman*; Thomas Harper and Richard Hodgkinson, London, 1639

Ducasse, C. J. — 'The Animal with Red Cheeks' (in *American Scholar*, July 1938)

Duties of a Lady's Maid; with Directions for Conduct, and Numerous Receipts for the Toilette; James Bulcock, London, 1825

Hole, Christina — *The English Housewife in the Seventeenth Century*; Chatto and Windus, London, 1953

Hubbard, Elizabeth — *Helpful Advice to Women Who Would Be Beautiful*; Mrs Hubbard's Salon, New York, 1910

Hunt, Leigh — *Men, Women, and Books*; Smith, Elders and Co., London, 1847

Hygeia

i-D

Jameson, Helen Follett — *The Beauty Box*; McLoughlin Brothers, Inc., Springfield, Mass., 1931

Johnstone, Justine — 'Wrong Roads to Beauty' (in the *Ladies' Home Journal*, June 1926)

Jonson, Ben — *The Works of Ben Jonson*; printed for D. Midwinter and others, London, 1756

Juvenal — *The Satires of Decimus Junius Juvenalis*; printed for Jacob Tongon, London, 1711

Knickerbocker, Elizabeth — 'Beauty of Face and Form as Achieved in New York' (in the *Delineator*, October 1915)

Knight, Charles — *Pictorial Gallery of the Arts*; Charles Knight and Co., London, 1845

Koller, Dr Theodor — *Cosmetics*; Scott, Greenwood and Son, London, 1911

Lacroix, Paul — *The XVIII*[th] *Century, Its Institutions, Customs, and Costumes*; Bichars and Son, London, 1876

Ladies Dictionary, The; John Dunton, London, 1694

Lady's Magazine

LaWall, Charles H. — *Four Thousand Years of Pharmacy*; J. B. Lippincott Co., Philadelphia, 1927

Layard, Austen H. — *Discoveries in the Ruins of Ninevah and Babylon*; G. P. Putnam and Co., New York, 1853

Le Camus, Antoine — *Abdeker: or, The Art of Preserving Beauty*; A. Millar, London, 1754

Le Gallienne, Richard — 'On the Use and Abuse of Complexions' (in *McClure's Magazine*, September 1916)

Lémery, Nicolas — *Curiosa Arcana: Being Curious Secrets, Artificial and Natural*; printed for J. N., London, 1711

Lémery, Nicolas — *Curiosities of Art and Nature*; Matthew Gilliflower and James Partridge, London, 1685

Lerner, Charles — 'Feminine Beautification' (in *Hygeia*, November 1933)

Lester, Katherine M. and Bess Oercke — *Accessories of Dress*; Manual Arts Press, Peoria, Illinois, 1942

Liébaut, Jean — *Trois Livres de L'Embellissement et Ornement du Corps Humain*; Libraire Juré, Paris, 1582

Lingua: or, the Combat of the Tongue and the Five Senses for Superiority; printed by G. Eld, for Simon Waterson, London, 1607

London Belles, The; Publishing Office in Dove Court, London, 1707

London Gazette

London Stage, The; Sherwood, Jones and Co., London, 1825

Long, Alice M. — *My Lady Beautiful or the Perfection of Womanhood*; Progress Co., Chicago, 1908

Mackay, Ernest J. — *Further Excavations at Mohenjo-Daro*; Government of India Press, New Delhi, 1938

Malmesbury, James Harris — *A Series of Letters of the First Earl of Malmesbury*; Richard Bentley, London, 1870

Malmstend, Lilyan — *Your Face and Figure*; Penn Publishing Co., Philadelphia, 1931

Markham, Gervase — *Countrey Contentments, or The English Huswife*; printed for R. Jackson, London, 1623

Marshall, Sir John (editor) — *Mohenjo-Daro and the Indus Civilization*; Arthur Probsthain, London, 1931

Martial — *The Epigrams of Martial*; George Bell and Sons, London, 1877

McClure's Magazine

Ménard, René — *La Vie Privée des Anciens*; A. Morel et Cie, Paris, 1880

Mennis, Sir John and Smith, Dr James — *Musarum Deliciae: or, The Muses Recreation (Facetiae)*; T. Davison, London. 1887 (from the 1640 edition)

Mirror of the Graces; I. Riley, New York, 1813

Miscellaneous — *The Fashion Book*; Phaidon Press, London, 1998

Monnier, Philippe — *Venice in the Eighteenth Century*; Chatto and Windus, London, 1910

Montaigne, Marie — *How to Be Beautiful*; Harper and Brothers, New York and London, 1913

Montez, Lola — *The Arts of Beauty: Or, Secrets of a Lady's Toilet*; Dick and Fitzgerald, New York, 1858

Mulvey, Kate and Melissa Richards — *Decades of Beauty: The Changing Image of Women 1880–1990s*; Hamlyn, London, 1998

Murray, Hannah — *The American Toilet*; Anthony Imbert, New York. 1827

Murray, Hannah — *The Toilet*; William Ballantyne, Washington, D.C., 1867

Napier, Lady Sarah — *The Life and Letters of Lady Sarah Lennox*; John Murray, London, 1901

Nars, François — *Makeup Your Mind*; PowerHouse Books, New York, 2002

Neuburger, Albert — *The Technical Arts and Sciences of the Ancients*; Macmillan, New York, 1930

Niccholes, Alex — *A Discourse of Marriage and Wiving*; printed by N.O. for Leonard Becket, in the Inner Temple, London, 1615

Nixon, Anthony — *A Straunge Foot-Post*; printed by E. A. ('dwelling neare Christ Church'), London, 1613

'Notions of Personal Beauty in Different Countries' (in *Penny Magazine*, 6 December 1845)

Nova

'Oldest Beauty Shop, The' (in *Current Opinion*, April 1901)

Orchamps, la Baronne d' — *Tous les secrets de la femme*; Bibliothèque des Auteurs Modernes, Paris, 1907

Outlook

'Paint, Powder, Patches' (in *Cornhill Magazine*, June 1863)

Palau, Guido — *Heads, Hair by Guido*; Booth-Clibborn Editions, London, 2000

Parker, Alan — *The Making of Evita*; Collins, London, 1997

Peacham, Henry — *The Worth of a Penny, or a Caution to Keep Money*; privately printed, 1641

Penny Magazine

Pictorial Review

Pierce, Anne Lewis — 'Dangerous Shortcuts to Beauty' (in *Good Housekeeping*, September 1912)

Piper, David — *The English Face*; Thames and Hudson, London, 1957

Plat, Sir Hugh — *Delightes for Ladies*; Humphrey Lownes, London, 1627

Porter, Sir Robert Ker — *Travels in Georgia, Persia, Armenia, Ancient Babylonia During the Years 1817, 1818, 1819, 1820*; Longman, Hurst, Rees, Orme, and Brown, London, 1821

Poucher, William A. — *Perfume, Cosmetics, and Soaps* (6th edition); Van Nostrand Co., Inc., New York, 1942

Prior, Matthew — *The Poetical Works of Matthew Prior*; printed for W. Straham, T. Payne, J. Rivington and Sons, J. Dodsley, T. Lowndes, T. Codell, T. Caslon, J. Nichols, and T. Evans, London, 1779

Purchas, Samuel — *Purchas his Pilgrimage;* printed by William Stansby for Henrie Featherstone, London, 1613

Puttenham, Richard — *The Arte of English Poesie*; R. Field, London, 1589

Queen's Closet Opened, The (11th edition); W. Taylor, London, 1713

Quennell, Marjorie and C. H. B. — *Everyday Things in Ancient Greece*; G. P. Putnam's Sons, New York, 1930

Rattner, Herbert — 'Cosmetics for Men' (in *Hygeia*, October 1946)

Rhead, G. Woolliscroft — *Chats on Costume*; T. Fisher Unwin, London, 1906

Rimmel, Eugene — *The Book of Perfumes*; Chapman and Hall, London, 1865

Rowlands, Samuel — *Look to It; For, Ile Stabbe Ye*; printed by E. Allde for W. Ferbrand and George Loftes, London, 1604

Rubinstein, Helena — *The Art of Feminine Beauty*; Horace Liveright, New York, 1930

Russell, Lillian — 'The Quest of Beauty' (in the *Delineator*, October 1911)

Salthe, Ole — 'Beauty and the Beast' (in *Independent Woman*, January 1940)

Saturday Book

Scavullo, Francesco — *Scavullo: Photographs Fifty Years*; Harry N. Abrams, Inc., New York, 1997

Schefer, Dorothy — *What Is Beauty?*; Thames and Hudson, London, 1997

Science News

Sévigné, Marie, Marquise de — *The Letters of Madame de Sévigné to Her Daughter and Friends*; Mason, New York, 1856

Shephard, Catherine — *My Lady's Toilette*; C. H. Graves, Philadelphia, 1911

Sozinskey, T. S. — *Personal Appearance and the Culture of Beauty, with Hints as to Character*; Allen, Lane, and Scott, Philadelphia, 1877

Spectator, The

Staffe, Baroness Blanche A. — *My Lady's Dressing Room*; Cassell, London, 1892

Stanhope, Philip Dormer — *Letters Written by the Late Right Honourable Philip Dormer Stanhope, Earl of Chesterfield, to His Son, Philip Stanhope, Esq.*; J. Nichols, London, 1800

Eddy, Kathleen — 'Nearly a Billion a Year for Beauty' (in the *Pictorial Review*, May 1924)

Edkins, Diana and Annette Tapert — *The Power of Style: The Women Who Defined the Art Of Living Well*; Crown Publishers, Inc., New York, 1994

Eifert, Virginia S. — 'The Ancient Art of Beautification' (in *Natural History*, November 1937)

'The Elaborate Coiffure' (in *Current Opinion*, April 1901)

England's Vanity; John Dunton, London, 1683

Ernst, Earle — *The Kabuki Theatre*; Oxford University Press, New York, 1956

Esten, John — *Why Don't You? Diana Vreeland Bazaar Years*; Universe Publishing, New York, 2001

Evelyn, John — *Diary and Correspondence*; Henry Colburn, London, 1850

Everybody's Magazine

The Face

Fairholt, F. W. — *Costume in England*; Chapman and Hall, London, 1846

Feld, Rose — 'The Cosmetic Urge' (in *Colliers*, 12 March 1927)

Feydeau, Ernst — *The Art of Pleasing*; G. W. Carleton and Co., New York, 1874

Firenzuola, Agnolo — *On the Beauty of Women*; James R. Osgood McIlvaine and Co., London, 1892

Fitzgeffrey, Henry — *Satyres And Satyricall Epigrams: With Certaine Observations at Black-Fryers*; printed by Edward Allde for Miles Patrich, London, 1617

Fletcher, Ella Adelia — *The Woman Beautiful*; Brentano, New York, 1900

Fleur, Marise de — 'The Accent of Make-up' (in *Sunset*, March 1926)

Fontanne, Lynn — 'Making the Most of Your Looks' (in *Ladies' Home Journal*, September 1927)

Fortune

Fosbroke, Thomas — *A Treatise on the Arts, Manufactures, Manners, and Institutions of the Greeks and Romans*; Longman, Rees, Brown, Green and Longman, London, 1833

Franklin, Alfred — *La Vie Privée d'Autrefois*; Librairie Plon, Paris, 1887

Garland, Madge — *The Changing Face of Beauty*; M. Barrows and Co., New York, 1957

Gentleman's Magazine, The

Gentleman's and London Magazine, The

Godey's Lady's Book

God's Voice Against Pride in Apparel

Goeckerman, William — 'Painting the Lily' (in *Hygeia*, November 1928)

Goldsmith, Oliver — *The Citizen of the World*; Wm. Otridge and Son, London, 1800

Good Housekeeping

Good Society; George Routledge, London, 1869

Goodman, Herman — 'Cold Cream' (in *Hygeia*, November 1944)

Gosson, Stephen — *Pleasant Quippes for Upstart Newfangled Gentlewomen*; Richard Johnes, London, 1595

Gower, F. Leveson — *Letters of Harriet Countess Granville*; Longmans, Green and Co., London, 1894

Grand-Carteret, John — *XIXe Siècle*; Librairie de Firmin-Didot et Cie, Paris, 1893

Griffith, Ivor — 'The Cosmetic Urge' (in *Popular Science Talks*, Volume 7, 1929)

Gross, Michael — *Model: The Ugly Business of Beautiful Women*; Bantam Press, London, 1995

Habits of Good Society: A Handbook of Etiquette for Ladies and Gentlemen; J. Hogg and Sons, London, 1859

Haden-Guest, Anthony — *The Last Party: Studio 54, Disco and the Culture of the Night*; William Morrow and Co., Inc., New York, 1997

Hall, Joseph — *Satires*; printed by C. Whittingham for R. Triphook, Chiswick, London, 1824

Hall, Thomas — *Comarum, the Loathsomnesse of Long Haire*; N. Webb and W. Grantham, London, 1654

Harleian Miscellany; R. Dutton, London, 1809

Harper's Bazaar

Harris, James — *Diaries and Correspondence of James Harris, First Duke of Malmesbury*; Richard Bentley, London, 1844

Haweis, Mary — *The Art of Beauty*; Harper and Brothers, New York, 1878

Historical Digest of the Provincial Press; Society for Americana, Boston, 1911

Stanley, Louis — *The Beauty of Woman*; W. H. Allen, London, 1955

Stevenson, Burton Egbert — *The Home Book of Verse*; Henry Holt, New York, 1926

Stevenson, Nils and Ray Stevenson — *Vacant: A Diary of the Punk Years 1976–1979*; Thames and Hudson, London, 1999

Stewart, James — *Plocacosmos, or the Whole Art of Hairdressing*; London, 1782

Strutt, James — *A Complete View of the Dress and Habits of the People of England*; Henry G. Bohn, London, 1842

Stubbes, Philip — *The Anatomie of Abuses*; Richard Jones, London, 1583

Sunset Magazine

Taylor, I. A. — 'Powder and Paint' (in *Living Age*, 9 December 1899)

Taylor, Jeremy (?) — *Several Letters Between Two Ladies: Wherein the Lawfulness and Unlawfulness of Artificial Beauty in Point of Conscience Are Nicely Debated*; Thomas Ballard, London, 1701

Tetlow, Henry — 'War Paint' (in *American Mercury*, July 1925)

Thomson, Gladys Scott — *Life in a Noble Household*; Jonathan Cape, London, 1937

Thomson, Gladys Scott — *The Russells in Bloomsbury 1669–1771*; Jonathan Cape, London, 1940

Thornley, Betty — 'Miss and Makeup' (in *Colliers*, 2 November 1929)

Thurston, Joseph — *The Toilette*; printed for Benj. Motte, at the Middle Temple Gate, in Fleet Street, London, 1730

Time

Toilet, The: A Dressing-Table Companion; S. Lingham, London, 1839

Toilet of Flora; J. Murray, London, 1784

Toilette of Health, Beauty, and Fashion, The; Allen and Ticknor, Boston, 1833

Tomes, Robert — *The Bazar Book of Decorum*; Harper and Brothers, New York, 1877

Tuke, Thomas — *A Treatise Against Painting and Tincturing of Men and Women*; printed by Creed and Allsope for Edw. Merchant, London, 1616

Twigg, Phyllis — *A Little Booke of Conceited Secrets and Delightes*; Medici Society, London and Boston, 1928

Vail, Gilbert — *A History of Cosmetics in America*; Toilet Goods Association, Inc., New York, 1947

Vanity Fair

Verney, Frances P. — *Memoirs of the Verney Family*; Longmans, Green, and Co., London, 1892

Verrill, Alpheus — *Perfumes and Spices*; L. C. Page and Co., Boston, 1940

Vogue

Vogue's Book of Beauty; Condé Nast Publications, New York, 1933

W

Walker, Alexander — *The Book of Beauty* (5th edition); Holland and Glover, New York, 1843

Walker, Mrs A. — *Female Beauty*; Scofield and Voorhies, New York, 1840

Warner, William — *Albion's England* (revised edition); William Warncr, London, 1596

'When Women Go to Beauty Parlors' (in the *Ladies' Home Journal*, November 1912)

White, Paul W. — 'Our Booming Beauty Business' (in *Outlook*, 22 January 1930)

'Why I Stopped Being a Beauty Specialist' (in the *Ladies' Home Journal*, 1 September 1910)

Wilkinson, Sir J. Gardner — *A Popular Account of the Ancient Egyptians*; John Murray, London, 1854

Williams, Mary Brush — 'How to Look Artificially Natural' (in the *Ladies' Home Journal*, September 1925)

Wolf, Annie — *The Truth About Beauty*; Lovell, Coryell, and Co., New York, 1892

Wright, Thomas — *Archaeological Album*; Chapman and Hall, London, 1845

Wright, Thomas — *Caricature History of the Georges*; Chatto and Windus, London, 1898

Wright, Thomas — *Womankind in Western Europe from Earliest Times*; Groombridge, London, 1869

'Wrinkles in the Wrinkle Lotion Business' (in *Everybody's Magazine*, December 1915)

Wycherly, William — *Love in a Wood*; printed for W. Peaks, A. Bettesworth, F. Clay, R. Wellington, C. Corbet, and J. Brindley, London, 1735

Wykes-Joyce, Max — *Cosmetics and Adornment*; Peter Owen, London, 1961

Index

Note: Italic numerals refer to illustrations

626